Maynooth Library
00378696

D1585413

The ELISA Guidebook

Second Edition

Series Editor
John M. Walker
School of Life Sciences
University of Hertfordshire
Hatfield, Hertfordshire, AL10 9AB, UK

For other titles published in this series, go to
www.springer.com/series/7651

METHODS IN MOLECULAR BIOLOGY™

The ELISA Guidebook

Second Edition

by

John R. Crowther

International Atomic Energy Agency, Animal Production & Health Section, Vienna, Austria

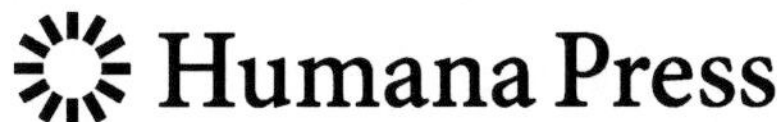

John R. Crowther
International Atomic Energy Agency
Animal Production & Health Section
Wagramer Str. 5
1400 Vienna
Austria

ISBN: 978-1-60327-253-7 e-ISBN: 978-1-60327-254-4
ISSN: 1064-3745 e-ISSN: 1940-6029
DOI: 10.1007/978-1-60327-254-4

Library of Congress Control Number: 2008940983

Cover illustration:

Printed on acid-free paper

springer.com

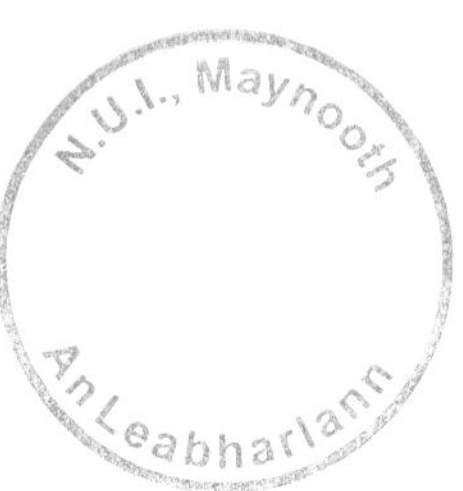

Preface

There have been very few developments that markedly affect the need to greatly revise the text from the last version of this book. This is testament to the fact that heterogeneous enzyme-linked immunosorbent assays (ELISA) provide ideal systems for dealing with a wide range of studies in many biological areas. The main reason for this success is test flexibility, whereby reactants can be used in different combinations, either attached passively to a solid phase support or in the liquid phase. The exploitation of the ELISA has been increased through continued development of specifically produced reagents, for example, monoclonal and polyclonal antibodies and peptide antigens coupled with the improvement and expansion of commercial products such as enzyme-linked conjugates, substrates and chromogens, plastics technology and design of microwell plates, instrumentation advances and robotics. However, the principles of the ELISA remain the same. There has been some rearrangement of chapters plus addition of three new ones dealing with charting methods for assessing the indirect ELISA, ruggedness and robustness of tests-aspects of kit use and validation, and internal quality control and external quality management of data, respectively. These reflect the need to control what you are doing with ELISA and to exploit the method to its full extent. I do not apologize for dealing with the same areas in different ways a number of times, as it is imperative that principles are understood to allow planning, operation, and control of ELISA.

A brief scan of the literature involving ELISA can be used to illustrate the continued success of ELISA. The number of publications with ELISA mentioned in all science areas from 1976 to 2004 is shown in Table 1. A fairly constant increase in the number of research works using ELISA methods is indicated. A breakdown of publications according to the areas of science in 5 yearly periods from 1980 given in Table 2 illustrates the versatility in the use of ELISA, as well as highlights the major areas of use in medicine and dentistry; immunology and microbiology, molecular biology, and genetics and biotechnology. It is interesting to note that the earliest exploitation of ELISA was in immunology and microbiology and molecular Biology and biotechnology, probably reflecting the greatest research areas. Medicine and dentistry (associated by the search engine) shows the greatest rate of increase in use (probably in the medical sphere only) from the 1990s.

The search results indicate the continued expansion of ELISA in science, and there is no reason to believe that this will change even in the face of modern technologies exploiting molecular methods. The analytical and systematic characteristics of ELISA are ideally suited to diagnosis at the screening level, for surveillance where larger scale sample handling is required, and for research. Many of the accepted standard assays in many scientific fields are ELISA-based and have replaced other "gold standard" assays. In conjunction with the rapidly evolving use of molecular methods centering on the polymerase chain reaction (PCR) technologies, there is a need to use serological confirmatory methods in a dual approach to directly identify and characterize disease agents and to assess disease prevalence through the measurement of specific antibodies or other chemical factors as a result of infection. The use of ELISA methods in testing the environment and animal or plant products as safe for human and animal consumption is also a rapidly evolving area for ELISA.

Table 1
Literature search in ScienceDirect database for ELISA

Year	Number
1976	6
1977	13
1978	14
1979	31
1980	45
1981	95
1982	125
1983	216
1984	257
1985	367
1986	420
1987	547
1988	565
1989	640
1990	682
1991	743
1992	774
1993	820
1994	870
1995	1,016
1996	1,093
1997	1,119
1998	1,099
1999	1,144
2000	1,118
2001	1,120
2002	1,198
2003	1,253
2004	1,591

ELISA, therefore, has been used in all fields of pure and applied aspects of biology. In particular, it forms the backbone of diagnostic techniques. The systems used to perform ELISAs make use of antibodies. These are proteins produced in animals in response to antigenic stimuli. Antibodies are specific chemicals that bind to the antigens used for their production; thus they can be used to detect the particular antigens if binding can be demonstrated. Conversely, specific antibodies can be measured by the use of defined antigens, and this forms the basis of many assays in diagnostic biology.

Table 2
Breakdown of literature search in science groups

Subject	1980–1984	1985–1989	1990–1994	1995–1999	2000–2004
Agriculture and biological sciences	87	274	615	804	827
Molecular biology, genetics, and biotechnology	374	1,329	1,762	1,845	2,096
Chemistry	8	29	77	208	279
Environmental science	4	13	52	125	162
Immunology and microbiology	514	1,584	2,128	2,450	2,772
Medicine and dentistry	280	971	1,639	2,875	3,372
Neurosciences	21	124	198	380	484
Pharmacology and toxicology	24	108	247	397	497
Veterinary sciences	71	219	522	769	853

The book describes the methods involved in ELISAs, where one of the reagents, usually an antibody, is linked to an enzyme and where one reagent is attached to a solid phase. The systems allow the examination of reactions through the simple addition and incubation of reagents. Bound and free reactants are separated by a simple washing procedure. The end product in an ELISA is the development of color, which can be quantified using a spectrophotometer. These kinds of ELISA are called heterogeneous assays and should be distinguished from homogeneous assays where all reagents are added simultaneously. The latter assays are most suitable for detecting small molecules such as digoxin or gentamicin.

The development of ELISA stemmed from investigations of enzyme-labeled antibodies *(1–3)*, for use in identifying antigens in tissue. The methods of conjugation were exploited to measure serum components in the first true ELISAs *(4–6)*. By far the most exploited ELISAs use plastic microtitre plates in an 8 × 12-well format as the solid phase *(7)*. Such systems benefit from a large selection of specialized commercially available equipment, including multichannel pipets for the easy simultaneous dispensing of reagents and multichannel spectrophotometers for rapid data capture. There are many books, manuals, and reviews of ELISA and associated subjects, which should be examined for more detailed practical details *(8–21)*.

The purpose of developing ELISAs is to solve problems. These can be divided into pure and applied applications, although the two are interdependent. Thus, a laboratory with a strong research base is essential in providing scientific insight and valuable reagents to allow more routine applications. The methods outlined show the flexibility of the systems. Their effective use is up to the ingenuity of scientists. Recent advances in science have given the immunoassayist greater potential for improving the sensitivity and specificity of assays, including ELISA. In particular the development of MAb technology has given us single chemical reagents (antibodies) of defined specificity, which can be standardized in terms of activity as a function of their weight. The development of gene expression systems has also given the possibility of expressing single genes as proteins for use in raising antibodies or acting as pure antigens. This technology goes hand-in-hand with developments in the polymerase chain reaction (PCR) technologies, which enables the very rapid identification of genes and their manipulation. In turn, improvements in the fields of rapid sequencing and X-ray crystallographic methods has led to a far more intimate understanding of the structure–function relationship of organisms in relation to the immunology of disease. The ELISA fits in rather well in these developments, since it is a binding assay requiring defined antibodies and antigens, all of which can be provided. Table 3 illustrates some applications of ELISA with relevant references.

Table 3
Applications of ELISA

General	Specific	References
Confirmation of clinical disease	Titration of specific antibodies	*(21–35)*
	Single dilution assays	*(27, 30–34, 36)*
	Relationship of titer to protection against disease	*(29, 37)*
	Kits	*(28, 32, 33)*
Analysis of immune response to whole organisms, purified antigens extracted from whole organisms, expressed proteins (e.g., vaccinia, baculo, yeast, baceteria), measurement, polypeptides, peptides	Antibody quantification	*(25, 26, 32, 34, 36, 38–40)*
	Antibody class measurement (IgM, IgG, IgA, IgD, IgE)	*(41–44)*
	Antibody subclass measurement (IgG1, IgG2b, IgG3)	*(42)*
	Antibody IG2a, affinity	*(28, 45, 46)*
Antigenic comparison	Relative binding antibodies	*(25, 26, 34, 40, 47)*
	Affinity differences in binding of antibodies	*(40, 45, 48–50)*
	Measurement of weight of antigens	*(28, 34, 46, 48, 51–56)*
	Examination of treatments to antigen (inactivation for vaccine manufacture, heating, enzyme treatments)	*(46)*

(continued)

Table 3 (continued)

General	Specific	References
	Identification of continuous and discontinuous epitopes by examination of binding of polyclonal and MAbs to denatured and nondenatured proteins	*(28, 55, 57, 58)*
	Antigenic profiling by MAbs	*(28, 57, 59–61)*
	Comparison of expressed and native problems	*(5, 55, 62, 63)*
	Use of MAbs to identify paratopes in polyclonal sera	*(58, 62, 64)*
Monoclonal antibodies	Screening during production	*(57, 59)*
	Competitive assay-antibody assessment	*(62)*
	Comparison of antigens	*(28, 32, 57, 58, 60, 62)*
	Use of MAbs to orientate antigens	*(55)*
Novel systems	High-sensitivity assays (Amplified-ELISA)	*(65)*
	Fluorogenic substrates	*(66)*
	Biotin–avidin systems	*(67)*
More recent references	Food analysis	*(68–70)*
	Fish	*(71–75)*
	AIDS	*(75–77)*
	SARS	*(78)*
	Bird flu	*(79, 80)*
	Allergens	*(81, 82)*
	Emerging diseases	*(83)*
	Psychiatry	*(84)*
	Review	*(85, 86)*
	Snakes	*(87)*
	Environment	*(88)*
	Chemoluminescence	*(89)*

The ability to develop ELISAs depends on as closer understanding of the immunological/serological/biochemical knowledge of specific biological systems as possible. Such information is already available with reference to literature surveys. Basic skills in immunochemical methods are also a requirement and an excellent manual for this is available *(90)*. References *(91, 92)* are excellent text books on immunology. An invaluable source of commercial immunological reagents is available in *(69)*. The references from 70 onwards are more recent and reflect newer fields into which ELISA has expanded and also the new problems arising as, for example, Avian influenza and SARS. It is difficult to see that there will be a significant reduction in the rate of use of ELISA directly or as part of other molecular systems, but this can only be assessed when the next edition of this book is written. The main danger is methods involving ELISA are now regarded easy to develop. This, as for all tests, is not true and good training in ELISA is even more important nowadays, since there is an incredible spectrum of reagents available for the development of tests. The linking of molecular methods to ELISA and other detection systems based on solid phase assays is exciting and full of potential, but there is a great need to attend to the basic understanding and principles of ELISA.

John R. Crowther
Vienna, Austria

References

1. Avrameas, S. and Uriel, J. (1966) Methode de marquage d'antigenes et d'anticorps avec des enzymes et son application en immunodiffusion. *Comptes Rendus Hendomadairesdes Seances de l'Acadamie des Sciences: D: Sciences naturelles (Paris)*, 262, 2543–2545.
2. Nakane, P.K. and Pierce G.B. (1966) Enzyme-labelled antibodies: preparation and application for the localization of antigens. *J. Histochem. Cytochem.* 14, 929–931.
3. Avrameas, S. (1969) Coupling of enzymes to proteins with gluteraldehyde. Use of the conjugates for the detection of antgens and antibodies. *Immunochemistry* 6, 43–52.
4. Avrameas, S. and Guilbert, B. (1971) Dosage enzymo-immunologique de proteines a l'aide d'immunosadorbants et d'antigenes marques aux enzymes. *Comptes Rendus Hendomadaires des Seances de l'Acadamie des Sciences: D: Sciences naturelles (Paris)* 273, 2705–2707.
5. Engvall, E. and Perlman, P. (1971) P. Enzyme-linked immunosorbent assay (ELISA).Quantitative assay of immunoglobulin G. *Immunochemistry* 8, 871–874.
6. Van Weeman, B.K. and Schuurs, A.H.W.M. (1971) Immunoassay using antigen enzyme conjugates. *FEBS Lett.* 15, 232–236.
7. Voller, A., Bidwell, D.E., Huldt, G., and Engvall, E. (1974) A microplate method of enzyme linked immunosorbent assay and its application to malaria. *Bull. Wld. Hlth. Org.* 51, 209–213.
8. Burgess, G. W., ed. (1988) *ELISA Technology in Diagnosis and Research.* Graduate School of Tropical Veterinary Science, James Cook University of North Queensland, Townsville, Australia.
9. Collins, W. P. (1985) *Alternative Immunoassays.* Wiley, Chichester, UK.
10. Collins, W. P. (1985) *Complimentary Immunoassays.* Wiley, Chichester, UK.
11. Crowther, J. R. (1995) *ELISA: Theory and Practice.* Humana, Totowa, NJ.
12. Ishikawa, E., Kawia, T., and Miyai, K. (1981) *Enzyme Immunoassay.* Igaku-Shoin, Tokyo, Japan.
13. Kemeny, D. M. and Challacombe, S. J. (1988) *ELISA and Other Solid-Phase Immunoassays. Theoretical and Practical Aspects.* Wiley, Chichester, UK.
14. Maggio, T. (1979) *The Enzyme Immunoassay.* CRC, New York.
15. Ngo, T.T. and Leshoff, H.M. (1985) *Enzyme-Mediated Immunoassay.* Plenum, NewYork.
16. Voller, A., Bidwell, D.E., and Bartlett, A. (1979) *The Enzyme-Linked Immunosorbent Assay (ELISA).* Dynatech Europe, London, UK.
17. Avrameas, S., Ternynck, T., and Guesdon, J.L. (1978) Coupling of enzymes to antibodies and antigens. *Scand. J. Immunol.* 8 (Suppl. 7), 7–23.
18. Blake, C. and Gould, B. J. (1984) Use of enzymes in immunoassay techniques. A review. *Analyst* 109, 533–542.
19. Guilbault, G. G. (1968) Use of enzymes in analytical chemistry. *Anal. Chem.* 40, 459.
20. Kemeny, D.M. and Challacombe, S.J. (1986) Advances in ELISA and other solid-phase immunoassays. *Immunol. Today* 7, 67.
21. Voller, A., Bartlett, A., and Bidwell, D.E. (1981) *Immunoassays for the 80s.* MTP, Lancaster, UK.
22. Kemeny, D.M. (1987) Immunoglobulin and antibody assays, in *Allergy an International Text-*

book (Lessoff, M.H., Lee, T. H., and Kemeny, D.M., eds.). Wiley, Chichester, UK, 319.

23. Kemeny, D.M. and Chantler, S. (1988) An introduction to ELISA, in *ELISA and Other Solid Phase Immunoassays. Theoretical and Practical Aspects.* (Kemeny, D. M. and Challacombe, S. J., eds.). Wiley, Chichester, UK.
24. Kemeny D.M. and Challacombe, S.J. (1988) Micrototitre plates and other solid-phase supports, in *ELISA and Other Solid-Phase Immunoassays. Theoretical and Practical Aspects* (Kemeny, D. M. and Challacombe, S. J., eds.). Wiley, Chichester, UK.
25. Abu Elzein, E.M.E. and Crowther, J.R. (1978) Enzyme-labelled immunosorbent assay technique in FMDV Research. *J. Hyg. Camb.* 80, 391–399.
26. Abu Elzein, E.M.E. and Crowther, J.R. (1979) Serological comparison of a type SAT2 FMDV isolate from Sudan with other type SAT2 strains. *Bull. Anim. Hlth. Prod. Afr.* 27, 245–248.
27. Crowther, J.R. (1986) Use of enzyme immunoassays in disease diagnosis, with particular reference to rinderpest, In *Nuclear and Related Techniques for Improving Productivity of Indigenous Animals in Harsh Environments.* International Atomic Energy Agency, Vienna, Austria, pp. 197–210.
28. Crowther, J.R. (1996) ELISA, in *FMD Diagnosis and Differentiation and the Use of Monoclonal Antibodies.* Paper pres. 17th Conf. OIE. Comm. FMD., Paris, pp. 178–195.
29. Denyer, M.S., Crowther, J.R., Wardley, R.C., and Burrows, R. (1984) Development of an enzyme-linked immunosorbent assay (ELISA) for the detection of specific antibodies against H7N7 and an H3N3 equine influenza virus. *J. Hyg. Camb.* 93, 609–620.
30. Hamblin, C. and Crowther, J.R. (1982) Evaluation and use of the enzyme-linked immunosorbent assay in the serology of swine vesicular disease. in *The ELISA: Enzyme- Linked Immunosorbent Assay in Veterinary Research and Diagnosis*(Wardley, R.C. and Crowther, J.R., eds.), Martinus Nijhoff, The Netherlands, pp. 232–241.
31. Hamblin, C. and Crowther, J.R. (1982) A rapid enzyme-linked immunosorbent assay for the serological confirmation of SVD, in *The ELISA: Enzyme-Linked Immunosorbent Assay in Veterinary Research and Diagnosis* (Wardley, R.C. and Crowther, J.R., eds.), Martinus Nijhoff, The Netherlands, pp. 232–241.
32. Sanchez Vizcaino, J.M., Crowther, J.R. and Wardley, R.C. (1983) A collaborative study on the use of the ELISA in the diagnosis of African swine fever. In: *African Swine Fever.* (CEC/ FAO Research Seminar, Sardinia, Sept. 1981). Wilkinson P.J., ed. Commission of the European Communities Publication EUR 8466 EN, 297–325.
33. The sero-monitoring of rinderpest throughout Africa. Phase two. Results for 1993. Proceedings of a Research Coordination Meeting of the FAO/IAEA/SIDA/OAU/IBAR/ PARC Coordinated Research Programme organized by the Joint FAO/IAEA Division of Nuclear Techniques in Food and Agriculture, Cairo, Egypt, 7–11, November 1993.
34. Wardley, R.C., Abu Elzein, E.M. E., Crowther, J.R., and Wilkinson, P.J. (1979) A solid-phase enzyme linked immunosorbent assay for the detection of ASFV antigen and antibody. *J. Hyg. Camb.* 83, 363–369.
35. Immunogens, Ag/Ab Purification, Antibodies, Avidin-Biotin, Protein Modification: PIERCE Immunotechnology Catalogue and Handbook, Pierce and Warriner, UK. Published yearly.
36. Armstrong, R.M.A., Crowther, J.R., and Denyer, M.S. (1991) The detection of antibodies against foot-and-mouth disease in filter paper eluates trapping sera or whole blood by ELISA. *J. Immunol. Methods* 34, 181–192.
37. Hamblin, C., Barnett, I.T.R., and Crowther, J.R. (1986) A new enzyme-linked immunosorbent assay (ELISA) for the detection of antibodies against FMDV. II. *Appl. J. Immun. Methods* 93, 123–129.
38. Crowther, J.R. and Abu Elzein, E.M.E. (1980) Detection of antibodies against FMDV using purified Staphylococcus A protein conjugated with alkaline phosphatase. *J. Immunol. Methods* 34, 261–267.
39. Hamblin, C., Mertens, P.P.C., Mellor, P.S., Burroughs, J.N., and Crowther, J.R. (1991) A serogroup specific enzyme linked immunosorbent assay (ELISA) for the detection and identification of African Horse Sickness Viruses. *J. Vir. Methods* 31, 285–292.
40. Rossiter P.B., Taylor W.P., and Crowther, J.R. (1988) Antigenic variation between three strains of rinderpest virus detected by kinetic neutralisation and competition ELISA using early rabbit antisera. *Vet. Microbiol.* 16, 195–200.
41. Kemeny, D.M. (1988) The modified sandwich ELISA (SELISA) for detection of IgE anantibody isotypes, in *ELISA and Other Solid-Phase Immunoassays. Technical and Practical Aspects.* (Kemeny, D. M. and Challacombe, S. J., eds.). Wiley, Chichester, UK.
42. Abu Elzein, E.M E. and Crowther, J.R. (1981) Detection and quantification of IgM, IgA, IgG1 and IgG2 antibodies against FMDV from bovine sera using an enzyme-linked immunosorbent assay. *J. Hyg. Camb.* 86, 79–85.

43. Anderson, J., Rowe, L.W., Taylor, W.P., and Crowther, J.R. (1982) An enzyme-linked immunosorbent assay for the detection of IgG, IgA and IgM antibodies to rinderpest virus in experimentally infected cattle. *Res. Vet. Sci.* 32, 242–247.
44. Bongertz, V. (2003) Anti-HIV-1 humoral immune response in Brazilian patients. *Clin. Appl. Immunol. Rev.* 3, 6, 307–317.
45. Abu Elzein, E.M.E. and Crowther, J.R. (1982) Differentiation of FMDV-strains using a competition enzyme-linked immunosorbent assay. *J. Virol. Methods* 3, 355–365.
46. Curry, S., Abrams, C.C., Fry, E., Crowther, J.R., Belsham, G., Stewart, D., and King, A.Q. (1995) Viral RNA modulates the acid sensitivity of FMDV capsids. *J. Virol.* 69, 430–438.
47. Sunwoo, H.H., Wang, W.W., Sim, J.S. (2006) Detection of Escherichia coli O157: H7 using chicken immunoglobulin Y. *Immunol.Lett.*106, 2,15, 191–193.
48. Crowther, J.R. (1986) FMDV, in *Methods of Enzymatic Analysis, 3rd ed.* (Bergmeyer, J. and Grassl, M., eds.), VCH, Weinheim, Germany, pp. 433–447.
49. Denyer, M.S. and Crowther, J.R. (1986) Use of indirect and competitive ELISAs to compare isolates of equine influenza A virus. *J. Virol. Meth.* 14, 253–265.
50. Goldberg, M.E. and Djavadi-Ohaniance, L. (1993). Methods for measurement of antibody/ antigen affinity based on ELISA and RIA. *Curr. Opin. Immunol.* 5, 278–281.
51. Yolken, R.H. (1982) Enzyme immunoassays for the detection of infectious antigens in fluids: current limitations and future prospects. *Rev. Infect. Dis.* 4, 35.
52. Abu Elzein, E.M.E. and Crowther, J.R. (1979) The specific detection of FMDV whole particle antigen (140S) by enzyme labelled immunosorbent assay. *J. Hyg. Camb.* 83, 127–134.
53. Crowther, J.R. and Abu Elzein, E.M.E. (1979) Detection and quantification of FMDV by enzyme labelled immunosorbent assay techniques. *J. Gen. Virol.* 42, 597–602.
54. Crowther, J.R. and Abu Elzein, E.M.E. (1979) Application of the enzyme-linked immunosorbent assay to the detection of FMDVs. *J. Hyg. Camb.* 83, 513–519.
55. Crowther, J.R. (1995) Quantification of whole virus particles (146S) of foot-and-mouth disease viruses in the presence of virus subunits (12S) using monoclonal antibodies in an ELISA. *Vaccine* 13, 1064–1075.
56. Hamblin, C., Mellor, P., Graham, M.S., and Crowther, J.R. (1990) Detection of african horse sickness antibodies by a sandwich competition ELISA. *Epid Infect.* 104, 303–312.
57. Crowther, J.R., Rowe, C.A., and Butcher, R. (1993) Characterisation of MAbs against type SAT 2 FMD virus. *Epidemiol. Infect.* 111, 391–406.
58. McCullough, K.C., Crowther, J.R., and Butcher, R.N. (1985) A liquid-phase ELISA and its use in the identification of epitopes on FMDV antigens. *J. Virol. Methods* 11, 329–338.
59. Crowther, J.R., McCullough, K.C., Simone E.F.DE., and Brocchi, E. (1984) Monoclonal antibodies against FMDV: applications and potential use. *Rpt. Sess. Res. Gp. Stand. Tech. Comm. Eur. Comm. Cont. FMD* 7, 40–45.
60. Crowther, J.R. (1986) ELISA, in *FMD Diagnosis and Differentiation and the Use of Monoclonal Antibodies.* Paper pres. 17th Conf. OIE Comm. FMD., Paris, pp. 153–173.
61. Samuel, A., Knowles, N.J., Samuel, G.D., and Crowther, J.R. (1991) Evaluation of a trapping ELISA for the differentiation of foot-and-mouth disease virus strains using monoclonal antibodies. *Biologicals* 19, 229–310.
62. Crowther, J.R., Reckziegel, P.O., and Prado, J.A. (1993) The use of MAbs in the molecular typing of animal viruses. *Rev. Sci. Tech. Off. Int. Epiz. 12,* 2, 369–383.
63. Pullen, M.A., Laping, N., Edwards, R., Bray J. (2006) Determination of conformational changes in the progesterone receptor using ELISA-like assay. *Steroids* 71, 9, 792–798.
64. Carlos, O.et-al. (2006) Evaluation of murine monoclonal antibodies targeting different epitopes of the hepatitis B virus surface antigen by using immunological as well as molecular biology and biochemical approaches. *J. Immunol. Methods* 313, 1–2, 30,38–47.
65. Johannsson, A., Ellis, D.H., Bates, D.L., Plumb, A.M., and Stanley, C.J. (1986) Enzyme amplification for immunoassays-detection of one hundredth of an attomole. *J. Immunol. Methods* 87, 7–11.
66. Crowther, J.R., Anguerita, L., and Anderson, J. (1990) Evaluation of the use of chromogenic and fluorigenic substrates in solid phase ELISA. *Biologicals*18, 331–336.
67. Linscott's Directory of Immunological and Biological Reagents. Linscott's Directory, Santa Rosa, CA.
68. Unusan, N. (2006) Occurrence of aflatoxin M1 in UHT milk in Turkey. *Food Chem.Toxicol.* 44, 11, 1897–1900.
69. Watanabe, E.et-al. (2006) Evaluation of performance of a commercial monoclonal antibody–based fenitrothion immunoassay and application to residual analysis in fruit samples. *J. Food Prot.* 69, 1, 191–198.

70. Carlin, F., Broussolle, V., Perelle, S., Litman, S., Fach, P. (2004) Prevalence of Clostridium botulinum in food raw materials used in REP-FEDs manufactured in France. *Int. J. Food Microbiol.* 91, 2, 141–145.

71. Rogers-Lowery, C.L., Dimock, R.V., Kuhn, R.E. Jr., (2007) Antibody response of bluegill sunfish during development of acquired resistance against the larvae of the freshwater mussel Utterbackia imbecillis. *Dev. Comp. Immunol.* 31, 2, 143–155.

72. Tsutsumi, T.et-al. (2006) Application of an ELISA for PCB 118 to the screening of dioxin-like PCBs in retail fish. *Chemosphere* 65, 3, 467–473.

73. Liu, W.et-al. (2006) Immune response against grouper nervous necrosis virus by vaccination of virus-like particles *Vaccine* 24, 37–39, 6282–6287.

74. Liao, T.et-al. (2006) An enzyme-linked immunosorbent assay for rare minnow (Gobiocypris rarus) vitellogenin and comparison of vitellogenin responses in rare minnow and zebrafish (Danio rerio). *Sci. Total Environ.* 364, 1–3, 284–294.

75. Pucci, B., Coscia, M.R., Oreste, U. (2003) Characterization of serum immunoglobulin M of the Antarctic teleost Trematomus bernacchii. *Comp. Biochem. Physiol. B, Biochem. Mol. Biol.* 135, 2, 349–357.

76. Neumann, J.et-al. (2006) Retroviral vectors for vaccine development: induction of HIV-1-specific humoral and cellular immune responses in rhesus macaques using a novel MLV(HIV-1) pseudotype vector. *J. Biotechnol.* 124, 3, 615–625.

77. Caterino-de-Araujo, A.et-al. (1998).Sensitivity of two enzyme-linked immunosorbent assay tests in relation to western blot in detecting human T-Cell lymphotropic virus types I and II infection among HIV-1 infected patients from São Paulo, Brazil. *Diag. Microbiol. Infect. Dis.* 30, 3, 173–182.

78. Huang, J., Ma, R., Wu, C.Y. (2006) Immunization with SARS-CoV S DNA vaccine generates memory CD4+ and CD8+ T cell immune responses. *Vaccine* 24, 23, 4905–4913.

79. Al-Natoura, Q.M., Abo-Shehada, M.N. (2005) Sero-prevalence of avian influenza among broiler-breeder flocks in *Jordan Prev. Vet. Med.* 70, 1–2, 45–50.

80. Dundon, W.G., Milani, A., Cattoli, G., Capua, I. (2006) Progressive truncation of the Non-Structural 1 gene of H7N1 avian influenza viruses following extensive circulation in poultry. *Virus Res.* 119, 2, 171–176.

81. Jennifer, M., Maloney, M.D., Martin, D., Chapman, P., Scott, H., Sicherer, M.D. (2006) Peanut allergen exposure through saliva: Assessment and interventions to reduce exposure. *J. Allergy Clin. Immunol.*118, 3, 719–724.

82. Dearman, R.J.et-al. (2003) Induction of IgE antibody responses by protein allergens: inter-laboratory comparisons. *Food Chemi. Toxicol.* 41, 11, 1509–1516.

83. Huestis, M., Gustafson, R., Moolchan, E., Barnes, A., Bourland, J., Sweeney, S., Hayes, E., Carpenter, P., Smith, M. Cannabinoid concentrations in hair from documented cannabis users. *Forensic Sci. Int.*169, 2–3, 129–136.

84. Huang, T.L., Lee, CT. (2006) Associations between serum brain-derived neurotrophic factor levels and clinical phenotypes in schizophrenia patients. *J. Psychiatr. Res.* 40, 7, 664–668.

85. Baker, K.N.et-al. (2002) Rapid monitoring of recombinant protein products: a comparison of current technologies. *Trends Biotechno.* 20, 4, 1, 149–156.

86. Crowther, J. R. (2000)The ELISA Guidebook. *Methods Mol Biol.*;149: 1–413III–IV, Humana, Totowa, NJ.

87. Rial, A., Morais, V., Rossi, S., Massaldi, H. (2006) A new ELISA for determination of potency in snake antivenoms. *Toxicon* 48, 4, 462–466.

88. Speight, S.E., Hallis, B.A., Bennett, A.M., Benbough, J.E. (1997) Enzyme-linked immunosorbent assay for the detection of airborne microorganisms used in biotechnology. *J Aerosol Sci.* 28, 3, 483–492.

89. March, C.et-al. (2005) Rapid detection and counting of viable beer-spoilage lactic acid bacteria using a monoclonal chemiluminescence enzyme immunoassay and a CCD camera. *J Immunol. Methods* 303, 1–2, 92–104.

90. Harlow, E. and Lane, D. (eds.) (1988) *Antibodies. A Laboratory Manual.* Cold Spring Harbor Laboratory, Cold Spring Harbor, NY.

91. Roitt, I. (1991) *Essential Immunology.* Blackwell, Oxford, UK.

92. Roitt, I., Brostoff, J., and Male, D. (eds.) (1993) *Immunology.* Mosby, Edinburgh.

93. Landon, J. (1977) Enzyme-immunoassay: techniques and uses. *Nature* 268, 483.

94. ZAvrameas, S., Nakane, P.K., Papamichail, M., and Pesce, A.J., eds. (1991) 25 Years of immunoenzymatic techniques. International Congress, Athens, Greece, September 9 12. *J. Immunol. Methods*150, 1–220.

95. Van Weemen, B.K. (1985) ELISA: highlights of the present state of the art. *J. Virol. Methods* 10371.

Contents

Chapter 1

Overview of ELISA in Relation to Other Disciplines

This chapter examines what areas of science are needed to allow optimal use of ELISA and notes their relationships. This information is useful for students and those instructing students. Diagrams, with brief descriptions of key points, are used to illustrate such relationships. Inherent in this exercise are considerations of the exact requirements by the operators in using the ELISA. Attention to increasing knowledge in those areas highlighted is essential both in developmental work to produce a working ELISA and in the ultimate value of any test devised. A good deal of attention should be directed at defining, as clearly as possible, the objectives for the ELISA. The development of a diagnostic test for a specific disease requires that all other data pertaining to the biology of that disease, e.g., antigenicity and structure of the agent, antibody production in different animals following infection, qualitative assessment of antibodies by different assays, and availability of standard or control sera, are known. Some attention must be paid to the laboratory facilities available, e.g., equipment, reagents already developed, small laboratory animals, experimental large animals, cash to buy commercial products, and trained personnel. In this way, the chances of producing a sustainable test to solve the defined problem are significantly greater than when a test is developed by a dabbling technique with poor or no forward planning.

Figure 1 emphasizes that we are considering the heterogeneous ELISA involving separation steps and a solid phase. Four major advantages of ELISA are promoted, all of which add to the reasons that this form of ELISA has been, and will continue to be, successful.

Figure 2 deals with the systematics of the ELISA and shows the various stages needed and factors important in those stages.

John R. Crowther, *Methods in Molecular Biology, The ELISA Guidebook, Vol. 516*

DOI: 10.1007/978-1-60327-254-4_1

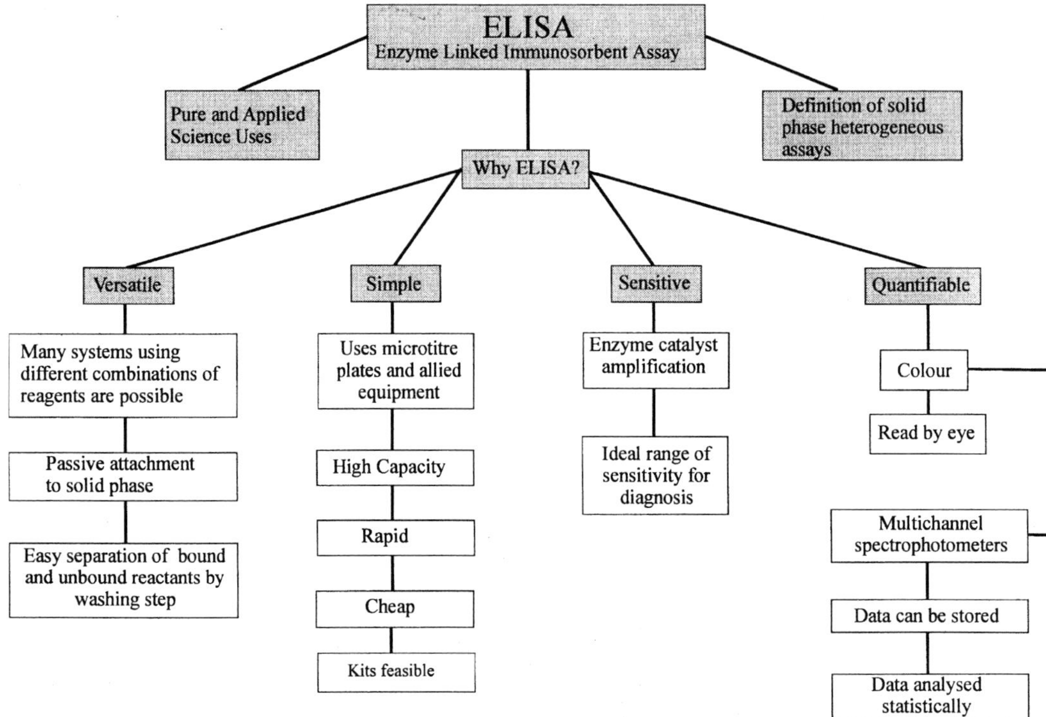

Fig. 1. Scheme showing features of ELISA that make it advantageous for a wide range of applications.

Figure 3 emphasizes that using the equipment to perform ELISAs requires skills, and that both physical and mental processes are needed. **Figure 3** also indicates that instruments need to be maintained for optimal performance.

Figure 4 deals with some of the enzymatic systems in the ELISA, and illustrates areas that need to be understood in order to allow optimal performance to be maintained. Understanding enzyme kinetics, catalysis reactions, hazards, and buffer formulation (pH control) are all essential.

Figure 5 illustrates the use of ELISAs in binding and inhibition/competition interactions to allow an understanding of a problem. It is essential that the chemical and physical nature of antibodies and antigens are understood, particularly in cases of developmental work. A full understanding of the antigenic properties of agents being examined is needed to allow maximum exploitation of ELISA, particularly if the results are ever to be understood.

Figure 6 deals with data processing and analysis. Various essential statistical parameters must be elucidated, if data are to be interpreted. This is true in understanding how to calculate the variance in a result, and also for examining populations. Such studies actually define any ELISA's performance, allowing

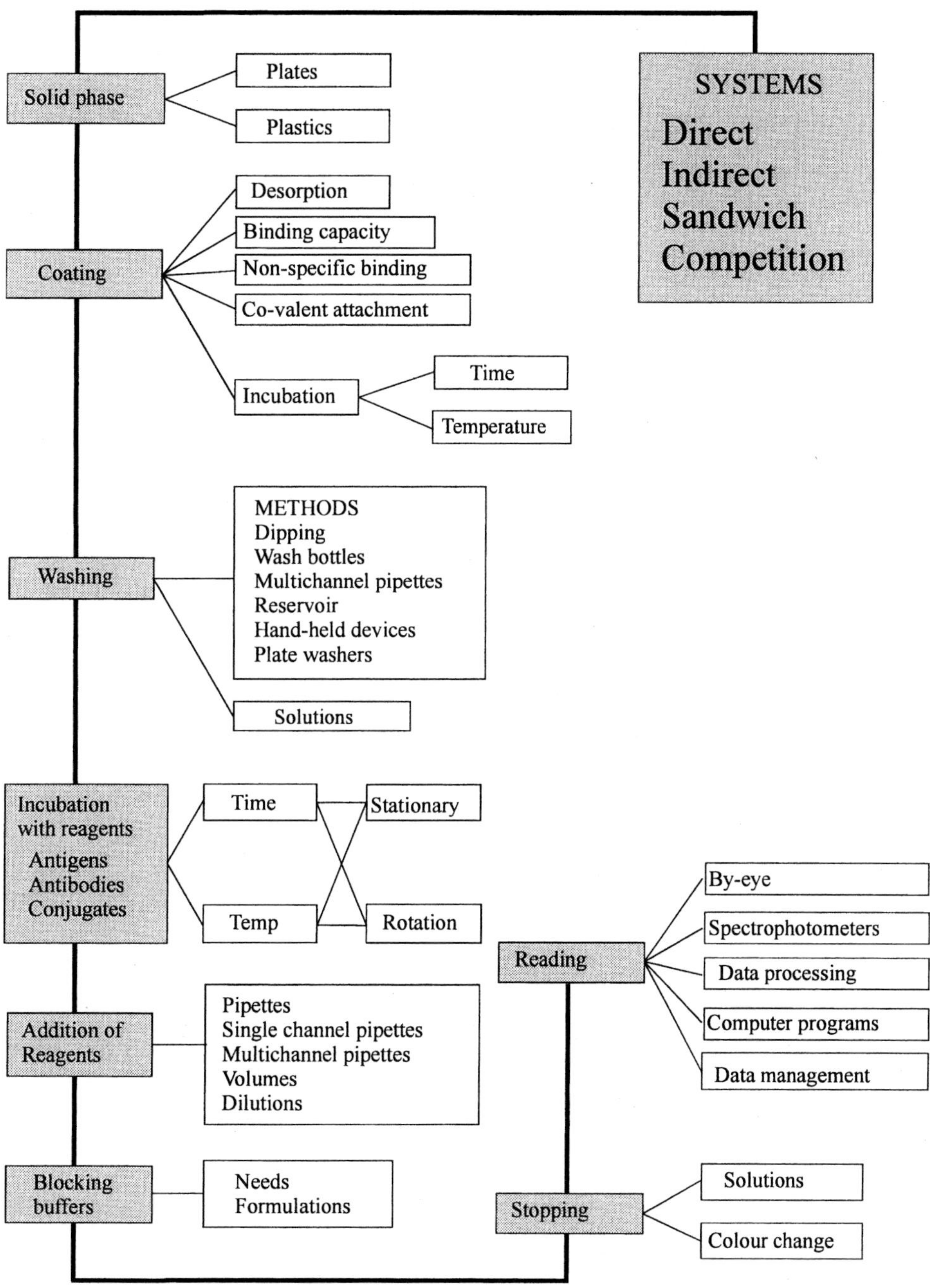

Fig. 2. Scheme relating stages in ELISA. Specific stages vary according to the system utilized.

confidence in results to be measured, thereby allowing a meaning to be placed on results. The concepts of controlling assays with references to standards is also needed.

Figure 7 extends the use of statistical understanding into epidemiological needs. A common use of ELISA is to provide data

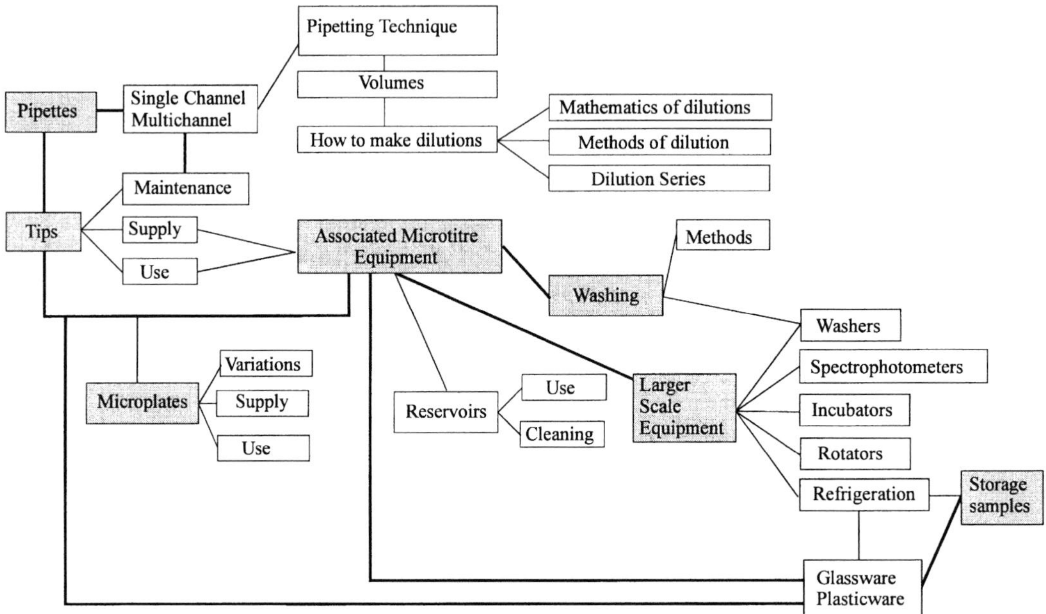

Fig. 3. Scheme relating equipment needs and skills for ELISA.

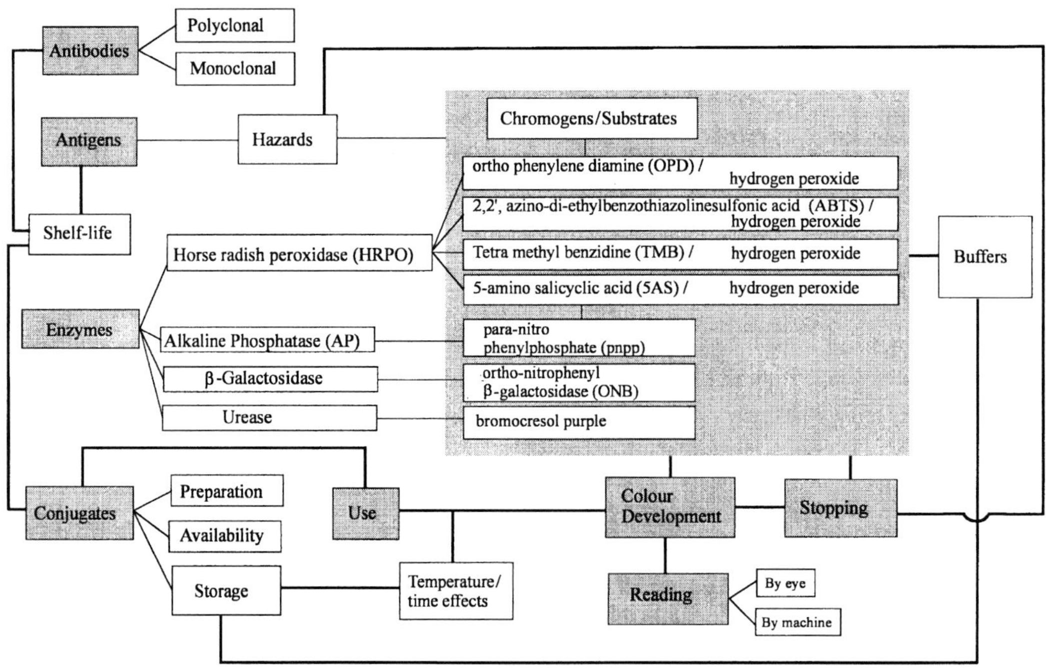

Fig. 4. Relationships of enzyme systems to components of ELISA.

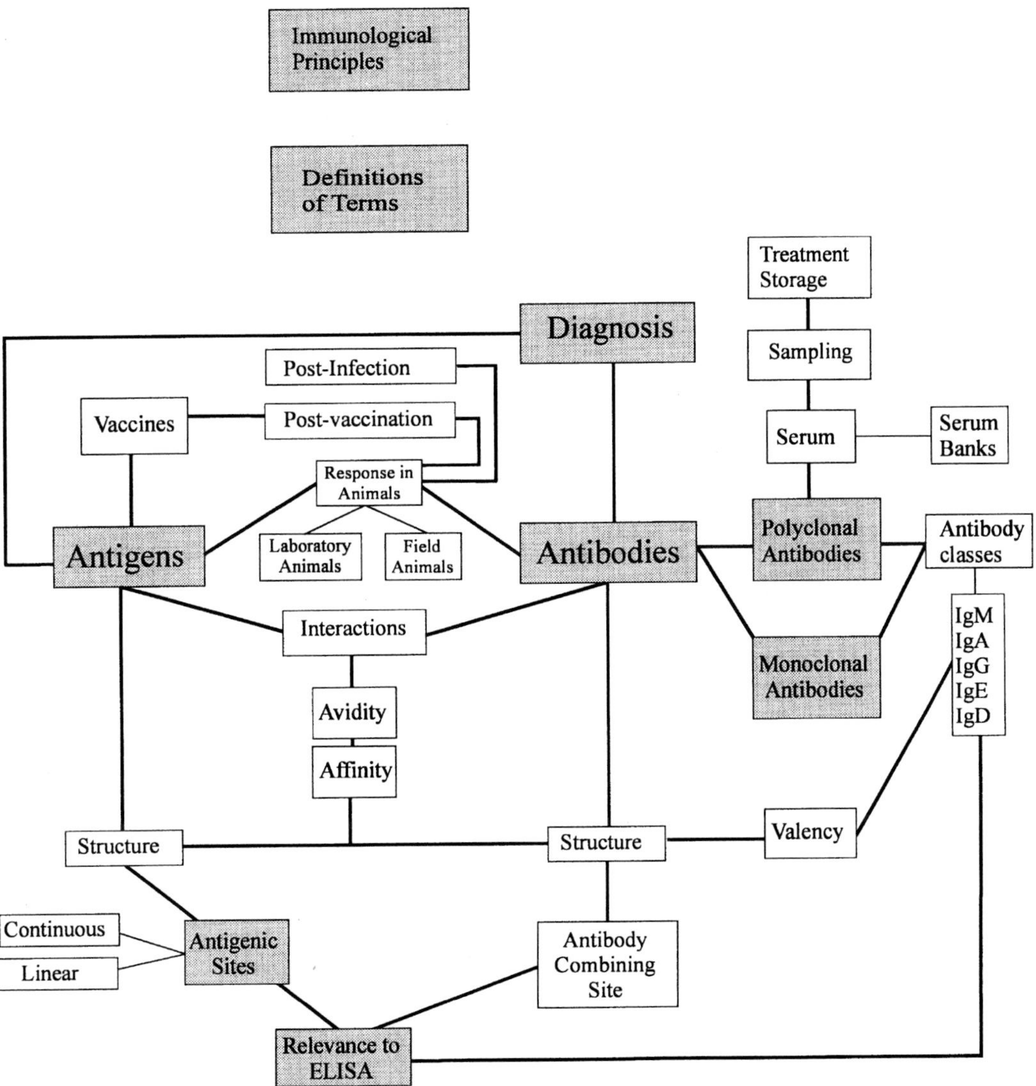

Fig. 5. Requires features in immunological understanding in order to establish ELISA.

on populations studied. The areas of sampling (size, number, and so forth) are vital when planning disease control strategies.

These simplified overviews should be used as reference points when considering the development and specific use of any ELISA. They should help readers with limited exposure to ELISA, particularly after studying the details in later chapters. They are also useful for trainers in establishing areas of competence in students.

These are the key points to keep in mind at this early stage when considering then use of ELISA:

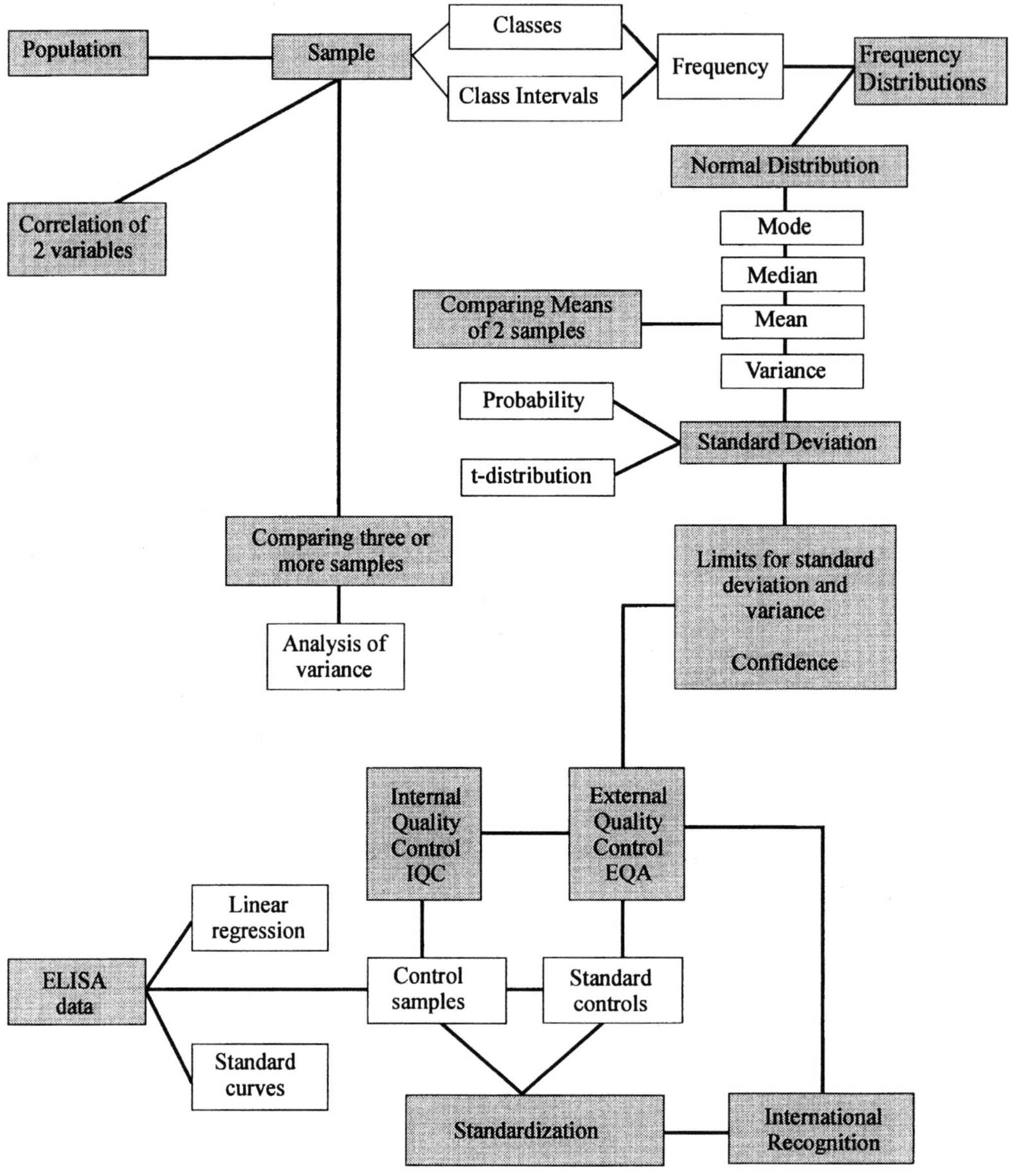

Fig. 6. Important statistical factors needed to make use of ELISA. Note the links to quality control (internal) and the establishment of confidence in test results. Increasingly, assays need international recognition.

1. The ELISA is a tool to solve a problem.
2. Any problem should be defined, as clearly as possible, with reference to all previous work defining the specific agent involved and related agents.
3. Other methods for analyzing the problem should be reviewed, particularly when tests are already established. This has implications if the ELISA is to replace existing tests.

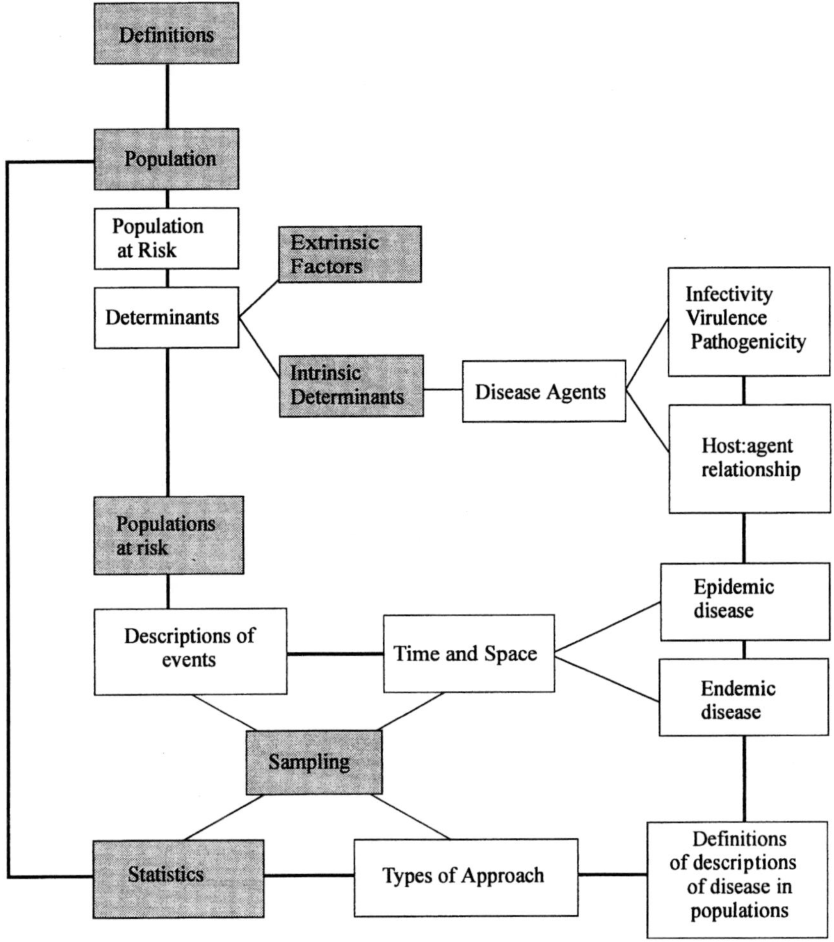

Fig. 7. Scheme relating basic areas in epidemiology that need to be understood in the context of data obtained from ELISA. Note the strong link with statistics/sampling, which is inherent in the test design.

4. The capacity for testing has to be addressed. For example, when an ELISA may be used on a large scale (kit), then sufficient reagents, standard sera, conjugates (batches), and antigen preparations must be available. Research leading to successful assays in which reagents are difficult to prepare on a large scale require extensive expertise to formulate, or are reliant on a specific limited batch of a commercial reagent are not sustainable.
5. When a test may be of use to a wider group of scientists, the possible conditions (laboratory facilities, expertise) should be considered when developing assays. Such technology transfer factors are relevant, particularly in laboratories in developing countries.

The knowledge and skills required to both perform ELISA and make use of the data have to be gained through a variety of sources, including textbooks. As with all other techniques, the ultimate benefit is not the technique in itself, but the meaningful gathering and analysis of the data. One factor not included in all these examples is that of common sense: The ability to really consider what one is doing, and why, and not to overlook the simplicity of what is needed by being blinded by the technology for its own sake. Most problems are relatively simple to examine after some clear thought. Thus, a good ELISA person will consider the problem first, obtain the necessary technical skills and equipment to perform a test, and then obtain data that is from a planned perspective. As much data from all other tests and the scientific literature should also be sought. This is true for an assay developer, as well as a person using a supplied, predetermined kit. The skills required by the use of a kit are no less than those of the developer; indeed, a kit in the hands of an unskilled worker is often useless. The majority (90%) of problems observed in the practice of ELISA are operator faults caused by lack of common sense, failure to appreciate the need to stick to instructions, sloppy technique, or poorly maintained equipment. Most of the remaining percentage is caused by poor-quality water.

Chapter 2

Systems in ELISA

This chapter defines the terms and examines the configurations used for most applications of ELISA. Such a chapter is important because the possibilities inherent in the systems of ELISA must be understood in order to maximize their versatility in assay design. All heterogeneous systems have three basic parameters:

1. One reactant is attached to a solid phase, usually a plastic microtiter plate with an 8 × 12-well format.
2. Separation of bound and free reagents, which are added subsequently to the solid phase-attached substance, is by a simple washing step.
3. Results are obtained through the development of color.

1. Definition of Terms

Immunoassays involve tests using antibodies as reagents. Enzyme immunoassays make use of enzymes attached to one of the reactants in an immunoassay to allow quantification through the development of color after the addition of a suitable substrate/chromogen.

As indicated, ELISAs involve the stepwise addition and reaction of reagents to a solid phase-bound substance, through incubation and separation of bound and free reagents using washing steps.

An enzymatic reaction is utilized to yield color and to quantify the reaction, through the use of an enzyme-labeled reactant. **Table 1** gives the definitions of terms used in ELISA. These terms are greatly amplified throughout the subsequent text.

John R. Crowther, *Methods in Molecular Biology, The ELISA Guidebook, Vol. 516*

DOI: 10.1007/978-1-60327-254-4_2

Table 1
Brief defination of terms

Term	Definition
Solid phase	Usually a microtiter plate well. Specially prepared ELISA plates are commercially available. These have an 8×12- well formatand can be used with a wide variety of specialized equipment designed for rapid manipulation of samples, including multichannel pipets.
Adsorption	The proces of adding an antigen or antibody, diluted in buffer, so that it attaches passively to the solid phase on incubation. This is a simple way for immobilization of one of the reactants in the ELISA and one of the main reasons for its success.
Washing	The simple flooding and emptying of the wells with a buffered solution to separate bound (reacted) from unbound (unreacted) reagents in the ELISA. Again, this is a key element to the successful exploitation of the ELISA.
Antigens	A protein or carbohydrate that when injected into animals elicits the production of antibodies. Such antibodies can react specifically with the antigen used and therefore can be used to detect that antigen.
Antibodies	Produced in response to antigenic stimuli. These are mainly protein in nature. In turn, antibodies are antigenic.
Antispecies antibodies	Produced when proteins (including antibodies) from one species are injected into another species. Thus, -guinea pig serum injected into a rabbit elicits the production of rabbit anti-guinea pig antibodies.
Enzyme	A substance that can react at low concentration as a catalyst to promote a specific reaction. Several specific enzymes are commonly used in ELISA with their specific substrates.
Enzyme conjugate	An enzyme that is attached irreversibly to a protein, usually an antibody. Thus, an example of antispecies enzyme conjugate is rabbit antiguinea linked to horseradish peroxidase.
Substrate	A chemical compound with which an enzyme reacts specifically. This reaction is used, in some way, to produce a signal that is read as a color reaction (directly as a color change of the substrate or indirectly by its effect on another chemical).
Substrate	A chemical that alters color as a result of an enzyme interaction with substrate.
Stopping	The process of stopping the action of an enzyme on a sub-strate. It has the effect of stopping any further change in color in the ELISA.
Reading	Measurement of color produced in the ELISA. This is quantified using special spectrophotometers reading at specific wavelengths for the specific colors obtained with particular enzyme-chromophore systems. Tests can be assessed by eye.

2. Basic Systems of ELISA

This section describes the principles involved in the many configurations possible in ELISA. The terminology used here may not always agree with that used by others, and care is needed in defining the assays by name. The specific assay parameters must always be examined carefully in the literature. The following set of definitions attempts to clear up the myriad of published approaches to describing the systems used in a few words such as "double-sandwich competitive ELISA" and "indirect sandwich inhibition ELISA." The aim is to have a clear approach. Three main methods form the basis to all ELISAs:

1. Direct ELISA
2. Indirect ELISA
3. Sandwich ELISA

All three systems can be used to form the basis of a group of assays called competition or inhibition ELISAs.

The systems (arrangement and use of reagents in the test) are illustrated herein through the use of symbols (as defined in **Table 2**) as well as terms. In this way, it is hoped that the reader will gain

Table 2
Defination of Symbols or terms used to describe assays

Symbol/term	Definition
▤	Solid-phase microtiter well
---	Attachment to solid phase by passive adsorption
Ag	Antigen
Ab	Antibody
AB	Antibody (different species donor than Ab)
Anti-Ab	Antispecies antiserum against species from donor Ab
Anti-AB	Antispecies antiserum against species from donor AB
**Enz	Enzyme liked to reactant
S	Substratelchroihophore system
WASH	Washing step
°C	Incubation
READ	Read color in spectrophotometer
+	Addition of reagents
**	Binding of reagents
STOP	Stopping of color development

a clear idea of the various systems and their relative advantages and disadvantages. A key feature of the flexibility of ELISA is that more than one system can be used to measure the same thing. This allows some scope to adapt assays to suit available reagents as well as to note areas of improvement through the identification of the need to prepare additional reagents – e.g., that monoclonal antibodies (mAbs) may be needed to give an assay the required specificity, or that a particular anti-species conjugate against a subclass of immunoglobulin (Ig) is required.

Practical details of the various stages, e.g., solid phase, buffers, incubation, and conjugates, are dealt with in detail in Chapters 3 and 4.

2.1. Direct ELISA

Direct ELISA can be regarded as the simplest form of ELISA, and is illustrated in **Fig. 1** and in **Diagram 1**.

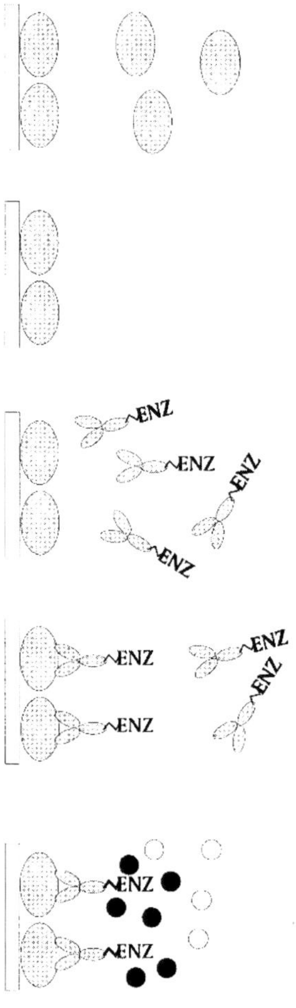

(i)

Antigen is added to the solid phase and adsorbs passively on incubation.

(ii)

After incubation, any non-bound antigen is washed away leaving the 'coated' solid phase.

(iii)

ENZ
ENZ
ENZ
ENZ

Antibodies specific for the antigen and labeled with an enzyme (conjugate) are added, and incubated.

(iv)

ENZ
ENZ
ENZ
ENZ

The conjugate binds with antigen on solid phase.

Any unbound (free) conjugate is washed away.

(v)

ENZ
ENZ

A substrate/chromophore solution is added and the enzyme catalyses the reaction to give a colored product.

The reaction is terminated after a certain time (Stopped) and the colour quantified (read) using a spectrophotometer.

Fig. 1. Direct ELISA. Antigen is attached to the solid phase by passive adsorption. After washing, enzyme-labeled antibodies are added. After an incubation period and washing, a substrate system is added and color is allowed to develop.

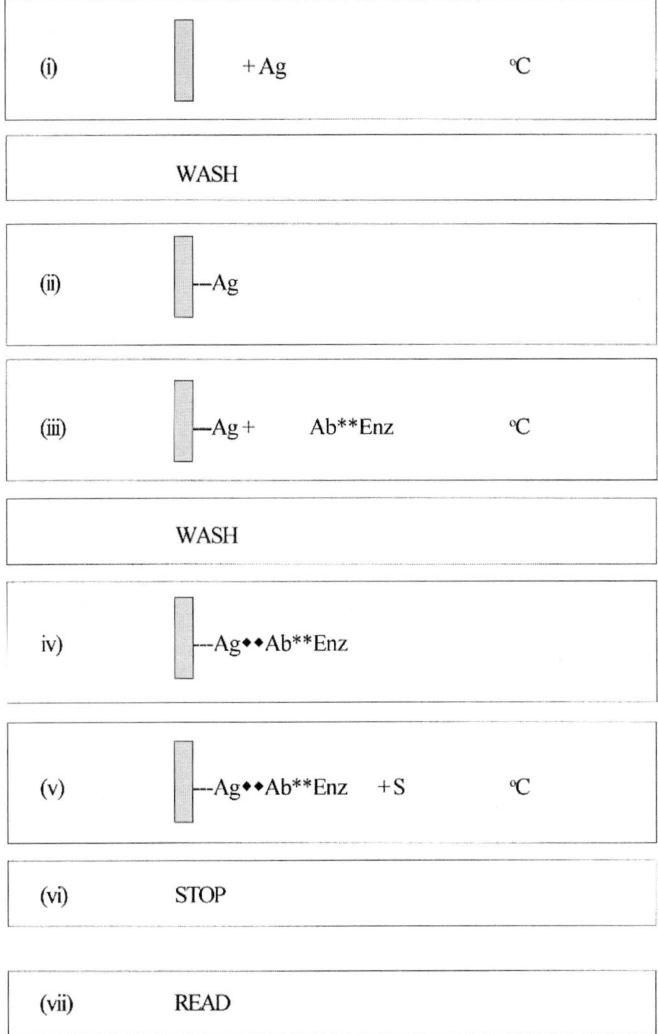

Diagram 1. Direct ELISA.

Antigen is diluted in a buffer (stage i), commonly a high pH (9.6) carbonate or bicarbonate buffer or neutral phosphate-buffered saline (PBS). The key is that the buffer contains no other proteins that might compete with the target antigen for attachment to the plastic solid phase. Antigens are mainly protein in nature and will attach passively to the plastic during a period of incubation. The temperature and time of incubation are not so critical, but standardization of conditions is vital, and the use of incubators at 37°C is favored (since they are widely available in laboratories). After incubation, any excess antigen is removed by a simple washing step (stage ii), by flooding and emptying the wells, using a neutral buffered solution (e.g., PBS). Antibodies conjugated with an enzyme can now be added (stage iii), and are directed specifically against antigenic sites on the solid phase-bound reagent. The conjugated antibodies are diluted in a buffer containing some substance that inhibits passive adsorption of protein, but that still allows immunological binding. Such substances either are other proteins, which are added at a high concentration to compete for the solid-phase sites with the antibody protein, or are detergents at low concentration termed *blocking agents*, and the buffers they help formulate, which are termed *blocking buffers*.

On incubation, antibodies bind to the antigen. Again, a simple washing step is then used to remove unbound antibodies (stage iv). Stage v involves the addition of a suitable substrate or substrate/chromogen combination for the particular enzyme attached to the antibodies. The objective is to allow development of a color reaction through enzymatic catalysis. The reaction is allowed to progress for a defined period, after which the reaction is stopped (stage vi) by altering the pH of the system, or by adding an inhibiting reactant. Finally, the color is quantified by the use of a spectrophotometer reading (stage vii) at the appropriate wavelength for the color produced.

This kind of system has severe limitations when used only in this form but has assumed great importance as the "target" system in competition and inhibition assays, particularly when mAbs are conjugated and/or highly defined antigens are used.

2.2. Indirect ELISA

Indirect ELISA is illustrated in **Diagram 2** and in **Fig. 2**. Stages i and ii are similar to the direct system. Stage iii involves the addition of unlabeled detecting antibodies, which are diluted in a buffer to prevent nonspecific attachment of proteins in antiserum to solid phase (blocking buffer). This is followed by incubation and washing away of excess (unbound) antibodies, to achieve specific binding (stage iv). Stage v is the addition of the conjugate (enzyme-labeled), anti-species antibodies, diluted in blocking buffer, again followed by incubation and washing to achieve binding of the conjugate (stage vi). Substrate/chromophore is then added to the bound conjugate (stage vii) and color develops, which is then stopped (stage viii) and read (stage ix) in a spectrophotometer.

The indirect system is similar to the direct system in that the antigen is directly attached to the solid phase and targeted by added antibodies (detecting antibodies). However, these added antibodies are not labeled with enzyme but are themselves targeted by antibodies linked to enzyme. Such antibodies are produced against the immunoglobulins of the species in which the detecting antibodies are produced and are termed anti-species conjugates. Thus, if the detecting antibodies were produced in rabbits, the enzyme-labeled antibodies would have to be anti-rabbit Igs in nature. This allows great flexibility in the use of anti-species conjugates in that different specificities of conjugate

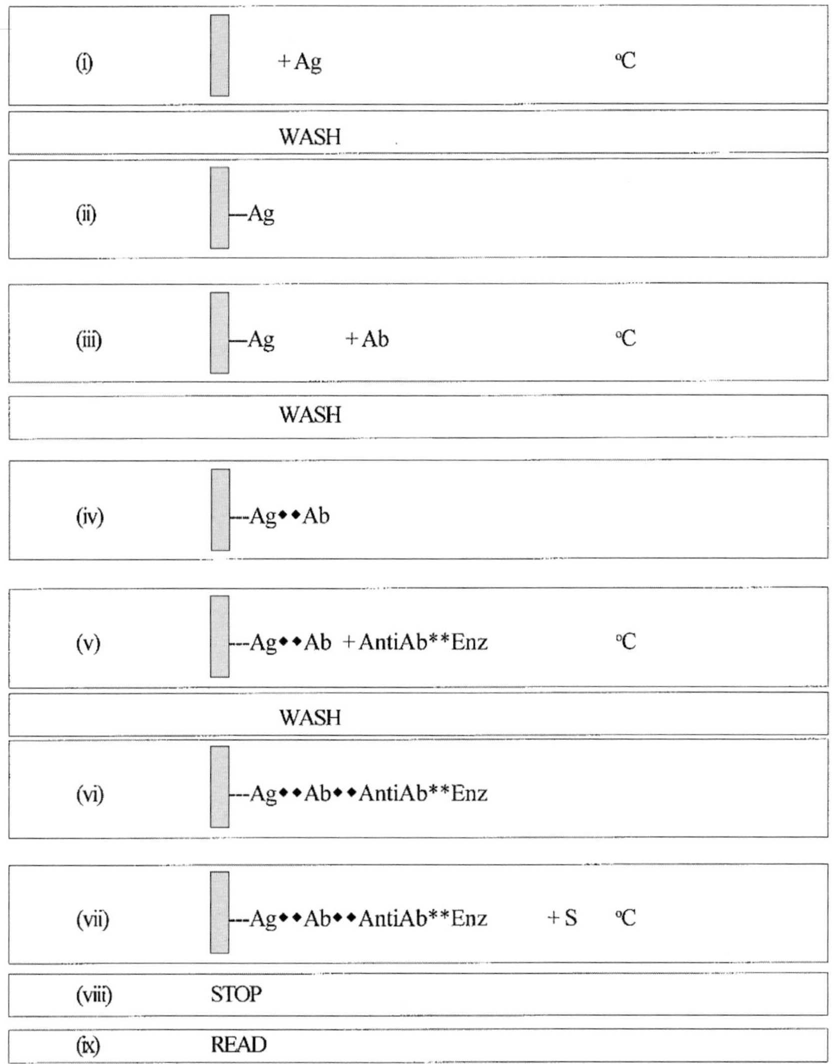

Diagram 2. Indirect ELISA.

can be used to detect particular immunoglobulin's binding in the assay, and there are literally thousands of conjugates available commercially. For example, the anti-species conjugate could be anti-IgM, anti-IgG_1, anti-IgG_2, and so on.

The indirect system offers the advantage that any number of antisera can be examined for binding to a given antigen using a single anti-species conjugate. Such systems have been heavily exploited in diagnostic applications, particularly when examining (screening) large numbers of samples. One problem that such systems have is the varying degree of nonspecific binding in individual sera. This tends to widen the dispersion (variability) in assay results and, therefore, increases the need to process many sera to assess confidence.

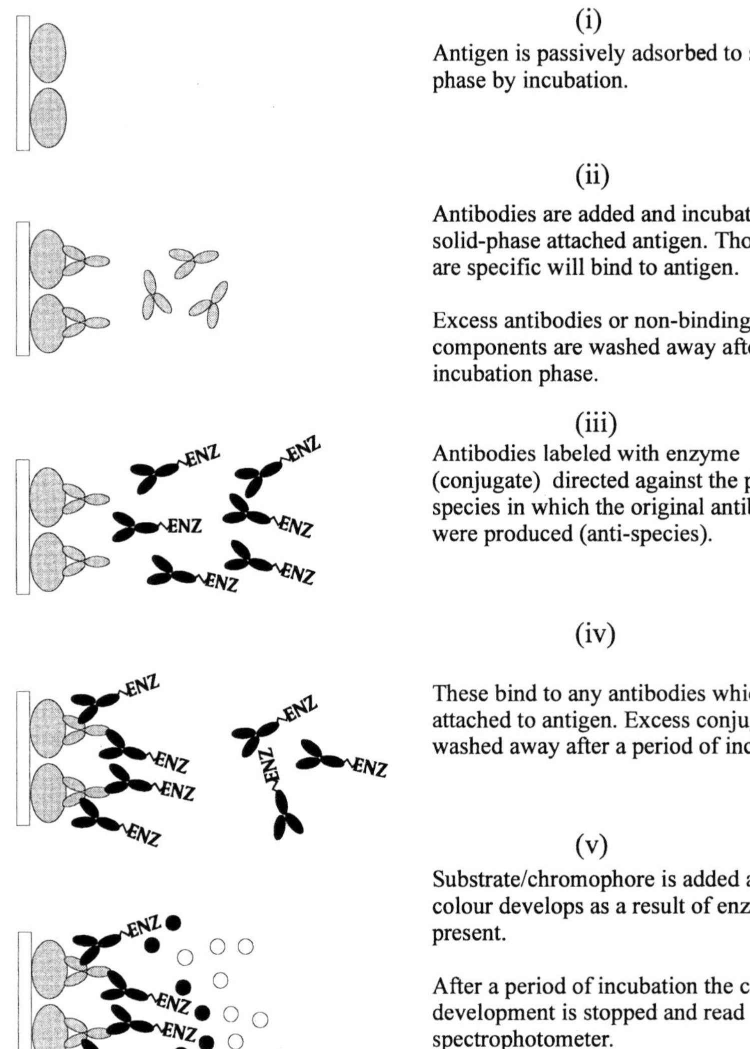

Fig. 2. Indirect ELISA. Antibodies from a particular species react with antigen attached to the solid phase. Any bound antibodies are detected by the addition of an anti-species antiserum labeled with enzyme. This is widely used in diagnosis.

2.3. Sandwich ELISA

Sandwich ELISA can be divided into two systems, which have been named the direct sandwich ELISA and the indirect sandwich ELISA.

2.3.1. Direct Sandwich ELISA

The direct sandwich ELISA is illustrated in **Diagram 3** and in **Fig. 3**.

The direct sandwich ELISA involves the passive attachment of antibodies to the solid phase (stages i and ii). These antibodies (capture antibodies) then bind antigen(s) that are added in stage

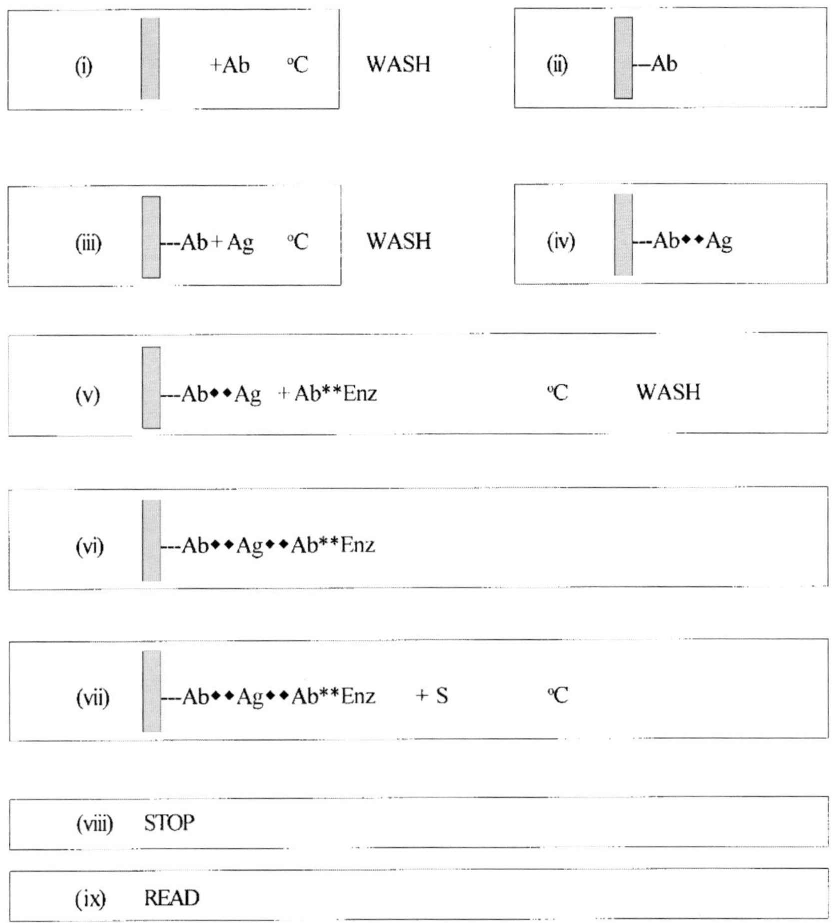

Diagram 3. Direct sandwich ELISA.

iii. The antigen(s) are diluted in a blocking buffer to avoid nonspecific attachment to the solid phase. Here, the components of the blocking buffer should not contain any antigens that might bind to the capture antibodies. After incubation and washing, an antibody–antigen complex is attached to the solid phase (stage iv).

The captured antigen (sometimes referred to as trapped) is then detected by the addition and incubation of enzyme-labeled specific antibodies in blocking buffer (stage v). Thus, this is a direct conjugate binding with the antigenic targets on the captured antigen. This second antibody can be the same as that used for capture, or be different in terms of specific animal source or species in which it was produced. After incubation and washing (stage vi), the bound enzyme is developed by the addition of substrate/chromogen (stage vii), then stopped (stage viii), and finally read using a spectrophotometer (stage ix).

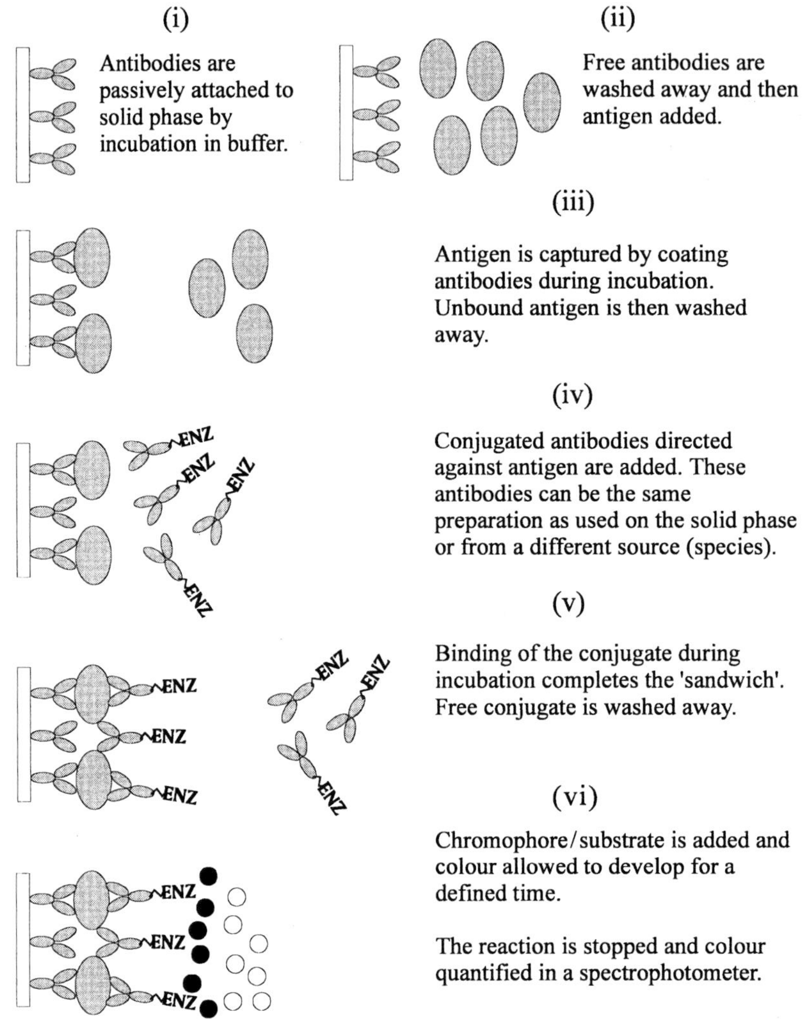

Fig. 3. Direct sandwich ELISA. This system exploits antibodies attached to a solid phase to capture antigen. The antigen is then detected using serum specific for the antigen. The detecting antibody is labeled with enzyme. The capture antibody and the detecting antibody can be the same serum or from different animals of the same species or from different species. The antigen must have at least two different antigenic sites.

Since a single enzyme-conjugated antibody is used, the system is limited to the specificities and properties inherent in that particular antibody set. This limits the versatility of the test – e.g., each antibody preparation used must be labeled (for different antigens) – in the same way as the direct ELISA was limited to single antibody preparations.

The system also is limited in that antigens must have at least two antigenic sites (epitopes), since both the capture and the detecting antibodies need to bind. This can limit the assay to relatively large antigenic complexes.

The capture antibody (on the solid phase), and the detecting antibody, can be against different epitopes on an antigen complex. This can be helpful in orienting the antigenic molecules so that there is an increased chance that the detecting antibodies will bind. It can also be an advantage when investigating small differences between antigenic preparations by the use of different detecting antibodies and a common capture antibody, and more versatile and hence appropriate systems are dealt with in **Subheading 2.3.2** The use of exactly the same antibodies for capture and detection (e.g., mAbs) can lead to problems, whereby there is a severe limitation of available binding sites for the detector. The size and the spatial relationship (topography) of the epitopes on the antigenic target are also critical and can greatly affect the assay.

2.3.2. Indirect Sandwich ELISA

Indirect sandwich ELISA is illustrated in **Diagram 4** and in **Fig. 4**. In indirect sandwich ELISA assay, stages i–iv are quite similar to

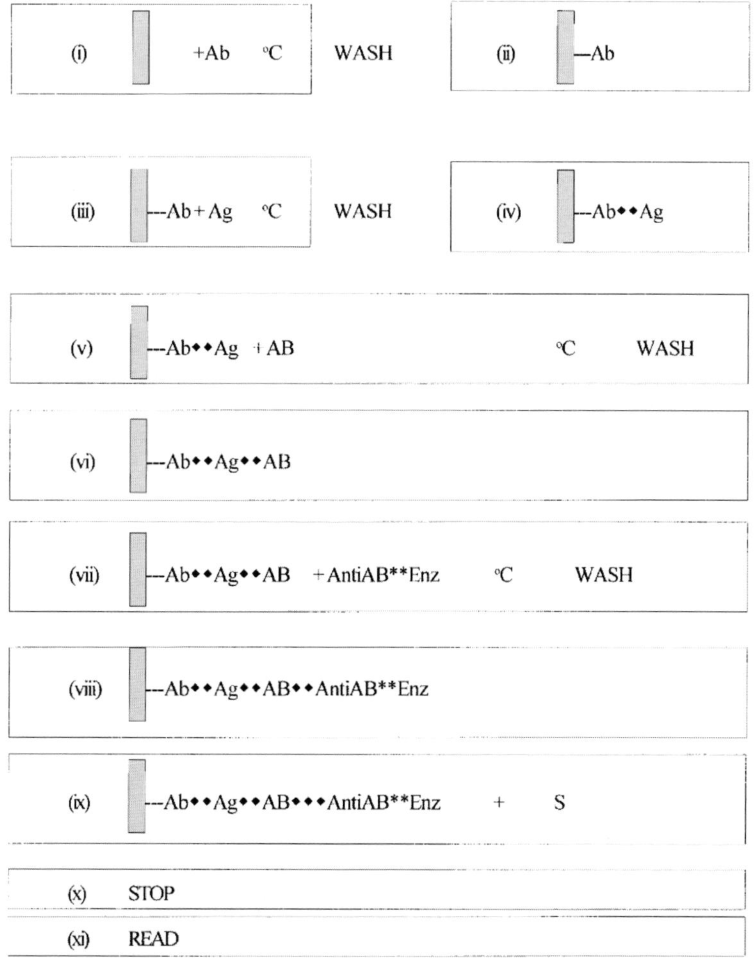

Diagram 4. Indirect sandwich ELISA.

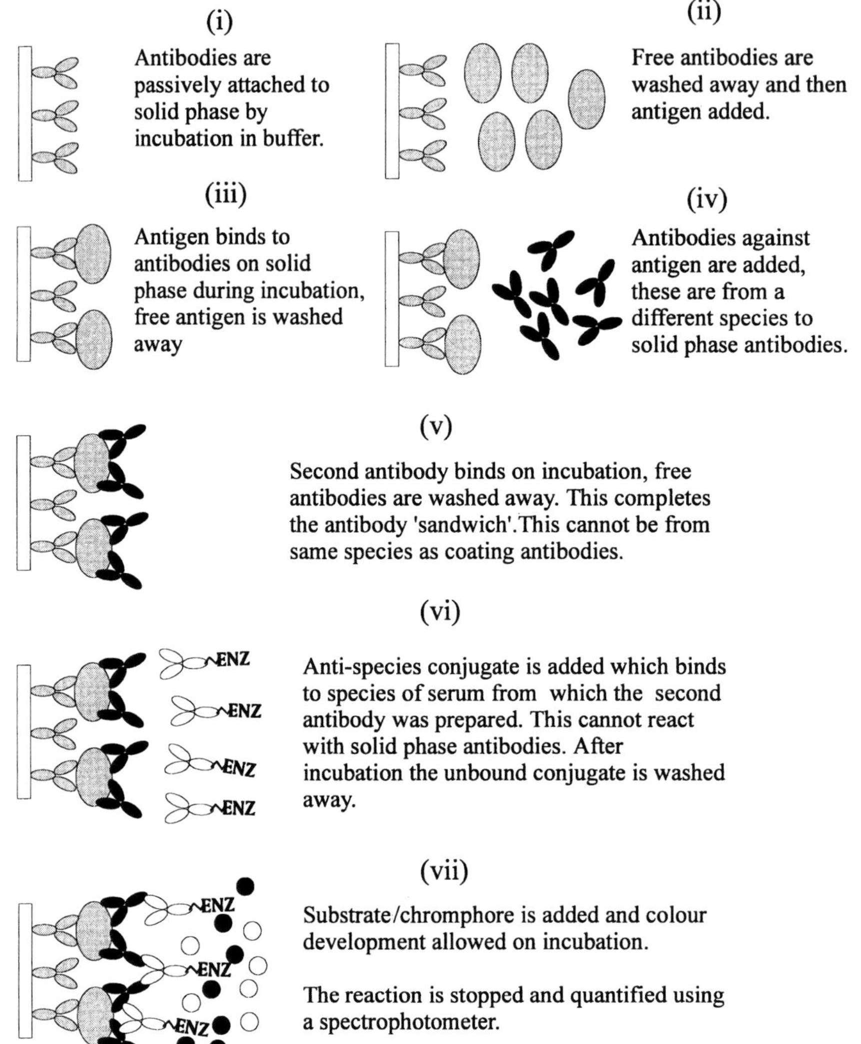

Fig. 4. Indirect sandwich ELISA. The antigen is captured by a solid-phase antibody. Antigen is then detected using antibodies from another species. This in turn is bound by an anti-species conjugate. Thus, the species of serum for the coating and detecting antibodies must be different; the anti-species conjugate cannot react with the coating antibodies.

those of the direct sandwich ELISA. Thus, antibodies are passively attached to the solid phase and antigen(s) are captured. However, stage v involves the addition of detecting antibodies. In this case, the antibodies are not labeled with enzyme. After incubation and washing (stage vi), the detecting antibodies are themselves detected by addition and incubation with an anti-species enzyme conjugate (stage vii). The bound conjugate is then processed as described in the other systems (stages xiii–ix).

The advantage of this assay is that any number of different sources of antibodies (samples) can be added to the captured antigen, provided that the species in which it was produced is not the same as the capture antibody. More specifically, the enzyme conjugated anti-species antibody does not react with the antibodies used to capture the antigen. It is possible to use the same species of antibody if immunochemical techniques are used to select and produce particular forms of antibodies and with attention to the specificity of the enzyme conjugate used. Thus, as an example, the capture antibody could be processed to a bivalent molecule without the Fc portion (also called $F(ab')_2$ fraction). The detecting antibodies could be untreated. The enzyme conjugate could then be an anti-species anti-Fc portion of the Ig molecule. Thus, the conjugate would react only with antibodies containing Fc (and therefore not the capture molecules). The need to devise such assays depends on the reagents available.

It may be that a mAb is available that confers a desired specificity as compared with polyclonal sera or that one wishes to screen a large number of mAbs against an antigen that must be captured (it may be at a low concentration or in a mixture of other antigens). In this case, the use of $F(ab')_2$ polyclonal sera is unsuccessful; therefore, the preparation of fragments for the capture antibody is worthwhile, and in fact, relatively easy-to-use kits are available for this purpose. The use of a commercially available anti-mouse Fc completes the requirements.

2.4. Competition/ Inhibition Assays

The terms *competition* and *inhibition* describe assays in which measurement involves the quantification of a substance by its ability to interfere with an established pretitrated system. The systems involve all the other ELISA configurations already described. The assays can also be used for the measurement of either antibody or antigen. The terminology used in the literature can lead to confusion; the term blocking-ELISA is also frequently used to describe such assays. This section describes the possible applications of such methodologies, indicating the advantages and disadvantages. C-ELISA (competition ELISA) and I-ELISA (inhibition ELISA) are used to describe generally the assays involving the elements described in **Subheading 2.1–2.3** and the particular application of competitive or inhibition assay dealt with specifically for each different system examined. Reference should be made to the preceding descriptions of the basic systems for direct, indirect, and sandwich ELISAs, which are the basis of the C–I assays.

2.4.1. Direct C-ELISA: Test for Antigen

Direct C-ELISA testing for antigen is described and shown in **Diagram 5** and in **Fig. 5**. A pretitrated, direct system is challenged by the addition of antigen. The effect of the addition is measured by a decrease in expected color of the pretitrated system (used as a control). Thus, the competition stages proper start at stage iii, in which a sample is added to a solid phase that has the system antigen already passively attached. This sample is diluted in blocking buffer to prevent antigen binding to the solid phase nonspecifically. At this stage, nothing should happen in terms of binding. The pretitrated dilution of labeled antibody (specific for the solid-phase antigen) is then added. The competitive phase now begins where, if the test antigen introduced is the same or similar to the solid-phase antigen, it will bind with the introduced labeled antibodies (stage ii a). The degree of competition in time depends on the relative concentration of molecules of the test and solid-phase antigen (and to the degree of antigenic similarity). After incubation and washing, the amount of labeled antibodies in the test is quantified after the addition of substrate, and so forth. When there is no antigen in the test sample, or when the antigenic similarities are limited, there is no binding with the labeled antibodies (stage ii b); thus, there is nothing to prevent (compete with) the binding of the labeled antibodies (stage iii). The net result is that, for samples containing antigen, there is

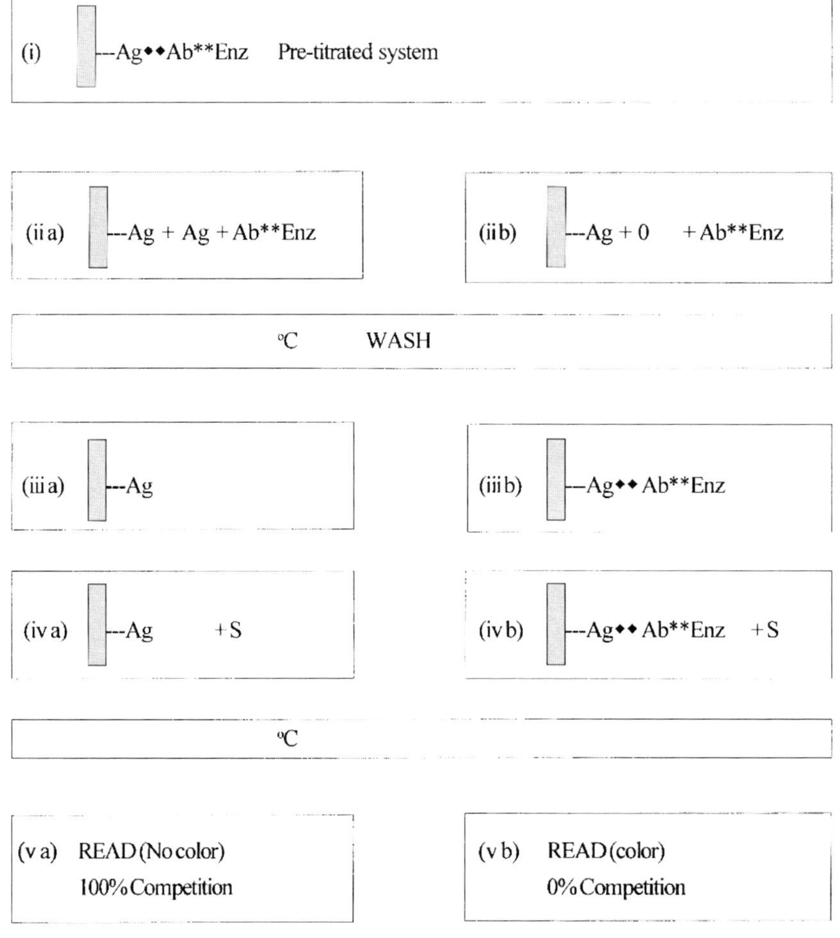

Diagram 5. Direct C-ELISA test for antigen.

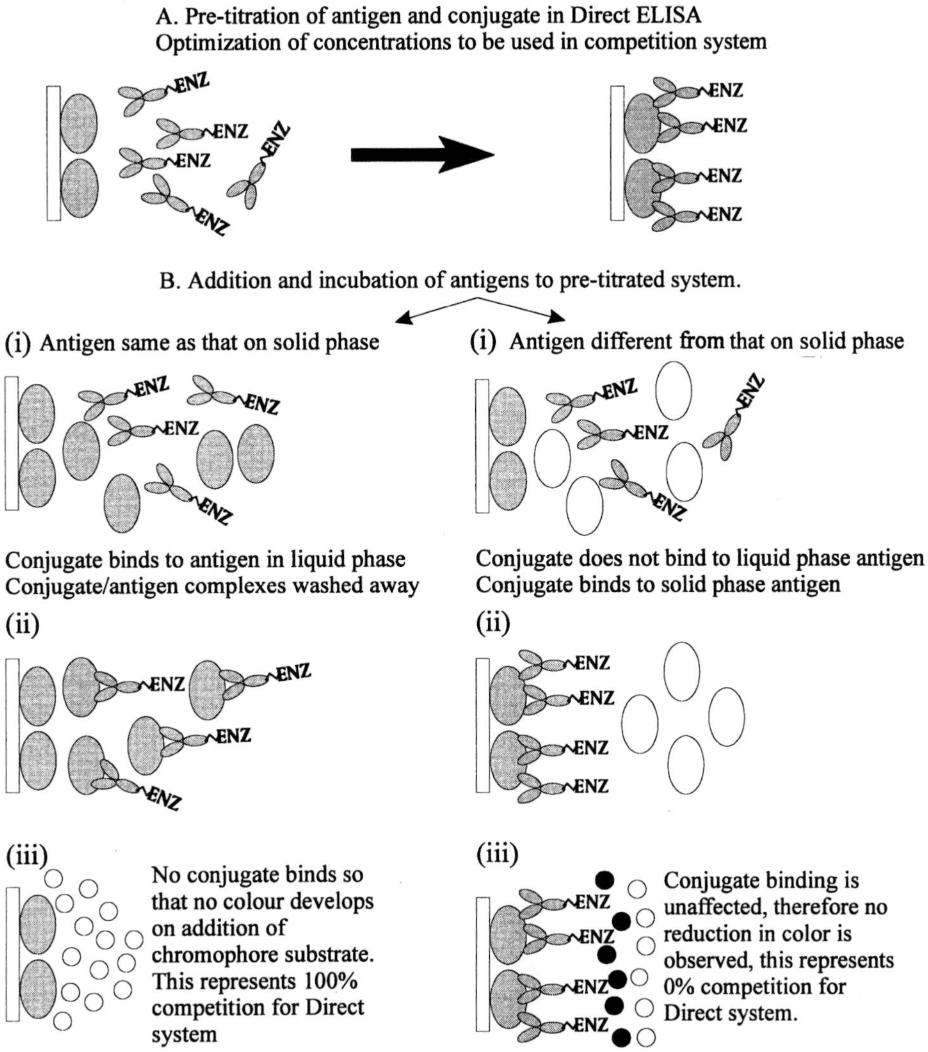

A. Pre-titration of antigen and conjugate in Direct ELISA
Optimization of concentrations to be used in competition system

B. Addition and incubation of antigens to pre-titrated system.

(i) Antigen same as that on solid phase

Conjugate binds to antigen in liquid phase
Conjugate/antigen complexes washed away

(ii)

(iii) No conjugate binds so that no colour develops on addition of chromophore substrate. This represents 100% competition for Direct system

(i) Antigen different from that on solid phase

Conjugate does not bind to liquid phase antigen
Conjugate binds to solid phase antigen

(ii)

(iii) Conjugate binding is unaffected, therefore no reduction in color is observed, this represents 0% competition for Direct system.

Fig. 5. Direct C-ELISA for antigen. Reaction of antigen contained in samples with the enzyme-labeled antibody directed against the antigen on the solid phase blocks the label from binding to the solid-phase antigen. If the antigen has no cross-reactivity or is absent, then the labeled antibody binds to the solid-phase antigen and a color reaction is observed on developing the test.

competition affecting the pretitrated expected color, whereas in negative samples there is no effect on the pretitrated color.

2.4.2. Direct C-ELISA: Test for Antibody

Direct C-ELISA testing for antibody is illustrated in **Diagram 6** and in **Fig. 6**. The system here is the same as that for the test of antigen; however, the measurement or comparison of antibodies is being made.

Again there is a requirement to titrate the direct ELISA system, which is then challenged by the addition of test antibodies.

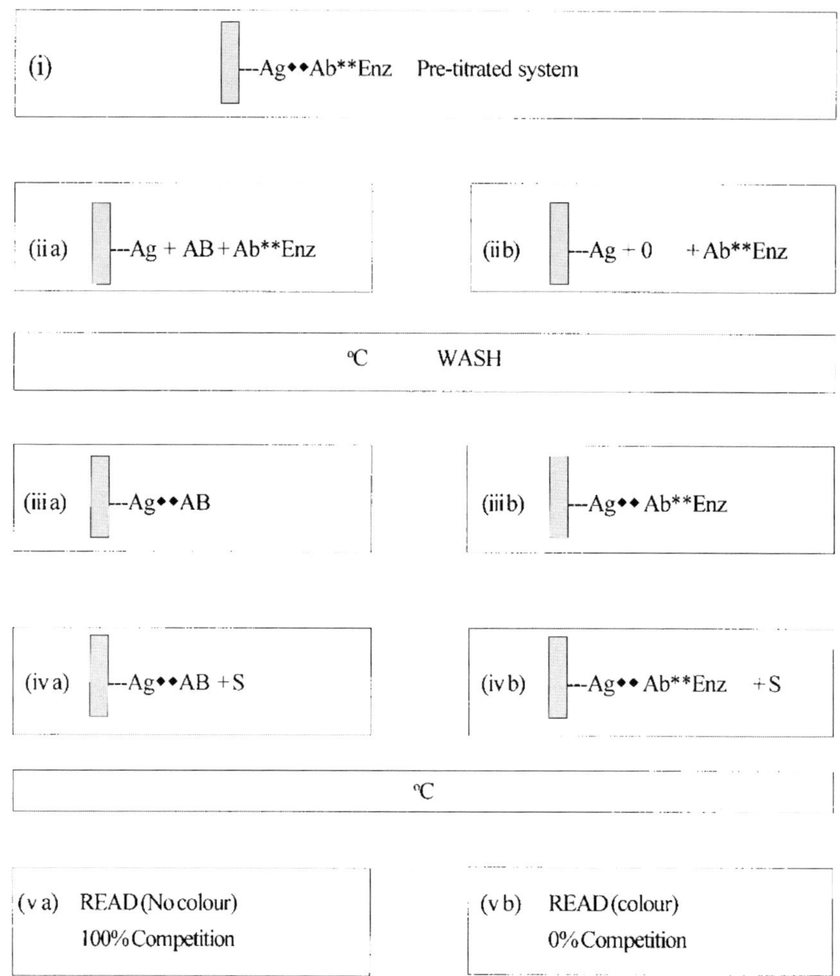

Diagram 6. Direct C-ELISA testing for antibody.

The competitive aspect here is between any antibodies in the test sample and the labeled specific antibodies for antigenic sites on the solid-phase bound antigen. The test sample and pretitrated labeled antibodies are mixed before adding to the antigen-coated plates.

2.4.3. Direct I-ELISA: Test for Antigen

Direct I-ELISA for antigen testing is not an available alternative, since test antigen has to be mixed with pretitrated labeled antibody. Thus, competitive conditions apply. One variation is that test antigen can be premixed with the labeled antibody and incubated for a period before the mixture is applied to the antigen-coated plates. In practice, this makes no difference to the assays in which antigen is added to the coated plates initially.

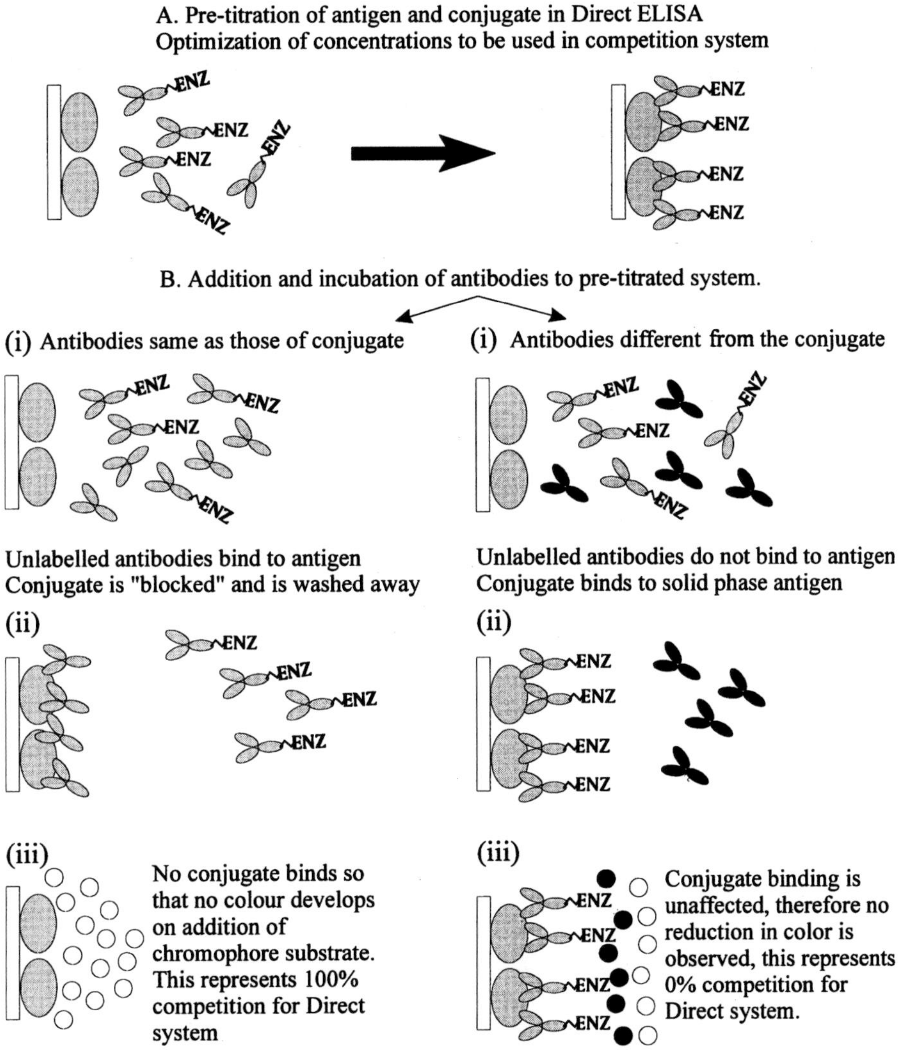

A. Pre-titration of antigen and conjugate in Direct ELISA
Optimization of concentrations to be used in competition system

B. Addition and incubation of antibodies to pre-titrated system.

(i) Antibodies same as those of conjugate

Unlabelled antibodies bind to antigen
Conjugate is "blocked" and is washed away

(ii)

(iii) No conjugate binds so that no colour develops on addition of chromophore substrate. This represents 100% competition for Direct system

(i) Antibodies different from the conjugate

Unlabelled antibodies do not bind to antigen
Conjugate binds to solid phase antigen

(ii)

(iii) Conjugate binding is unaffected, therefore no reduction in color is observed, this represents 0% competition for Direct system.

Fig. 6. Direct C-ELISA for antibody. The degree of inhibition by the binding of antibodies in a serum for a pretitrated enzyme-labeled antiserum reaction is determined.

2.4.4. Direct I-ELISA: Test for Antibody

The test sample possibly containing antibodies specific for the antigen on the plates is added and incubated for a period. There are then two alternatives: (1) the wells can be washed and then the pretitrated labeled antibody can be added, or (2) pretitrated labeled antibody can be added to the wells containing the test sample. In these ways, the advantage in terms of binding to the antigen on the wells is given to the test sample. Bound antibodies then inhibit or block the binding of the subsequently added labeled antibodies.

2.5. Competitive and Inhibition Assays for Indirect ELISA

2.5.1. Indirect C-ELISA Antigen Measurement

Indirect C-ELISA antigen measurement is illustrated in **Diagram 7** and in **Fig. 7**.

2.5.2. Indirect C-ELISA Antibody Measurement

Indirect C-ELISA antibody measurement is illustrated in **Diagram 8** and in **Fig. 8**.

Note that the same pretitrated system can be used for both antigen and antibody titration. The respective analytical sensitivities of the systems as adapted for antigen and antibody measurement can be altered with respect to the initial titration of the reagents in the pretitration phase. Thus, by using different concentrations of antibody, the effective sensitivity for competition or inhibition by antigen or antibody can be altered to favor

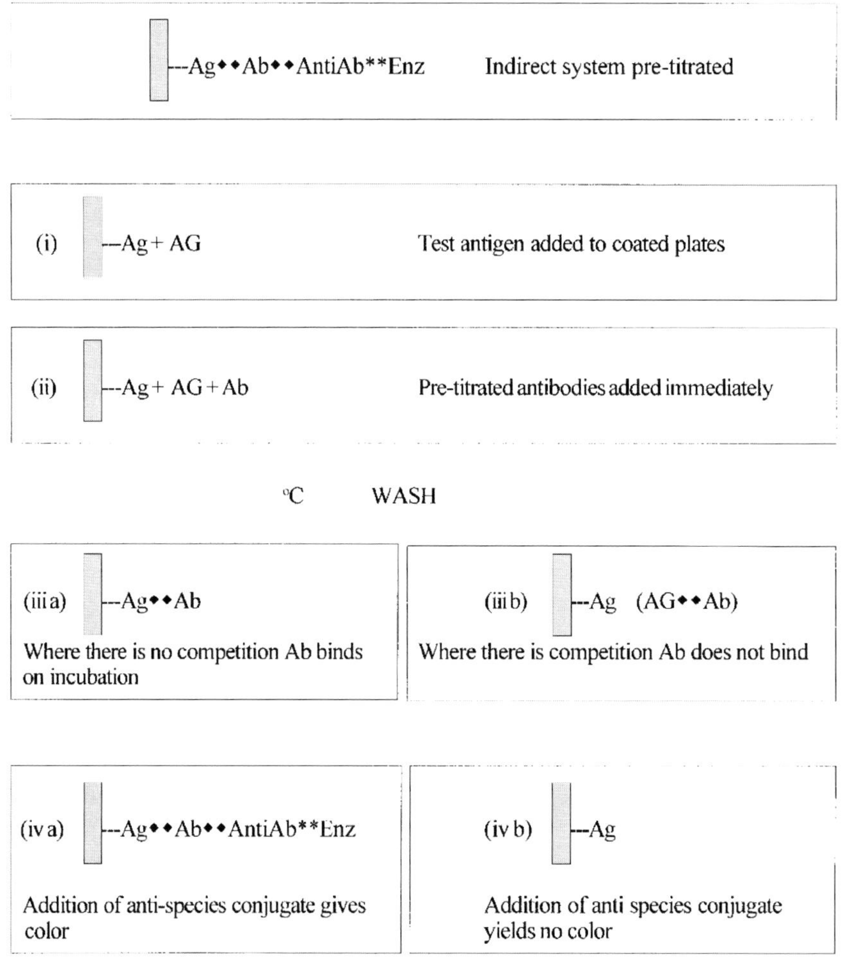

Diagram 7. Indirect C-ELISA antigen measurement.

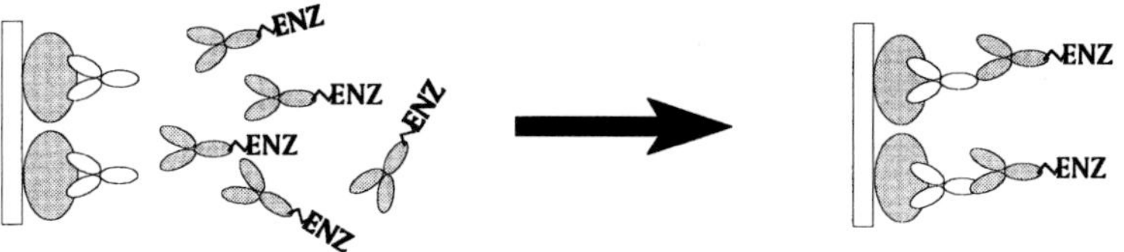

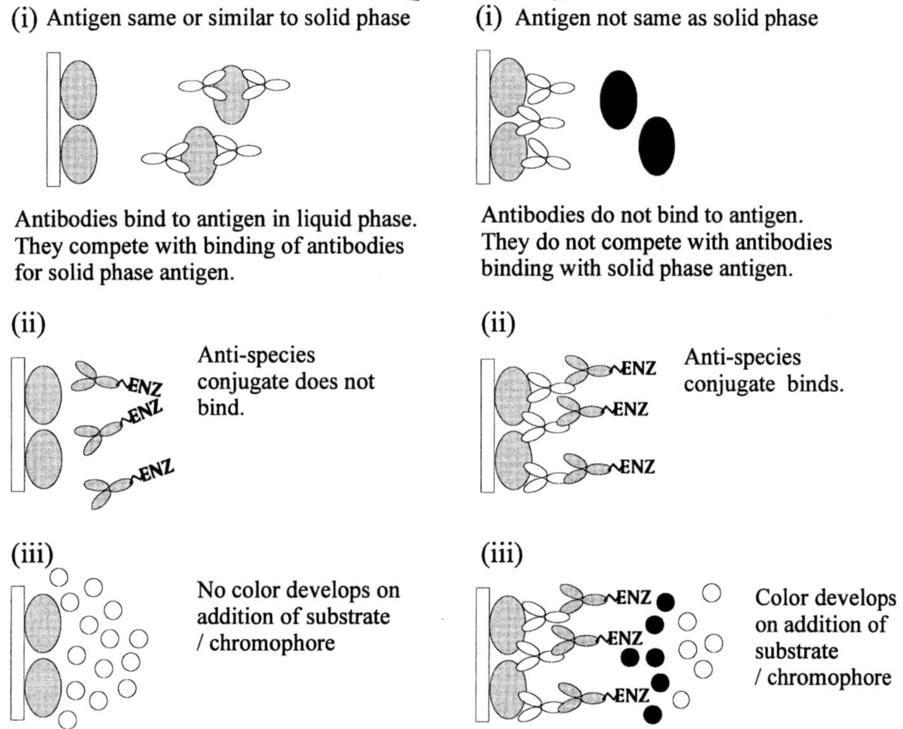

Fig. 7. Indirect C-ELISA antigen measurement. The degree of competition by the binding of antigens in a sample for a pretitrated enzyme-labeled antiserum reaction is determined.

either analytical sensitivity or specificity. It is important to realize this when devising assays based on competition or inhibition, whereby they can be adapted to be used to measure either antigen or antibody. Alterations in the concentrations of reactants can offer more idealized tests to suit the analytical parameters needed (degrees of required specificity and sensitivity). This is particularly important when devising assays based on polyclonal antibodies, which are markedly affected through the use of different dilutions of sera (alterations in quality of serum depending on relative concentrations of antibodies against specific antigenic determinants).

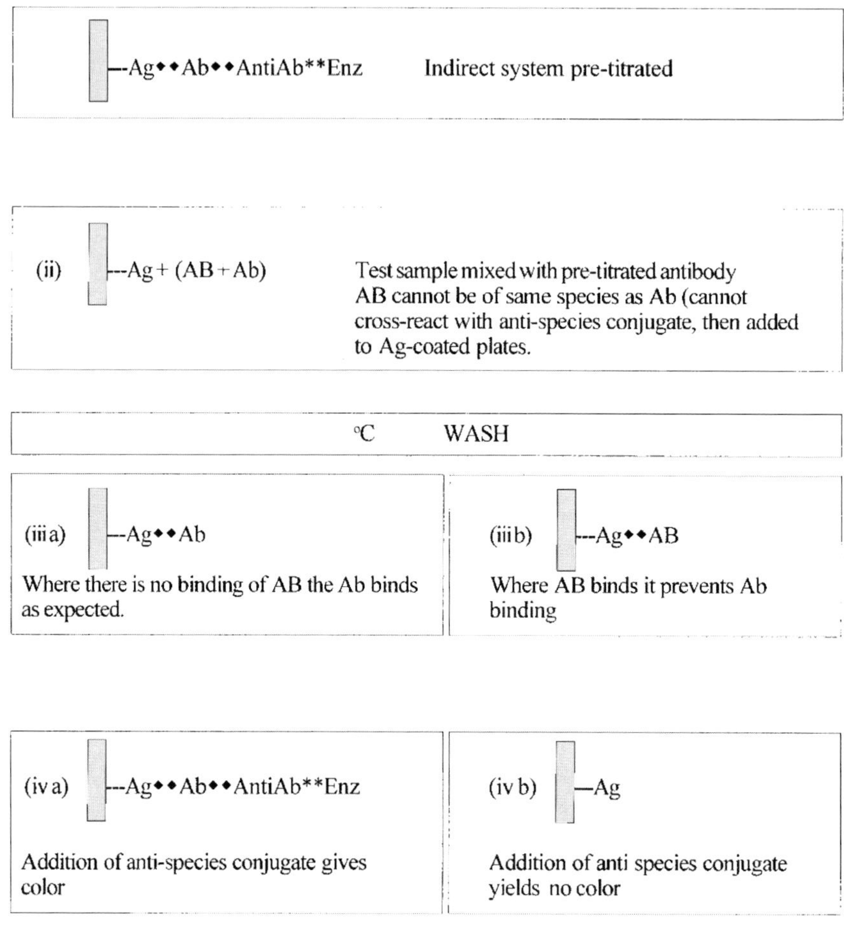

Diagram 8. Indirect C-ELISA antibody measurement.

2.5.3. Indirect I-ELISA Antigen Measurement

The test sample containing antigen can be premixed with the pretitrated antibody and incubated. The mixture can then be added to antigen-coated plates. The advantage of binding with the antibody is then in favor of the test sample. This is illustrated in **Diagram 9**.

2.5.4. Indirect I-ELISA Antibody Measurement

Principles of indirect I-ELISA antibody measurement are shown diagrammatically as follows. The sample containing AB is added to the antigen-coated plates and incubated. There are then two alternatives: (1) a washing step followed by the addition of pretitrated antibody, or (2) no washing step and the addition of pretitrated antibody to the mixture. This is illustrated in **Diagram 10**. Once again the advantage of binding is afforded to the sample.

A. Pre-titration of Indirect ELISA
Optimization of concentrations to be used in competition system

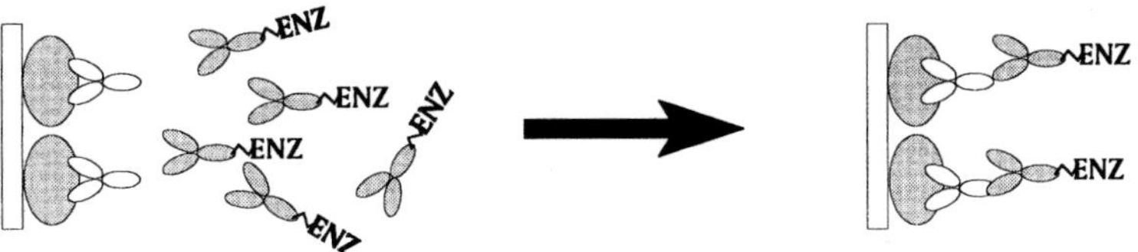

B. Mix pre-titrated and test antibodies. Add to coated plates.

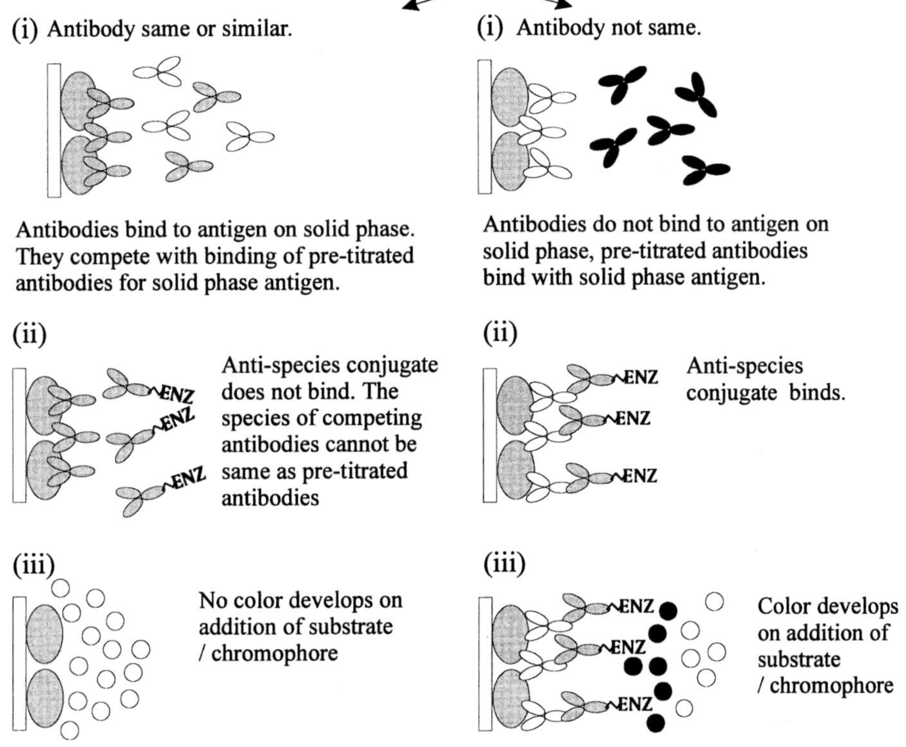

Fig. 8. Indirect C-ELISA antibody measurement. The degree of competition by the binding of antibodies in a sample for a pretitrated enzyme-labeled antiserum reaction is determined.

2.6. Competition and Inhibition Assays for Sandwich ELISAs

Reference to previous sections reminds us that sandwich ELISAs are performed with both direct and indirect systems; that is, both involve the use of an immobilized antibody on the solid phase to capture antigen. For the direct sandwich ELISA, the detecting antibody is labeled with enzyme, whereas in the indirect system the detecting antibody is not labeled, which is in turn detected using an anti-species conjugate.

Both systems are more complicated than those described previously in that there are more stages involved. Consequently,

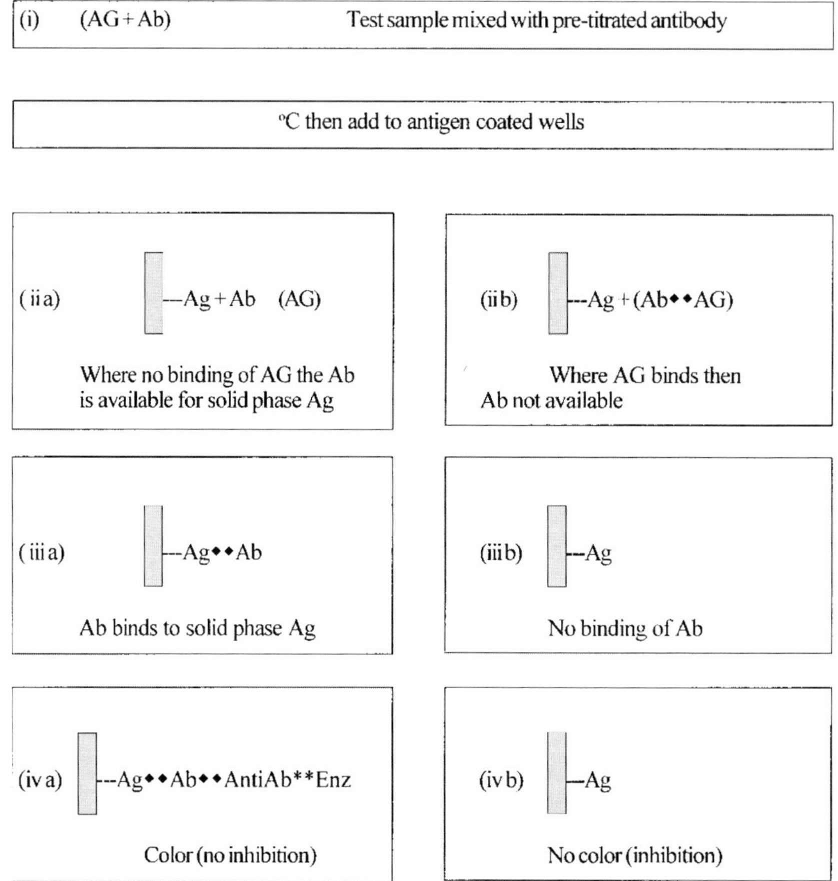

Diagram 9. Indirect I-ELISA antigen measurement.

the possibilities for variation in competing or inhibiting steps are increased. Attention must be focused on why a certain system is used as compared with others.

The main point about using sandwich assays is that they may be essential for presentation of antigen, usually by concentrating the specific antigen from a mixture through the use of a specific capture serum. Thus, the advantages of competitive/inhibitive techniques rely on antigen capture. Whether direct or indirect measurement of detecting antibody is used depends on exactly what kind of assay is being used. This section covers the principles, which in turn highlight the problems that must be addressed. Unsuitable systems are also illustrated.

The assays are described under direct sandwich and indirect sandwich headings. Direct sandwich involves assays utilizing a capture and a directly labeled detecting antibody (two antibody systems), and indirect sandwich involves assays utilizing

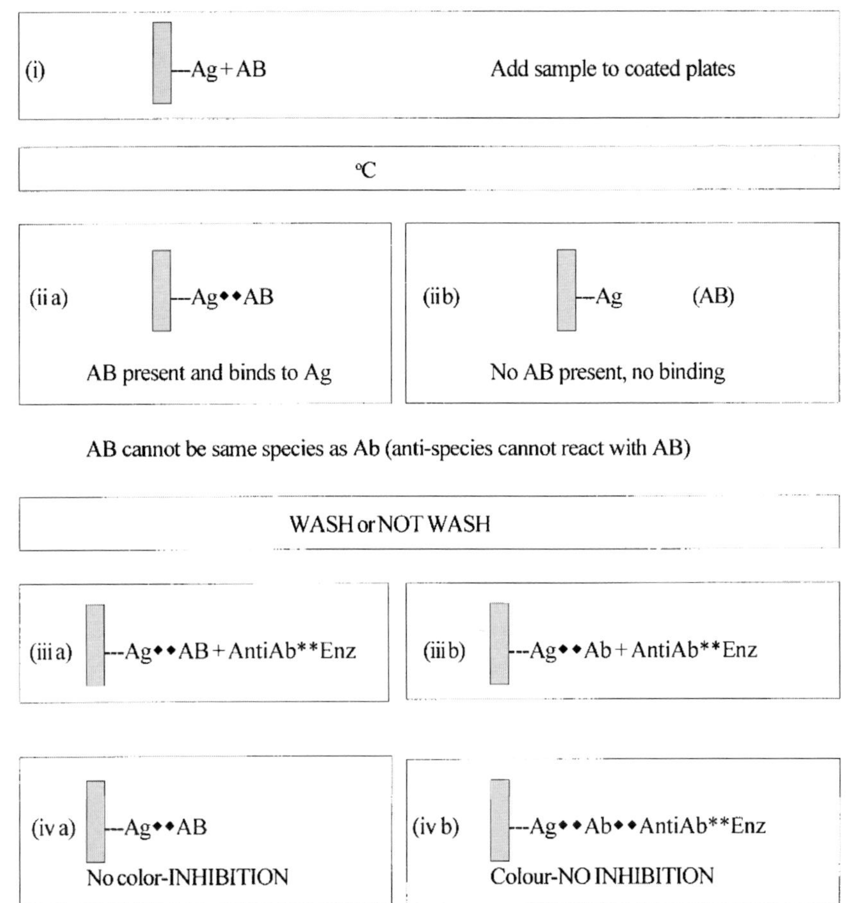

Diagram 10. Indirect I-ELISA antibody measurement.

three antibody systems (anti-species conjugate used to measure detecting serum). They are described for detecting antigen or antibody, as in the previous sections. The use of competition (C) and inhibition (I) assays is also described. Care should be taken to revise the basic sandwich systems since each must be titrated to optimize conditions before being applied in the competition/inhibition assay.

2.6.1. Direct Sandwich C-ELISA for Antibody

Direct sandwich C-ELISA for antibody is illustrated in **Diagram 11** and in **Fig. 9**.

2.6.2. Direct Sandwich I-ELISA for Antibody

The direct sandwich I-ELISA for antibody is as described for the previous competitive system except that the sample under test is added to the captured antigen for a time preceding the addition of the labeled antibodies. Following this incubation step, there are two alternatives. The first is to add the pretitrated labeled

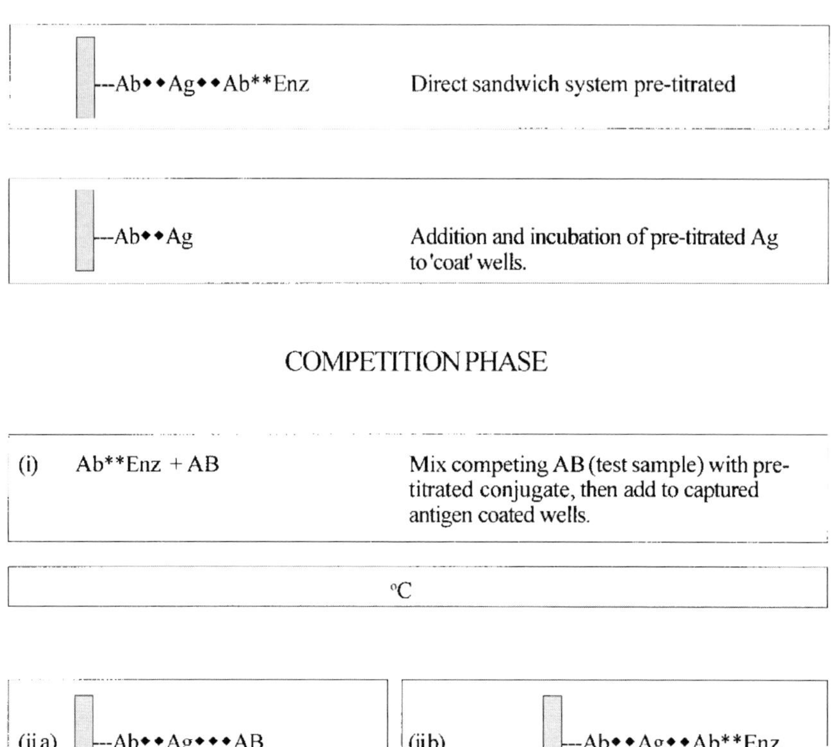

Diagram 11. Direct sandwich C-ELISA for antibody.

antibodies directly to the reaction mixture followed by incubation. The second is to wash the wells, thereby washing away any excess test antibodies before the addition of labeled antibodies. For each alternative, there is an incubation step for the labeled antibodies followed by washing and then addition of substrate/chromophore solution. The results are read according to the reduction in color as seen in controls in which no test sample was added. The greater the concentration of test antibodies that bind, the greater the degree of inhibition of the labeled antibodies.

The number of components for the indirect sandwich ELISAs is increased and consequently the number of reagent combinations. The reader should by now be familiar with the descriptions in diagrammatic form so that the next series of assays exploiting the indirect sandwich ELISAs can be examined more briefly, with the principles involved being highlighted.

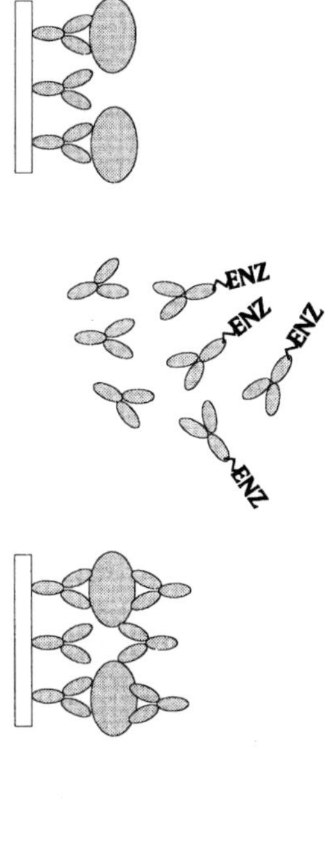

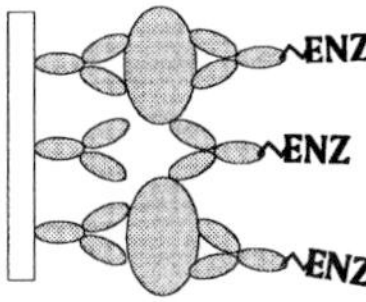

(i) System titrated to capture antigen. Detected by specific antibodies conjugated to enzyme.

(ii) Mixture of pre-titrated conjugate and test antibodies is made.This is added to antigen on coated plates.

(iii) Where the test antibodies are in large excess, they bind to antigen, preventing binding of conjugate.Competition.

(iv) Where there is no binding of test antibodies, the conjugate is free to bind. NO competition.

Fig. 9. Direct sandwich competition ELISA for antibody. This system exploits the competition of antibodies in a sample for the binding of a pretitrated quantity of labeled antibody specific for the antigen captured by the coating antibodies on the wells. The extent of competition depends on the relative concentrations of the test and labeled antibodies.

2.6.3. Direct Sandwich C- and I-ELISA for Antigen

The direct sandwich C- and I-ELISA for antigen is not suitable for the examination of antigen contained in test samples.

2.6.4. Indirect Sandwich C-ELISA for Antibody

The reader should reexamine the components of the indirect sandwich ELISA. Here, as in the direct sandwich system, antigen is captured by antibodies bound to the wells. The difference is that the antigen is detected first with an unlabeled antibody, which in turn, is detected and quantified using an anti-species conjugate. The exact time at which reagents/samples are added determines whether the system is truly examining competition or inhibition. **Diagram 12** illustrates where sample can be added to compete with the pretitrated indirect sandwich system.

It is critical that the antibody (AB) enzyme conjugate does not bind with the antibodies present in the test sample. The degree of competition is proportional to the amount of antibodies present

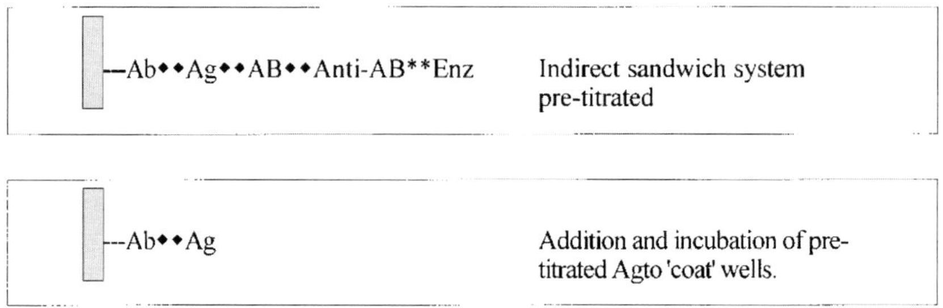

COMPETITION PHASE

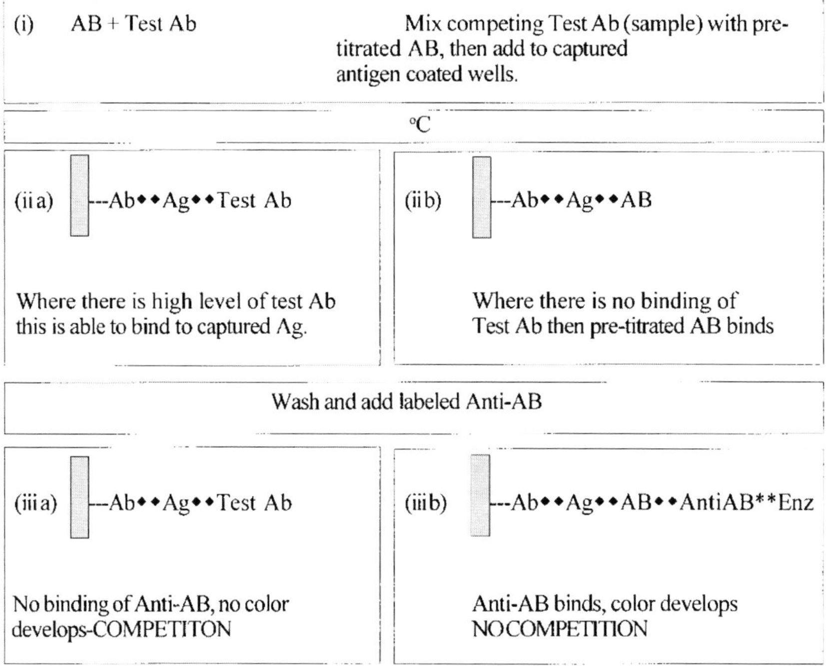

Diagram 12. Indirect sandwich C-ELISA for antibody addition on reagents.

in the test sample. The system offers greater flexibility in the use of different detecting antibodies (AB) for the captured antigen as compared with the direct sandwich assay. The system avoids producing specific conjugates for each of the sera used as detecting antibody (AB). Intrinsically, this also favors a more native reaction, since the introduction of enzyme molecules directly onto antibodies can affect their affinities (hence overall avidity of detecting AB). Thus, such a system is ideal in which the antigen must be captured and in which a number of detecting sera must be analyzed without chemical or physical modification. This also applies to the ELISA system described next.

2.6.5. Indirect Sandwich I-ELISA for Antibody

The indirect sandwich I-ELISA for antibody is similar to that of C-ELISA except that the time of addition of reagents is altered to allow a greater chance for reaction. This is illustrated in **Diagram 13**.

2.6.6. Indirect Sandwich C-ELISA for Antigen

The main problem with this form of antigen assay (indirect sandwich I-ELISAs) is that the wells are coated with antibodies that capture

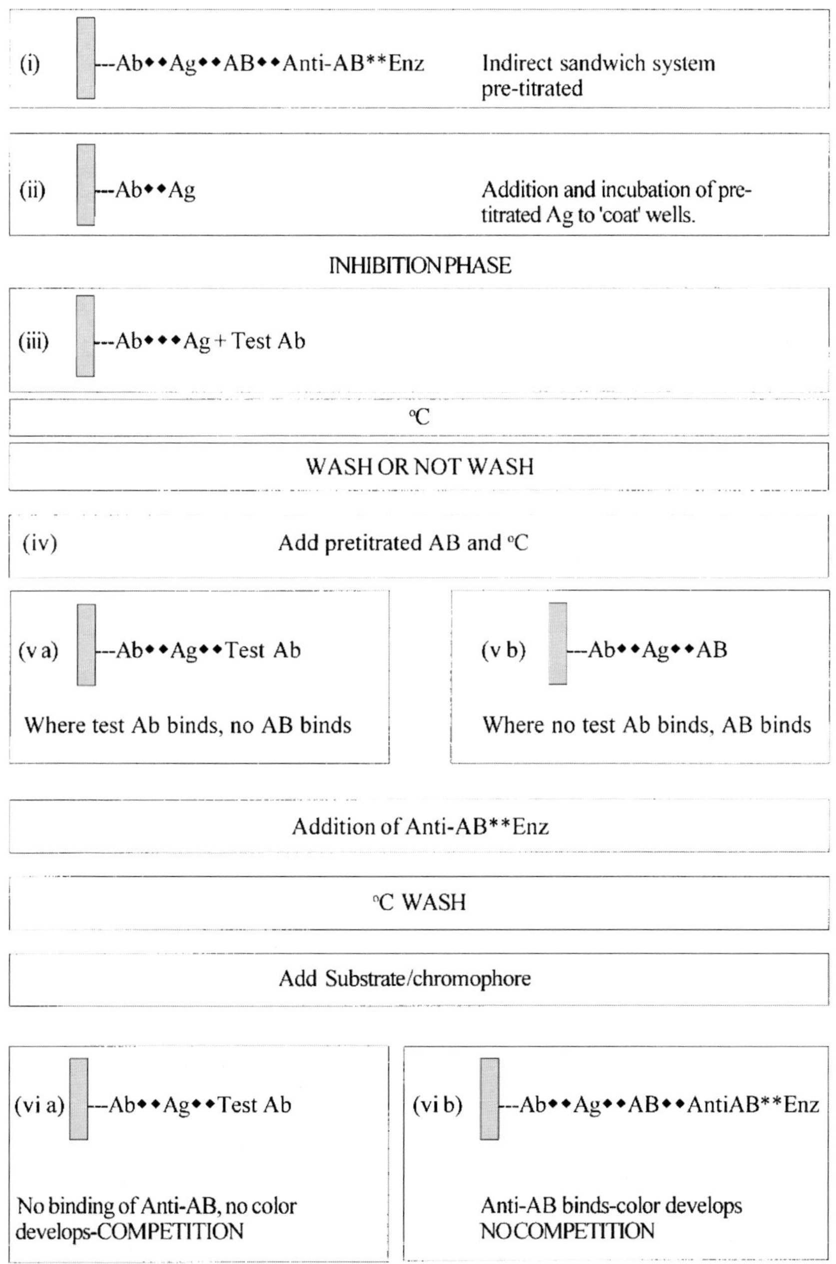

Diagram 13. Indirect sandwich I-ELISA for antibody.

antigen. Thus, any subsequent addition of antigen in a test sample will be bound to the wells if it is not fully saturated with the initially added coating antigen. The pretitration of the system then requires that there be no free antibodies coating the wells. Hence, the exact conditions for pretitration may differ from that for the antibody assays examined in **Subheadings 2.6.4** and **2.6.5**. The antigen has to be in excess, as shown in **Diagram 14**

The competitive phase occurs between the added test sample possibly containing antigen and the detecting second antibodies (AB), as shown in **Diagram 15**

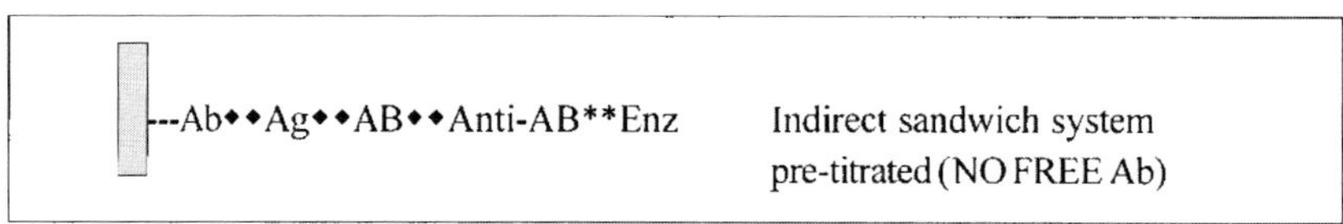

Diagram 14. Indirect sandwich C-ELISA for antigen.

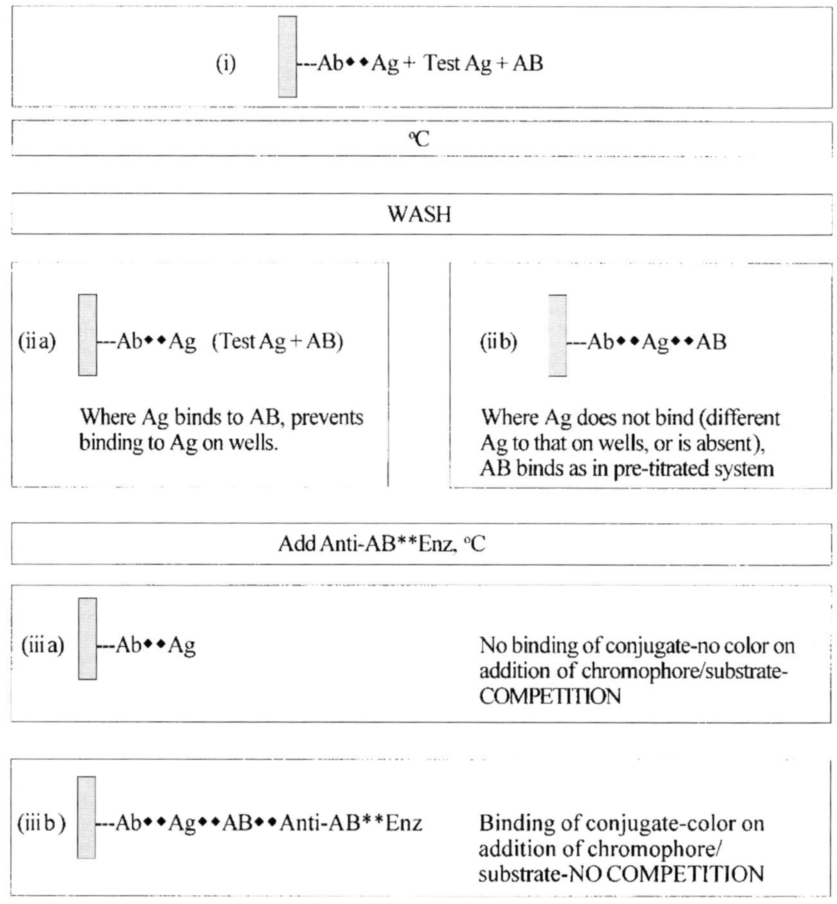

Diagram 15. Competitive phase between sample and antibodies.

2.6.7. Indirect Sandwich I-ELISA for Antigen

The indirect sandwich I-ELISA for antigen is essentially similar to that of C-ELISA except that the AB and the test antigen are mixed and incubated separately before being added to the wells containing captured antigen.

2.7. Choice of Assays

The most difficult question to answer when initiating the use of ELISAs is which system is most appropriate? This section attempts to investigate the relationships among the various systems to aid in assessing their suitability. The following questions must be addressed:

1. What is the purpose of the assay?
2. What reagents do I have?
3. What do I know about the reagents?
4. Is the test to be developed for a research purpose to be used by me alone, or for applied use by other workers?
5. Is the test to be used in other laboratories?
6. Is a kit required?

These questions have a direct effect on the phases that might be put forward as a general rule for the development of any assay. For example:

1. Feasibility – proof that a test system(s) can work (phase 1).
2. Validation – showing that a test(s) is stable and that it is evaluated over time and under different conditions (phase 2).
3. Standardization – quality control, establishment that a test is precise and can be used by different workers in different laboratories. At this stage a generalized examination of the availability of reagents and the effect this has on setting up a variety of systems will be made (phase 3).

2.7.1. Assessing Needs

It is assumed that there is some interest in the field in which an ELISA has to be developed. This infers that there is an understanding of the problem being addressed in terms of the biology involved and an appreciation of the literature concerning the target antigens and possible interactions of any agent with animals. If such knowledge is lacking, it should be sought through contact with other workers and by reading literature relevant to the field and associated areas, which includes the critical assessment of previously developed assays (including any ELISAs). Although this may seem obvious, unfortunately, information that is readily available to allow more rapid development of "new" assays and also comparative data assessment is often neglected.

For example:

1. We may have an antigen and may know a great deal or very little about it.
2. We may have a high concentration of a defined protein/polypeptide/peptide of known amino acid sequence or have

a thick soup of mixed proteins containing the antigen(s) at a low concentration contaminated with host cell proteins.

3. We may have an antiserum against antigen. This could be against purified antigen or against the crude soup. The antibody may have been raised in a given species, e.g., rabbit. We may have an IgG fraction of the antiserum (or could easily make one).
4. We may have field sera against the antigen (bovine sera). We may have a mAb. We may have antisera from different species, e.g., rabbit and guinea pig sera. ELISAs for similar systems may have been developed and can be found in the literature.
5. We may require an enzymatic reaction in the assay, and therefore will need an anti-species conjugate (commercial most probably) or will have to label an antigen-specific serum with enzyme (are there facilities to do this?). We must decide which commercial conjugate to buy. This will depend on the desired specificity of the conjugate (anti–whole molecule IgG, anti–H-chain IgG, anti–H chain IgM, and so on). The choice is somewhat determined by the aims of the assay and its design. Thus, we may wish to determine the IgM response of cattle to our antigen, which will require an anti-IgM (specific) somewhere in the ELISA protocol.

Obviously the basic needs for performing the ELISA must be addressed in terms of plates, pipets, buffers, reader, and so forth. In addition, if there is a need to develop a set of reagents that might be used as a universal assay, an assessment as to the scale of requirements is needed as early as possible. Thus, an estimate as to the likely usage of an assay should be made in terms of test units required in a defined time. This is translated into needed volumes of antigen, antisera, and conjugate (plates, pipet tips, and so forth). This need can be compared with what has been developed (or what needs to be produced).

For example, a test may be developed that is dependent on a single rabbit antiserum. The final volume may be 30 mL. The titer used in an assay may be 1/1,000. The test volume used is 50 μL. Therefore the maximum number of samples that can be run as single tests is 30 × 1,000 × 20 = 600,000.

This may be enough for universal testing for ten laboratories (60,000 samples per year) for one year, or if it runs tests on 6,000 samples a year, the reagent is satisfactory for 10 years. However, if the rabbit serum titer was 1/100, this effectively gives only enough reagent for testing 60,000 samples, which may be too little for a universal test.

Although this is a simplistic approach, early recognition as to why an ELISA is being developed is essential, which is often forgotten until the universal demands are examined. This approach should also be taken with considerations of antigen production, particularly when this may be difficult. Such considerations can also modify the selection of specific systems used. Thus, although a successful indirect ELISA using purified antigen may be obtained, the yield of the antigen may be low and the processing laborious and expensive, such that any larger-scale use of the test is prohibitive. This problem may be alleviated through the use of capture antibodies and crude (more easily obtained) antigen preparations in the development of sandwich assays.

This approach extends to conjugates in which there may be certain commercial products or locally produced reagents that define the success of ELISAs. This is to ensure continuity of supply and standardization of reagents; sufficient quantities must be available to meet long-term needs.

2.7.2. Examination of Possible Assays with Available Materials

Obviously the reagents available must be examined first, as previously stated. This section examines some extremes so as to illustrate the relationship of the assays available and their particular advantages. Scenarios are described (A–C) in which different reagents are available, and these will probably cover most of those that are met in practice. Let us assume that there are sera to test from infected and noninfected animals. Further subtleties can be examined by defining the specificities of the conjugates (anti-IgG, IgM, or whether they are H-chain specific). The increase in choice of reagents and the possibilities for performing different ELISA configurations are given below.

1. Scenario A
   - (a) Crude antigen (multiple antigenic sites)
   - (b) Antibody raised against crude antigen in rabbits
   - (c) Anti-cow conjugate
   - (d) Postinfected and day 0 (uninfected) cow sera
2. Scenario B
   - (a) Purified antigen (small amount, e.g., 100 μg)
   - (b) Crude antigen (large amount)
   - (c) Antibody raised in rabbits against pure antigen
   - (d) Anti-rabbit conjugate
   - (e) Anti-cow conjugate
   - (f) Postinfected and day 0 (uninfected) cow sera
3. Scenario C
   - (a) Crude antigen (as in A)
   - (b) Antibody against pure antigen (rabbit)
   - (c) Antibody against pure antigen (guinea pig)
   - (d) Anti–guinea pig conjugate
   - (e) Postinfected and day 0 (uninfected) cow sera
   - (f) Anti-cow conjugate
   - (g) Anti-rabbit conjugate

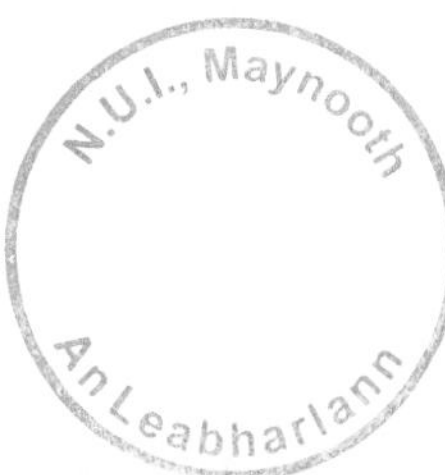

Scenario A

The use of crude antigen directly in an ELISA might be unsuccessful since it may be at a low concentration relative to other proteins and thus attach only at a low concentration. This would make unavailable the ELISA approaches as shown in **Subheadings 2.1** and **2.2** and thus competitive methods based on these as in **Subheadings 2.4** and **2.5**

Since a rabbit serum against the antigen is available, this may be used as a capture serum (or as capture IgG preparation), coated on the wells to capture the crude antigen to give a higher concentration to allow the bind. Thus, systems in **Subheadings 2.3** and **2.6** become available.

Any bound test antibody would be from cows and thus detected using an anti-bovine conjugate. This may cause problems since the crude antigen was used to raise the rabbit serum. Hence, antibodies against contaminating proteins may be produced in the rabbit. The cow sera being tested may react with such captured contaminants. However, when the antigen is an infectious agent, antibodies against the contaminating proteins may not be produced, thus eliminating the problem.

When the antigen is used as a vaccine, whereby relatively crude preparations similar to the crude antigen are used to formulate the vaccine, then this problem will be present. Attempts can be made to make the rabbit serum specific for the desired antigenic target.

Solid-phase immunosorbents involving the contaminating crude elements (minus the desired antigen) can be used to remove the anticrude antibodies from the rabbit serum, which could then be titrated as a capture serum. An example can be taken from the titration of foot-and-mouth disease virus antibodies. The virus is grown in tissue culture containing bovine serum. Even when virus is purified from such a preparation, minute amounts of bovine serum contaminate the virus. When this purified virus is injected into laboratory animals as an inactivated preparation, a large amount of anti-bovine antibodies as well as anti-virus antibodies are produced. This serum cannot be used in a capture system for specifically detecting virus grown as a tissue culture sample (containing bovine serum) because it also captures bovine serum. The capture serum is also unsuitable for capturing relatively pure virus for the titration of bovine antibodies from bovine serum samples because the capture antibodies react strongly with the detecting cow serum. Thus, the capture serum has to be adsorbed with solid-phase immunosorbents produced through the attachment of bovine serum to agarose beads.

Once the specificity of the capture serum is established, the optimization of the crude antigen concentration can be made using a known or several known positive cow sera in full dilution ranges. Inclusion of dilution ranges of negative sera allows

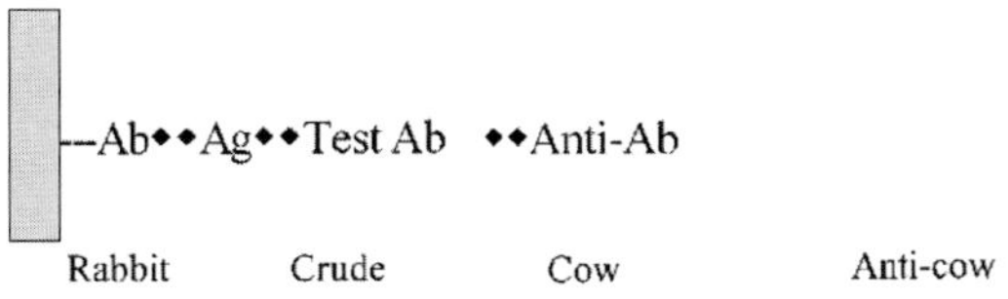

--Ab••Ag••Test Ab ••Anti-Ab

Rabbit Crude Cow Anti-cow

Diagram 16 Use of reagents to set up a sandwich ELISA

assessment of the difference between negative and positive sera at different dilutions of serum. Diagram 2.16<COMP: Insert Diagram 2.16 near here> illustrates the use of the reagents to set up a sandwich ELISA. The assay is made possible through the specific capture of enough antigen by the solid-phase rabbit serum.

Scenario B

This scenario is not so different from scenario A; however, there are more reagents. The antigen is available purified for use in raising antibodies in rabbits. Thus, with due reference to the reservations already described for scenario A, there is a basis for setting up a capture ELISA since the rabbit antibodies may capture the antigen at a high concentration from the crude antigen preparation, which is present in a large amount. The developmental system of the capture ELISA is as shown earlier.

The availability of the anti-rabbit conjugate may allow the development of competitive assays if enough specific antigen binds to plates, although this is unlikely, as already indicated. The antigen and rabbit serum could be titrated in an indirect ELISA (*see* **Subheading 2.2**) in a checkerboard fashion enabling the optimization of the antigen and serum. These optimal dilutions could be used to set up competitive ELISAs (*see* **Subheading 2.5.2**) in which cow sera would compete for the pretitrated antigen/rabbit/anti-rabbit conjugate system. Again, it must be emphasized that this is unlikely since the antigen is crude and some form of capture system will be needed to allow enough antigen to be presented on the wells.

Because scenario B has some purified antigen, it could be used in the development of a similar competitive assay. This will depend on the availability of this antigen, which can be determined after the initial checkerboard titrations in which the optimal dilution of antigen is calculated. The chief benefit of obtaining purified antigen is to obtain a more specific serum in rabbits allowing specific capture of antigen from the crude sample. In many cases, there is enough antigen of sufficient purity to be used in assays.

Scenario C

Here, all the possibilities of the first two situations plus the production of a second species (guinea pig) of serum against the purified antigen are present.

This allows the development of sandwich competitive assays (*see* **Subheading 2.6**) using either the rabbit or guinea pig as capture serum or detector with the relevant anti-species conjugate.

Different species may have better properties for acting as capture reagents and also show varying specificities. This can be assessed in chessboard titrations and is relevant because we require results on the detection and titration of cattle sera so that the competitive phase relies on the interruption of a pretitrated antibody as close to the reaction of cattle serum with antigen as possible. Rabbit or guinea pig serum may differ in their specificities as compared with cattle sera.

Further Comments

The assays shown in **Subheading 2.4.2** (competition for direct ELISA) are probably inappropriate owing to the possession of crude antigen (for reasons described earlier). However, if it can be shown that enough antigen can attach and that cattle sera react specifically (and not through excess antibodies directed against contaminants in the crude antigen), then we can set up assays based on this system. This requires identification of a positive cow serum and labeling of this serum with an enzyme.

Of more practical value could be the use of a positive cow serum labeled with enzyme. The serum can then be used both as capture, particularly as an IgG fraction) and for detection. In this way the competitive assay shown in **Subheading 2.6.1** is feasible and may have an advantage in that the reaction being competed against is homologous (cow antibody against antigen). This avoids complications through the use of second-species antisera produced by vaccination. The system is suitable for measuring the competition by other cow sera because the detecting antibody is labeled. Thus, a worker with relatively few reagents and the ability to label antibodies with an enzyme may have enough materials to develop assays. This brief description of system possibilities has concentrated on antibody detection. Note that most of these comments are relevant to antigen detection.

Chapter 3

Stages in ELISA

This chapter gives general information on essential practical features of ELISAs. These can be summarized as follows:

1. Adsorption of antigen or antibody to the plastic solid phase
2. Addition of the test sample and subsequent reagents
3. Incubation of reactants
4. Separation of bound and free reactants by washing
5. Addition of enzyme-labeled reagent
6. Addition of enzyme detection system (color development)
7. Visual or spectrophotometric reading of the assay

1. Solid Phase

The most widely exploited solid phase is the 96-well microtiter plate manufactured from polyvinyl chloride (flexible plates) or polystyrene (inflexible rigid plates). Many manufacturers supply plates designed for ELISA and provide a standardized product. The use of a wide variety of plates from different manufacturers has been reported for a broad spectrum of biological investigations. It is impossible to recommend one product as a universally accepted plate. In cases in which specific assays have been developed, it is prudent to use the recommended plate; however, because, in practice, there is relatively little difference between plates, it is possible to perform the same test using different plates provided that suitable standardization is performed. In this respect, laboratories that deal with large numbers of ELISAs

John R. Crowther, *Methods in Molecular Biology, The ELISA Guidebook, Vol. 516*

DOI: 10.1007/978-1-60327-254-4_3

involving different antigens and antibodies can perform standardized assays using the same type of plate. Ideally, flat-bottomed wells are recommended, in which spectrophotometric reading is employed to assess color development. However, round-bottomed wells can be used in which visual (by eye) assessment of the ELISA is made. Such plates can be read by a spectrophotometer but are not ideal.

The performance of plates should be examined for given assays on a routine basis, since it cannot be automatically assumed that the plates will not vary in performance. This is particularly important when different batches of plates are received. The batch number usually can be obtained from the boxes in which the plates are provided and from documentation accompanying the plates. Some plates also have codes embossed onto the plastic to identify the particular stamps used in their manufacture. In practice, sometimes poor-quality plates are sent out even when a certificate of guarantee is provided.

1.1. Immobilization of Antigen on Solid-Phase Coating

A key feature of the solid-phase ELISA is that antigens or antibodies can be attached to surfaces easily by passive adsorption. This process is commonly called coating. Most proteins adsorb to plastic surfaces, probably as a result of hydrophobic interactions between nonpolar protein substructures and the plastic matrix. The interactions are independent of the net charge of the protein, and thus each protein has a different binding constant. The hydrophobicity of the plastic–protein interaction can be exploited to increase binding, since most of proteins' hydrophilic residues are at the outside and most of the hydrophobic residues orientated toward the inside *(1)*.

Partial denaturation of some proteins results in exposure of hydrophobic regions and ensures firmer interaction with the plastic. This can be achieved by exposing proteins to low pH or mild detergent and then dialysis against coating buffers before coating.

The rate and extent of the coating depends on these factors:

1. Diffusion coefficient of the attaching molecule
2. Ratio of the surface area being coated to the volume of the coating solution
3. Concentration of the substance being adsorbed
4. Temperature
5. Time of adsorption

These factors are linked. It is most important to determine the optimal antigen concentration for coating in each system by suitable titrations. A concentration range of 1–10 μg/mL of protein, in a volume of 50 μL, is a good guide to the level of protein needed to saturate available sites on a plastic microtiter plate. This can be reliable when relatively pure antigen (free of other proteins other than the target for immunoassay) is available. Thus, the concentration can be related to activity. However, when coating solutions contain relatively small amounts of required antigen(s), the amount attaching to a well is reduced according to its proportion in the mixture. Other contaminating proteins will take up sites on the plastic. Because the plastic has a finite saturation level, the use of relatively crude antigens for coating may lead to poor assays.

Care must be taken to assess the effects of binding proteins at different concentrations, since the actual density of binding may affect results. High-density binding of antigen may not allow antibody to bind through steric inhibition (antigen molecules are too closely packed). High concentrations of antigen may also increase stacking or layering, which may allow a less stable interaction of subsequent reagents. Orientation and concentration of antibody molecules must also be considered because these factors affect the activity of assays. **Figures 1** and **2** reveal the elements of adsorption.

1.2. Coating Time and Temperature

The rate of the hydrophobic interactions depends on the temperature: the higher the temperature, the greater the rate. There are many variations on incubation conditions. It must be remembered that all factors affect the coating, and thus a higher concentration of protein may allow a shorter incubation time as compared with a lower concentration of the antigen for a longer time. The most usual regimes involve incubation at 37°C for 1–3 h or overnight at 4°C, or a combination of the two, or incubation (more vaguely) at room temperature for 1–3 h (*see* **ref. 2** for a typical study). There are many more variations, and ultimately, each scientist must titrate a particular antigen to obtain a standardized regime. Increasing the temperature may have a deleterious effect on antigen(s) in the coating stage, and this may be selective, so that certain antigens in a mixture are affected whereas others are not. Rotation of plates can considerably reduce the time needed for coating by increasing the rate of contact between the coating molecules and the plastic.

1.3. Coating Buffer

The coating buffers most used are 50 mM carbonate, pH 9.6; 20 mM Tris-HCl, pH 8.5; and 10 mM phosphate-buffered saline (PBS), pH 7.2 *(2)*. Different coating buffers should be investigated when problems are encountered or compared at the beginning of assay development. From a theoretical point of view, it is best to use a buffer with a pH value 1–2 units higher than the isoelectric point (p*I*) value of the protein being attached. This is not easy to determine in practice since antigens are often complex mixtures of proteins. By direct study of the effects of different pHs and ionic strengths, greater binding of proteins may be observed. An increase in ionic strength to 0.6 M NaCl in combination with an optimal pH was found to give better results for the attachment of various herpes simplex viral peptides *(3)*. Proteins

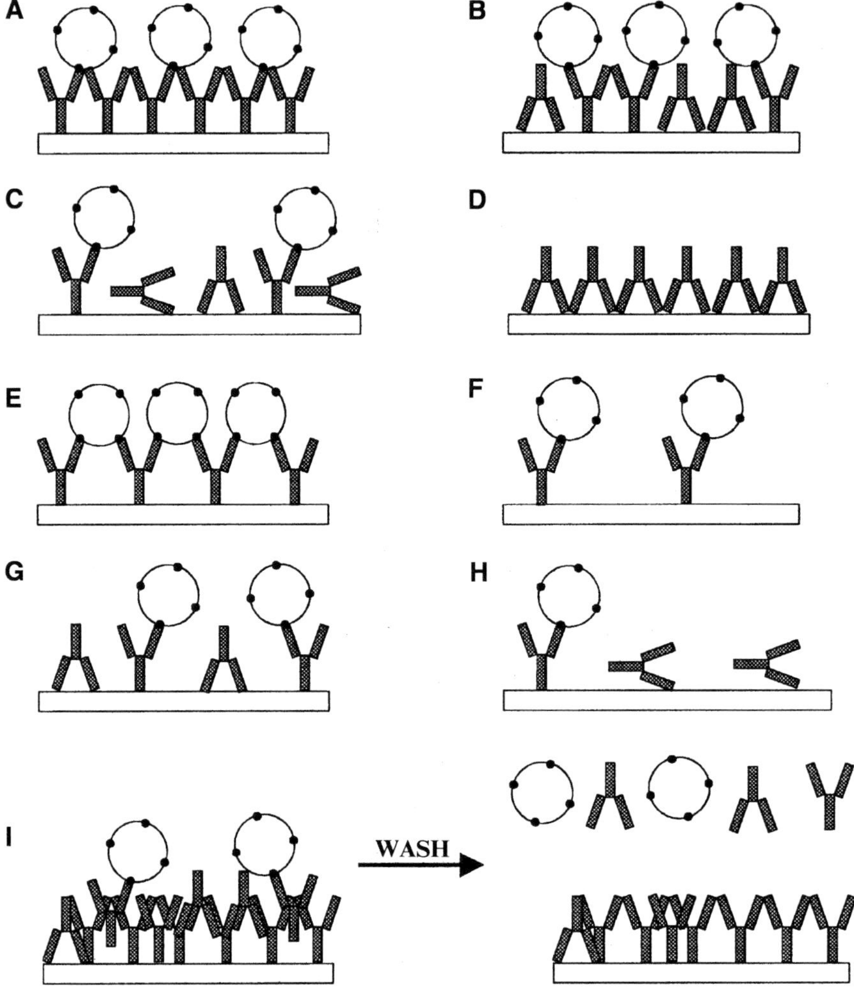

Fig. 1. Effects on antibodies of coating. **(A)** Antibody molecules packed evenly, orientation of Fc on plate, monovalent interaction of multivalent Ag; **(B)** antibody molecules packed evenly, orientation Fc and Fab on plate, monovalent binding of multivalent Ag; **(C)** antibody binding in all orientations, monovalent binding of multivalent Ag; **(D)** antibody binding via Fab, no binding of Ag; **(E)** antibody spaced with orientation to allow bivalent interaction between adjacent antibody molecules; **(F)** antibody spaced too widely to allow adjacent molecules to bind bivalently via Fc; **(G)** as in **(E)** except that orientation is via Fc or Fab; **(H)** more extreme case of **(C)** with less antibody and more molecules inactive owing to orientation; **(J)** multilayered binding in excess leading to binding but elution on washing.

with many acidic proteins may require a lower pH to neutralize repulsive forces between proteins and the solid phase, as shown in **ref. 3**, in which the optimal coating for peptides was pH 2.5–4.6. PBS, pH 7.4, is also suitable for coating many antigens. Coating by drying down plates at 37°C using volatile buffers (ammonium carbonate) and in PBS is often successful, particularly when relatively crude samples are available. Some antigens pose particular problems, including some polysaccharides, lipopolysaccharides, and glycolipids. In cases in which it proves impossible to directly

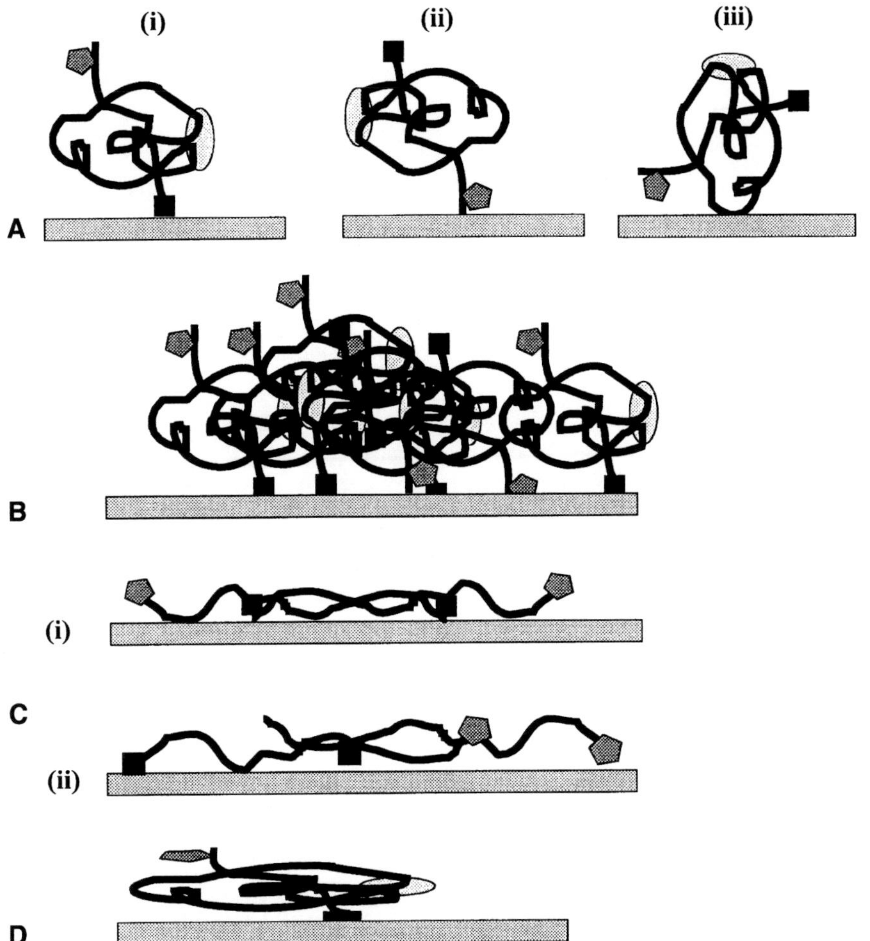

Fig. 2. Possible effects on soluble protein of immobilization. Protein is shown as having three antigenic sites (epitopes). Two are linear (*solid box* and shaded pentagon), and one is conformational dependent (*shaded oval*). **(A)** (i–iii) The orientation of the molecule on the well affects the presentation of the individual epitopes. This is true of passive and covalent binding to plastic. **(B)** Aggregation of the antigen can complicate presentation and also lead to leaching following binding with detecting antibody. **(C)** The antigen may be altered through treatment before attachment. In both (i) and (ii) the conformational epitope has been destroyed. Note also that the orientation of the molecules affects the presentation and spacing between individual epitopes. **(D)** Nondenatured protein can also alter its conformation by passive adsorption to plastic.

coat wells with reagent, initial coating of the wells with a specific antiserum may be required. Thus, sandwich (trapping) conditions must be set up. Passive adsorption has several theoretical, although not necessarily practical, drawbacks. These include desorption, binding capacity, and nonspecific binding.

1.4. Desorption

Because of the noncovalent nature of the plastic–protein interactions, desorption (leaching) may take place during the stages of the assay. However, if conditions are standardized, leaching does not affect the viability of the majority of tests. There are some reports that the vigorousness of washing at the various stages of assays (including that after coating) affects the assays through stripping of protein; however, I have not encountered this problem.

1.5. Binding Capacity

It is important to realize that plastic surfaces have a finite capacity for adsorption. The capacity for proteins to attach to microplate wells is influenced by the exact nature of the protein adsorbed to the specific plate used. Saturation levels of between 50 and 500 ng per well have been found valid for a variety of proteins when added as 50-µL volumes. The effective weight of protein per well can be increased if the volume of the attaching protein is increased, effectively increasing the surface area of the plastic in contact with the coating antigen. In cases in which there is an obvious discrepancy between the actual concentration of protein added (where known) and the values just given, the titration of the ELISA should be re-examined. Thus, if concentrations of, e.g., 1–10 mg/mL (or greater) of sample are needed to coat the wells, this will not have an ideal situation.

1.6. Nonspecific Binding

Unlike antigen–antibody interactions, the adsorption process is nonspecific. Thus, it is possible that any substance may adsorb to plastic at any stage during the assay. This must be considered in assay design because reagents may react with such substances. High levels of nonspecific binding can be alleviated through alteration of systems relying on direct adsorption of antigen and the use of sandwich techniques, in which specific antibodies capture and concentrate specific antigens.

1.7. Covalent Antigen Attachment

A variety of chemicals that couple protein to plastic have been used to prevent desorption, the antigen being covalently bound. These include water-soluble carbodiimines, imido- and succinimidylesters, ethanesulfonic acid, and glutaraldehyde. Precoating of plates with high molecular weight polymers such as polyglutaraldehyde and polylysine is another alternative *(4, 5)*. These bind to plates with a high efficiency and act as nonspecific adhesive molecules. This method is particularly useful for antigens with a high carbohydrate content since these normally bind poorly to plastic.

Generally, successful assays can be obtained without the need to link antigens to plates covalently. Specially treated activatable plates are now available. The use of covalently attached proteins does offer the possibility that plates could be reused. After an assay, all reagents binding to the solid-phase attached protein could be washed away after using a relatively severe washing procedure, e.g., low pH. The covalent nature of the bonds holding the solidphase antigen would prevent this from being eluted. Provided this procedure did not destroy the antigenicity of the solid-phase attached reagent, the plates might be exploited after equilibration with normal washing buffers.

2. Washing

The purpose of washing is to separate bound and unbound (free) reagents. This involves the emptying of plate wells of reagents followed by the addition of liquid into wells. Such a process is performed at least three times for every well. The liquid used to wash wells is usually buffered, typically with PBS (0.1 M, pH 7.4), so as to maintain isotonicity, since most antigen–antibody reactions are optimal under such conditions. Although PBS is most frequently used, lower-molarity phosphate buffers (0.01 M) may be used, provided that they do not influence the performance of the assay. These buffers are also more cost-efficient.

In some assays tap water has been used for washing. This is not recommended because tap water varies greatly in composition (pH, molarity, and so forth). However, assays may be possible provided the water does not markedly affect the components of the test. Generally, the mechanical action of flooding the wells with a solution is enough to wash wells of unbound reagents. Some investigators leave washing solution in wells for a short time (soak time) after each addition (1–5 min). Sometimes detergents, notably Tween-20 (0.05%), are added to washing buffers. These can cause problems: excessive frothing takes place producing poor washing conditions since air is trapped and prevents the washing solution from contacting the well surface. When using detergents, care must be taken that they do not affect reagents adversely (denature antigen), and greater care is needed to prevent frothing in the wells. The methods used for washing are given next.

2.1. Dipping Methods

The whole plate is immersed in a large volume of buffer. This method is rapid but is likely to result in cross-contamination from different plates. It also increases the cost of washing solution.

2.2. Wash Bottles

Fluid is added using a plastic wash bottle with a single delivery nozzle, which is easy and inexpensive. Here the wells are filled individually in rapid succession and then emptied by inverting the plate and flicking the contents into a sink or suitable container filled with disinfectant. This process is repeated at least three times. Wells filled with washing solution may also be left for about 30 s before emptying.

2.3. Wash Bottles Plus Multiple Delivery Nozzles

This is essentially as in **Subheading 2** except that a commercially multiple delivery (usually 8) device is attached to the outlet of the bottle. This enables 8 wells to be filled at the same time.

2.4. Multichannel Pipets

The multichannel pipets used in the ELISA can be used to fill the wells carefully. The washing solution is contained in reservoirs.

2.5. Large Reservoir

The use of a large reservoir of washing solution is convenient. Here, a single or multiple nozzle can be connected to the reservoir via tubing so that the system is gravity fed. Care must be taken so that large volumes of solution do not become microbially contaminated.

2.6. Special Hand-Washing Devices

Hand-washing devices are available commercially and involve the simultaneous delivery and emptying of wells by a handheld multiple-nozzle apparatus. These are convenient to use but require vacuum-creating facilities. In washing the plates manually, the most important factor is that each well receives the washing solution so that, e.g., no air bubbles are trapped in the well, or a finger is not placed over the corner wells. After the final wash in all manual operations, the wells are emptied and then blotted free of most residual washing solution. This usually is accomplished by inverting the wells and tapping the plate on to an absorbent surface such as paper towels, cotton towels, or sponge material. Thus, the liquid is physically ejected and absorbed to the surface, which is soft and therefore avoids damage to the plate.

2.7. Specialist Plate Washers

Specialty plate washers are relatively expensive pieces of apparatus that fill and empty wells. Various washing cycles can be programmed. These are of great advantage when pathogens are being examined in ELISA because they reduce aerosol contamination. Most of the methods involving manual addition of solutions and emptying of plates by flicking into sinks or receptacles must be regarded as potentially dangerous if human pathogens are being studied, particularly at the coating stage if live antigen is used. Also, remember that live antigens can contaminate laboratories where tissue culture is practiced. The careful maintenance of such machines is essential because they are prone to machine errors such as a particular nozzle being blocked.

3. Addition of Reagents

Immunoassays involve the accurate dispensing of reagents in relatively small volumes. The usual volumes used in ELISA are in the range of 50 or 100 μL per well for general reagents, and 2–10 μL for samples. It is essential that the operator be fully aware of good pipetting technique and understand the relationships of grams, milligrams, micrograms, nanograms, and the equivalent for volumes, e.g., liters, milliliters, and microliters. Thus, assays cannot be performed when there is no knowledge of how to make up, e.g., 0.1 M solutions. The ability to make accurate dilutions is also extremely important so that problems can be solved before you attempt ELISA or any other biological studies (e.g., having a 1/50 dilution of antiserum but needing to make up a 1.3500 dilution in a final volume of 11 mL).

3.1. Pipets

The microtiter plate system is ideally used in conjunction with multichannel microtiter pipets. Essentially they allow the delivery of reagents via 4, 8, or 12 channels and are of fixed or variable volumes of 25–250 μL.

Single-channel micropipets are also required that deliver in the range of 5–250 μL. Samples are usually delivered by microtiter pipets from suitably designed reservoirs (troughs) that hold about 30–50 mL. General laboratory glasswares are needed such as 5- and 25-mL glass or plastic bottles, and 10-, 5-, and 1-mL pipets.

3.2. Evaluating Pipet Performance

Pipetting errors are often a major cause of nonreliable test results in a diagnostic laboratory. A simple control technique is hereby proposed to circumvent this problem. At the beginning of each workday, the pipet should be checked for dust and dirt on the outside surfaces. Particular attention should be paid to the tip cone. No other solvent except 70% ethyl alcohol should be used to clean the pipet.

3.2.1. Short-Term Performance Evaluation: Control of Pipet Calibration Using Graduated Tips

The exercise will take only a few minutes, but it will make you absolutely confident of preventing pipetting errors related to the function of the pipet.

1. Set the volume of the pipet as indicated in the accompanying manufacturer's instructions.
2. Place a graduated tip firmly on the tip cone.
3. Aspirate the specified volume of distilled water into the tip.
4. Hold the filled tip in a vertical position for a few seconds.
5. Check for leakage.
6. Check that the aspirated volume corresponds to the specified volume as indicated by tip graduation.
7. Repeat **steps 1–6** at least five times.
8. Practice the reversed and nonreversed pipetting techniques.

3. 2.2. Long-Term Performance Evaluation: Control of Pipet Calibration Using Gravimetric Calibration Method

If the pipet is used daily, it should be checked every 3 months. By means of the gravimetric calibration method (*see* **Table 1**), the pipet should be examined for leakage, accuracy, and precision.

Accuracy and precision can easily be calculated by the formulae in **Subheadings 2.2.1** and **2.2.2**. In contrast to commercial pipet calibration computer software, the conversion factor for calculating the density of water suspended in air at the test temperature and pressure is not considered. For calibration of multichannel pipets, examine each channel separately.

Table 1
Example of gravimetric calibration method used for three specified volumes pipet (40–200 µL)

	Nominal volume		
	5:1	25:1	50:1
Measurement 1	5.12	25.08	50.21
Measurement 2	4.91	25.01	50.01
Measurement 3	5.07	25.27	50.19
Measurement 4	5.01	25.01	50.12
Measurement 5	4.98	24.89	50.00
Average	5.02	25.07	50.11
Accuracy (%)	0.36	0.28	0.21
Precision (%)	1.62	0.55	0.20

Accuracy (As Defined for This Exercise)

A pipet is accurate to the degree that the volume delivered is equal to the specified volume. Accuracy is expressed as the mean for replicate measurements:

$$E\% = [(V - V_0)/V_0] \times 100$$

where $E\%$ = accuracy; V = mean volume; and V_0 = nominal volume.

Precision (As Defined for This Exercise)

Precision refers to the repeatability of dispensed samples. It is expressed as the coefficient of variation (CV%).

$$\text{CV}\% = (S / W) \times 100$$

in which S = standard deviation and W = mean weighing.

Equipments Needed

The following equipments are needed:

1. Calibrated thermometer; to measure water temperature
2. Distilled water
3. Glass vessel with a volume 10–50 times that of the test volume
4. Analytical balance (calibrated?)
5. Pipet (labeled) and tips

Conduct the test on a vibration-free surface covered with a smooth, dark, nonglared material. Work in an area that is free of dust.

Procedure

1. Set the volume of the pipet as indicated in the accompanying manufacturer's instructions.
2. Place a pipet tip firmly on the tip cone.

3. Aspirate the specified volume of water into the tip.
4. Hold the filled tip in a vertical position for a few seconds and check for leakage.
5. Dispense the distilled water into a preweighed beaker and record the weight to the nearest tenth of a milligram. Repeat at least five times.
6. Calculate the results (accuracy, precision).
7. Record the results over time.

In theory, optimum accuracy and precision values approach zero. Note that the smaller the specified volume chosen for evaluation, the greater the effect of volume variation on accuracy and precision. Therefore, it is good laboratory practice to plot the results of accuracy and precision for a pipet's specified volume on a data chart over time.

Finally, you must decide which level of accuracy and precision can be met in your laboratory. This depends on what the pipet is used for. For the preparation of aliquots of serum bank samples, the pipetting error will not significantly matter. For ELISA, however, pipetting of a small, e.g., 10-μL volume for preparation of working conjugate dilutions requires the best accuracy and precision; bear this in mind because if you are pipetting 5 rather than 10 μL, you will obtain a double-diluted working conjugate dilution and, consequently, an unreliable assay result. As a rule, a volume error of 1% for volumes 10 μL is still acceptable in a serodiagnostic laboratory.

Recalibration of Pipets

To recalibrate pipets, refer to the manufacturer's detailed instructions or contact the service representative.

2.3. Pipet Troubleshooting

Table 2 provides the most common problems encountered with pipetting, possible causes, and solutions.

3. Tips

After the microplate, the tips are the most important aspect of ELISA and also an expensive component. Many thousands of tips might be needed to dispense reagents. Many manufacturers supply tips; therefore, care must be taken to find tips that fit the available microtiter pipets.

Multichannel pipet tips are best accessed by placing them in special boxes holding 96 tips in the microplate format. The tips can be purchased in boxes (expensive), and then the boxes can be refilled by hand with tips bought in bulk. Sterile tips are available in the box format. Generally, tips should not be handled directly by hand. When restocking boxes or putting the tips on pipets, plastic gloves should be worn to avoid contaminating the tips.

Tips for dispensing in single-channel pipets have to be carefully considered. In cases in which small volumes (5–20 μL) are

Table 2
Troubleshooting of pipetting errors

Problem	Cause	Solution
Leakage	Tips are not compatible Tips are incorrectly attached Foreign bodies are between the piston O-ring and cone Insufficient grease is on the tip cone and O-ring	Choose compatible tips Attach firmly Clean the tip cone, and attach new tips Clean and grease the O-ring and tip cone Apply grease
Innaccurate dispensing	The pipet is incorrectly operated Tips are incorrectly attached High-viscosity fluids are not present	Follow instructions Attach tips firmly Recalibrate the pipet using high-viscosity fluids

pipeted, the pipet manufacturer's recommended tips should be used. It is essential that the tips fit securely on the pipets and that they can be pressed on firmly by hand (avoiding their end). Particular care is needed when multichannel pipets are used to pick up tips from boxes, since often one or two tips are not as securely positioned as the rest, which causes pipetting errors. The operator should always give a visual check of the relative volumes picked up.

When cost-efficiency is a factor, tips may be recycled after washing. However, it is not recommended that tips that have been in contact with any enzyme conjugate be recycled and these should not be placed with other tips used for other stages in ELISA. The washing of tips should be extensive, preferably in extensive acid or strong detergent solutions, followed by rinsing in distilled water. The cost/benefit of washing must be examined carefully, because the production of sufficient quantities of distilled water can be expensive. Tips should be examined regularly and damaged ones should be discarded. **Figure 3** illustrates some practical aspects of pipetting in ELISA. Note that the training in pipetting techniques is extremely vital to the successful performance of ELISA.

3.4. Other Equipment

Several manufacturers supply microtiter equipment to aid multichannel pipetting, including tube and microtip holders. The former consists of a plastic box that carries 96 plastic tubes with a capacity of about 1 mL. The tubes are held in exactly the same format as a microtiter plate so that samples can be stored or diluted in such tubes and multichannel pipets can then be used for rapid transfer from the tubes. The tip holders involve the same principle, whereby tips for the multichannel pipets are stored in

Avoid dripping from tips. When taking sample ensure that any excess liquid on outside of tip is conducted away by touching tip on side of container.

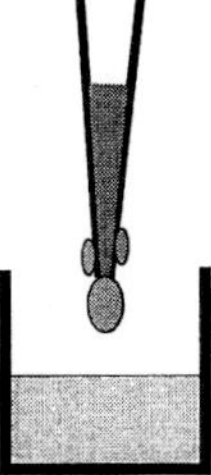

Do not press tips into wells, this bends the points of the tips and introduces error when expelling liquid by pipetting action.

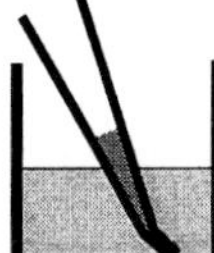

Do not put tips in wells at the wrong angle; this can leave sample on side of wells.

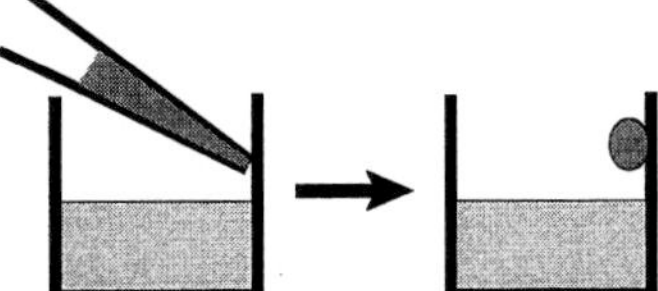

Make sure that tips touch sides of wells and liquid when adding sample, and when tip is leaving wells after expulsion of sample.

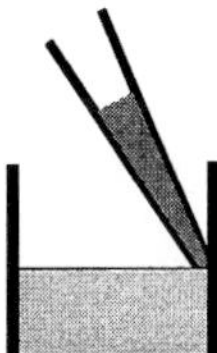

Fig. 3. Factors influencing proper dispensing of samples into microtiter plate wells.

the 96-well format so that they can be placed on to multichannel pipets rapidly in groups of 8 or 12. Various reservoirs with 8 or 12 channels for separation of reagents are also available. These are useful for the simultaneous addition of separate reagents.

4. Incubation

The reaction between antigens and antibodies relies on their close proximity. During ELISA, this is affected by their respective concentrations, distribution, time and temperature of incubation, and pH (buffering conditions). In any interaction, the avidity of the antibodies for the particular antigen(s) is also important. Two types of incubation conditions are common: (1) incubation of rotating plates (with shaking) and (2) incubation of stationary plates. These conditions affect the times and temperatures required for successful ELISAs and are therefore discussed separately.

4.1. Incubation of Reagents While Rotating Plates

The effect of rotating plates is to mix the reactants completely during the incubation step. Since the solid phase limits the surface area of the adsorbed reactant, mixing ensures that potentially reactive molecules are continuously coming into contact with the solid phase. During stationary incubation, this is not true and mixing takes place only owing to diffusion of reagents. Thus, to allow maximum reaction from reagents in stationary conditions, greater incubation times may be required than if they are rotated. This is particularly notable when highly viscous samples, e.g., 1/20 serum, are being examined. This represents 5% serum proteins, and diffusion of all antibodies on to the solid phase may take a long time. This can be avoided if mixing is allowed throughout incubation. Similarly, when low amounts of reactant are being assayed, the contact time of the possibly few molecules that have to get close to the solid-phase reactant is greatly enhanced by mixing throughout incubation. Simple and very reliable rotating devices are available with a large capacity for plates. Shakers with limited capacity (e.g., four plates) are also available.

Figure 4 gives the advantages of rotation. Rotation allows ELISAs to be performed independently of temperature considerations. The interaction of antibodies and antigens relies on their closeness, which is encouraged with the mixing during rotation. Stationary incubation relies on the diffusion of molecules, and thus is dependent on temperature. Therefore, standardization of temperature conditions is far more critical than when rotation is used.

The effect of temperature also has implications when many plates are stacked during incubation, since the plates heat up at different rates depending on their position in the stack. The wells on the inside may take longer to equilibrate than those on the outside, which has a direct effect on the diffusion conditions, which in turn, affects the ELISA. This is negated by rotation because there is the same chance of molecular contact in all wells.

4.2. Stationary Incubation Conditions

Assays may be geared to stationary conditions, although the exact times and temperatures of incubation may vary. The temperatures for incubation are most commonly 37°C, room temperature (on the bench), and 4°C. Usually the time of incubation under stationary conditions reflects which incubation temperature is used. Therefore, at 4°C, a longer incubation might be given (overnight). In general, most incubations for stationary assays involving the reaction of antigen and antibodies are 1–3 h at 37°C. Sometimes these conditions are combined so that one reagent is added for, say, 2 h at 37°C followed by one overnight at 4°C, usually because this produces a convenient work schedule. When

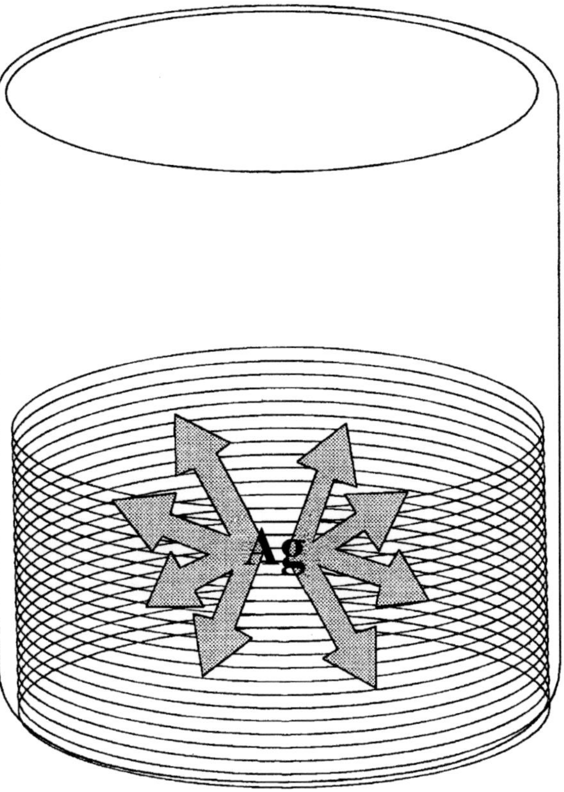

Fig. 4. Continuous mixing enables maximum contact of molecules in liquid phase with those on solid phase. This alleviates the following problems: temperature – the close approximation of antigen and antibody is necessary to allow binding (Increasing temperature under stationary conditions increases diffusion rate of molecules and variations in temperature will affect rate and variation in the test, e.g., stacking plates.); variation in handling – plates may be unequally moved during incubation causing unequal mixing (Different operators use different techniques that are not controllable, e.g.., plates may be tapped or other operators may move the pates.); viscosity effects – when samples are of different viscosities, this may affect diffusion of molecules under stationary conditions; times of incubation – these can be reduced under rotationary conditions; and detection of low concentrations – this is increased by rotation.

incubation is performed at room temperature, care must be taken to monitor possible seasonal variations in the laboratory, since temperatures can be quite different, particularly in nontemperate countries. Direct sunlight should also be avoided, as must other sources of heat, such as from machinery in the laboratory. As already stated, how the plates are placed during stationary incubation should be considered. Ideally, they should be separated and not stacked.

In assays, the plates should also be handled identically and there should be no tapping or shaking of the plates (including accidental nudging or movement by other personnel), because this will allow more mixing and interfere with the relative rate of diffusion of molecules in different plates. Regular handling can be a primary cause of operator-to-operator variation.

Under mixing conditions, most antigen–antibody reactions are optimum after 30 min at 37°C, so that assays can be greatly speeded up with no loss in sensitivity. This is not true under stationary conditions. Care must be taken to consider the types of antibodies being measured under various conditions since ELISAs rarely reach classical equilibrium conditions. **Figure 5** illustrates the factors affecting ELISA under stationary conditions.

Fig. 5. Effects when incubating stationary plates.

Stacking plates leads to uneven heating

Outside wells heat up quicker than inside wells

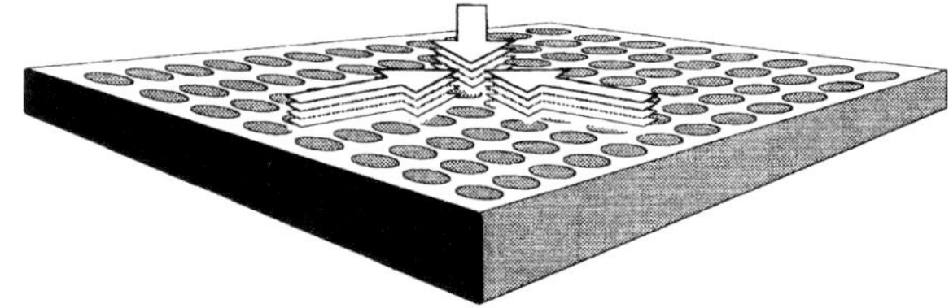

Any variation in moving plates alters mixing of reagents

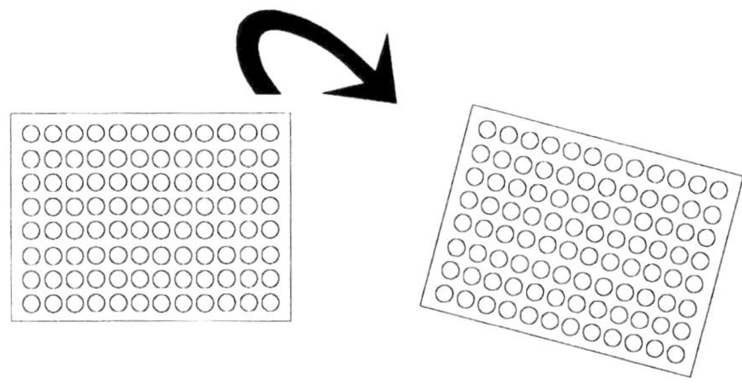

5. Blocking Conditions and Nonspecific Reactions

Measures must be taken to prevent nonspecific adsorption of proteins to wells from samples added after the coating of the solid phase before, during, or as a combination of both times. Nonspecific adsorption of protein can take place with any available plastic sites not occupied by the solid-phase reagent. Thus, if one is assessing bovine antibodies in bovine serum, and bovine proteins other than specific antibodies bind to the solid phase, anti-bovine conjugate will bind to these and give a high background color.

Two methods are used to eliminate such binding. One is the addition of high concentrations of immunologically inert substances to the dilution buffer of the added reagent. Substances added should not react with the solid-phase antigen nor the conjugate used. Commonly used blocking agents are given in **Table 3**, and they act by competing with nonspecific factors in the test sample for available plastic sites. The concentration used often

Table 3
Commonly used ELISA blocking agents

Protein	Reference
Normal rabbit serum	*(6)*
Normal horse serum	*(7)*
Human serum albumin	*(8)*
Bovine serum albumin	*(9)*
Fetal calf serum	*(10)*
Casein	*(11)*
Casein hydrolysate	*(12)*
Gelatin	*(13)*
Detergents	
Tween-20	*(9)*
Tween-80	*(14)*
Triton X-100	*(15)*
Sodium dodecyl sulfate	*(15)*
Other	
Dextran sulfate	*(7)*
Coffee mate	*(16)*
Nonfat dried milk	*(17)*

depends on the dilutions of the test samples; thus, if 1/20 serum is being tested (5% protein) then blocking agents have to be at high concentration to compete successfully, or have an increased binding potential as compared with the nonspecific substance. Such blocking agents can also be added as a separate step before the addition of the sample; this increases the competing ability of the blocker. Nonionic detergents have also been used to prevent nonspecific adsorption. These are used at low concentration so as to allow interaction of antigen and antibody. Occasionally, both detergents and blocking substances are added together.

The best conditions for individual assays are only assessed in practice; however, the cost of such reagents should be taken into account. Skimmed milk powder (bovine source), has been used successfully in many assays and is quit inexpensive. But, certain blocking agents may be unsuitable for different enzyme systems. For example, skimmed milk cannot be used in urease-directed ELISA, or when biotin–avidin systems are used. Contaminating substances such as bovine immunoglobulin (IgG) in bovine serum albumin (BSA) may eliminate the use of certain blocking agents from different suppliers. Most assays are validated under stated blocking conditions. However, investigators may adapt assays for use with other blocking reagents in which prescribed substances prove unobtainable or expensive.

5.1. Nonspecific Immunological Mechanisms

Reactions between solid-phase, positively charged basic proteins and added reagents owing to ionic interactions have been described *(15)*. This was removed by the addition of heparin or dextran sulfate in the diluent. The positive charges could also be removed by the addition of a low concentration of an anionic detergent sodium dodecyl sulfate (SDS). Such interactions have been noted for conjugates, which, although they do not bind to uncoated plates, do bind strongly to those containing antigens. The addition of a variety of blocking buffers, e.g., containing BSA, Tween-20, or casein, does not overcome the problem. Usually a high concentration of nonimmune serum from the same species as that in which the conjugate was prepared is necessary to prevent such a reaction.

5.2. Immunological Mechanisms

There are a large number of reports in which antibody–antigen reactions have been noted where they should not have occurred. These can be termed *aspecific reactions* and are of an immunological nature. These are antibodies that are naturally present in serum, which bind to antibodies from other species. They are not present in all sera, and consequently, cause problems in ELISA. For example, human heterophilic antibodies have been demonstrated against a common epitope on the F(ab')^2 fragment of IgG from bovine, ovine, equine, guinea pig, rat, and monkey species *(18)*. Methods of overcoming such antibodies include the use of F(ab')^2 as capture antibody in which the heterophilic reaction is against the Fc portion of IgG, or the use of high levels of normal serum obtained from the same species as the ELISA antibody in the blocking buffer. A review of heterophilic antibodies is given in **ref. 18**.

5.3. Interference by Rheumatoid Factor

Rheumatoid factor (RF) can cause a high level of false positives in the indirect ELISA. The factors are a set of the IgM class of antibodies that are present in normal individuals but are usually associated with pathological conditions. They bind to the Fc portion of IgG antibodies that either are complexed with their respective antigen or are in an aggregated form. Thus, any solid-phase/IgG/RF will be recognized by conjugates that recognize IgM and produce a false positive. Conversely, the binding of the RF to the antigen–IgG complex has been shown to interfere with the binding of IgG-specific conjugates, producing a lower or false reaction in ELISAs.

5.4. Miscellaneous Problems

Many sera contain antibodies specific for other animal serum components; for example, anti-bovine antibodies are commonly present in human sera *(19)*. Care must be taken when dealing with conjugates that may have unwanted cross-reactions of this type. Many conjugates are pretreated to adsorb out such unwanted cross-species reactions. Reagents are available for this purpose in which various species serum components are covalently linked, e.g., to agarose beads. These are added to sera, incubated for a short time, and then centrifuged into a pellet. Such beads can be reused after a treatment, which breaks the immunological bonds between the antigen and serum component with which it reacted. Such solid-phase reagents are more advantageous than methods in which normal sera are added to absorb out activities because the antibody molecules are totally eliminated from the solution.

5.5. Treatment of Samples

Many laboratories routinely heat sera to 56°C. This can cause problems in ELISA and should not be pursued. Heating can cause large increases in nonspecific binding to plates (*see* **ref. 8**).

6. Enzyme Conjugates

Intrinsic to the ELISA is the addition of reagents conjugated to enzymes. Assays are then quantified by the buildup of colored product after the addition of substrate or a combination of substrate and dye. Usually antibodies are conjugated to enzymes; some methods are given subsequents. Other commonly used systems involve the conjugation of enzymes to pseudoimmune reactors such as proteins A and G (which bind to mammalian IgGs), and indirect labeling using biotin–avidin systems. Four commonly used enzymes will be described. **Tables 4** and **5** give the properties of enzymes, substrates, and stopping conditions.

6.1. Horseradish Peroxidase Plus Hydrogen Peroxide Substrate

Horseradish peroxidase (HRP) plus hydrogen peroxide substrate is widely used. HRP is a holoenzyme of molecular weight 40,200, containing one ferritprotoprotein group per molecule. The apoenzyme is a glycoprotein of 308 amino acids and eight neutral carbohydrate side chains attached through asparigine residues. The polypeptide chain alone has a molecular weight of 33,890 and it has four disulfide linkages. The covalent structure consists of two compact domains sandwiching the hemin group. Seven isoenzymes of HRP have been isolated. Isoenzyme C (p*I* 8.7– 9.0) apoprotein (6.8) is the main cationic form constituting about 50% of the commercially available highly purified HRP. The reaction mechanism and spectral changes of peroxidase catalysis are complex, involving peroxidatic, oxidatic, catalytic, and

Table 4
Substrates and chromophores commonly used in ELISA

Enzyme label (mol wt)	Substrate	Chromophore	Buffer
HRP(40,000)	Hydrogen peroxide(0.004%)	OPD	Phosphate/citrate, pH 5.0
	Hydrogen peroxide(0.004%)	TMB	Acetate buffer, 0.1M, pH 5.6
	Hydrogen peroxide(0.002%)	ABTS	Phosphate/citrate, pH 4.2
	Hydrogen peroxide(0.006%)	5-AS	Phosphate, 0.2 M, pH 6.8
	Hydrogen peroxide(0.02%)	Diaminobenzidine	Tris or PBS, pH 7.4
AP(100,000)	pnpp(2.5 mM)	pnpp	Diethanolamine (10mM) and magnesium chloride (0.5 mM), ph9.5
-Galactosidase (540.000)	ONPG(3 mM)	ONPG	Magnesium choloride and 2-mercaptoethanol in PBS, pH 7.5
Urease (480.000)	Urea	Bromocresol	pH 4.8

Table 5
Enzyme labels, chromophores, and stopping conditions in ELISA

		Color		Reading (nm)		
Enzyme label	System	Not stopped	Stopped	Not Stopped	Stopped	Stop solution
HRP	OPD	Green/ orange	Orange/ brown	450	492	1.25 M sulfuric acid
	TMB	Blue	Yellow	650	450	SDS(1%)
	ABTS	Green	Green	414	414	No stop
	5-AS	Brown	Brown	450	450	No stop
	Diaminobenzidine	Brown	Brown	N/A	N/A	No stop
AP	pnpp	Yellow/ green	Yellow/ green	405	405	2 M sodium carbonate
β-Galactosidase	ONPG	Yellow	Yellow	420	420	2 M sodium carbonate
Urease	Urea bromocresol	Purple	Purple	588	588	Merthiolate(1%)

hydroxylactic activities. For a full explanation see **ref. 20**. The substrate hydrogen peroxide is also a powerful inhibitor, and so defined concentrations must be used. The reduction of peroxide by the enzyme is achieved by hydrogen donors that can be measured after oxidation as a color change. The choice of converted substrates that remain soluble is essential in ELISA so that optimal spectrophotometric reading can be made. Commonly used chemicals are given next.

6.1.1. Ortho-Phenylenediamine

Ortho-phenylenediamine (OPD) is prepared as a solution of 40 mg of donor per 100 mL of 0.1 M sodium citrate buffer, pH 5.0. Preweighed tablets are available commercially.

6.1.2 2,2′-Azino Diethylbenzothiazoline Sulfonic Acid

2,2′-Azino diethylbenzothiazoline sulfonic acid (ABTS) is prepared at the same concentration as OPD but in 0.1 M phosphate/citrate buffer, pH 4.0. Tablets are available.

6.1.3. 5-Aminosalicylic Acid

Commercial 5-aminosalicylic acid (5-AS) is dissolved in 100 mL of distilled water at 70°C for about 5 min with stirring. After cooling to room temperature, the pH of the solution is raised to 6.0 using a few drops of 1 M sodium hydroxide.

6.1.4 .Tetramethyl Benzidine

The optimum substrate (hydrogen peroxide) concentration of tetramethyl benzidine (TMB) depends on the hydrogen donor and the solid phase. This is usually established in preliminary tests, but concentrations between 0.010 and 0.0005% are adequate. Hydrogen peroxide is available as 30% commercially. The development of the colored product is measured at different wavelengths. The optimum wavelength may also shift if the reaction is stopped by a blocking reagent to prevent change in the optical density (OD) after a reaction period. The stopping reagents involving HRP are solutions of hydrochloric or sulfuric acid for OPD and TMB, SDS for ABTS. The optimal wavelengths for reading are 415 nm for ABTS; 492 nm for acidified OPD (420 nm for nonacidified OPD); 492 nm for 5-AS; and 655 nm for TMB (unstopped), 450 nm (acidified).

6.2. Alkaline Phosphatase Plus p-Nitrophenylphosphate

Alkaline phosphatase (ALP) used in immunoassays generally comes from bovine intestinal mucosa or from *Escherichia coli*, and these sources differ considerably in their properties. ALPs are dimeric glycoproteins, and all their zinc metalloenzymes contain at least two Zn (II) per molecule. *See* **ref. 20** for a detailed explanation of their structure and reaction mechanisms. ALPs are assayed in buffer depending on the source of the enzyme. For bacterial enzyme, 0.1 M Tris-HCl buffer, pH 8.1, containing 0.01% magnesium chloride is used. For intestinal mucosal enzyme a 10% (w/w) diethanolamine (97 mL in 1 L of a 0.01% magnesium chloride solution) buffer pH 9.8

(adjusted with HCl) is used. *p*-Nitrophenylphosphate (pnpp) is added just before use (available as preweighed pellets) to 1 mg/mL. The production of nitrophenol is measured at 405 nm. The reaction is stopped by the addition of 0.1 volume of 2 M sodium carbonate. Note that inorganic phosphate has a strong inhibitory effect on AP and therefore PBS or similar buffers are to be avoided.

Other chromogenic substrates can also be exploited, including phenolphthalein monophosphate, thymophthalein monophosphate, β-glycerophosphate, and uridine phosphate. Fluorigenic substrates can also be used such as β-naphthyl phosphate, 4-methylumbelliferyl phosphate, and 3-*o*-methylfluorescein monophosphate *(21)*.

6.3. β-Galactosidase Plus O-Nitrophenyl-β-d-Galactopyranoside

The reagent is prepared by the addition of a solution containing 70 mg of *o*-nitrophenyl-β-d-galactopyranoside (ONPG) per 100 mL of 0.1 M potassium phosphate buffer, pH 7.0, containing 1 mM magnesium chloride and 0.01 M 2mercaptoethanol. The reaction may be stopped by the addition of 0.25 volume of 2 M sodium carbonate.

6.4. Urease, pH Change, and Bromocresol Purple Indicator

The reagent is prepared by the addition of a weakly buffered solution of urea (pH 4.8) in the presence of bromocresol purple. The urea is hydrolyzed to liberate ammonia in the presence of urease, which raises the pH of the solution, resulting in a color change from yellow to purple. The reaction can be stopped by the addition of 10 μL of a 1% solution of merthiolate® (thimerosal) to each well. **Tables 4** and **5** summarize the properties of various enzyme systems.

7. Availability of Conjugates

Conjugates may be obtained commercially or made in individual laboratories. Great care must be exercised in using the appropriate reagent in any assay. Thus, the immunological implications of various reagents must be considered and information sought. Many conjugates are directed against different species serum components. These are some of their features:

1. The species in which the antiserum is produced can be important. Thus, donkey anti-cow IgG denotes that a donkey has been used to prepare antiserum against cow IgG. Other examples are rabbit anti-pig and pig anti-dog.
2. The preceding description must be refined since both the donating serum and the immunogen are probably subjected to immunochemical treatments. Thus, the donating serum can be crudely fractionated before conjugation (which is usual), or

may be affinity purified, so that the conjugate is 100% reactive against the immunogen. Examples are donkey IgG anti-cow IgG or donkey IgG (affinity purified) anti-cow IgG.

These descriptions deal with the processing of the donor serum after production and before conjugation. The description of the immunogen is also sometimes critical. Using the last example, the cow IgG may have itself been affinity purified before injection of the donkey, or specific parts of the Ig purified to raise a subclass-specific antiserum, for example, heavy-chain IgG may have been injected into the animal so that the conjugate only reacts with IgG. Remember that all Ig classes share antigens, so that it is highly likely that an antiserum raised against IgGs of any species will detect IgA, IgM, as well as IgG. Thus, the specificity of the conjugate has to be considered in any assay.

3. Different sources and batches of conjugates from the same manufacturer may vary. Thus, in large-scale applications, it is good practice to obtain a successful batch sufficient for all future testing. The anti-IgG one obtained from commercial company A may give different results from that obtained from company B.

Conjugates must be titrated to optimum conditions and not used in excess. This is vital to obtain reliable results.

8. Conjugation with Enzymes

The analytical sensitivity of the ELISA depends on the ability of the antibody to bind and the specific enzyme activity of the labeled immunoreactant, the conjugate. The linkage of an enzyme to an antigen or antibody may affect the specificity of an assay if any chemical modification of the moieties involved alters the antigenic determinants or the reactive sites on antibody molecules. Thus, chemical methods that do not affect these parameters have been chosen. Most of the techniques are straightforward and can be readily used by nonspecialists interested in developing their own enzyme immunoassays.

Not only must the immunoreactivities be maintained after conjugation, but also the catalytic activity of the enzyme. Following conjugation it is necessary to test the immunoreactivity to determine whether it has the desired specification. Before use in ELISA, it may be necessary to purify the conjugates to remove unconjugated antigen or antibody and free enzyme. Reagents used to produce conjugates are numerous and their mode of action is to modify the functional groups present on proteins. Antigens that are nonproteinaceous (e.g., steroids) can be conjugated with different means and are not dealt with here. Enzymes are covalently bound to reagents either directly by reactive groups on both the enzyme and reagent or after introduction of reactive groups (e.g., thiol or maleimid groups) indirectly via homo- or heterobifunctional reagents in two-step procedures *(22)*. The requirements for optimal conjugation are as follows:

1. Simplicity and rapidity
2. Reproducibility (obtaining constant molar ratio of enzyme and reagent)
3. High yield of labeled reagent and low yield of polymers of enzyme and reagent
4. Low-grade inactivation of reagent and enzyme
5. Simple procedures f or separation of labeled and unlabeled reagents
6. Long-term stability without loss of immunological and enzymatic activities

9. Development of Label

The substrate is usually chosen to yield a colored product. The rate of color development will be proportional, over a certain range, to the amount of enzyme conjugate present. On a kinetic level, reactions are distinguished by their kinetic order, which specifies the dependence of reaction rate on the concentration of reactants. Under the conditions generally employed in ELISA, the reaction exhibits zero order with respect to the substrate. Too little substrate will limit the rate of production of product. Thus, sufficient substrate must be present to prevent the substrate and/or cofactors from being rate limiting. In cases in which substrate and chromogenic hydrogen donors are necessary for color development, the concentrations of both must be assessed to obtain optimum conditions.

The product must be stable within a defined time, and products that are unstable in bright light or at temperatures at which the assay is performed should be avoided. The physicochemical parameters that affect the development of color include the following:

1. Buffer composition and pH
2. Reaction temperature
3. Substrate and/or cofactor concentration and stability, product stability, and enzyme stability
4. Substrate and product stability

9.1. Horseradish Peroxidase

HRP is active over a broad pH range with respect to its substrate, hydrogen peroxide; however, the optimum pH for the development of label in the ELISA will vary depending on the chromogenic donor. Changing the pH will reduce the reaction rate, but will not affect the reaction kinetics; for example, increasing the pH to 5.0 for ABTS will slow down the rate of reaction (pH optimum 4.0), but will not affect the linearity of the kinetics. The majority of the buffers used in substrate formulation are of low-molarity citrate base. Because the reaction kinetics are dependent on pH, a stable buffering capacity is essential. The stability of HRP varies in different buffers, being more stable in 0.1 M citrate than in 0.1 M phosphate buffer. High-molar phosphate buffer can be particularly damaging to HRP at low pH. Nonionic detergents exert a stabilizing effect on the enzymic activity of HRPO, and this can be enhanced by increasing reaction temperatures. Detergents have also been demonstrated as having a stabilizing effect on the enzymes.

9.2. Alkaline Phosphatase

AP is active at alkaline pH, optimum above pH 8.0. The buffer used with the substrate pnpp is diethanolamine/HCl, pH 9.6. Inorganic Mg^{2+} is essential for enzymatic activation. Nonionic detergents appear to have no effect on enzyme activation, substrate catalysis, or product development. Inactivation of the enzyme on contact with microplates does not occur.

9.3. Urease

Urease is enzymatically active over a broad pH range. The specificity of urease for its substrate (urea) is almost absolute. The urease substrate solution contains urea and a pH indicator, bromocresol purple, at pH 4.7. The urease catalyzes the urea into ammonia and bicarbonate, and the released ammonia causes an increase in pH that changes the color of the indicator from yellow to purple. The generation of color is not directly related to the amount of urea catalyzed. Because the color development is dependent on pH, it is essential to check that the pH is accurate before addition to wells in a test. It is also essential that no alkaline buffers remain after, e.g., washing (pH 7.4, PBS) because this will cause a change in color, and plates must be washed finally in water if PBS is the usual washing buffer.

9.4. Reaction Temperature

Between-well variation in an assay can cause differential rates of color development. Similarly, varying temperatures in the performance of the assay can cause variation. It is advisable, therefore, that substrates be added at a defined temperature and that plates be incubated under uniform conditions – normally room temperature. Note that this definition is rather loose and that each laboratory should be assessed since temperature can vary greatly in different countries. The best practice is to add substrate solutions at a defined temperature obtained by using solutions heated to (or cooled) to that defined temperature. This is particularly important when attempting to standardize assays among operators and laboratories in which a fixed time for stopping an assay is used.

9.5. Substrate/ Cofactor Concentration and Stability

As already stated, substrate concentrations must be optimized. This is usually stated for particular systems (literature, kits, and so forth). Certain solutions can be made and stored. As an example, OPD can be made up in buffer, stored frozen in well-sealed vials, and then be thawed and used (after the addition of H_2O_2). This negates the need to weigh out small amounts of OPD for small volumes of substrate solution and aids standardization of assays. The use of preweighed chemicals in the form of tablets available commercially also greatly improves the accuracy and convenience of producing substrate solutions, although these tablets are expensive.

9.6. Product Stability

Once the substrate has been catalyzed and a colored product achieved, it is essential that the color remains stable. In the majority of ELISAs, positive results are read by eye or by spectrophotometer as the intensity of color (OD) as compared with a series of previously worked out negative values. An unstable colored product would affect the buildup of color. For spectrophotometric reading of results, it is vital that the product color remains stable without shifting the absorption spectrum, as the microplate readers assess the absorbance of the colored addition of a reagent preventing further enzymatic activity. This is dealt with in the next section.

9.7. Enzyme Stability

The enzymes used in the ELISA are stable with respect to their activity with defined substrates. Thus, a high degree of consistency is found using the same batch of conjugate under defined conditions.

9.8. Substrate and Product Stability

Substrates are only soluble to a limited extent in aqueous buffers. The use of mixed aqueous/organic buffers is possible. These solvent systems can allow significantly greater amounts of substrates to be incorporated into solution and also allow their use in microplate ELISAs. Partially or totally insoluble products can be used in variants of ELISA, e.g., in the staining of sections in immunohistochemistry in which insoluble products localize the area of antigen or antibody reaction.

10. Stopping Reactions

Reagents are added to prevent further enzymatic reaction in ELISA. This is performed at a time as determined for the specific assay. This process is usually called stopping and the reagent used is the stopping reagent. Stopping is usually done at a time when the relationship between the enzyme–substrate–product is in the linear phase. Molar concentrations of strong acids or strong bases stop enzymic activity by quickly denaturing enzymes. Other stopping reagents are enzyme specific. Sodium azide is a potent inhibitor of HRP, whereas EDTA inhibits AP by the chelation of metal ion cofactors.

Since the addition of stopping agents may alter the absorption spectrum of the product, the absorption peak must be known. For example, OPD/ELISAs stopped by sulfuric acid are read at 492 nm (450 nm before stopping). **Table 5** gives the wavelengths for reading the appropriate substrates before or after the addition of stopping agents. The addition of stopping agents can also increase the sensitivity of an ELISA. In the addition of stopping reagent, the volumes must be kept accurate, since photometric readings are affected if the total volume of reactants varies.

11. Reading

As the product of substrate catalysis is colored, it can be read in two ways:
(1) by eye inspection or (2) using a spectrophotometer.

11.1. Reading by Eye

ELISAs can be designed for use with either reading by eye or a spectrophotometer although different conditions and controls may have to be included. The principles of ELISA must be thoroughly understood before either system is adopted. In particular testing by eye is not necessarily simpler to standardize. However, when correct standardization is used, it offers sensitive assays. When a correct plate template is used, the range of color product will be from full through partial color to no color.

Known, strong positive samples will give strong color, weak positives will give partial color, and negatives will give no color, or that of negative wells. Controls of this sort must be incorporated into the intended assays. Some difficulties arise in differentiating weak positives from negatives by eye. The interpretation of tests by eye can vary from operator to operator, and, hence, results are more subjective than by using a spectrophotometer. Some substrate–enzyme combinations favor reading by eye.

In cases in which tests have to be read by eye (when instrumentation is not available), the best assays can be produced in other laboratories that can quantify reagents using machine reading and evaluate the parameters of the reading by eye. As an example, a negative population of sera can be examined, and control negative sera, reflecting different parts of the negative OD distribution, can be adopted for controls by eye. Thus, a serum having the highest OD value may be selected as the negative control. Any sera giving discernible results by eye higher than this serum would therefore be assessed with high confidence as being positive. Assays that require comparison of closely related data, such as competition assays, are not suitable for interpretation by eye, e.g., in which the competition slope is compared.

11.2. Spectrophotometric Reading

The product of the substrate catalysis by enzyme is measured by transmitting light of a specific wavelength through the product and measuring the amount of adsorption of that light, if any, with a machine. Because different products are produced in ELISA, care must be taken to select appropriate filters for the detection of the correct wavelengths. Although microcuvets and conventional spectrophotometers can be used for this purpose, these are laborious in cases in which large numbers of samples are measured. Special machines are available for the reading of colored products in microplates. These read the absorbance of each well at a preselected wavelength of light. Either one well can be read at a time (manual readers), or more suitably, a column of eight wells can be read simultaneously (semiautomatic or automatic multichannel spectrophotometers).

For semiautomatic readers, the wavelength filters are added manually, whereas for automatic readers, the wavelength filter(s) are contained as an internal filter wheel and can be selected from a control panel. In the main, the results from such machines are expressed as absorbance units and are recorded on paper rolls, or through interfacing with a computer. Various (limited but useful) ways of processing the data is usually available, such as the expression of the absorbance values as a matrix or as plus and minus against control wells or values given to the machine. Most readers can be connected to computers, and a range of software (commercial and private) is available to manipulate and store data. This is important in large-scale sample handling, or in which complicated arithmetic routines are performed on the data. An important feature of the ELISA having a colored product that can be examined by eye is that tests can be rapidly assessed before machine reading; one can see that a test has or has not worked at a glance. Thus, extensive reading time is not wasted if a careless mistake has occurred, unlike radioimmunoassay, in which it is essential to count samples before results are obtained. Such assessment by eye is also convenient when "sighting" experiments are being conducted during the development of assays.

12. Practical Problems

This section discusses problems associated with the practical aspects of ELISAs that have been observed under different laboratory conditions.

12.1. Overall Observations on Running ELISA

The major cause of problems in running an ELISA is the scientist(s) involved. This has been demonstrated graphically through my involvement in training and supplying kit reagents to many laboratories worldwide. The main problem is lack of close contact training in the fundamentals of ELISA so that the scientist has the experience to identify and then solve problems in the use of reagents. There is no substitute for good training.

12.1.1. Problems Caused by Lack of General Scientific Knowledge

The biological implications of results cannot be assessed without general knowledge of several fields of science, such as epidemiology, immunochemistry, biochemistry, and immunology, as indicated in Chapter 1.

12.1.2. Problems Are Caused by Sloppy Technique

The reproducibility of any assay relies, in part, on the accuracy of the investigators involved. This is further complicated when many people perform the assay (e.g., in a laboratory concerned with large-scale testing of sera on a routine basis). Attempts should be made to provide individual assessments to improve reliability of techniques (e.g., accurate pipetting and timing). Quality control and quality assurance protocols should be developed, as discussed in Chapter 9.

12.1.3. Common Problems of Instrumentation and Reagents

Not all problems can be blamed directly on the operator. Although the individual steps of ELISAs are relatively simple, assays can be regarded as complex in that several steps with different reagents (all of which have to be standardized) must be made. This increases the likelihood of problems in any methodology. Reagents also have to be stored and are subject to contamination by microorganisms or from other operators introducing unwanted reagents through the use of contaminated pipet tips. A surprisingly common error is the reading of wells at the wrong wavelength. Operators must learn to read the color by eye as well as to read the OD. In cases in which operators have never seen an ELISA, then this can be excused, although when a plate does show "decent" color, the OD readings should be giving a range of values for any substrate of about 1 OD. If plates showing a strong to moderate color as assessed by eye, but only low OD readings (0.1–0.3 maxima), then the wavelength should be checked. Confusion about the filter can be the result of other operators placing filters in machines for other systems as well as not knowing where a particular wavelength filter is on a filter-wheel machine. Often software programs also indicate a wavelength on the readout that is not associated with the machine, but merely the wavelength at which the test should be read.

12.1.4. Water

Water can be a major problem in the standardization of assays among different laboratories even when identical reagents are used. Thus, some kits supply water, at least for the initial dilutions of the stock reagents. The reasons why water affects the ELISA have not been extensively examined and no single factors have emerged as being most important. It is a good idea to use triple-distilled water, but it is not always available to less well-equipped laboratories. The type of problem encountered is that of readings higher than expected using control sera as well as plate blanks. The supply of tested water for the preparation of buffers for the initial dilutions of reagents will solve this problem. Operators should also obtain supplies from other laboratories to examine whether they solve observed problems.

12.1.5. Laboratory Glassware

Laboratory glassware should be clean and well rinsed in glass-distilled water. This avoids the introduction of contaminants or adverse pH conditions into ELISA reagents, especially when initial dilutions of conjugate are concerned. The use of acids can cause problems if sufficient rinsing is not done, since enzymes are destroyed.

12.1.6. Micropipet Tips

Micropipet tips are expensive and can be in short supply in some laboratories. They can be washed, but the following steps should be taken:

1. Never wash and reuse tips that have delivered conjugate or conjugate solution.
2. Check that the ends of the tips are not damaged during use and washing.
3. Always rinse the tips very well in distilled water.
4. Dry the tips before use.
5. Get the appropriate tips to fit your micropipets. A poor fit causes problems with pipetting, which leads to inaccuracy.

5. 12.1.7. Micropipets

Because micropipets are the instruments that deliver volumes of liquid, they are fundamentally important to the accuracy of the ELISA. They should be checked regularly for precision and accuracy of delivery volumes. Instructions on how to do this are usually included with the pipets; if not, ask the manufacturer how they are to be checked. Limited maintenance of the pipets should be made with attention to the plungers in multichannel pipets, which get contaminated. Care should be taken to make sure that liquids are not pulled into the pipet; if so, they must be cleaned. Corrosion can occur when, e.g., sulfuric acid stopping reagent is taken into the body of a pipet.

12.1.8. Plates

1. If a particular plate is recommended, then use that plate unless you retitrate given reagents in another manufacturer's plate.
2. Never use a tissue culture grade plate for ELISA. Sometimes these plates can be made to work, but they give much more variability than those specifically made for ELISA.
3. Always report which plate and which treatment of the plate has been made.
4. Reuse of plates after washing is problematic and high variability is observed. However, if economic and supply reasons deem it necessary, use 2 M NaOH overnight after washing the plates in tap water, and then rinse thoroughly in distilled water. You should use washed plates with many more controls than for new plates to measure variability.

4. 12.1.9. Troughs (Reservoirs)

1. Use specific troughs only for conjugate and substrate to avoid cross contamination.
2. After use, wash the troughs in tap water, followed by distilled water and then leave them soaking in a mild detergent. For use, rinse in tap water, distilled water, and then dry with towel.
3. Never leave reagents in troughs for a long time after they have been used in an assay; rinse immediately if possible.

12.1.10. Substrate Solution

The temperature of the substrate solution is important because this affects the rate of color reaction. Therefore, try to perform the addition with the substrate always at the same temperature. This can easily be achieved if buffer tablets are used by keeping the water used at a constant temperature, or preincubating the substrate in a water bath. When substrate solution is kept frozen, you must ensure that on thawing the same temperature is achieved for every test (again by using a water bath). A range of 20–30°C is recommended. The variation in temperature of the substrate solution will be the greatest factor in causing differences among assays performed with the same reagents.

12.1.11. Timing of Steps

Generally, individual steps should be timed accurately; thus, for a 1-h incubation step, no more than 5 min either way should be tolerated. For assays that recommend specific times, there is no reason that they cannot be met. Timing is less important when plates are rotated, although it is good practice to follow protocols accurately.

12.1.12. Incubation

We have already considered stationary vs. rotated plates. The conclusion is that rotation of plates for incubation steps is highly recommended to eliminate viscosity effects; time differences; and temperature effects, including edge-well differences caused when plates are stacked and incubated stationary. However, when a rotator is not available, provided that standardization of methods is used, stationary plate assays are not a problem. The following tips are helpful when incubating plates that are not rotated:

1. Avoid stacking the plates; keep them separated.
2. Incubate at 37°C.
3. Always use the same procedure for addition of reagents; that is, do not tap one plate, pick another up three times, or examine one or two plates during the incubation and not others. Using different procedures mix the reagents over the solid phase to different degrees, thereby altering the interaction in the wells. Thus, take more care handling the plates identically in one test and from day to day.
4. If incubation has to be done at room temperature make a note of the temperature and its variation during the year. This may explain variation in results at different times.

12.1.13. Conjugates

Care must be taken with conjugates because they are the signal suppliers of the whole assay.

1. Make sure you understand what the conjugate is (species made, specific antibody activity, and so forth).
2. Store at recommended temperatures.
3. Never store diluted conjugate for use at a later time.
4. Always make up the working dilution of conjugate just before you need it.
5. Always use clean tips, preferably previously unused, to dispense conjugates.
6. If the recommended dilution or titrated dilution of conjugate is very high (e.g., 1/10,000), add 1 μL–10 mL to make 10 mL at working strength. You may have difficulty in making small volumes of working strength. Thus, a small dilution should be made to allow feasible pipetting of the conjugate without waste. Dilute in 50% glycerol/50% PBS to, say, 1/10 of the original. Store at –20°C if possible.
7. Never leave conjugates on the bench for an excessive time.
8. Preferably add sterile glycerol (equal volume) for conjugates stored at –20°C.

12.1.14. Addition of Stopping Solution

Because the multichannel spectrophotometer reads through a thickness of liquid, any change in the volume in a well will result in an alteration of OD reading for the same colored solution. Thus, it is important to add stopping solution accurately to achieve the same volume in each well and limit the effect of volume changes (This, of course, is also true of addition of conjugate solution and concerns the blotting of plates to eliminate residual washing solution, all of which affect the final volume per well.)

12.1.15. Addition of Samples

An accurate and consistent pipetting technique is a prerequisite for limiting pipetting error. Major problems are caused by the following factors:

1. Failure to put sample into the buffer in the well, leaving it on the side of the plate (particularly when plates are incubated stationary).
2. Frothing on addition of samples.
3. Lack of concentration when adding a large number of samples, causing missed wells and duplication of samples in the same well.
4. Poorly maintained pipets and tips.
5. Improperly thawing out sera (protein tends to collect at the bottom of the tubes on freezing) so that adequate mixing to ensure homogeneity is essential.

5. 12.1.16. Reading Plates/Data

The advantage of ELISA is that the plates can be read quickly and a large amount of data can be generated that can lead to several problems:

1. Computerization whereby the plate data are processed and the results given (e.g., ±56%) must be checked quickly from examination of plate data by eye. This is essential since some programs do not give warnings to check highly suspect results probably caused by a major sampling error. Thus, mean values may be calculated from the plate data by the computer and use these to ascribe positive or negative for particular samples. Unless safety features to screen for extremely different OD values in a pair are included in the program, false results are obtained (e.g., two values for a serum are 0.40 and 0.42, mean = 0.41 = positive; two values for a serum are 0.02 and 0.74, mean = 0.41?). Personal examination of initial plate data would easily spot this serum result as nonsense, whereas the sole reference to the computer printout of positive/negative would not. This is a facile example, but more complex analytical programs have similar hidden problems.
2. Large databases set up to store data from large-scale screening. This is related to the checking factor in which results read directly into a database are taken as reliable without examination by eye of the feasibility of those results. Researchers often wish to have results from several laboratories, and therefore

programs have been supplied to facilitate this need. Such programs can easily dehumanize the diagnostic process by controlling results and denying the ability to backcheck data.

3. Cables that connect computers to spectrophotometers and printers that do not work. These are general hardware problems that must be conquered.

12.2. Troubleshooting ELISA

Table 6 presents some of the problems commonly seen in ELISA development and practice and highlights areas that should be examined first when assays are proving difficult.

Table 6
Problems and solutions in ELISA

Problem	Solution
No/very little color even after 30-min incubation with substrate/chromophore	
No hydrogen peroxide added	Check
Hydrogen peroxide stock inactivated	Retitrate
Added blocking buffer in adsorption step for antigen	Check
Wrong dilution of hydrogen peroxide	Check
Color all over plate	
Too strong conjugate	Cheek dilution
Conjugate reacts with something other than target species	Cheek with suitable controls
Serum factors in heated sera	Do not heat sera routinely
Patchy color	
Poor and variable coating of plates with reagents	Check coating buffer and homogeneity of preparation
Bubbles in multichannel pipet tips	Aviod overvigorous pipeting and detergents
Poor pipeting technique	Practice more care
Plates faulty or non-ELISA plates	Contact manufacturer; try alternative plates
Incubated plates in stacks	Keep plates separated during stationary incubation
Poor mixing of reagents including test sample	Ensure mixing on sampling
Dilution series poorly done	Practice pipeting; examine pipets for wear; recalibrate pipets

(continued)

Table 6 (continued)

Problem	Solution
Poor washing	Avoid detergents in wash solution; ensure no air bubbles are trapped in wells
Color develops very quickly	
Conjugate too strong	Retitrate
One reagent at too high concentation	Check dilutions
Color develops too slowly	
Conjugate too weak	Check dilutions used; retitrate
Contamination inhibits enzyme activity (e.g., sodium azide for peroxidase)	Avoid wrong preservatives
Low temperature of incubation	Make sure temperature of substrate is correct
pH of substrate incorrect	Check
Totally unexpected results	
Plate format incorrect	Check
Dilution series in test protocol	Check
Gross error in test protocol	Check
Visual estimation of color does not match ELISA reader results	Check for contaminated damaged filter; inappropriate filter (wrong wavelength)
High background color	
Nonspecific attachment of antibodies	check for unsuitable blocking conditions or omission of blocking buffer
Antispecies conjugate reacts whether any reagent	Set up controls to assess with reagent on plate nonspecifically to any binds other in test

References

1. Cantarero, L. A., Butler, J. E., and Osborne, J. W. (1980) The binding characteristics of proteins for polystyrene and their significance in solid-phase immunoassays. *Analyt. Biochem.* 105, 375–382.
2. Kurstak, E., Tijssen, P., Kurstak, C., and Morisset, R. (1986) Enzyme immunoassay in diagnostic medical virology. *Bull. W. H. O.* 64(3), 465–479.
3. Geerligs, H. G., Weijer, W. J., Bloemhoff, W., Welling, G. W. and Welling-Wester, S. (1988) The influence of pH and ionic strength on the coating of peptides of herpes simplex virus type I in an enzyme-linked immunosorbent assay. *J. Immunol. Methods* 106, 239–244.
4. Rembaum, A., Margel, S., and Levy, A. (1978) *J. Immunol. Methods* 24, 239.

5. Gabrilovac, J., Pachmann, K., Rodt, H., Gager, G. and Thierfelder, S. (1979) Par-ticle-labelled antibodies I. Anti-Tcell antibodies attached to plastic beads by poly-l-lysine. *J. Immunol. Methods* 30, 161–170.
6. Kohno, T., Hashida, S., and Ishikawa, E. (1985) A more sensitive enzyme immunoassay of anti-insulin IgG in guinea pig serum with less non-specific binding of normal guinea pig serum. *J. Biochem.* 98, 379–384.
7. Meegan, J. M., Yedloutsenig, R. J., Peleg, B. A., Shy, J., Peters, C. J.,Walker, J. S., and Shope, R. E. (1987) Enzyme-linked immunosorbent assay for detection of antibodies to Rift Valley Fever Virus in ovine and bovine sera. *Am. J. Vet. Res.* 48, 1138–1141.
8. Husby, S., Holmskov-Neilsen, U., Jensenius, J. C., and Erb, K. (1982) Increased non-specific binding of heat treated proteins to plastic surfaces analyzed by ELISA and HPLC-fractionation. *J. Immunoassay* 6, 95–110.
9. Herrmann, J. E., Hendry, R. M., and Collins, M. F. (1979) Factors involved in enzyme-linked immunassay and evaluation of the method of identification of enteroviruses. *J. Clin. Microbiol.* 10, 210–217.
10. Harmon, M. W., Russo, L. L., and Wilson, S. Z. (1983) Sensitive enzyme immunoassay with b-D-galactosidase-Fab conjugate for detection of type A influenza virus antigen in clinical specimens. *J. Clin. Microbiol.* 17, 305–311.
11. Kenna, J. G., Major, G. N., and Williams, R. S. (1985) Methods for reducing nonspecific antibody binding in enzyme-linked immunosorbent assays. *J. Immunol. Methods* 85, 409–419.
12. Robertson, P. W., Whybin, L. R., and Cox, J. (1985) Reduction in non-specific binding in enzyme imunoassays using casein hydrolysate in serum diluents. *J. Immunol. Methods* 76, 195–197.
13. Gary, W. G. J. R., Kaplan, E. J., Stine, E. S., and Anderson, J. L. (1985) Detection of Norwalk Virus antibodies and antigen with a biotin/avidin system. *J. Clin. Microbiol.* 22, 274–278.
14. Hatfield, R. M., Morris, B. A., and Henry, A. (1987) Development of and enzyme-linked immunosorbent assay for the detection of humoral antibodies. *Avian Pathol.* 16, 123–140.
15. Dietzen, R. G. and Francki, R. I. B. (1987) Nonspecific binding of immunoglobulins to coat proteins of certain plant viruses in immunoblots and indirect ELISA. *J. Virol. Methods* 15, 159–164.
16. York, J. J. and Fahey, K. J. (1988) Diagnosis of Infectious Laryn gotracheitis using a monoclonal antibody ELISA. *Avian Pathol.* 17, 173–182.
17. Vogt, R. F., Phillips, D. L., Henderson, L. O., Whitfield, W., and Spierto, F. W. (1987) Quantitative differences among various proteins as blocking agents for ELISA microtiter plates. *J. Immunol. Methods* 101, 43–50.
18. Boscato, L. M. and Stuart, M. C. (1988) Heterophilic antibodies: a problem for all immunoassays. *Clin. Chem.* 33, 27–33.
19. Dise, T. and Brunell, A. P. (1987) Anti-bovine antibody in human sera as a cause of nonspecificity in enzyme immunoassay. *J. Clin. Microbiol.* 25, 987–990.
20. Deshpand, S. S. (1996) Enzyme Immunoassays from Concept to Product Development. Chapman & Hall, New York.
21. Ngo, T. T. (1991) Immunoassay. *Curr. Opin. Biotechnol.* 2, 102–109.
22. Ishikawa, E., Imagawa, M., Hashide, S., Yoshatake, S., Hagushi, Y.,and Ueno, E. (1983) Enzyme labelling of antibodies and their fragments for enzyme immunoassays and immunological staining. *J. Immunoassay* 4, 209.

Chapter 4

Titration of Reagents

This chapter examines in detail the necessary practical skills needed to facilitate the development and sustainability of ELISAs. Basic methodologies to set up all systems are discussed so that the reader can both investigate the possibilities of tests using his or her reagents and use with confidence the reagents obtained from other sources. As with all other tests, it is vital that scientists realize the principles of the methods to allow good judgement based on quantifiable and controllable features. In other words, there should be a full understanding of what is being performed in the laboratory. The intention of this training is to produce new skills and understanding as well as to encourage critical assessment. Such a mentality is necessary and supported through the application of statistical criteria to results and to continuous monitoring of performance.

1. Chessboard or Checkerboard Titrations

The many ELISA systems described previously require that the reagents used be optimized. In other words, the working concentration of each component of the test must be assessed. **Table 1** gives a simplified overview of the systems, indicating the number of reagents needed to be optimized, as a reminder.

A key feature in helping this process is through the use of chessboard or checkerboard titrations (CBTs). The use of microtiter plates is an important feature of ELISAs. This chapter describes this type of format. CBTs can be accomplished in any format in which reagents can be diluted, but the microtiter plate, with its associated equipment for ease of pipetting, is ideal. It will become clear that CBT is not the only method for optimizing

John R. Crowther, *Methods in Molecular Biology, The ELISA Guidebook, Vol. 516*

DOI: 10.1007/978-1-60327-254-4_4

Table 1
Basic ELISA system components requiring titration

ELISA	Reagents involved	Number titrated
Direct	Antigen; antibody conjugated to enzyme	2
Indirect	Antigen; antibody; antispecies conjugate	3
Direct sandwich	Capture antibody; antigen; conjugated second antibody	3
Indirect sandwich	Capture antibody; antigen; second antibody; antispecies conjugate against second antibody	4

reagents, and that often concentrations must be adjusted with reference to actual test conditions.

The process of CBT involves the dilution of two reagents against each other to examine the activities inherent at all the resulting combinations. The maximum number of reagents that can be titrated on a plate is two, and this is illustrated in the direct ELISA (*see* **Subheading 1.1**). The use of CBT in some other systems with more than two reagents is also illustrated. The descriptions of pipetting and diluting techniques are also fundamental to the performance of ELISAs in general. As the reader becomes familiar with the methods, fewer details will be necessary to describe the tests.

1.1. Direct ELISA CBT

Figure 1 shows diagrammatically the dilution scheme. The upper part of **Fig. 1** illustrates the typical numbering and lettering associated with microtiter plates. Thus, columns are labeled 1–12 and rows are labeled A–H. This nomenclature is used henceforth to identify locations on the plates.

1.1.1. Stage (i) of Direct ELISA CBT

Stage (i) involves diluting the antigen in a coating buffer. The volumes usually used in ELISA are 50 or 100 μL. In this chapter, we use 50 μL as the standard volume added to wells. A twofold dilution range is usual at this stage, e.g., one volume taken from one well and added to the same volume in the next well, and so on. The most practical way of performing the test is as follows:

1. Add the diluent (in this stage the coating buffer) in 50-μL volume to all wells of the plate using a multichannel pipet.
2. Add 50 μL of a dilution of the antigen to all wells in column 1.
   a. The initial dilution can be made in a small bottle to result in a volume necessary for addition to column 1; that is, you

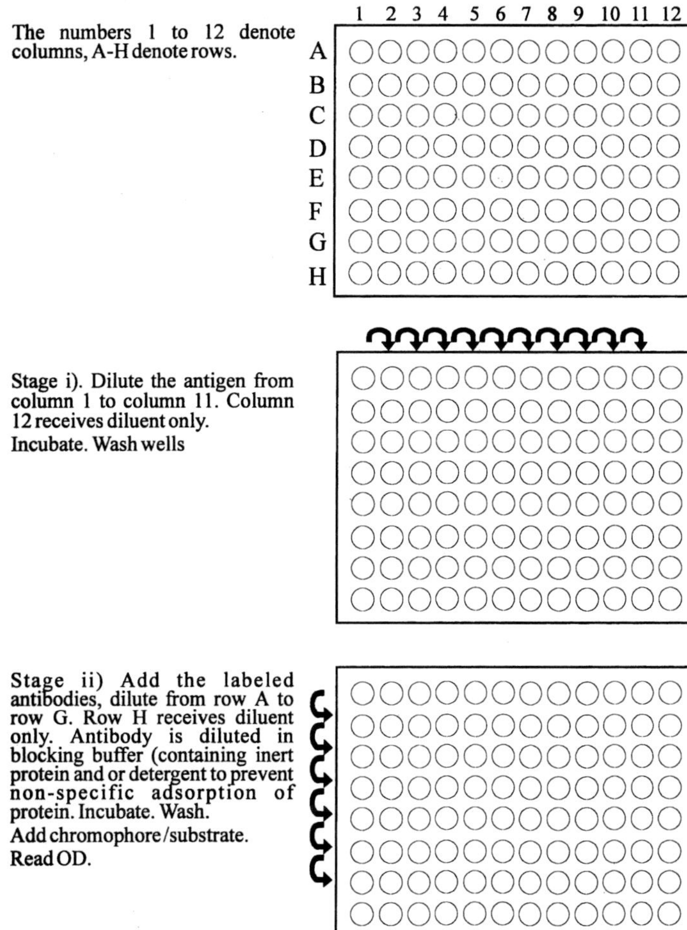

Fig. 1. Plate layout and CBT of antigen against conjugated antibody for direct ELISA.

will need eight wells × 50 μL = 400 μL of antigen dilution. It is advisable to make slightly more of the initially diluted antigen than is theoretically needed to allow for material adhering to bottles, and so forth; in this case, 500 μL (0.5 mL) should be made.

b. Assessment of the initial dilution is based on any knowledge of the likely antigen concentration (e.g., as assessed from other tests). With the CBT there is going to be a direct assessment of activity in the ELISA at a range of concentrations, and therefore, if there is a gross under- or overestimate of antigen, another CBT can be made accounting for such problems. The likely purity of the antigen (concentration of specific antigens as compared with contaminants) and the availability of antigen must be considered. A useful starting dilution for all antigens might be 1/10–20 in coating buffer. Let us assume that we add 1/20.

3. Add 50 μL of the prediluted antigen to all wells in column A. Mix with a multichannel pipet fitted with eight tips. The mixing implies that the liquid in the well is pipeted up and down in the tip at least five times. This should not be done too vigorously.
4. After the final mixing, take 50 μL of the diluted antigen from the eight wells in column A and transfer to column B. Mix as before. Repeat the procedure until column 11. Note that this means there is no antigen in column 12, and this will serve as one control (development of color with conjugate dilutions on wells containing no antigen).
5. After the final mixing action in column 11, take out 50 μL and discard. In the wells we have created a twofold dilution series of antigen in coating buffer, beginning at 1/20 in column A and ending at 1/20,480 in column 11.
6. Incubate the plate to allow time for the adsorption of antigen to the wells. The nature and time of the incubation should be the same as that used in the test proper. Most antigens will attach, with incubation under stationary conditions at 37°C in 2 h. However, it may be more convenient to allow overnight incubation at 4°C. Whatever conditions are applied, they must be followed in the subsequent development of the test, since alteration in times, temperatures, or regimes of shaking or tapping plates will alter the kinetics of adsorption.
7. Now wash the plate by flooding and emptying the wells with phosphate-buffered saline (PBS), as described in Chapter 3.

1.1.2. Stage (ii) of Direct ELISA CBT

Stage (ii) involves making a similar dilution range of the conjugated antibody made against the antigen. In this case the dilution range is made from row A to G. The added buffer is blocking buffer (containing a relatively high concentration of inert protein to prevent nonspecific binding of proteins (*see* Chapter 3)). In this case, the blocking buffer might be PBS (0.1 M, pH 7.6) containing skimmed milk powder (5%) and 0.05% Tween-20.

The dilution range is made using the multichannel pipet with 12 tips, directly in the wells. Again, there must be mixing between each addition. Note that there is no dilution of conjugate into row H; this acts as a control for only substrate and antigen (since the wells contain a dilution range of antigen). The initial dilution should be in the region of 1/50 for a direct conjugate.

1. Incubate the plate under rotation (best) at 37°C for 1 h or stationary at 37°C for 2 h. Wash the wells.
2. Add chromophore/substrate. This could be any of the ones described in Chapter 3 added with due care as to accuracy and checks on the pHs of the buffers involved. In this example, we shall assume we add H_2O_2/*ortho*-phenylenediamine (OPD) at 50 μL/well (in every well of the plate).

3. Leave the plate stationary for 15 min to allow color to develop. The exact timing of color development and conditions should be adhered to in subsequent assays. At this stage, it is good practice to observe the plate for the rate of color development.
4. Stop (depending on system).
5. Read the OD of color in a spectrophotometer.

1.2. Results

Table 2 presents stylized results that might be obtained. We are attempting to assess the optimal dilutions of antigen to coat the wells and the interaction of the conjugate.

Figure 2 shows the data plotted.

Table 2
Results of CBT (OD data)[a]

	1	2	3	4	5	6	7	8	9	10	11	12
A	2.1	2.2	2.1	2.1	2.0	2.1	1.9	1.7	1.5	1.3	1.0	0.6
B	2.1	2.0	1.9	2.0	1.9	1.8	1.7	1.5	1.3	0.9	0.5	0.3
C	2.1	2.0	1.9	1.9	1.8	1.7	1.7	1.5	1.2	0.9	0.5	0.3
D	1.8	1.8	1.7	1.8	1.5	1.2	1.0	0.7	0.5	0.3	0.2	0.1
E	1.8	1.8	1.7	1.5	1.3	1.1	0.9	0.7	0.5	0.3	0.2	0.1
F	1.5	1.5	1.4	1.3	1.1	0.9	0.7	0.5	0.3	0.2	0.1	0.1
G	0.7	0.7	0.7	0.6	0.6	0.5	0.3	0.2	0.1	0.1	0.1	0.1
H	0.2	0.1	0.1	0.1	0.1	0.1	0.1	0.1	0.1	0.1	0.1	0.1

[a]Note that rows D and E are highlighted and column 12 rows A–C are boxed

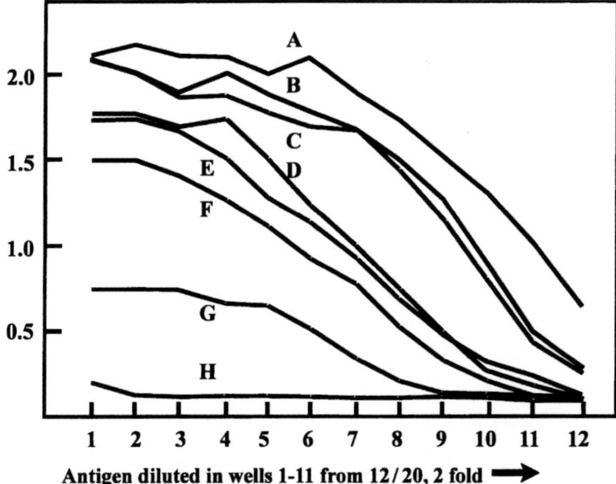

Fig. 2. Plots of OD values obtained relating different antigen concentrations to different dilutions of labeled antibody. Row 12 received no antigen. A–G indicate rows containing different dilutions of labeled antibody. Row H did not receive labeled antibody.

4.1.2.1 Analysis of Data

Each of the columns contains a constant but different dilution of antigen. Differences in color between the columns, where there is a constant addition of labeled antibody, reflects the effect of altering the concentration of antigen. The rows can be assessed for a maximum color in which there is a range of values that are similar. This can be regarded as a plateau and reflects areas where the antibody is in excess. In this area, where there is no decrease in color on dilution of the antigen, a maximum saturating level of antigen is coated to the plates. Thus, we can identify regions of excess antigen or antibody. Taking row A:

	1	2	3	4	5	6	7	8	9	10	11	12
A	2.1	2.2	2.1	2.1	2.0	2.1	1.9	1.7	1.5	1.3	1.0	0.6

The shaded values are similar, giving a plateau maximum value of about 2.0 OD units. There is no effect on color where antigen is coated at 1/20, 1/40, 1/80, 1/160, 1/320, or 1/640 (wells 1–6). This indicates that in the presence of a constant dilution of antibody, there is a similar amount of antigen coating the wells to a dilution of 1/640. Following further dilution, there is a decrease in OD values on dilution of the antigen.

Note that rows B and C give similar results showing a plateau from rows 1–6. Figure 2 shows graphically that the curves are similar, although there are slight reductions on dilution of the conjugate. Again, this indicates that antigen is in excess, certainly at the dilution added to column 5. Thus, increasing the concentration of antigen above that contained in dilution at 1/320 only wastes antigen.

	1	2	3	4	5	6	7	8	9	10	11	12
A	2.1	2.2	2.1	2.1	2.0	2.1	1.9	1.7	1.5	1.3	1.0	0.6
B	2.1	2.0	1.9	2.0	1.9	1.8	1.7	1.5	1.3	0.9	0.5	0.3
C	2.1	2.0	1.9	1.9	1.8	1.7	1.7	1.5	1.2	0.9	0.5	0.3

The OD values in column 12 should be considered since this column represents the color developing where there is no antigen. The values are high for A–C, relative to color for D–G, which are low and the same. This color can be presumed to be the result of nonspecific attachment of the conjugate to the wells. The higher the amount of protein added, the greater the chance of nonspecific events. Note that there is a reduction in color down each of the columns on dilution of conjugate even where an excess of antigen is shown (columns 1–5/6). This is owing to the reduction in concentration of the conjugate (diluting out of reactive enzyme-labeled antibodies).

To obtain the most controllable results in ELISA, maximum OD values should be about 1.5.–1.7 OD units. Values above this are inaccurate on instrumentational grounds. Thus, optimization involves assessment of assays in which plateau maxima are near these OD values. This is based on OPD/H_2O_2 and other systems that have their own optima, but these should never approach very high ODs with respect to each substrate/chromophore system. Let us now concentrate on rows D and E, where this is a plateau height of 1.8 in the region where antigen is in excess:

D	1.8	1.8	1.7	1.8	1.5	1.2	1.0	0.7	0.5	0.3	0.2	0.1
E	1.8	1.8	1.7	1.5	1.3	1.1	0.9	0.7	0.5	0.3	0.2	0.1

For row D, there is a titration of antigen (decrease in color from the maximum on dilution of antigen) beginning at column 5, and for row E starting at column 4. The titration curves for each seen in **Fig. 2** are not as "high" as for those in A–C; however, the background values for both are low (0.1 OD) and identical with controls in which there is no addition of antigen or conjugate (e.g., H-12).

On further dilution of conjugate (rows F–H), there is a distinct decrease in the color obtained in which antigen has been shown to be in excess and on dilution of the antigen. Here, there is a drop in the potential analytical sensitivity of the assay (ability to detect antigen) reflected in the decrease in plateau height OD and the area under the titration curves seen in **Fig. 2**.

This has been a rather long description of a relatively simple operation. However, remember that at the beginning of the test, it was not known whether antigen bound to a plate or whether the labeled antibody would bind to antigen. We can view the results of the plate by eye very quickly and almost instantly see that the test has worked and what the optimal areas are, without reference to the actual OD results. This can be important when performing initial experiments in which a relatively large amount of work is necessary to assess a more complex situation. The ability to assess tests very rapidly by eye is a distinct advantage over assays in which quantification relies on instrumentation alone.

We can summarize the results as follows:

1. The antigen coats plate to give maximum reaction where antibody conjugate is in excess to 1/320–1/640.
2. Conjugate dilutions in rows A–C are too strong and give plateau maxima that are too high.
3. Rows D and E give good titration curves for antigen and have ideal plateau height maxima.
4. There is a loss in analytical sensitivity if the conjugate is diluted as in rows F and G.

We have now completed the first sighting experiment evaluating the direct ELISA. At this stage, we can repeat the experiment with some alterations of reagent dilutions or conditions, depending on the results obtained. In the preceding example, we obtained ideal results with good activity for antigen and antibody conjugate. However, this is not always the case. Two examples of poor results necessitating alterations and reassessment are presented next.

1.2.2. Poor Results

Table 3 presents the results of an experiment identical to that described in **Subheading 4.1.1.** We now see that there is a good result in rows A and B and that after this dilution of antigen, very little color is produced. This indicates that there is little antigen attaching on dilutions greater than that used in row B. The conjugate appears to be usable to detect antigen until rows D and E since we obtain similar OD values where there is enough antigen coating the wells. In this case, the CBT could be repeated with a different dilution range of antigen to increase possibly the plateau maximum area in the presence of excess conjugate.

The next example (*see* **Table 4** for results) shows what may happen when the conjugate is of a low reactivity.

The results show that we have low color in the test. There is a rapid decrease in color on dilution of the labeled serum, rows A to B to C, and so on. There is, however, a plateau from columns 1 to 5 (A–C) indicating that there is antigen attaching at a similar level in these wells. In this case, one variation suggested from the initial CBT would be to coat plates with antigen at the dilution used in row 3 (the last dilution showing a plateau maximum value) and to titrate the conjugate, beginning at a higher concentration. In this way, a better estimate of conjugate activity would be obtained.

This situation is common to direct ELISA systems because production of good conjugates depends on the specific activity of the antibodies labeled, which is a function of the weight of enzyme attached to antigen-specific antibodies. Conjugation of

Table 3
Results of CBT (OD data) in which the antigen is limiting reaction

	1	2	3	4	5	6	7	8	9	10	11	12
A	1.7	1.3	0.7	0.4	0.3	0.2	0.1	0.1	0.1	0.1	0.1	0.1
B	1.7	1.3	0.5	0.3	0.2	0.1	0.1	0.1	0.1	0.1	0.1	0.1
C	1.7	1.2	0.4	0.3	0.2	0.2	0.1	0.1	0.1	0.1	0.1	0.1
D	1.6	1.8	0.3	0.3	0.2	0.1	0.1	0.1	0.1	0.1	0.1	0.1
E	1.5	1.8	0.3	0.2	0.2	0.1	0.1	0.1	0.1	0.1	0.1	0.1
F	1.4	1.5	0.2	0.2	0.1	0.1	0.1	0.1	0.1	0.1	0.1	0.1
G	0.9	0.7	0.2	0.2	0.1	0.1	0.1	0.1	0.1	0.1	0.1	0.1
H	0.1	0.1	0.1	0.1	0.1	0.1	0.1	0.1	0.1	0.1	0.1	0.1

Table 4
Results of CT (OD data) in which the labeled antibody is limiting reaction

	1	2	3	4	5	6	7	8	9	10	11	12
A	1.0	1.0	1.0	0.9	0.8	0.4	0.3	0.1	0.1	0.1	0.1	0.1
B	0.6	0.6	0.5	0.5	0.5	0.4	0.3	0.1	0.1	0.1	0.1	0.1
C	0.3	0.3	0.3	0.3	0.3	0.2	0.1	0.1	0.1	0.1	0.1	0.1
D	0.2	0.1	0.1	0.1	0.1	0.1	0.1	0.1	0.1	0.1	0.1	0.1
E	0.1	0.1	0.1	0.1	0.1	0.1	0.1	0.1	0.1	0.1	0.1	0.1
F	0.1	0.1	0.1	0.1	0.1	0.1	0.1	0.1	0.1	0.1	0.1	0.1
G	0.1	0.1	0.1	0.1	0.1	0.1	0.1	0.1	0.1	0.1	0.1	0.1
H	0.1	0.1	0.1	0.1	0.1	0.1	0.1	0.1	0.1	0.1	0.1	0.1

polyclonal sera usually results in the specific attachment of the enzyme to a relatively small percentage of the total protein content of the sample that is specific to the antibody. The rest of the protein is labeled, leading to problems with high backgrounds.

1.2.3. Plateau OD Values

The maximum color obtained in an assay in which reagents are in excess results from the following factors:

1. The amount of antigen that can passively attach to a well.
2. The number of antigenic sites available for antibody binding.
3. The density of the antigenic components on the wells.
4. The specific activity of the conjugate in terms of how much enzyme is attached to particular antibody species in the whole serum and their respective affinities.

These factors are examined later. However, the CBT allows a rapid estimate of the feasibility of assays whose results may indicate problems associated with these factors.

2. More Complicated Systems

After the simplest case of the direct ELISA we must consider situations in which there are three or more components to titrate. These are shown in **Table 5**. Remember that only two components can be varied by dilution in any test. The criteria for assessment of each of the stages in CBT are similar to those described extensively for the direct ELISA. Remember also that the CBT aims to

Table 5
Possible combinations for titrations[a]

	Indirect EL ISA (three components) antigen + antibody + antispecies conjugate	
1. Antigen D	Antibody D	Antispecies conjugate C
2. Antigen C	Antibody D	Antispecies conjugate D
	Optimized reagents in 1 and 2 checked in 3	
3. Antigen C	Antibody C	Antispecies conjugate D
	Direct Sandwich ELISA (three components)antibody + antigen + labeled antibody	
1. Antibody D	Antigen D	Labeled antibody C
2. Antibody C	Antigen D	Labeled antibody D
	Optimized reagents in 1 and 2 checked in 3	
3. Antibody C	Antigen C	Labeled antibody D
	Indirect Sandwich ELISA (four components)antibody + antigen + antibody + anti-antibody conjugate	
1. Antibody D	Antigen D antibody C	Anti-antibody C
2. Antibody C	Antigen C antibody D	Anti-antibody D
	Optimized reagents in 1 and 2 checked in 3 and 4	
3. Antibody C	Antigen C antibody D	Anti-antibody C
4. Antibody C	Antigen C antibody C	Anti-antibody D

[a]constant amount (no dilution series); *D* dilution series

indicate optimal conditions and is quite useful in arriving rapidly at a feasible concentration range for all components in the desired assay. The objective is to examine reagents for their usefulness and lead to conditions for a fully defined test to perform a specific task.

Competition assays involve the interruption of these systems. They have to be titrated in the same way to allow competitive or inhibition techniques.

2.1. Indirect ELISA

The indirect assay is used mainly to measure antibodies against a specific antigen either through the full titration of a sample or as a single dilution. Thus, we need a test with an optimal amount of antigen coated to wells that will successfully bind to antibodies, which, in turn, can be detected with an optimal amount of anti-species conjugate. We can only titrate two of these variable in one assay. The most important aspects to consider are (1) that enough antigen is available for antibody binding – we do not wish to waste antigen by adding concentrations that are too high such that the wells receive a large excess of antigen compared with the amount needed to fill available plastic sites; and (2) that we have optimal amounts of conjugate to avoid high nonspecific backgrounds and to allow the detection of all bound antibody molecules to give the required analytical sensitivity to be achieved. We also need to assess the effect of diluting negative sera (from same species as test samples) on an assay to obtain an idea as to the possible backgrounds of such sera at various dilutions. Thus, we can modify the needs for setting up this assay:

1. We need a sufficient amount of antigen coating to the wells to capture antibodies.
2. We need at least one serum positive for the antigen.
3. We need at least one negative serum from the same species as the test samples.
4. We need an anti-species conjugate.

2.1.1. Initial CBT

The initial test should be a CBT relating antigen dilutions to the positive and negative sera, using a commercial conjugate diluted to the recommended level. However, the individual laboratory estimation of optimal titers of anti-species conjugates is relatively easily made using the direct ELISA format. Either whole serum from the particular animal species target or a fraction (e.g., IgG) from the serum can be used to coat plates in stage (i) of the direct assay. When whole serum is used, 1/200 should be the initial dilution from rows 1 to 11. When IgG is prepared the weight can be measured spectrophotometrically and a starting concentration of 10 μg/mL used.

The second stage involves dilution of the conjugate in blocking buffer. Estimation of the optimal amount of conjugate is as already described. A dilution yielding a plateau maximum or about 1.8 OD units with a good titration curve should be used in indirect ELISA assessment. The dilution used can be altered later as a result of examination of results from the titration. This may be necessary since the exact nature and concentration of the specific immunoglobulins binding in the indirect ELISA to the specific antigen(s) may differ from those in the serum or serum fraction preparations.

2.1.2. Stage (i) of Indirect ELISA CBT

Figure 3 presents the stage (i) CBT for the indirect ELISA. This stage titrates the antigen against the positive and negative sera and can be regarded as a "sighting" exercise. Remember that conditions can be changed in a repeat CBT. Typical results might be those in **Table 6**.

In this example, we have used a titration of antigen from 1/50, twofold, and a titration of serum from 1/50, twofold. The controls for the test are shown in column 12, which contains no

Stage i)

Dilute the antigen from column 1 to column 11. Column 12 receives diluent only.

Incubate.

Wash wells

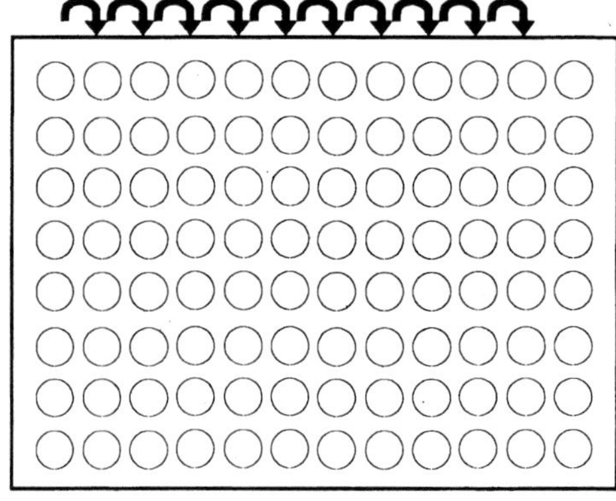

Stage ii)
Add the serum containing antibodies against antigen (one plate) or negative serum (second plate), dilute from row A to row G. Row H receives diluent only. Antibody is diluted in blocking buffer (containing inert protein and or detergent to prevent non-specific adsorption of protein.
Incubate.

Wash.

Add anti-species conjugate (given or pre-titrated) at single dilution in blocking buffer. Incubate. Wash.
Add chromophore / substrate.

Incubate. Stop reaction.

Read OD.

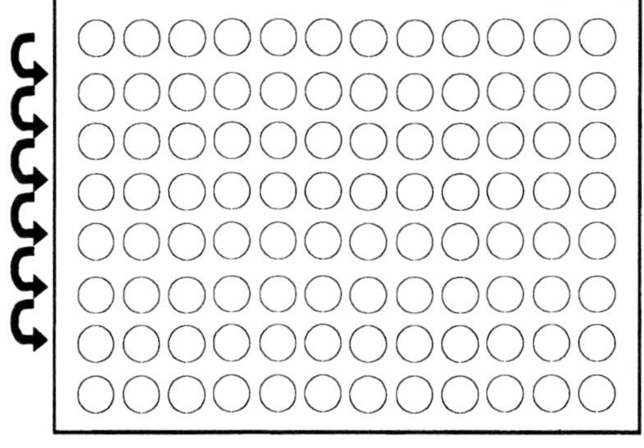

Fig. 3. Plate layout and CBT of antigen against positive and negative sample sera for indirect ELISA. Constant dilution of anti-species conjugate was used.

antigen but contains a dilution range of antibody and row H, which contains a dilution range of antigen, but no antibody. The results can be regarded as good, since we have color development at high levels and a corresponding titration as we reduce antigen or antibody. **Table 7** shows the area in gray, where there is an optimal amount of antigen coating allowing antibodies to be titrated maximally.

Thus, antigen can be diluted to the levels in columns 5 and 6 before there is a loss in color. Note that the plateau height maxima do decrease particularly after row E, indicating that there is a reduction in antibodies binding owing to the decrease in amount of antigen coating the wells.

Examination of column 12 indicates that in the absence of antigen, the positive serum at dilutions of 1/50, 1/100, and 1/200 does bind to the plate-producing background. This is typical of serum in the indirect assay, and such nonspecific

Table 6
Results of Stage 1 titration of altigen and positive antibody containing sample for indirect ELISA

	1	2	3	4	5	6	7	8	9	10	11	12
A	2.2	2.3	2.2	2.1	2.0	2.0	1.9	1.6	1.5	1.3	0.8	0.6
A	2.2	2.3	2.2	2.1	2.0	2.0	1.9	1.6	1.5	1.3	0.8	0.6
B	2.2	2.0	1.9	2.0	1.9	1.8	1.7	1.5	1.3	0.8	0.5	0.3
C	2.1	2.0	1.9	1.9	1.8	1.7	1.6	1.5	1.2	0.7	0.5	0.3
D	1.9	1.9	1.7	1.8	1.5	1.2	1.0	0.7	0.5	0.3	0.2	0.1
E	1.8	1.8	1.7	1.5	1.3	1.1	0.8	0.6	0.5	0.3	0.2	0.1
F	1.3	1.3	1.2	1.2	1.1	0.8	0.6	0.5	0.3	0.2	0.1	0.1
G	0.7	0.7	0.7	0.6	0.6	0.5	0.3	0.2	0.1	0.1	0.1	0.1
H	0.4	0.3	0.3	0.3	0.2	0.2	0.2	0.1	0.1	0.1	0.1	0.1

Table 7
Optimal coating region for titrating antibodies

	1	2	3	4	5	6	7	8	9	10	11	12
A	2.2	2.3	2.2	2.1	2.0	2.0	1.9	1.6	1.5	1.3	0.8	0.6
B	2.2	2.0	1.9	2.0	1.9	1.8	1.7	1.5	1.3	0.8	0.5	0.3
C	2.1	2.0	1.9	1.9	1.8	1.7	1.6	1.5	1.2	0.7	0.5	0.3
D	1.9	1.9	1.7	1.8	1.5	1.2	1.0	0.7	0.5	0.3	0.2	0.1
E	1.8	1.8	1.7	1.5	1.3	1.1	0.8	0.6	0.5	0.3	0.2	0.1
F	1.3	1.3	1.2	1.2	1.1	0.8	0.6	0.5	0.3	0.2	0.1	0.1
G	0.7	0.7	0.7	0.6	0.6	0.5	0.3	0.2	0.1	0.1	0.1	0.1
H	0.3	0.2	0.1	0.1	0.1	0.1	0.1	0.1	0.1	0.1	0.1	0.1

backgrounds have to be considered carefully when adapting the indirect ELISA for screening of test samples at single dilutions, since they influence the effective analytical sensitivity of assays. The same color develops in the titration of the negative serum (**Table 8**), indicating that this background stems from an interaction of the serum proteins contained in the serum.

Table 8 shows the results of titrating the negative serum. There is generally much lower color development, expected when there is no antibody binding to the antigen. There is, however, some color at various combinations, particularly when

Table 8
CBT of antigen and negative serum

	1	2	3	4	5	6	7	8	9	10	11	12
A	0.7	0.7	0.3	0.3	0.3	0.3	0.3	0.3	0.3	0.3	0.3	0.6
B	0.4	0.3	0.3	0.2	0.2	0.2	0.2	0.2	0.2	0.2	0.2	0.2
C	0.2	0.1	0.1	0.1	0.1	0.1	0.1	0.1	0.1	0.1	0.1	0.1
D	0.1	0.1	0.1	0.1	0.1	0.1	0.1	0.1	0.1	0.1	0.1	0.1
E	0.1	0.1	0.1	0.1	0.1	0.1	0.1	0.1	0.1	0.1	0.1	0.1
F	0.1	0.1	0.1	0.1	0.1	0.1	0.1	0.1	0.1	0.1	0.1	0.1
G	0.1	0.1	0.1	0.1	0.1	0.1	0.1	0.1	0.1	0.1	0.1	0.1
H	0.1	0.1	0.1	0.1	0.1	0.1	0.1	0.1	0.1	0.1	0.1	0.1

the concentrations of the negative serum are high. This color is owing to nonspecific attachment of the serum components from the species of animal being tested. Thus, the background needs to be examined and can be reassessed when retitrating the conjugate as described in stage (ii). As already indicated, there is color in A12, and it is almost as high as that seen in A1. The latter well contains antigen, indicating that there is a slight increase in binding, although it is not great. The serum dilutions of 1/50 and 1/100 do show some background, and as already indicated, this is mainly owing to interaction of the serum proteins with the plate nonspecifically. **Figure 4** plots the data for positive and negative sera.

2.1.3. Stage (ii) of Indirect ELISA CBT

From the first CBT, we can estimate an antigen dilution in which there is good color development as a result of the binding with antibodies. Because we do not wish to waste antigen by adding in excess (which is washed away in the coating phase), we can select the last dilution of antigen, which gives a good titration curve for the antiserum (i.e., high plateau height maxima and high end point). **Table 7** indicates that columns 5–6 have enough antigen to fulfill these criteria. Thus, wells could be coated at this single dilution, and it would be expected that the positive serum would titrate with a maximum OD (in which antibodies were in excess) of ~2.0, and that antibodies would still be detected (on dilution) to row G.

Titration of Sera

For titration of sera, the positive serum dilution range is not extensive enough to allow titration of antibodies to an endpoint (where OD in the presence of antibodies equals background OD). This can be addressed by altering the dilution range of the positive antiserum in stage (ii). Assuming we have taken the

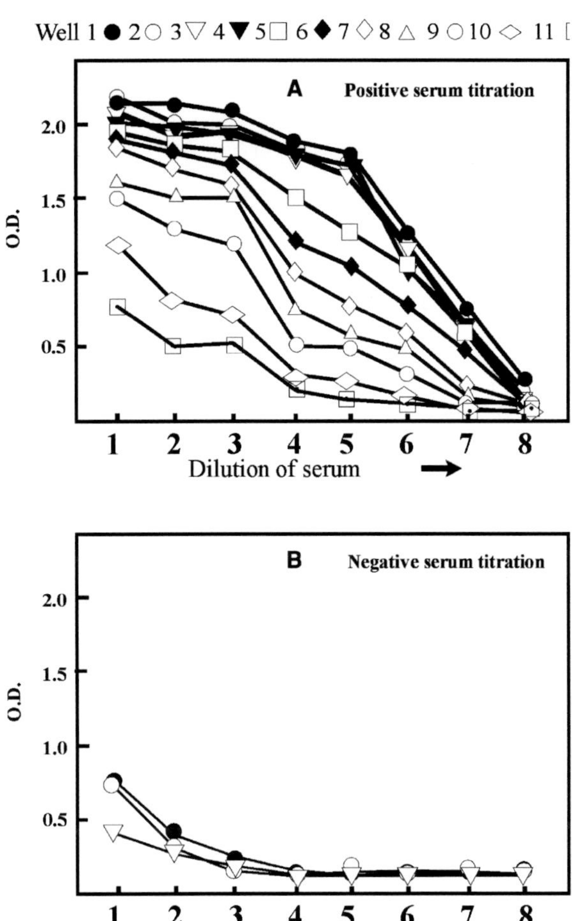

Fig. 4. Graph relating OD values for different antigen concentrations against dilution series of antibody in CBT. Curves show titration of antiserum at different antigen dilutions from wells 1 to 11. Points for 4–12 not shown as all are identical to dilution for 3.

antigen dilution as that in column 5, then the first operation in stage (ii) involves the following:

1. Coat wells of two plates with antigen at a dilution equivalent to that in column 5 (1/800). Incubate for the same times as in stage (i). Wash the wells.
2. Add a dilution range of positive or negative antisera as used in stage (i). Incubate and wash the wells. Here, as previously indicated, we can alter the range since in stage (i) we did not find the end point of the positive serum because we used a too-limited range of dilutions. We can increase the range in any of three ways:
   a. Diluting the serum beginning at column 1 and diluting to column 11.
   b. Starting at a higher initial dilution, e.g., 1/200.
   c. Altering the dilution range to threefold (rather than twofold).

The best method has to be assessed with reference to the initial CBT. When the dilution range is far too low and high color is obtained across the plate with indication of a titration only in the last two rows, then the use of a threefold range is recommended.

In the present example, the dilution of positive serum began at 1/50 and was diluted twofold, in a seven-well series. Thus, we obtained dilutions of 1/50, 1/100, 1/200, 1/400, 1/800, 1/1,600, and 1/3,200. At the last dilution, we had not obtained an end point, and by examination of the curves, we can predict that at least another four similar dilution steps would be needed before the color would be reduced to background (because the antibodies were diluted out). Thus, in stage (ii) we can use the coated plate and dilute the positive serum from 1/50 [as in stage (i)] by 11 steps to 1/51,200, using columns 1–11.

Titration of Anti-species Conjugate

In stage (i) we estimated the appropriate conjugate dilution either from information given by the producers or from a preliminary CBT of the conjugate against serum coated to wells. Titration of the conjugate at this point offers an examination of its activity under the indirect assay conditions proper, allowing refinement of the dilution to maximize analytical sensitivity as a result of identifying areas where excess conjugate produces high backgrounds.

1. Add a twofold dilution range of conjugate from row A to H. Incubate and then wash. Again, we have the opportunity of adjusting the starting dilution based on stage (i) results. When the commercial company recommendation is used, it is good practice to begin the conjugate dilution approximately fourfold higher than recommended and to dilute to at least fourfold lower. As an example, if the recommended dilution is 1/2,000, then the conjugate should be titrated from 1/500 in twofold steps to 32,000. When there is an initial CBT against relevant serum, then the same procedure should be adopted around the initially found optimum.
2. Add relevant chromophore/substrate to the system and incubate.
3. Stop the reaction as in stage (i) and read the OD in a spectrophotometer.

2.1.4. Results

Tables 9 and **10** shows the results for the CBTs. **Table 9** shows that there is a high background of 0.5 in row A, column 12. In this row, 1/500 conjugate was used, which indicates that it is binding nonspecifically with the antigen-coated plates. This finding is confirmed in **Table 10**, where the background value is maintained on dilution of the negative serum from A2 to A12. Although these are idealized results, they do illustrate a common phenomenon. The background is reduced in row B (dilution of conjugate 1/1,000 with reference to the value in column 12 of

Table 9), but **Table 10** shows that there is still a higher background in B3–B12, indicating some nonspecific complications.

In row C for both plates, the background in column 12 is low (0.1) and remains constant for the rest of the dilutions of the conjugate. This can be regarded as the minimum background for the test (plate background). **Table 9** indicates that there is a "good" titration of serum in row C, where there is a plateau (region of maximum OD), indicating a region of excess antibody. Thus, the conjugate at the dilution in row C (1/2,000)

Table 9
Result of CBT for positive serum[a]

	1	2	3	4	5	6	7	8	9	10	11	12
A	1.8	1.8	1.8	1.8	1.6	1.2	1.1	0.9	0.6	0.5	0.5	0.5
B	1.8	1.8	1.8	1.8	1.6	1.2	1.1	0.9	0.6	0.5	0.3	0.2
C	1.7	1.7	1.7	1.7	1.6	1.1	0.9	0.7	0.5	0.4	0.2	0.1
D	1.6	1.6	1.5	1.3	1.1	0.9	0.7	0.5	0.3	0.2	0.2	0.1
E	1.2	1.1	0.9	0.8	0.7	0.6	0.5	0.4	0.3	0.2	0.1	0.1
F	0.8	0.7	0.6	0.5	0.4	0.3	0.2	0.2	0.1	0.1	0.1	0.1
G	0.5	0.5	0.5	0.4	0.3	0.2	0.1	0.1	0.1	0.1	0.1	0.1
H	0.3	0.2	0.1	0.1	0.1	0.1	0.1	0.1	0.1	0.1	0.1	0.1

[a]Antigen was constant. Serum was diluted at 1/50, twofold, from column 1 to 11. Conjugate was diluted at 1/500, twofold, rows A–G

Table 10
Result of CBT for negative serum[a]

	1	2	3	4	5	6	7	8	9	10	11	12
A	0.6	0.5	0.5	0.5	0.5	0.5	0.5	0.5	0.5	0.5	0.5	0.5
B	0.4	0.3	0.2	0.2	0.2	0.2	0.2	0.2	0.2	0.2	0.2	0.2
C	0.1	0.1	0.1	0.1	0.1	0.1	0.1	0.1	0.1	0.1	0.1	0.1
D	0.1	0.1	0.1	0.1	0.1	0.1	0.1	0.1	0.1	0.1	0.1	0.1
E	0.1	0.1	0.1	0.1	0.1	0.1	0.1	0.1	0.1	0.1	0.1	0.1
F	0.1	0.1	0.1	0.1	0.1	0.1	0.1	0.1	0.1	0.1	0.1	0.1
G	0.1	0.1	0.1	0.1	0.1	0.1	0.1	0.1	0.1	0.1	0.1	0.1
H	0.1	0.1	0.1	0.1	0.1	0.1	0.1	0.1	0.1	0.1	0.1	0.1

[a]Antigen was constant. Serum was diluted at 1/50, twofold, from column 1 to 11. Conjugate was diluted at 1/500, twofold, rows A–G

can detect the bound antibodies and an optimal OD reading can be obtained. The end point (with reference to the OD obtained in the absence of serum [C12]) has not been obtained, but there is a gradual reduction in OD as the serum is diluted (titration curve). This can be contrasted to the idealized results for row C in **Table 10**. Here, no titration is observed at any dilution of the negative serum.

Reduction in the concentration of the anti-species conjugate has two effects. One is to reduce the plateau maximum color, and the other is to effectively reduce the end point of the titration. Thus, in **Table 9** we see a small reduction in plateau in row D, which becomes marked when we further dilute.

By row G, we have a low OD even where we know that there is enough antibody binding to give a strong signal in the presence of excess antibody (as seen in A–D, columns 1–4/5). The optimal dilution of the conjugate at this stage is therefore taken from assessing the plateau maximum color and the titration end point with reference to the backgrounds in the controls. In this case, a dilution of conjugate of 1/2,000 to 1/4,000 appears optimal with the serum dilutions used. At this dilution, there is no OD measured in the negative serum.

Binding Ratios

Another way of examining the results is to calculate the binding ratios (BRs) relating the positive and negative titrations. This is simply the OD value at a given dilution for the positive serum divided by that of the negative serum. **Table 11** gives the BRs for the data in **Tables 9** and **10**. This process gives a clearer picture of the best conditions for setting up assays and is a feature used when tests are used for diagnostic purposes.

Table 11
BRs positive and negative sera from table 9 and 10

	1	2	3	4	5	6	7	8	9	10	11	12
A	3.0	3.6	3.6	3.6	3.2	2.4	2.2	1.8	1.2	1.0	1.0	1.0
B	4.5	6.0	9.0	9.0	8.0	6.0	5.5	4.5	3.0	2.5	1.5	1.0
C	17.0	17.0	17.0	17.0	16.0	11.0	9.0	7.0	5.0	4.0	2.0	1.0
D	16.0	16.0	15.0	13.0	11.0	9.0	7.0	5.0	3.0	2.0	2.0	1.0
E	12.0	11.0	9.0	8.0	7.0	6.0	5.0	4.0	3.0	2.0	1.0	1.0
F	8.0	7.0	6.0	5.0	4.0	3.0	2.0	2.0	1.0	1.0	1.0	1.0
G	5.0	5.0	4.0	3.0	2.0	1.0	1.0	1.0	1.0	1.0	1.0	1.0
H	3.0	2.0	1.0	1.0	1.0	1.0	1.0	1.0	1.0	1.0	1.0	1.0

Table 11 illustrates the highest BRs in rows C and D, despite the OD values for the positive serum being higher in A and B. This results from the relatively low OD values for the negative serum at higher dilutions of conjugate. Note that the BRs at 1/50 and 1/100 positive serum in A1, B1, and 2 are lower than in subsequent wells. This is typical and results from the effect of high nonspecific binding at these dilutions with negative sera. In fact, it is usual for this effect to be more exaggerated in practice.

Care is needed in interpreting best conditions by this method because where there are extremely low OD values for binding with negative sera, even low OD values for positive sera can appear to give best results. However, the lower the OD values being examined, the higher the potential variation in results, and therefore a compromise between what seems to be the highest BR values and obtaining a reasonable OD value in the positive sample is required. The assessment of end points can also be made using this method. The last dilution of serum that gives a BR of >1.0 can be judged as the end point.

In our idealized example, the end points for the various dilutions of conjugate are shown as a line in **Table 12**. Here, we can see that the effect of diluting conjugate is to reduce the end points (E–G). In B–D, the final end point has not been found, although the indication from examination of the BR data is that the conjugate dilution in C gives the highest potential analytical sensitivity since it has a BR of 4.0 at the dilution in column 10, as compared with the other results. The only controls not discussed are those in row H. These are antigen-coated wells (constant), with antibody dilutions of 1/50 twofold, but no conjugate. In this example, there is some color in the 1/50 and 1/100 positive serum wells despite the lack of conjugate. This can affect the

Table 12
End points of serum titrations

	1	2	3	4	5	6	7	8	9	10	11	12
A	3.0	3.6	3.6	3.6	3.2	2.4	2.2	1.8	1.2	1.0	1.0	1.0
B	4.5	6.0	9.0	9.0	8.0	6.0	5.5	4.5	3.0	2.5	1.5	1.0
C	17.0	17.0	17.0	17.0	16.0	11.0	9.0	7.0	5.0	4.0	2.0	1.0
D	16.0	16.0	15.0	13.0	11.0	9.0	7.0	5.0	3.0	2.0	2.0	1.0
E	12.0	11.0	9.0	8.0	7.0	6.0	5.0	4.0	3.0	2.0	1.0	1.0
F	8.0	7.0	6.0	5.0	4.0	3.0	2.0	2.0	1.0	1.0	1.0	1.0
G	5.0	5.0	4.0	3.0	2.0	1.0	1.0	1.0	1.0	1.0	1.0	1.0
H	3.0	2.0	1.0	1.0	1.0	1.0	1.0	1.0	1.0	1.0	1.0	1.0

estimation of which serum dilution should be used in an indirect assay involving testing of samples at a single dilution. This effect disappears at 1/200 positive serum and is not observed for the negative serum.

2.1.5. Conclusion

Although the use of CBT may seem a laborious process, the principles are easy. Initially the antigen was titrated against the antisera using an estimate of the conjugate dilution. This indicated that there was a significant difference between the two sera in the OD values obtained. The approximate antigen concentration that coated the plates was then taken and used to relate the antisera and conjugate dilutions. Thus, we can conclude the following:

1. The antigen can be used at 1/800.
2. The conjugate can be used at 1/2,000–1/4,000.
3. There is a good discrimination of positive serum from negative serum using these conditions, and a dilution of serum at 1/400 could be suggested for a test involving single dilutions of sample.

2.1.6. Developing Indirect ELISAs

The tests just described can be made in 2 days, and further refinements can be made using the reagents in additional tests in which smaller changes in dilutions can be assessed. However, as with all ELISAs, it is imperative that the ultimate purpose of the test be addressed as early as possible.

In cases in which the test is to be used to screen hundreds or thousands of sera according to positivity, based on a single dilution (in duplicate or triplicate), the titration phase must include a reasonable amount of work to recognize the factors inherent in examination of a varied population of antisera. The previous example centered on the use of a single positive and negative serum. This is patently not going to reflect differences in the population of sera to be examined. Thus, at the stage where we have a working dilution of the antigen and conjugate, we must now include more positive and negative sera (when possible) to further test the parameters for optimizing analytical sensitivity. The problem then is to assess these factors:

1. Whether the optimal antigen holds for a number of negative and positive sera.
2. The optimal antiserum dilution to use for single-sample screening. This is a balance between achieving maximum analytical sensitivity and maximal specificity.
3. The mean OD value of a negative population (and its variability). This allows the designation of positivity at different confidence levels and its variation.

The indirect assay may be used in a competitive or inhibition assay. In these cases, the problem is to screen positive sera for characteristics that best match those for field or experimental sera in terms of antibody populations reacting with specific determinants on the antigen used. It may be necessary to screen a number of positive sera under test conditions to identify a single serum with the best properties.

Indirect assays also offer a relatively easy and rapid method of end point titration of many sera. Relatively simple titrations can give confidence in the properties of sera to be used in other tests (i.e., they can confirm positivity or negativity). This is examined next in the worked examples of the use of indirect ELISAs.

2.2. Direct Sandwich ELISA

Direct sandwich ELISA is a three-component assay. We have to titrate the following:

1. The capture antibody
2. The antigen that is captured
3. The detecting conjugate

Only two components can be varied in any one test, and so the same criteria as indicated in the indirect ELISA apply. Probably the most variable area in this assay is the activity of the labeled conjugate, which is usually produced in the laboratory developing the assay. Such conjugates can have quite different properties owing to the intrinsic amount of enzyme that is attached to specific antibodies within a polyclonal serum produced against the antigen. Thus, no assumptions as to the activity can be made as in the case of anti-species conjugates from commercial sources, and the initial titrations require possibly more cycles to fine-tune concentrations.

2.2.1. Aids in Developing Assays

One aid to developing such assays can be the use of indirect ELISAs to assess the relationship of antigen and antibody binding. However, the need to develop a capture ELISA (antibody on wells as reagent to capture antigen) usually stems from the need to concentrate a weak antigen (unsuitable for indirect ELISA) or to capture a specific component of an antigenic mixture. The selection of an antiserum for labeling and conjugation for use in the sandwich ELISA could be based on estimation of the titer of a number of sera by the indirect ELISA, where the antigen can be coated in a sufficient quantity. Thus, high-titer sera can be identified. Such titrations can be made by other methods, leading to the selection of sera with the highest activities.

2.2.2. Stage (i): Titration of Capture Antibody and Antigen

Figure 5 shows the scheme for stage (i) of direct sandwich ELISA. Whole serum is used as the capture reagent, a dilution of 1/100 should be used in column 1. When IG (e.g., IgG) has been prepared from the antiserum, the concentration of protein can be easily found through reading absorbance in an ultraviolet spectrophotometer. In this case, a starting concentration of 10 µg/mL should be used (we are still using a 50-µL volume as the

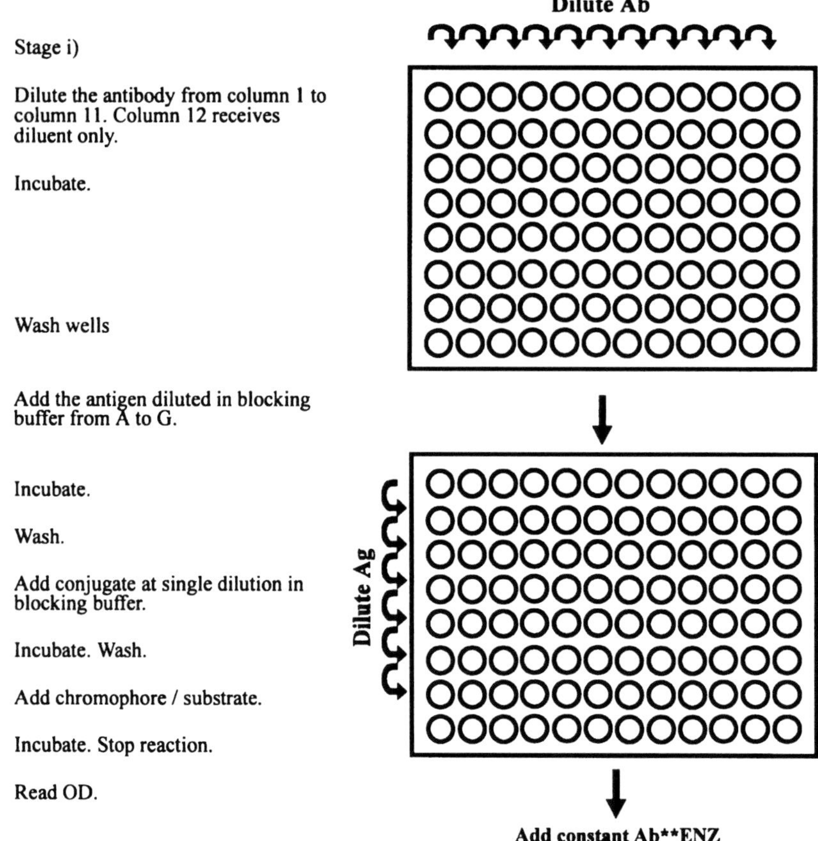

Fig. 5. CBT of capture antibody against antigen for direct sandwich ELISA.

constant in this example). At this level of protein, the wells will be saturated so that the activity of the capture antibody relies on the relative concentration of the specific antibodies in the IgG fraction as compared with the other IgG molecules in the serum. The addition of any higher concentration is a waste and will not improve the capturing ability of the coating reagent. The dilution range should be twofold and serum diluted to column 11. The usual diluents for antibodies are PBS, pH 7.2, or carbonate/bicarbonate buffer, pH 9.6.

After incubation (e.g., 1–2 h at 37°C), the wells are washed. Next, the antigen is diluted from row A to row G. When there is no indication from other assays as to the likely concentration of the antigen, then the dilution range should be started at 1/50.

The assumption here is that there is a sufficient volume of antigen to allow such a dilution. When there are very small volumes of antigen of unknown concentration, then you must decide whether there is enough antigen to develop any test or whether it is of a high concentration and that 1/50 will be enough to titrate originally. The results of stage (i) will indicate whether the antigen is of a high or low concentration. For a 1/50 dilution in a 50-μL volume test, we will require 12 wells at 1/50 for row A plus 12 wells at 1/50 for dilution in row B (a total of 1,200 μL [1.2 mL]) for the test. This equals 24 μL of undiluted antigen for a single stage (i) CBT. Remember to allow a little extra volume than that exactly required. Thus, 30 μL will be a more realistic volume diluted to 1,500 μL. The antibody is diluted in a suitable blocking buffer to prevent nonspecific attachment of proteins to the wells. After incubation and washing, a constant dilution of the labeled detecting serum is added. Since we have no idea as to the effective activity, then add conjugate diluted to 1/200. Thus, we need a volume of 96 wells × 50 μL = 4,800 μL (4.8 mL), say, 5,000 μL (5.0 mL) to allow for losses. This means that we need 5,000/200 μL of undiluted conjugate for a plate in stage (i) = 25 μL. The calculations are included here to remind operators to pay attention to the availability of reagents. After incubation, the relevant chromophore/substrate solution is added and the color development read with or without stopping (depending on the system).

Results of Stage (i)

Table 13 gives an example of good results. The columns contain dilutions of capture serum, and the rows contain dilutions of captured antigen. Row A contains the highest amount of antigen and examination of the OD values shows that there is a plateau of OD values from column 1 to 4. This indicates that detecting serum is in excess and that there is enough antigen to allow for a significant signal (1.9 OD units). A similar plateau is observed in row B, indicating that dilution of antigen has no significant effect on the titration of the serum. The data in A and B are identical, indicating that there is the same amount of captured antigen present in the rows. Row C shows a slightly reduced plateau OD value but the extent of the plateau (to column 4) is the same as

Table 13
Example of good test result from stage (i)

	1	2	3	4	5	6	7	8	9	10	11	12
A	1.9	1.9	1.9	1.9	1.8	1.3	1.1	0.9	0.6	0.5	0.3	0.1
B	1.9	1.9	1.9	1.9	1.8	1.3	1.1	0.9	0.6	0.5	0.3	0.1
C	1.8	1.8	1.8	1.8	1.6	1.1	0.9	0.7	0.5	0.4	0.2	0.05
D	1.6	1.6	1.6	1.5	1.2	1.0	0.9	0.7	0.5	0.3	0.1	0.05
E	1.2	1.1	0.9	0.8	0.7	0.6	0.5	0.4	0.3	0.2	0.05	0.05
F	0.8	0.7	0.6	0.5	0.4	0.3	0.2	0.2	0.05	0.05	0.05	0.05
G	0.5	0.5	0.5	0.4	0.3	0.2	0.1	0.05	0.05	0.05	0.05	0.05
H	0.2	0.1	0.05	0.05	0.05	0.05	0.05	0.05	0.05	0.05	0.05	0.05

for A and B. This reduction indicates that there is a slight reduction in the amount of captured antigen. This is also reflected by examination of the full titration range values; however, the background OD (column 12) is lower in C (0.05) than in A and B (0.1). The continued reduction in antigen concentration (D–G) exaggerates the loss of ability of the detecting serum to be titrated where both the plateau height maxima and the end points are reduced significantly. These data can be expressed as BRs, relating the values in the presence of serum to the control values in column 12. **Table 14** shows these values.

Examination of BR exaggerates the advantage of using the antigen at lower concentrations than those used to obtain maximum OD, since the background OD values (antigen plus only conjugate) are lower. From the data in **Tables 13** and **14**, we can estimate an optimal dilution of antigen to be that used in row C and the optimal dilution of capture antibody to be that used in column 4. This is highlighted in **Table 14**. Assuming we started the dilutions of capture serum at 1/200 and antigen at 1/50, we have optimal values for each of 1/1,600 (serum) and 1/200 (antigen), respectively.

2.2.3. Stage (ii): Titration of Antigen and Labeled Antibody

We can now fix the concentration of one of the reactants. Stage (i) used a constant dilution of labeled detecting serum (1/200) that gave successful results. However, we need to know the optimal titration of this reagent so as not to waste a valuable resource (by underestimation of the concentration) and to examine the effects on the ultimate analytical sensitivity of the assay. The idea is to optimize the dilution of conjugate in detecting the captured antigen.

Stage (ii) involves coating plates with a constant amount of capture serum as determined in stage (i) (equivalent to dilution in

Table 14
Binding ratios of serum

	1	2	3	4	5	6	7	8	9	10	11	12
A	19	19	19	19	18	13	11	9	6	5	3	1
B	19	19	19	19	18	13	11	9	6	5	3	1
C	36	36	36	36	32	22	18	14	10	8	4	1
D	32	32	32	30	24	20	18	14	10	6	2	1
E	24	22	18	16	14	12	10	8	6	4	1	1
F	16	14	12	10	8	6	4	4	1	1	1	1
G	10	10	10	8	6	4	2	1	1	1	1	1
H	4	5	1	1	1	1	1	1	1	1	1	1

column 4 = 1/1,600). After incubation and washing, the antigen is added at a twofold dilution range from a value two- to fourfold higher than found to be optimal in stage (i) from row A to G. After incubation and washing, the detecting conjugate is diluted from column 1 to 11 starting at a dilution two to fourfold higher than that used in stage (i), i.e., 1/50–100. After incubation and washing and addition of substrate/chromophore, the test is read. **Table 15** presents idealized data.

Reference to the rows in **Table 15** shows that at 1/50 conjugate we have a good titration range of antigen but there is a high background (0.4). On dilution, we obtain similar results in rows B–D indicating that the detecting conjugate is in excess until the dilution used in row D. Note also that there is a significantly lower background (column D12) than in C12 and B12. On further dilution (rows E–G), we lose the plateau height and end points for titrating the antigen. Again the BRs can be plotted relating the antigen concentration to conjugate concentration to clarify the impact of the observed differences in background (**Table 16**). The data indicate that the optimal conjugate dilution for use in detecting available antigen is that observed in row D (1/400). The dilution in row E (1/800) gives quite similar results and could be used to detect the antigen when the availability of the conjugate is a strong consideration.

4.2.2.4. Further Refinement

Stages (i) and (ii) enable a good estimate of the concentrations of each reactant to be made. The idealized example is when the tests work well. Even here we may require further CBTs to establish

Table 15
Titration of antigen and detection of labeled serum with constant capture antibody[a]

	1	2	3	4	5	6	7	8	9	10	11	12
A	2.1	2.1	2.1	2.1	2.0	1.9	1.8	1.7	1.2	0.6	0.4	0.4
B	1.9	1.9	1.9	1.9	1.8	1.3	1.1	0.9	0.6	0.5	0.3	0.2
C	1.9	1.9	1.9	1.9	1.8	1.3	1.1	0.9	0.6	0.5	0.3	0.1
D	1.9	1.9	1.9	1.9	1.8	1.3	1.1	0.9	0.6	0.5	0.3	0.05
E	1.8	1.8	1.8	1.7	1.5	1.3	1.1	0.8	0.5	0.3	0.2	0.05
F	0.8	0.7	0.6	0.5	0.4	0.3	0.2	0.2	0.05	0.05	0.05	0.05
G	0.5	0.5	0.5	0.4	0.3	0.2	0.1	0.05	0.05	0.05	0.05	0.05
H	0.2	0.1	0.05	0.05	0.05	0.05	0.05	0.05	0.05	0.05	0.05	0.05

[a]Constant capture antibody was 1/1,600. Antigen was diluted from 1–11, beginning 1/50, twofold. Labeled antibody was diluted fro A to G, beginning 1/50, twofold

Table 16
BRs for data in table 15[a]

	1	2	3	4	5	6	7	8	9	10	11	12
A	5	5	5	5	5	5	5	4	3	2	1	1
B	10	10	10	10	9	7	6	5	3	3	2	1
C	10	10	10	10	9	7	6	5	3	3	2	1
D	38	38	38	38	36	26	22	18	12	10	6	1
E	36	36	36	34	30	26	22	16	10	6	4	1
F	16	14	12	10	8	6	4	4	1	1	1	1
G	10	10	10	8	6	4	2	1	1	1	1	1
H	4	2	2	1	1	1	1	1	1	1	1	1

[a]Data are rounded up to one decimal piacei

more precise conditions; for example, a CBT of dilutions of capture antibody against constant antigen and dilutions of conjugate could be examined. The initial CBTs also give an opportunity to set up limited studies on field samples. Thus, if you wish to titrate antigen in samples, you could coat plates with antibody, add serial dilutions of test antigens, and then detect these with the conjugate. This would investigate how proper field samples behave in a test and possibly give clues as to the need to modify conditions.

The titration of all three reactants also allows them to be used in similar assays with other reagents. Thus, we may wish to examine another antigen in the assay. The capture serum and detecting conjugate can be used at the dilutions found from CBTs, but the new antigen titrated. Similarly, other capture antibody preparations can be used in tests involving the antigen and conjugate used at the optimal dilutions, as found by CBTs.

As for the description of the direct ELISA, the purpose for which the assay is being developed should always be the strongest factor in test reagent optimization. Ultimately, the test will have to be proved to perform on particular samples and under specific conditions, and validation of ELISAs must meet such conditions.

2.2.5. Bad Results

The idealized example is typical of good results in which all reactants perform well, i.e., can be used at high dilution and give OD values that are relatively high. When one or more of the reactants is at a low concentration or has poor binding characteristics in the assay, the CBT soon indicates where the problems reside.

Although the number of examples cannot be exhaustive, demonstration of a few bad results is probably far more informative than giving the ideal situation.

Low Color Generally over Plate

Table 17 gives the results of a similar CBT for stage (i) of the direct sandwich ELISA (results shown in **Table 13**).

Generally there is low color. There is a plateau corresponding to a maximum value of 0.4 OD units, from column 1 to 5 (highest concentrations of capture antibody), which indicates that the antigen is being captured. There are several reasons for the low OD value in this region:

1. The capture antibodies specific for the antigen are at a low concentration with respect to other serum proteins or do not bind as well as other proteins. Thus, the amount of antigen captured is limited. In this situation, there is no observed increase in OD on increasing the capture antibody concentration.
2. The amount of antigen available for capture is low. This is unlikely since dilution of antigen (from A to B to C, and so on) does not decrease the OD observed in columns 1–4, indicating that there is an excess of antigen to row F (after which we observe a reduction in OD).
3. The activity of the conjugate is low.

The CBT can be repeated using increased starting concentrations of the titrated components. Thus, we could begin the capture antibody concentration at 10×, which was used in the first CBT. It is unlikely, however, that this will increase the OD values since we did observe that there was an extensive (columns 1–5) plateau maximum indicating that there was maximal activity being measured that did not alter on dilution of the antigen.

Table 17
CBT, low OD data stage (i) direct sandwich ELISA[a]

	1	2	3	4	5	6	7	8	9	10	11	12
A	0.4	0.4	0.4	0.4	0.4	0.3	0.3	0.2	0.2	0.1	0.1	0.1
B	0.4	0.4	0.4	0.4	0.4	0.3	0.3	0.2	0.2	0.1	0.1	0.1
C	0.4	0.4	0.4	0.4	0.4	0.3	0.3	0.2	0.2	0.1	0.1	0.1
D	0.4	0.3	0.4	0.4	0.4	0.4	0.4	0.4	0.3	0.3	0.2	0.1
E	0.4	0.4	0.4	0.3	0.3	0.2	0.2	0.2	0.1	0.1	0.1	0.1
F	0.4	0.4	0.3	0.2	0.2	0.2	0.1	0.1	0.1	0.1	0.1	0.1
G	0.3	0.2	0.2	0.2	0.1	0.1	0.1	0.1	0.1	0.1	0.1	0.1
H	0.1	0.1	0.1	0.1	0.1	0.1	0.1	0.1	0.1	0.1	0.1	0.1

[a]Capture serum diluted is in columns 1–11, antigen diluted is in rows A–H, and the constant was conjugate

In cases in which there is an observed increase in OD on increasing capture antibody, the CBT can be reassessed and a stage (ii) CBT can be performed. When there is no increase in OD values with increased concentrations of antigen or conjugate, the strongest candidate for replacement is the capture antibody. When this antibody is the same as that used for conjugation, both should be replaced.

Extremes of Color

When there is a very high color in the majority of the wells, the CBT must be repeated with lower concentrations of reactants. **Table 18** gives data from such a plate. The reagent responsible for the high readings may be directly identified from the CBT. Close examination of background values is also necessary because the results may be owing to a very high nonspecific binding of one of the reactants.

The data in **Table 18** shows a high background for the conjugate in the absence of capture serum (column 12). Row H indicates that there is no color obtained in which there is antigen and capture antibody in the absence of conjugate. Thus, there is unwanted nonspecific color through attachment of the enzyme conjugate to the wells. This could indicate that the conjugate is being used at far too high a concentration, so that the blocking buffer conditions are not preventing nonspecific adsorption of the enzyme-labeled proteins. There is a titration of antigen on diluting the capture serum, indicated in the backgrounds in column 12; for example, in row G, which has a background of 0.9, a plateau of ~2.0 is observed with an OD above background observed in column 11 and a reduction in color gradually from columns 3 and 4 to column 11.

Table 18
High color in CBT[a]

	1	2	3	4	5	6	7	8	9	10	11	12
A	2.5	2.6	2.5	2.7	2.7	2.1	2.0	1.9	1.7	1.6	1.6	1.6
B	2.8	2.6	2.5	2.8	2.7	2.1	2.0	1.9	1.7	1.6	1.6	1.6
C	2.7	2.5	2.4	2.6	2.7	2.1	2.0	1.9	1.7	1.6	1.6	1.6
D	2.6	2.7	2.4	2.6	2.7	2.1	2.0	1.9	1.7	1.6	1.5	1.4
E	2.2	2.3	2.3	2.6	2.7	2.1	2.0	1.9	1.7	1.6	1.5	1.3
F	2.1	2.2	2.2	2.6	2.7	2.1	2.0	1.9	1.7	1.6	1.5	1.0
G	2.0	2.0	1.9	1.9	1.8	1.7	1.4	1.3	1.2	1.6	1.3	0.9
H	0.1	0.1	0.1	0.1	0.1	0.1	0.1	0.1	0.1	0.1	0.1	0.1

[a]Capture antibody titrated is in columns 1–11, and constant antigen A12–H12, conjugate diluted is in rows A–GJ*Readings are out of accurate range for reader

A further CBT can be made using the conjugate beginning with that used in row F in the first attempt. **Table 19** gives idealized results. Here, the background is eliminated by row D (results are the same in D12, E12, F12, and G12). The effect of diluting the capture antibody is to titrate the antigen after an initial plateau (region of excess capture antibody or antigen). The conjugate dilution up to row D is not suitable owing to the high backgrounds obtained. Thus, a dilution of conjugate at about that in rows D and E can be assessed in the second stage of the CBT, in which the capture antibody and antigen can be varied.

Very Weak Reactions

In cases in which little color is observed, we run into more difficulties because there is no obvious indicator of whether one or all the reagents are not functioning.

A special case is when there is no color development even after a significant time of incubation of the substrate/chromophore. Then the most likely culprit is the operator who forgets to add substrate to the reaction mixture. This can be tested by dipping a microtip into a conjugate and putting the tip into the remaining substrate/chromophore solution. This should show a rapid color change; if not, the operator should repeat the test making sure that the proper substrate/chromophore mixture is correct.

When there is color, the CBT can be repeated. Should very low color then be obtained, the initial CBT should be repeated beginning with much higher concentrations of the two reagents being titrated. This can be a relatively futile operation since we know the dilutions of reactants and have usually added these at a

Table 19
Repeat of CBT in which high color was obtained using more dilute conjugate[a]

	1	2	3	4	5	6	7	8	9	10	11	12
A	2.1	2.2	2.2	2.6	2.7	2.1	2.0	1.9	1.7	1.6	1.5	1.0
B	2.0	2.0	1.9	1.9	1.8	1.7	1.4	1.3	1.2	1.6	1.3	0.9
C	1.9	1.9	1.9	1.9	1.8	1.6	1.3	1.1	0.9	0.5	0.3	0.3
D	1.8	1.8	1.8	1.8	1.8	1.5	1.1	0.8	0.6	0.4	0.2	0.1
E	1.6	1.6	1.6	1.6	1.6	1.3	1.1	0.7	0.5	0.3	0.2	0.1
F	1.2	1.1	1.1	1.1	1.1	1.0	0.9	0.6	0.4	0.2	0.1	0.1
G	0.9	0.9	0.8	0.8	0.7	0.6	0.5	0.4	0.3	0.2	0.1	0.1
H	0.1	0.1	0.1	0.1	0.1	0.1	0.1	0.1	0.1	0.1	0.1	0.1

[a]Capture antibody titrated is in columns 1–11, constant antigen is in A12–H12, and conjugate diluted is in rows A–G (beginning with dilution used in row F in the initial CBT)

high concentration in the initial CBT. Obviously, the third reactant (conjugate) can be critical, and so a higher concentration can be added. Once again, when conjugates are not reacting at dilutions from 1/100 and below, there is little practical value in pursuing their use.

Thus, low color can result from an error such as failing to add proper reagents, making a mistake in the original dilution, or having all the reactants of inadequate strength.

It is easier to assess the reason for low color when there is an indication that one of the reagents is active. This is illustrated in **Table 20**, in which there is some color development in one area of the plate associated with column 1 and rows A–E. Since we have a constant amount of antigen and 1.5 OD units in column 1 is observed, this indicates that both the antigen and conjugate can function although the activity of the conjugate is also rapidly diminished after row C.

The fault here lies with the capture antibody, whose ability to capture rapidly dilutes out by column 3. The CBT could be repeated with higher concentrations in column 1. As already indicated, since the capture antibodies are present as a small component of the total serum proteins, and its capture activity resides in the ability of these specific antibodies to bind to the wells, it may be impossible to achieve a better capture reagent with this serum.

2.2.6. CBT for Other Systems

The last examples are meant to indicate the first developmental steps in analyzing the suitability of available reagents. In all cases, there is always going to be the need to make adjustments to allow

Table 20
Results where one or more reagents are week[a]

	1	2	3	4	5	6	7	8	9	10	11	12
A	1.5	0.5	0.3	0.1	0.1	0.1	0.1	0.1	0.1	0.1	0.1	0.1
B	1.5	0.4	0.2	0.1	0.1	0.1	0.1	0.1	0.1	0.1	0.1	0.1
C	1.2	0.3	0.1	0.1	0.1	0.1	0.1	0.1	0.1	0.1	0.1	0.1
D	0.8	0.1	0.1	0.1	0.1	0.1	0.1	0.1	0.1	0.1	0.1	0.1
E	0.4	0.1	0.1	0.1	0.1	0.1	0.1	0.1	0.1	0.1	0.1	0.1
F	0.2	0.1	0.1	0.1	0.1	0.1	0.1	0.1	0.1	0.1	0.1	0.1
G	0.1	0.1	0.1	0.1	0.1	0.1	0.1	0.1	0.1	0.1	0.1	0.1
H	0.1	0.1	0.1	0.1	0.1	0.1	0.1	0.1	0.1	0.1	0.1	0.1

[a]Capture antibody titrated is in columns 1–11, constant antigen is in A12–U12, and conjugate diluted is in rows A G

establishment of defined test protocols. The CBT allows only a rough estimate of activities.

More complicated systems (e.g., those relying on four reactants) rely on establishing rough parameters for two of the reagents and examining the affect of diluting the other two. Such assays can be helped greatly through the developmental work with other ELISA systems using the same reagents. Examples are given next.

Developing an Indirect Sandwich ELISA

We have already titrated capture antibodies for use in a direct sandwich ELISA. Thus, the effective concentrations of capture antibodies, antigen, and conjugate are known. Now we wish to develop an indirect sandwich ELISA replacing the labeled antibodies directly prepared against the target antigen by a nonlabeled detecting serum and an anti-species conjugate. A good reason to do this would be to allow the use of many different animal sera for examination. A good starting point would be to perform a CBT using constant capture antibodies and antigen and titration of the detecting serum and conjugate. The species of the detecting serum would have to be different from that of the capture antibodies since we are adopting an anti-species conjugate (the anti-species conjugate has to be tested for non-ELISA activity against the coating antibodies). Conditions for the optimal coating and antigen concentrations can be used initially. If the test is successful, adjustments can be made by altering any one of the reactant's concentrations.

The establishment of the concentrations of reagents in tests other than those finally used is not uncommon. In fact, pretitration in other systems could be used as a deliberate tool. In the majority of cases, laboratories are working with a limited range of antigens and antibodies, and their exploitation in different systems often results from the need to improve methods defined by a specific task at hand. The reagent link extends to developments in monoclonal antibodies (mAbs), in which polyclonal antibodies may be used at some stage to help production of a more specific or sensitive test. As an example, an indirect sandwich ELISA based on polyclonal sera is available, and we are investigating the use of a detecting mAb (possibly to see whether we can increase specificity for detecting captured antigen). Here, the initial CBT should involve constant capture antibodies and antigen, and titrate the mAb and anti-mouse conjugate. We know for certain (based on original polyclonal-based ELISA) that we can provide enough captured antigenic target for the mAb. Similarly, the activity of the mAb as a capture reagent can be assessed using the constant components of antigen, polyclonal detecting serum, and conjugate.

Chapter 5

Theoretical Considerations

This chapter examines the aspects of using ELISA to solve problems, definitions of terms met in serology, antibody structure, and the production of antibodies in animals, units, dilutions, and molarities. *Antibodies – A Laboratory Manual (1)* is an excellent manual of techniques relevant to ELISA, and all scientists involved in experimental work involving antibodies should have this manual. The manuals given in **refs.** *2* and *3* also provide extensive relevant practical information.

1. Setting Up and Use of ELISA

The main aim in the development or use of established ELISAs is to measure some reactant. The need to measure a substance is the major reason for the assay. ELISAs can be used in pure and applied fields of science, but the chief reason they are worth developing is their high sample-handling capacity, ideal analytical sensitivity, and ease of performance. Another factor is the ease of reading, so that time is not wasted when a test has gone wrong. Thus, ELISAs can be assessed by eye before machine reading; for example, time is not wasted in reading 1,000 sample points before this insight is obtained (as in radioimmunoassay). Care must be taken not to discard successful tests merely because ELISAs are in fashion. The relationship between ELISA results and other test system results must be established so that a large amount of comparative work using ELISA and one or more assays might be involved in setting up the ELISA as a standard assay.

John R. Crowther, *Methods in Molecular Biology, The ELISA Guidebook, Vol. 516*

DOI: 10.1007/978-1-60327-254-4_5

2. What Is Known Already

A body of knowledge is often available in the scientific literature on any problem faced by an investigator. Therefore, a survey is necessary. This would mainly involve the detailing of work concerning the biological agent (antigen) being examined and any work involved with its relationship to defined hosts in experimental (laboratory animals) and field studies. This knowledge can be divided into two categories: the biochemical/molecular biological aspects of the agent and the immunological aspects (serology and immunology per se).

The literature may deal with the exact agent the investigator wishes to study or a similar agent and also reveal whether ELISAs have been performed. Obviously the two aspects of biochemistry and serology are related via the host. The main task at the beginning of any study is to define the aims properly. Scientists should also examine published work with care since often assays have been poorly devised or have been validated with little data. Scientists should also seek advice from others in related fields and examine whether reagents have already been produced that might be applicable to their own problems. A particular area is the use of monoclonal antibodies (mAbs).

An excellent catalog of immunological reagents is available, Linscott's, that lists and updates reagents and suppliers of thousands of polyclonal and monoclonal reagents of direct relevance to ELISA. Much information is also available in catalogs of commercial firms that often have detailed technical descriptions of the use of their products.

3. Complexity of Problems

Complexity of problems is manifested throughout the interrelationship between the agent and host. The concept of the relationship between antigenicity/immunogenicity and protection should be examined in this light. Thus, the major dogmas of antibodies and antigens must be examined. This book does not investigate the theories surrounding immunology, and textbooks should be consulted for more details. This chapter highlights relevant knowledge to allow more information to be sought. The following definitions are helpful.

3.1. Antigenicity

Antigenicity is the ability of proteins and carbohydrates to elicit the formation of antibodies, which, by definition, bind specifically to the antigens used for injection into animals. Antibodies may be produced as a consequence of replication of an agent or by injection of inactivated whole or parts of that agent. This can further be refined so that defined peptides or polypeptides are used. The antigens used to elicit antibodies can, in turn, be used in tests such as the ELISA.

3.2. Immunogenicity

Immunogenicity is a measure of the effect of binding of antibodies elicited by any substance. More specifically, the effect is one of producing some degree of immunity against the disease agent. Generally, such measurements are made in vitro or in animal systems other than those being examined in the field.

3.3. Protection

Production of antibodies and demonstration of immunogenic responses does not necessarily mean that animals will be protected against the challenge of the disease agent. The relationship of immunoassay results to protection is never straightforward because of the many other factors involved in immunological response, e.g., cellular immunity.

4. Antigenic Considerations

Inherent to the understanding of what is being measured in any ELISA is the definition of terms involving antigens and antibodies and an understanding of the implications of the size, number of possible antigenic sites (epitopes), distribution of epitopes (distance between them), variability of epitopes, effect on variation in epitopes on different assay systems, and so forth. As the size (molecular weight) of disease agents increases, complexity increases.

4.1. Size Considerations

Immunoassays must be developed with as much knowledge as possible of all previous studies. The complexity of agents generally increases with their size. On theoretical grounds, the relationship of size to possible complexity can be demonstrated by examining spherical agents of different diameters, beginning at 25 nm (e.g., the size of a foot-and-mouth disease virus (FMDV) particle).

One can calculate that the area bound by an Fab molecule (single arm combining site of antibody without Fc) is ~20 nm^2. This can represent an antigenic site (epitope). Thus, the number of possible sites on the virus is the surface area of the virion divided by the surface area of the combining site. The surface area of a sphere is $4 \times \pi \times r^2$; therefore, for FMDV, $4 \times 3.14 \times 12.5^2 = 12.56 \times 156.25 = 1{,}962$ nm^2. By dividing this by 20, the maximum number of Fab sites possible is 98.

Table 1
Relationship of diameter of agents to number of binding sites

Diameter	Fab sites	IgG sites
25	98	32
250	9,800	3,200
2,500	980,000	320,000
25,000	98,000,000	32,000,000

If the diameter of the agent is increased by twofold to 50 nm, using the same calculation, the number of sites is 392. Another twofold increase in diameter gives 1,468. These are small agents. If the calculations are done for agents increasing in diameter by tenfold steps, for Fab and whole IgG (binding bivalently effective area 60 nm^2), the data would be as given in **Table (1)**.

The numbers in **Table 1** illustrate that the surface area increases as a square function of the diameter. Such a calculation is based on the facts that the whole surface is antigenic (rarely true) and that the molecules bind maximally. However, experimentally, relative figures close to the theoretical are obtained. This has implications in immunoassays since one can calculate how much antibody is needed to saturate any agent, or measure the level of antibody attachment as a function of available surface.

Since we know the molecular weight of IgG (and Fab), we can calculate the weight of a number of molecules. Thus, the molecular weight of IgG = 150,000. Using Avogadro's number ($\sim 6 \times 10^{23}$), we obtain the following results:

1. 1 g of IgG contains $\sim 6 \times 10^{23}/1.5 \times 10^{5} = 4 \times 10^{18}$ molecules.
2. 1 mg of IgG contains $\sim 4 \times 10^{18}/10^{3} = 4 \times 10^{15}$ molecules.
3. 1 μg of IgG contains $\sim 4 \times 10^{18}/10^{6} = 4 \times 10^{12}$ molecules.
4. 1 ng of IgG contains $\sim 4 \times 10^{18}/10^{9} = 4 \times 10^{9}$ molecules.
5. 1 pg of IgG contains $\sim 4 \times 10^{18}/10^{12} = 4 \times 10^{6}$ molecules.

Such a model calculation helps us to understand at the molecular level what we are dealing with when faced with different antigens.

4.2. Definitions

There may be some confusion concerning the terminology used in immunological and serological circles. This section provides some working definitions that will aid the understanding of the mechanisms involved in ELISAs.

4.2.1. Antigen

An antigen is a substance that elicits an antibody response as a result of being injected into an animal or as a result of an infectious process. Antigens can be simple (e.g., peptides of molecular weight about 5,000) to complex. Antibodies specific for the antigen are produced. The definition can be extended to molecules that evoke any specific immune response, including cell-mediated immunity or tolerance.

4.2.2. Antigenic Site

An antigenic site is a distinct structurally defined region on an antigen as identified by a specific set of antibodies usually using a polyclonal serum.

4.2.3. Epitope

An epitope is the same as an antigenic site, but in which a greater specificity of reaction has been defined, e.g., using tests involving mAbs in which a single population of antibodies identifies a single chemical structure on an antigen.

4.2.4. Epitype

An epitype is an area on an antigen that is identified by a closely related set of antibodies identifying very similar chemical structures (e.g., mAbs, which define overlapping or interrelated epitopes). An epitype can be regarded as an area identifying slightly different specificities of antibodies reacting with the same antigenic site.

5.4.2.5. Continuous Epitope

A continuous epitope is produced by consecutive atoms contained within the same molecule. Such epitopes are also referred to as linear epitopes and are not usually affected by denaturation (*see* **Fig. 1**).

4.2.6. Discontinuous Epitope

A discontinuous epitope is produced from the interrelationship of atoms from nonsequential areas on the same molecule or from atoms on separate molecules. Such sites are also usually conformational in nature (*see* **Fig. 2**).

4.2.7. Linear Epitope

A linear epitope is the same as a continuous epitope, with recognition of atoms in a linear sequence (*see* **Fig. 1**).

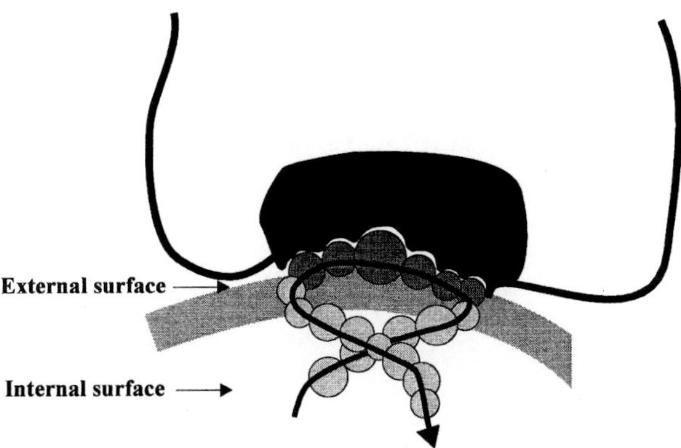

Fig. 1. Representation of a linear of continuous site. *Black area* shows paratope of antibody with specificity for site.

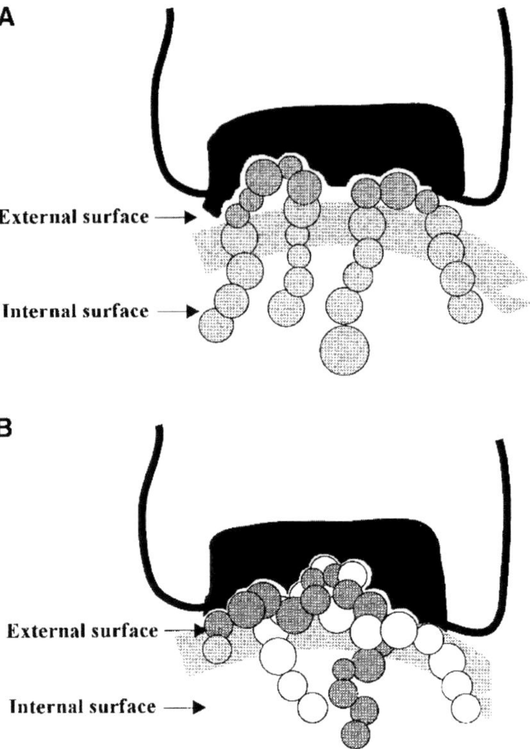

Fig. 2. Representations of two types of conformational epitopes. *Black area* shows papatope of antibody molecule with specificity for the sites. **(A)** Recognition of three-dimensional (3D) relationship of atoms from nonconsecutive atoms on same protein molecule; **(B)** recognition of 3D relationship of atoms on two different protein molecules.

4.2.8. Conformational Epitope

A conformational epitope is formed through the interrelationship of chemical elements combining so that the 3D structure determines the specificity and affinity. Such epitopes are usually affected by denaturation (*see* **Fig. 2**).

4.2.9. Antibody-Combining Site

An antibody-combining site is the part of the antibody molecule that combines specifically with an antigenic site formed by the exact chemical nature of the H and L chains in the antibody molecule.

4.2.10. Paratope

A paratope is the part of the antibody molecule that binds to the epitope. It is most relevant to mAbs in which a single specificity for a single epitope can be defined.

4.2.11. Affinity and Avidity

Affinity and avidity relate to the closeness of fit of a paratope and epitope. Considered in thermodynamic terms, it is the strength of close-range noncovalent forces. Mathematically it is expressed as an association constant (K, L/mol) calculated under equilibrium conditions. Affinity refers to the energy between a single epitope and paratope. Antisera usually contain populations of antibodies directed against the same antigenic site that have different affinities owing to their differences in exactness of fit. Antisera of multiple specificity (i.e., specific to many determinants on an antigen) cannot be assessed for affinity; however, they can be assessed for overall binding energy with an antigen in any chosen assay. This is termed the *avidity* of the serum. The avidity represents an average binding energy from the sum of all the individual affinities of a population of antibodies binding to different antigenic sites.

4.2.12. Polyclonal Antibodies

Polyclonal antibodies are the serum product of an immunized animal containing many different antibodies against the various mixtures of antigens injected. The antiserum is the product of many responding clones of cells and is usually heterogeneous at all levels. These levels include the specificity of the antibodies, classes and subclasses, titer, and affinity. The response to individual epitopes may be clonally diverse, and antibodies of different affinities may compete for the same epitope. This variation means that polyclonal antisera cannot be reproduced (*see* **Fig. 3**).

4.2.13. Monoclonal Antibodies

mAbs are antibodies derived from single antibody-producing cells immortalized by fusion to a B-lymphocyte tumor cell line to form hybridoma clones. The secreted antibody is monospecific in nature and thus has a single affinity for a defined epitope (*see* **Fig. 4**).

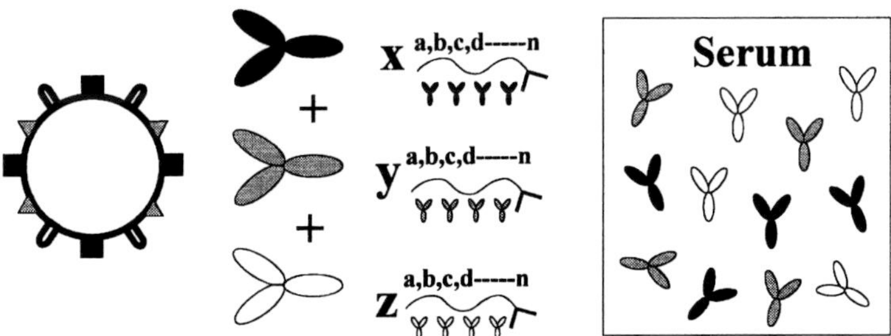

Fig. 3. Specific antibodies are produced against different sites and can vary in affinity against the same site. This, a,b,c,d-----n, represents a range of slightly different antibody populations recognizing antigenic sites x, y, and z. The antibodies have different affinities, classes, and isotypes. The resulting mixture is a polyclonal antiserum.

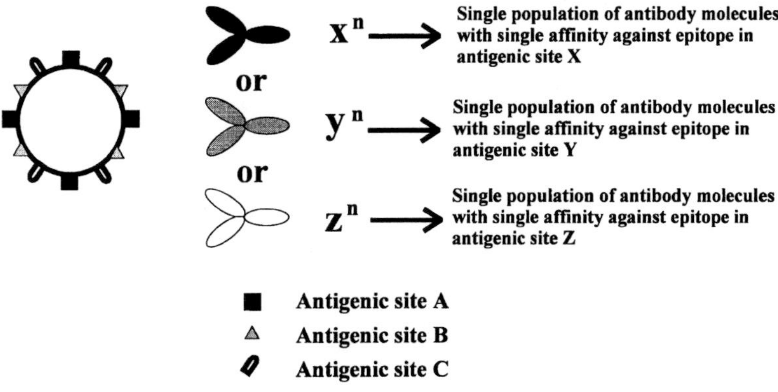

Fig. 4. mAbs are monospecific in terms of antigenic target and affinity.

5. Antibodies

Antibodies form a group of glycoproteins present in the serum and tissue fluids of all mammals. The group is also termed *immunoglobulins* (Igs) indicating their role in adaptive immunity. All antibodies are Igs, but not all Igs are antibodies, that is, not all the Ig produced by a mammal has antibody activity. Five distinct classes of Ig molecules have been recognized in most higher mammals. These are Ig, IgG, IgA, IgM, IgD, and IgE. These classes differ from each other in size, charge, amino acid composition, and carbohydrate content. There are also significant differences (heterogeneity) within each class. **Figure 5** shows the basic polypeptide structure of the Ig molecule.

5.1. Antibody Structure

The basic structure of all Ig molecules is a unit of two identical light (L) polypeptide chains and two identical heavy (H) polypeptide chains linked together by disulfide bonds. The class and subclass of an Ig molecule is determined by its heavy-chain type. Thus, in the humans, there are four IgG subclasses – IgG_1, IgG_2, IgG_3, IgG_4 – that have heavy chains called 1, 2, 3, and 4. The differences between the various subclasses within an individual Ig class are less than the differences between the different classes. Therefore, IgG_1 is more closely related to IgG_2, and so on than to IgA, IgM, IgD, or IgE. The most common class of Ig is IgG.

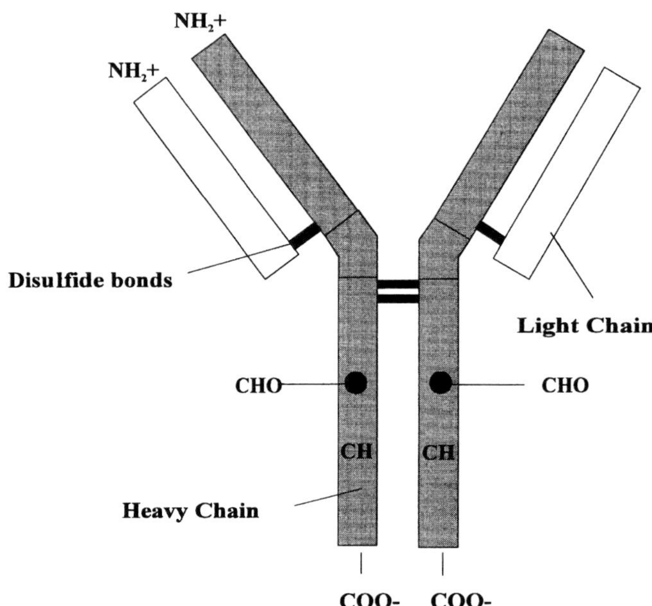

Fig. 5. Representation of basic structure of an IgG molecule.

IgG molecules are made up of two identical light chains of molecular weight 23,000 and two identical heavy chains of molecular weight 53,000. Each light chain is linked to a heavy chain by noncovalent association, and also by one covalent disulfide bridge. For IgG, each light-heavy chain pair is linked to the other by disulfide bridges between the heavy chains. This molecule is represented schematically in the form of a Y, with the amino (N-) termini of the chains at the top of the Y and the carboxyl (C-) termini of the two heavy chains at the bottom of the Y shape. A dimer of these light-heavy chain pairs is the basic subunit of the other Ig isotypes. The structures of these other classes and subclasses differ in the positions and number of disulfide bridges between the heavy chains, and in the number of L–H chain pairs in the molecule. IgG, IgE, and IgD are composed of one L–H chain pair. IgA may have one, two, or three light-heavy chain pairs. IgM (serum) has five light-heavy chain pairs, whereas membrane-bound IgM has one. In the polymeric forms of IgA and IgM, the light-heavy chain pairs are held together by disulfide bridges through a polypeptide known as the J chain.

In both heavy and light chains, at the N-terminal portion the sequences vary greatly from polypeptide to polypeptide. By contrast, in the C-terminal portion of both heavy and light chains, the sequences are identical. Hence, these two segments of the molecule are designated variable and constant regions. For the light chain, the variable (V) region is about 110 amino acid residues in length and the constant (C) region of the light chain is similarly about 110 amino acids in length.

The variable region of the heavy chain (V_H) is also about 110 amino acid residues in length, but the constant region of the heavy chain (C_H) is about 330 amino acid residues in length. The N-terminal portions of both heavy and light chain pairs comprise the antigen-combining (binding) sites in an Ig molecule. The heterogeneity in the amino acid sequences present within the variable regions of both heavy and light chains accounts for the great diversity of antigen specificities among antibody molecules. By contrast, the constant regions of the heavy chain make up the part of the molecule that carries out the effector functions that are common to all antibodies of a given class.

Figure 5 shows that there must be two identical antigen-binding sites (more in the case of serum IgM and secretory IgA); hence, the basic Y-shaped Ig molecule is bivalent. This bivalency permits antibodies to cross-link antigens with two or more of the same epitope. Antigenic determinants that are separated by a distance can be bound by an antibody molecule.

The antigen-combining site (active site) is a crevice between the variable regions of the light and heavy chain pair. The size and shape of this crevice can vary owing to differences in the relationship of V_L and V_H regions as well as to differences in variation in the amino acid-sequence. Thus, the specificity of antibody will result from the molecular complementarity between determinant groups (epitopes) on the antigen molecule and amino acid residues present in the active site.

An antibody molecule has a unique 3D structure. However, a single antibody molecule has the ability to combine with a range (spectrum) of different antigens. This phenomenon is known as multispecificity. Thus, the antibody can combine with the inducing antigenic determinant or a separate determinant with similar structures (cross-reacting antigen). Stable antigen–antibody complexes can result when there is a sufficient number of short-range interactions between both, regardless of the total fit. This is a problem for the immunoassayist, and care must be taken to ensure that the operator is assaying for the correct or desired antigen; therefore, careful planning of negative and positive controls is essential.

5.1.1. Antibody Digestion

Figure 6 demonstrates the digestion of IgG using papain or pepsin proteolytic enzymes. Mild proteolysis of native Ig at the hinge regions of the heavy chain by papain will cleave IgG into

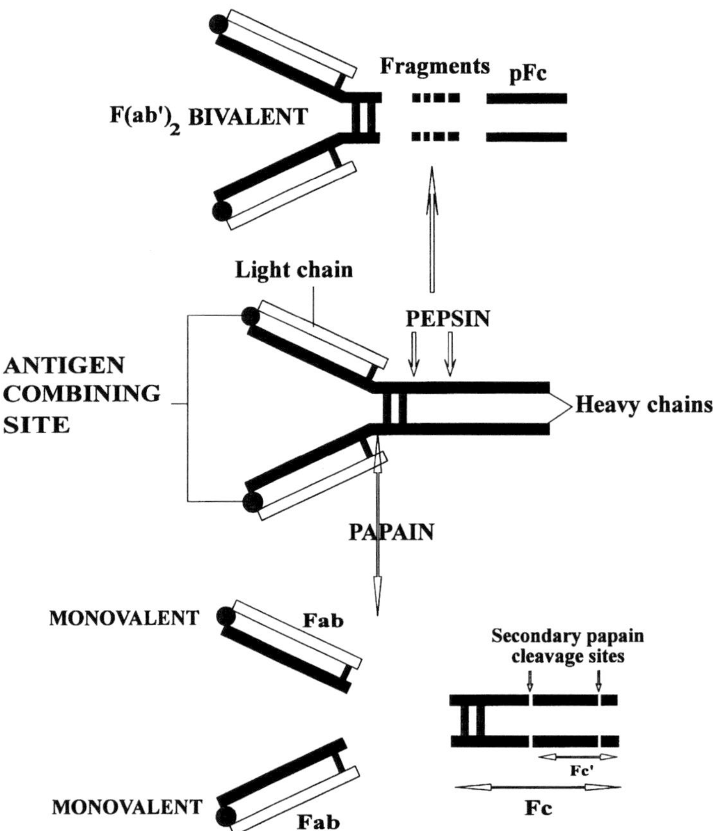

Fig. 6. Enzymatic cleavage of human IgG. Pepsin cleaves the heavy chain to give F(Ab') and o/Fc' fragments. Further action results in greater fragmentation of central protein to peptides. Papain splits the molecule in the hinge region to give two Fab_2 fragments and the Fc fragment. Further action on the Fc can produce Fc.'

three fragments. Two of these fragments are identical and are called fragment antigen binding or Fab. Each Fab consists of the variable and constant regions of the light chain and the variable part of the constant (ChI domain) regions of the heavy chain. Therefore, each Fab carries one antigen binding site. The third fragment, consisting of the remainder of the constant regions of the heavy chains, is readily crystallizable and is called fragment crystallizable or Fc.

Pepsin digestion cleaves the Fc from the molecule but leaves the disulfide bridge between the Fab regions. This molecule contains both antigen-combining sites and is bivalent.

5.1.2. Antibody Classes

The five immunological classes (isotypes) can be distinguished structurally by differences in their heavy chain constant regions (i.e., mainly the Fc portion). These heavy chain classes define the corresponding Ig classes IgA, IgG, IgD, IgE, and IgM. Some classes can be divided further into subclasses.

In addition, two major types of light chains exist, based on the differences in the constant region Cl and are known as kappa (κ) and lambda (λ). Igs from various mammals appear to conform to this format. However, the subclass designation and variety may not be the same in all species examined; for example, mice have IgG_1, IgG_{2a}, IgG_{2b}, IgG_3, and cows have IgG_1 and IgG_2.

5.2. Antibody Production in Response to Antigenic Stimulus

The antibodies produced in a humoral response to antigenic stimulus are heterogeneous in specificity and may include all Ig classes. This heterogeneous response is owing to the fact that most antigens have multiple antigenic determinants that trigger off the activation of different B-cells. Therefore, the serum of any mammal (vertebrate) contains a heterogeneous mixture of Ig molecules. The specificities of these Ig molecules will reflect the organism's past antigenic exposure and history.

The first antibody produced in response to a primary exposure of an immunogen is IgM. When the immunogen is persistent or the host (mammal) is reexposed to the immunogen, other classes of antibody may be produced as well as IgM. The body compartment in which the immunogen is presented can determine the predominant antibody isotype produced (e.g., IgA in the gastrointestinal (GI) tract). In general, primary exposure to an immunogen stimulates the production of IgM initially, followed by the appearance of IgG, as shown in **Fig.** 7.

If no further exposure occurs, or the immunogen is removed by the mammal, a low level of IgM and IgG can be detected. If reexposure occurs, a similar peak of IgM antibody is produced that declines in a similar kinetic manner to the primary IgM response, but the IgG response is not only more rapid (over time) but also reaches higher serum levels that persist for a longer period of time. This IgG response to reexposure is known as the anamnestic response. This is illustrated in **Fig.** 7.

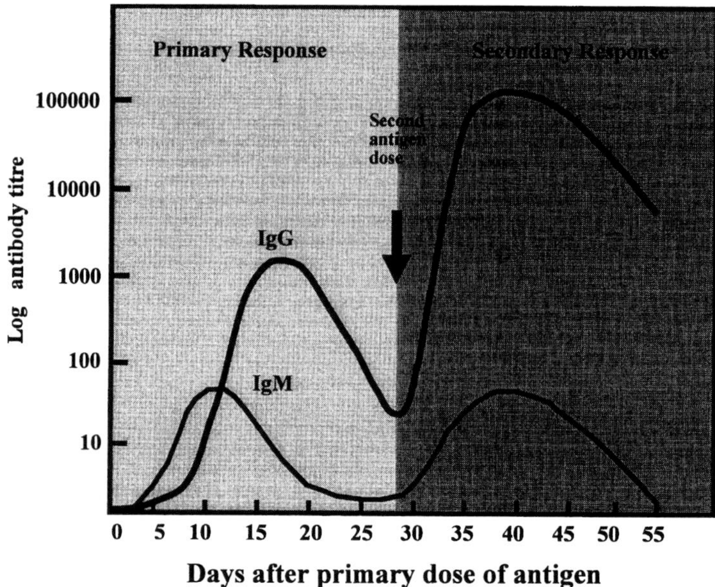

Fig. 7. Anamnestic response following second administration of antigen. Primary response following initial antigen dose has a lag phase in which no antibody is detected (4–5 days). This is followed by a lag phase in which antibody is produced. A plateau phase follows in which antibody titers stabilize, after which a decline in titer is observed. On secondary stimulation, there is an almost immediate rise in titer and higher levels of antibodies are achieved that are mainly IgG.

In cases in which complex antigens occur, as in infectious diseases, the dosage (infection level), type of antigen (viral, bacterial, protozoan, helminthic), route of infection (oral, respiratory, cutaneous), and species of mammal infected (cow, pig, camel, human) will all affect the degree and speed by which IgG replaces IgM.

These considerations are vital for the immunoassayist who is concerned with diagnosing infectious diseases of mammals, and great care and planning should be exercised before undertaking such immunoassays. Note also that at this stage, different infectious disease agents can stimulate different antibody isotypes. For example, certain viral pathogens stimulate predominantly IgM agglutinating responses, bacterial polysaccharides stimulate IgM (and IgG_2 in humans) antibodies, and helminthic infections stimulate the synthesis of IgE antibody.

In general, it can be stated that during the development of immunity to infectious disease agents, the antibodies produced become capable of recognizing antigens better, as demonstrated by improved antigen–antibody interaction. The multispecificity of antibody molecules (i.e., the ability to combine with a variety of epitopes containing similar molecular structures) is dependent not only on the heterogeneity of the epitope in question, but also on the molecular construction of the antigen-reactive sites (paratopes) of the antibody molecules.

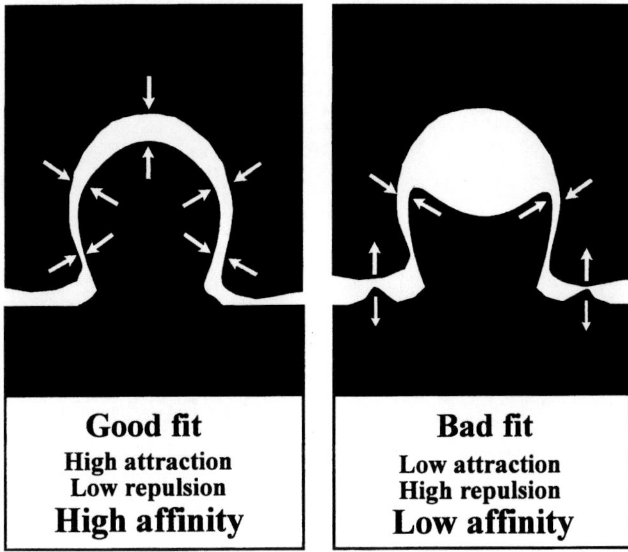

Fig. 8. A good fit between antigenic sites and antibody-combining sites creates as environment for the intermolecular attractive forces to be created and limits the chances of repulsive forces. The strength of the single antigen–antibody bond is the affinity that reflects the summation of the attractive and repulsive forces.

5.3. Affinity and Avidity

The binding energy between an antibody molecule and an antigen determinant is termed *affinity*. Thus, antibodies with paratopes that recognize epitopes perfectly will have high affinity (good fit) for the antigen in question, whereas antibodies with paratopes that recognize epitopes imperfectly will have low affinity (poor fit). Low-affinity antibodies in which the fit to antigen is less than perfect will have fewer noncovalent bonds established between the complex, and the strength of binding will be less, as shown in **Fig. 8**.

With simple immunogens containing few epitopes, as the antibody response develops (in response) to this immunogen, its recognition by antibody will become better or closer, that is, low-affinity antibodies will be replaced by high-affinity antibodies, which will cause the interaction between antigen and antibody to be more stable. Antibodies produced later during infection are generally of higher affinity than those produced early on during infection. Hence, the IgG antibodies produced in response to reexposure will be of higher affinity than those produced in response to initial exposure.

In a serum sample in which there has been polyclonal stimulation of antibody production by antigen, a variety of affinities will be present within the antibodies. The match (fit) between antibodies to that antigen will be variable, and the antibodies present in that serum sample will bind to antigen differentially. Thus, not only can an antigen stimulate different antibody isotypes but also antibodies with different affinities for the antigenic determinant.

Avidity can be regarded as the sum of all the different affinities between the heterogeneous antibodies contained in a serum and the various antigenic sites (epitopes). It is important to realize that the avidity of a serum may change on dilution because an operator may be diluting out certain populations of antibodies.

As an example, we could have a serum containing a low quantity of antibodies showing high affinity for a particular complex antigen and a high quantity of low-affinity antibody. Under immunoassay conditions in which that serum is not diluted greatly, we would have competition for antigenic sites between the high- and low-affinity antibodies, and the high-affinity antibodies would react preferentially. On dilution, however, the concentration of the high-affinity antibodies would be reduced until we would be left only with low-affinity antibodies. Such problems are important when an operator is using immunoassays to compare antigens by their differential activity with different antisera. The dilution of any serum can affect its ability to discriminate between antigens owing to the dynamics of the heterogeneous antibody population (relative concentrations and affinities of individual antibody molecules).

Such problems of quality and quantity do not apply to mAbs, because, by definition, the Ig molecules in the population are identical. They all have the same affinity and therefore the avidity equals affinity. Thus, the population reacts identically to any individual molecule in that population. On diluting the monoclonal population, there is no alteration in the affinity/avidity of the serum, and a change noted for reaction between the mAb and antigen must be from changes on the particular antigen.

Figure 9 illustrates cross-reactions between sera and different antigens. Here, specific reactions occur in which all the antibodies have "best fit." When two antigens share a similar antigen, cross-reactions will be observed. The two nonidentical sites may also contribute to the cross-reaction. When all the antibodies show no recognition of the antigens available, no reaction will be seen. It is important to understand the concepts of variability in (1) isotype production and (2) affinity and affinity maturation when developing immunoassays for infectious disease agents that are normally more chronic than acute in duration.

As antigens are introduced into different compartments of the mammalian body, they can stimulate the production of different antibody isotypes. Local antibody responses in the GI tract and the respiratory tree are predominantly IgA isotypes, whereas those in the other major compartments are predominantly IgG (IgM). Certain sites in the body (e.g., testes) are immunologically privileged and stimulate lower antibody responses to immunogens. Most infectious diseases are transmitted by aerosolization, close contact, or vectors; thus, their route of transmission is variable. In addition, their final location may be distant from their

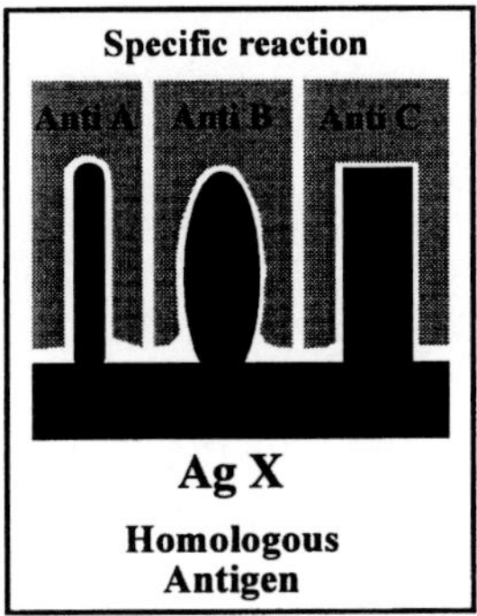

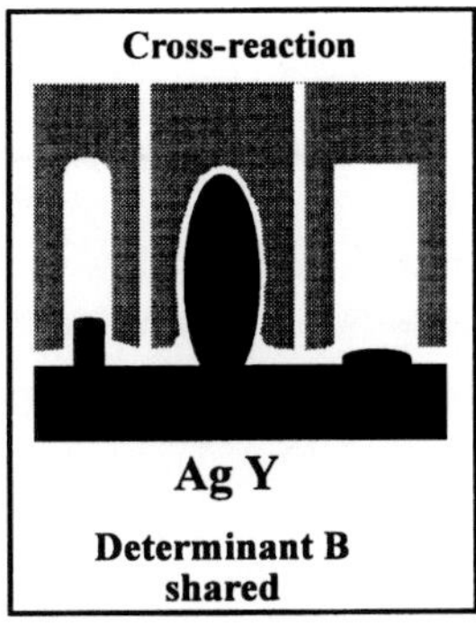

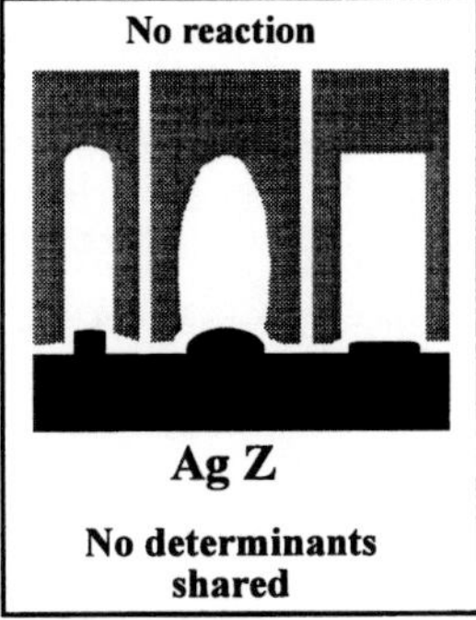

Fig. 9. Specificity, cross-reactivity, and nonreactivity. Antisera contain populations of antibodies. Each population is directed against a different determinant (A, B, and C). Antigen X and Y share a determinant (B); thus, antiserum against X will react with antigen Y (cross-react) as well as reacting specifically with antigen X. Antiserum against antigen X does not react with antigen Z since no determinants are shared.

point of deposition. Similarly, whereas some pathogens are capable of division within the host, others are incapable of division within the mammalian host (e.g., helminths).

5.4. Antibody Production in Response to Immunization/ Vaccination

Individuals can be rendered resistant to infectious agents by either passive immunization or active immunization. In general, the beneficial effects of immunization are mediated by antibodies, and therefore the effects of immunization can be monitored by the immunoassayist.

5.4.1. Passive Immunization

Passive immunization is accomplished by transferring antibodies from a resistant to a susceptible host. Passively transferred antibodies confer a temporary but immediate resistance to infection, but are gradually catabolized by the susceptible host. Once passive protection wanes, the recipient becomes susceptible to infection again. Passively transferred antibodies can be acquired by the recipient either transplacentally and transcolostrally as in neonates, or by injection of purified antibodies from a resistant donor into a susceptible recipient.

5.4.2. Active Immunization

Active immunization is accomplished by administering antigens of infectious agents to individuals so that they respond by producing antibodies that will neutralize the infectious disease agents, once contracted. Reexposure to such agents, following active immunization, will result in an anamnestic immune response, in which the antibodies or effector cells produced will be capable of neutralizing the effect of or destroying the inciting agents. Such antibodies are known as protective antibodies, and their complementary antigens as protective antigens. The protection conferred by active immunization is not immediate, as in passive immunization, because the immune system requires considerable time process such antigens and produce protective antibodies. However, the advantage of active immunization is that it is long lasting, and restimulation by the same antigens present in pathogens leads to an anamnestic response. It is important to recognize that the immunity produced to pathogens, following active immunization, is only as broad as the antigenic spectrum of the preparation used for immunization. Protection can be afforded using different approaches in the formulation of vaccines.

5.4.3. Live Vaccines

Live vaccines may be attenuated by the passage of agents (e.g., viruses) in an unusual host so that they become nonpathogenic to vaccinated animals. Usually these are good vaccines because they supply the same antigenic stimulus as the disease agent. There can be problems of reversion to the pathogenic agent and some replication of the agent usually occurs.

5.4.4. Modified Vaccines: Whole Disease Agent

Vaccines can be grown and then chemically modified (e.g., heat killed, nucleic acid modified (mutagens), or formaldehyde treated). These are potentially good vaccines in which full antigenic spectrum is given. The antigenic mass must be high, since there is no replication to challenge the immune system. Repeat vaccinations are common to elevate antibody levels.

5.4.5. Purified Antigens

Protective antigens can be identified and used as proteins, polypeptides, and peptides as immunogens, usually with adjuvants. Usually these vaccines are not as good as those in which total antigenic spectrum is used. They have the advantages of being able to synthesize products on large scale by chemical methods (e.g., as peptides) and are noninfectious.

5.4.6. DNA Technology Products

Genes producing particular immunogens can be inserted into replicating agents so that their products are expressed. Novel approaches include use of mammalian viruses, insect viruses (baculovirus expression), yeasts, and *E. coli*.

5.4.7. Generalities

Most vaccines are administered by either sc or im injections. When vaccinating large herds of animals, other techniques such as high-pressure jet injections may be employed. Obviously the risk of administering unwanted or contaminating organisms and antigens should be minimal; hence, sterile administration of vaccines is indicated. Subcutaneous or im vaccination should induce all antibody isotypes given the fact that the inciting antigens are capable of doing so. Therefore, the immunoassayist must consider whether total antibody assays, isotype-specific assays, or assays to detect antigen clearance are to be utilized to assess the effects of vaccination.

Some antigens may be administered orally (e.g., poliomyelitis vaccines in humans) by incorporation in food or drinking water (e.g., in poultry flocks) or by inhalant exposure of an aerosolized vaccine (e.g., diseases of the respiratory tract). In these instances, the production of local antibodies to prevent the ingress of pathogens through the GI or respiratory tree barriers should be sought. The immunoassayist must decide whether an assay for isotype-specific antibodies, notably IgA, may provide deeper insight into the benefits of vaccination than an assay for total antibody.

In some instances in which infectious disease agent is endemic and vaccination, especially of newborns, is indicated, it may prove difficult or impossible to differentiate the beneficial effects of vaccination because residual levels of antibody may be present in nonvaccinated stock. Such factors must be borne in mind when assays are developed to determine the immunological status of large groups of mammals.

5.5. Antibody Production in Response to Infectious Agents

It is beyond the scope of this book to catalog the humoral immune responses produced in mammals in response to the variety of infectious disease agents such as viruses, bacteria, fungi, protozoa, helminths, and arthropods. Such information may be obtained from textbooks and specialized review articles. This section deals with the general considerations of host–parasite relationships, with specific reference to the production of antibodies to pathogens. As already mentioned, most infectious diseases are transmitted by aerosolization, close contact, or vectors, and their final location may be distant from their point of deposition. Therefore, these pathogens involve multiple organs. Similarly, many pathogens, but not all, have the capacity to divide within the mammalian body, and in such instances, the numbers and amounts of antigens produced will increase over time and be proportional to the number of pathogens at the time of sampling. When pathogens do not divide or reproduce in the mammalian host, the amount of antigens produced may be directly proportional to the infective dose. Hence, in devising assays for infectious disease agents, the immunoassayist must take into account whether high or low concentrations of antigens and antibodies are to be sought. When antibody titers of less than 1:50 are anticipated, serum dilutions of less than 1:50 or possibly less than 1:10 for the test serum must be employed. Previous knowledge of specific host–parasite systems will prove invaluable in devising more specific and sensitive enzyme immunoassays.

Although many nonimmunological mechanisms exist for the removal of pathogens from the body (e.g., lysozyme, iron-binding proteins, myeloperoxidase, lactoperoxidase, complement, basic peptides, and proteins), it is generally recognized that the immune system plays a vital role in the control and destruction of pathogens. For this reason, the measurement of antibody or antigen by sensitive assays, such as ELISA, provides a useful indicator for the assessment of immune status. When an infectious agent enters the mammalian body, the first components recognized as foreign are surface components of that pathogen. This host–pathogen interface plays a vital role in the control of infectious diseases, not only in its involvement in stimulating the early humoral immune response but also in its involvement in mediating protective immune responses. Immune responses that reduce pathogen numbers by lysis, agglutination, or phagocytosis and that reduce the antigen load are normally regarded as protective responses. Such antibodies directed against specific epitopes on the pathogens can be sought by the immunoassayist in an effort to correlate protective responses with clinical betterment. However, insight into the molecular basis of such interactions is necessary before immunoassays can be developed to demonstrate protective responses (e.g., knowledge of the immunochemistry of the surface-exposed molecules and their epitopes, knowledge of specific antibody isotypes that mediate these responses). Because infectious disease agents stimulate antibody production, these antibodies can prove useful to the immunoassayist for detecting exposure to pathogens.

We have seen that when the antigens of pathogens are recognized by the host, an antibody response ensues, initially of the IgM isotype and followed by the IgG isotype, together with an increase in antibody affinity, over time. When a variety of antibody isotypes is produced in response to infection, this isotypic variation can be used to determine the chronicity of the infection since IgM antibody isotypes normally appear before IgG antibody isotypes. Similarly, increasing levels of antibodies can indicate current infections or exacerbations of infections, whereas decreasing antibody titers can indicate past infections or successful control of current infection. In the absence of detectable free circulating antibody, either free antigen or circulating immune complexes can be detected by ELISA. When antibodies specific to antigens of a pathogen are used to detect the presence of free antigen in the test sample, a direct correlation can be made between ELISA positivity and current infection. When protective mechanisms occur, destruction of the pathogen is the outcome. This is accompanied by the release of previously internal components, which, if antigenic, will stimulate the production of specific antibodies. Thus, the destruction of pathogens will lead to the production of antibodies against the antigen repertoire, both surface exposed and internal, of that pathogen. Owing to the commonness of some internal antigens (e.g., enzymes), the consensus of opinion indicates that the more specific antigens or pathogens (excluding endotoxins) are surface expressed at one time or another during development. The surface-exposed antigen mosaic is normally less complex than the internal antigen mosaic of pathogens.

5.5.1. Effect of Antibody in Viral Infection

Viruses as a group must enter a cell to proliferate, since they lack the biochemical machinery to manufacture proteins and metabolize sugars. Some viruses also lack the enzymes required for nucleic acid replication. The number of genes carried by viruses varies from 3 to about 250, and it is worth noting how small this is compared with the smallest bacterium.

The illnesses caused by viruses are varied and include acute, recurrent, latent (dormant but can recur), and subclinical. The immune response ranges from apparently nonexistent to lifelong immunity. The acute infection is probably most encountered by the immunoassayist who is interested in animal diseases, but it must be borne in mind that the total knowledge of a specific disease is needed in order to devise assays of relevance to specific problems.

Because the outer surfaces (capsids) of virus contain antigens, it is against these antigens and the envelope that the antiviral antibodies are mounted. The first line of defense (excluding interferon) is either IgM and IgG antibodies in which viruses are present in plasma and tissue fluids (vector transmitted) or secretory IgA antibodies where viruses are present on epithelial surfaces (airborne, close contact). Some viruses that replicate entirely on epithelial surfaces (e.g., respiratory tree, GI tract, genitourinary (GU) tract) and that do not have a viremic phase will be controlled by secretory IgA. Antibodies may destroy extracellular viruses, prevent virus infection of cells by blocking their attachment to cell receptors, or destroy virus-infected cells.

5.5.2. Effect of Antibody in Bacterial Infection

The role of antibody in combating bacterial infection is diverse. Antibody to bacterial surface antigens (fimbriae, lipotechoic acid, and some capsules) prevents the attachment of the bacterium to the host cell membrane by blocking receptor sites. Antibody can neutralize bacterial exotoxins (possibly by blocking the interaction between the exotoxin and the receptor site). Normally IgG antibodies are responsible for neutralization of toxins. Antibody to capsular antigens can neutralize the antiphagocytic properties of the capsule, or in organisms lacking a capsule, antibodies to somatic antigens may serve a similar function. IgG antibodies are regarded as more effective opsonins than IgM in the absence of complement than IgG. It is the most effective antibody isotype in the presence of complement. Thus, IgM antibodies are more effective in inducing complement-mediated lysis and bacterial opsonization prior to phagocytosis. Antibody can block transport mechanisms and bacterial receptors (e.g., for iron-chelating compounds), neutralize immunorepellants (which interfere with normal phagocytosis), and neutralize spreading factors that facilitate invasion (e.g., enzymes, hyaluronidase).

5.5.3. Effect of Antibody in Protozoan Infection

In general, antibodies serve to regulate parasites that exist in the bloodstream and tissue fluids, but they are ineffective once the parasite has become intracellular. Hence, the importance of antibody varies with the infection under study. The presence of encysted morphological forms in the host also reduces the efficacy of antibodies (e.g., Toxoplasma, Entamoeba, Giardia). Many protozoan parasites undergo development in the mammalian host, which is manifested in morphologically distinct form. Such developmental forms have often associated stage-specific surface antigens.

Antibodies can damage parasites directly, induce lysis, activate complement, agglutinate extracellular forms, stimulate antibody-dependent cellular cytotoxicity, and block their entry into their host cells. IgM, IgG, and IgA antibody isotypes are involved in these reactions. The isotype specificity not only depends on in which host compartment the parasite is residing (e.g., respiratory tree, GI tract, GU tract (IgA), bloodstream, lymphoid tissue (IgM, IgG)), but also on the antigens expressed during the different developmental stages and their chronicity.

Protozoan parasites can induce chronic infections in mammals, and therefore large amounts of antibody (IgM + IgG) are produced in response to infection. The external surfaces, and the antigens contained therein, are important in the control of protozoan infections and many effective/protective antibody mechanisms are directed against them.

Protozoan parasites are capable of the polyclonal stimulation of B-cells, and, hence, in some infections (e.g., trypanosomiasis) large quantities of nontrypanosomal IgM and IgG antibodies are produced. In such instances, the immunoassayist should have the capability of distinguishing parasite-specific from nonspecific antibody responses. Protozoan parasites are also capable of depressing the immune response (immunodepression) (e.g., Babesia), and in such instances circulating antibody levels are reduced. The above phenomena must be borne in mind when devising ELISAs for protozoan parasites.

5.5.4. Effect of Antibody in Helminth Infections

Helminths (trematodes, cestodes, nematodes, Acanthocephalans) normally have complicated life cycles, and their larger size and increased complexity cater for the increase in antigenic diversity found within them. In addition, when many developmental forms exist in the host, a stage specificity of antigens (restricted to each stage) has been demonstrated. Helminth parasites induce chronic infections, and such long-term antigen challenge exposure can produce elevated levels of circulating antibodies. Because helminth parasites are normally transmitted by close contact, vectors, water, and possibly aerosolization, they affect numerous tissues and organs of the host. Some helminths have a minimal migratory phase, but the majority are capable of migration throughout the host's soft tissues.

Antibodies of IgM, IgG, IgA, and IgE isotypes are produced in response to helminth antigens, and depending on in which physiological compartment of the host the parasite is residing, each isotype can be utilized in ELISAs for detecting antibody recognition (exposure) of parasite antigens. IgE Igs are elevated in helminth infections, and although only a proportion of the IgE Ig produced has antibody activity against parasite antigen(s), this class of Ig has been implicated in resistance to helminth. Both IgG and IgE antibodies are involved in antibody-dependent cellular cytotoxicity mechanisms against helminth parasites.

Helminth parasites are the most complex infectious disease agents infecting mammals, and hence the host's antibody responses to them are the most diverse. Unlike other infectious diseases, most helminths do not divide in the body of the final host, and therefore the antigenic load is dependent on the infective dose. Exceptions to this are *Echinococcus* spp. and *Strongyloides* spp. Antibodies are produced against antigens present within helminths (somatic antigens), antigens on helminth outer surfaces (surface antigens), and antigens in helminth excretions or secretions (excretory–secretory (ES) antigens). The ES antigens of helminths have been shown to confer the most specificity in immunoassays. Not all stages of the helminth life cycle occur in the mammalian host, and therefore it is vital that the immunoassayist consider the pathogen of interest with reference to this. Antigens collected or extracted from stages of the parasite that do not occur in the final host are unlikely to be of use for detecting antibodies to the parasite in that host. Similarly, because helminths develop within the host, the earlier mammalian stages of development stimulate antibodies against antigens of only that stage. Later developmental stages stimulate antibodies not only to their respective stages but also to previous stages if homologous or cross-reacting antigens occur in such stages. The humoral immune responses to helminths are complex and care is necessary in developing ELISAs for helminth infections in order that cross-reactions be minimized. Helminths are capable of modulating the immune response, and immunosupression of antibody responses occurs in some diseases (e.g., Haemonchus).

5.5.6. Overview on Antibody Production

In the previous sections, the complexity of the humoral response to infectious disease agents was demonstrated. As the agents become structurally more complex, a greater degree of antigenic diversity arises, which can complicate immunodiagnosis. However, it is apparent that infectious disease agents stimulate the production of specific antibodies in hosts, and these antibodies can be used in ELISAs to determine the exposure of a host to a pathogen. Similarly, interactions between host and pathogen cause the release of pathogen antigens into the host's bodily fluids. These antigens can be used in ELISAs to detect current infections. In endemic areas mammals may be infected with more than one pathogen. In cases in which antigens of each pathogen are non–cross-reactive with antibodies produced in response to each pathogen, diagnosis by immunoassay is straightforward. Difficulties will inevitably arise when cross-reacting antigens (possibly from closely related pathogens) and antibodies occur. Care must be taken when developing ELISAs for such systems, and basic research to define the problems of cross-reactions must be undertaken.

In considering antigens of potential usefulness in immunodiagnosis, it is apparent that the greater the number or variety of antigens used to detect circulating antibodies, the wider the antibody diversity detected will be, and hence the likelihood of detecting positive cases. However, owing to the complexity and cross-reactivity of antigens and antibodies, the immunoassayist must select the antigen or group of antigens that stimulate antibody production but do not produce cross-reactions.

5.5.7. Relationship Between Antigen and Antibody In Vivo

We have seen that the ingress of antigens into the host's body eventually leads to the production of circulating antibodies to them. In the case of complex antigens (e.g., infectious disease agent antigens), each antigen can stimulate the production of a variety of antibody isotypes with a variety of affinities, and these antibodies can be used in ELISA for the immunodiagnosis of infectious diseases. In certain infectious diseases (e.g., viruses, bacteria, protozoa) in which the pathogens divide in the host's body, as the pathogen burden increases, so does the antigenic load. Similarly, when pathogens are dealt with effectively (e.g., by lysis) the release of previously internalized antigens into the surrounding tissue occurs, thus increasing the free antigenic load in the host.

One function of antibodies is to mop up free antigen and cause the antigen–antibody complex produced to be removed from the system, normally by phagocytic cells. It is important to consider the kinetics of antigen and antibody appearance and disappearance when dealing with antibody responses to infectious disease agents.

In the early stages of a primary infection, very little circulating antibody is present. When the infectious disease antigens are processed by the host, antibody synthesis occurs and these antibodies, predominantly of the IgM isotype, recognize specific antigens. In this stage of the disease process, antigen levels would be expected to be higher than antibody levels in the fluid sampled, i.e., excess antigen. Because there are relatively higher concentrations of antigen than antibody, all available antibody will be bound to antigen to form immune complexes, leaving the residual antigen free to circulate in bodily fluids. As more antibody is produced in response to continuous antigen challenge, the relative concentrations of antibody and antigen become similar, and as this antibody binds to antigen, less free antigen is present. At a point where the amount of circulating antibody equals the amount of free antigen, following antigen–antibody interaction to produce immune complexes, neither free antibody nor free antigen remains, and at this point both reactants are equivalent. When the concentration of circulating antibody exceeds the concentration of circulating antigen, no free antigen will be present, but a residual amount of antibody will be present, i.e., excess antibody.

This is a simplistic account of the interaction between antibody and antigen, but it demonstrates that whenever specific antibodies to an antigen and that antigen interact, immune complexes are produced. The antibody isotype, antibody affinity, number of epitopes on an antigen molecule, and chronicity of antigen and antibody production are all important in determining the fate of immune complexes. In general, large complexes (those found by interaction of antibodies and antigen with numerous epitopes) are removed by phagocytic cells. Smaller complexes (antibodies and antigen with few epitopes) are removed slowly by phagocytes and remain in the circulation longer. The main sites for immune complex removal are the liver (Kupfer cells), spleen, and lungs. Low-affinity immune complexes are smaller than high-affinity complexes, and therefore persist longer in the circulation. Excess antigen and excess antibody immune complexes are normally smaller than antigen–antibody equivalent immune complexes and therefore remain in the circulation longer.

Some of the pathology associated with infectious diseases is owing to immune complex deposition. Thus, in certain instances the concentration of soluble (circulating) immune complexes in bodily fluids can provide insight into immune complex pathology. The immunoassayist should be capable of devising assays for soluble immune complexes. For example, in excess antigen complexes in which an antigen-specific antibody (preferably from a different species from the host) is available, the antigen can be trapped by adsorbing the specific antibody onto the ELISA plate. The reaction can be developed with an anti-host species-specific antibody enzyme conjugate.

Because infectious diseases are often chronic, immune complexes would be expected to be produced owing to persistent antigen and antibody production. In the early stages, excess antigen would be expected, and hence the immunoassayist could measure circulating antigen. Remember that the antigen chosen for measurement has to be specific for the pathogen in question. As the disease state progresses to chronicity, less free antigen will be available owing to increased antibody production and the immunoassayist should measure circulating antibodies or circulating immune complexes. It should be borne in mind that infectious disease organisms are antigenically complex, may or may not divide within the host, may reinfect the host, or may vary antigenically, and hence the balance previously described between antigen and antibody will vary from pathogen to pathogen. Because pathogens produce numerous antigens of different immunogenicity, many antigen–antibody interactions involving both low- and high-affinity antibodies will be present.

The most useful assays will be those that take into account the preceding considerations. The pathogen–host interactions should be examined as fully as possible before ELISAs are developed. Finally, as already mentioned, many infectious disease agents have immunomodulatory effects varying from immunodepression, including reduction in humoral antibody production, to the induction of T- or B-cell tolerance. Tolerance, in which an organism becomes unresponsive to a particular antigen, may occur in a variety of ways, but the outcome is that antibodies fail to be produced. Infectious disease agents can blockade receptors on antibody-forming cells or mature antigen-specific lymphocytes and make them unresponsive to that antigen. When high levels of antigen such as pneumococcal polysaccharide induce the event, a state of high zone tolerance exists. When low doses of monomeric antigen induce the event, a state of low zone tolerance exists. Thus, in designing ELISAs the effect of parasite antigens on the induction of tolerance must be considered.

5.8. Diagnostic Usefulness of Antigens and Antibodies in Infectious Diseases

Detection of both antigens and specific antibodies can prove useful in the laboratory diagnosis of infectious diseases. As we have seen, the production of specific antibodies in response to antigen challenge is multifactorial. Not only antigens and antibodies but also immune complexes can be detected by ELISA, and each will aid diagnosis. In general, free circulating antigen is present for shorter periods of time than free circulating antibody. Reinfection with the same pathogen or exacerbation will cause transient increases in free circulating antigen (antigenemia), followed by increased production of circulating antibodies. Both these events can be detected by ELISA, and the immunoassayist must be aware of this. Similarly, soluble immune complexes can be detected by ELISA, although the assay design is somewhat more complicated.

Because antigens of infectious disease agents stimulate the production of specific antibodies, the latter can be used in ELISAs as an indicator of infection. Normally the antibody response is long-lived and often is present in the absence of the inciting antigens. For this reason, the detection of antibodies in the host does not indicate the presence of a current infection, but does indicate exposure. Antibodies to some antigens are more persistent than are antibodies to other antigens and, in some instances, may persist for the lifetime of the individual. In such instances, the question, "is the host immune or refractory to reinfection?" cannot be answered by detecting antibodies to antigen mosaics of pathogens. Questions such as, "is the residual antibody effective in the prevention of reinfection?" can only be answered when the biological effects of these antibodies are known.

Effects such as neutralization, agglutination, attachment onto receptors to prevent intracellular localization, and lysis are well-known biological effects of antibodies on infectious disease agents. If the mechanism of immunity is known (i.e., the effect of antibody on the target antigens), and if the target antigens can be isolated, they can be used in ELISAs to monitor the rate of production and duration of protective antibody. Few of these assays are available at present, and therefore the immunoassayist must utilize other general phenomena associated with the development of the immune response. The following situations expand this idea.

5.8.1. Neonates

Maternal antibody of the IgG isotype is transmitted passively to neonates transplacentally and in the colostrum. Other isotypes are also found in colostrum and milk (IgA, IgM), but are not transmitted across the neonatal GI tract. Both IgM and IgG antibodies to antigen can be assayed for, and when IgG antibodies are present in the absence of IgM antibodies, the likelihood of them being passively transmitted is high. When humoral IgM antibodies occur, then the organism must be synthesizing them de novo. If antibodies are assayed for in other physiological compartments of the body (e.g., GI tract), these conclusions become invalid since both maternal IgM and IgA are secreted in milk and may still be biologically active as co-proantibodies.

5.8.2. Immunologically Competent Mammals

We have seen that IgM is the first isotype of humoral antibody produced in response to antigenic challenge and that if the challenge persists it is replaced by IgG isotype. If the infection is chronic and the antigen persists, or reexposure occurs, higher levels of IgG will be produced. This information is valuable to the immunoassayist because when total antibody (all isotypes) is assayed, an increase in antibody titer over time is indicative of a current infection. This is also true when isotype-specific second antisera are used. The comparison of IgM and IgG levels is also a useful indicator.

Persistent antigen induces an isotype switch in T-cell-dependent antigens, stimulating the production of IgG rather than IgM. If IgM and IgG levels to the same antigen are compared, the following can be deduced: IgM antibody in the absence of IgG antibody means there has been recent acquisition of infection in which no isotype switch has occurred as yet. IgM and IgG antibody present means prior acquisition of infection, in which isotype switch has occurred, with IgM response present but possibly declining. Prior acquisition of infection where isotype switch has occurred means that the host has become reexposed to the same antigen, stimulating the production of more IgM antibody.

IgG antibody in the absence of IgM antibody could mean the previous acquisition of infection, in which isotype switch has occurred, and the IgM response is below the assay detection level. In this case, the infection would be expected to be chronic.

When antigens are localized in the respiratory tract, the GI tract, or GU tract, stimulating local antibody responses, the detection of IgA antibody isotypes would be of value. Similarly, when it is known that pathogens stimulate isotype-specific responses (e.g., helminth), IgE-specific antibody responses can be assayed.

5.8.3. Herd Immunity

Each individual in a group has a varying potential to respond to antigens and hence to mount a protective immune response. The range of immune responses in a group follows a normal distribution pattern whereby the majority of individuals mount an average immune response, and a small proportion mount either a very effective immune response or an ineffective immune response. When vaccination or exposure to a pathogen is concerned, <100% of the population will be adequately protected, and for those individuals concerned, this lack of protection will be serious. This lack of protection may be owing to the inability to recognize antigens or to produce antibodies (agammaglobulinemia). These individuals can act as reservoirs of pathogens for future transmission to other susceptible individuals, and the seriousness of the situation will depend on the mode of transmission, the number of susceptible individuals, and in cases in which vaccination is common practice, the efficacy of vaccination.

Less than 100% protection may be sufficient to prevent the spread of the disease within the population, since the likelihood of a susceptible individual encountering an infected individual becomes reduced. This phenomenon is known as herd immunity and is an important consideration in assessing the potential of individuals in a population to succumb to infection.

Many factors can affect the quantity and quality of an immune response, most of which have been mentioned previously. Other factors that affect the immune response are stress, pregnancy, surgery, concomitant infections, extremes of temperature, and especially malnutrition. All these factors reduce the quantity and quality of the immune response, and when the immunoassayist performs seroepidemiological surveys to assess the herd immunity among various populations, these factors must be taken into account prior to determining levels of adequate protection within a population.

For each infectious disease, antibody levels (if any) in naive, subclinically infected, clinically infected, and immune individuals in the endemic population should be sought. Only in this way can the immunoassayist relate antibody levels to infection. Once these parameters are known, the effect of vaccination in these individuals can be assayed as well as the relationship between protective antibody and immunity.

One major problem is that individuals in an endemic area have had previous exposure of an infectious disease agent, or antigens thereof, and therefore ascribing an antibody titer or threshold above which protection occurs and below which reinfection occurs is difficult, if not impossible.

The situation becomes more complex when assessing the protective effects of vaccination in such a group of individuals. Often individual antibody levels are static owing to chronic exposure and variable owing to previously mentioned factors. In the instances in which naive individuals become immune, seroconversion occurs, but in the majority of instances where individuals have had previous exposure, increases in antibody levels are sought. These may be so small that they become statistically nonsignificant.

5.9. Antigenic Commonness

Because there is a limited number of amino acids and carbohydrates and so forth produced by living organisms, the number of combinations of these components is limited (for proteins and carbohydrates). Therefore, it is likely that different organisms will produce similar proteins, glycoproteins, and so on. When partial or complete similarities occur in the products of living organisms, a commonness in terms of antibody recognition occurs.

Structural proteins appear to be well conserved and would be expected to demonstrate immunological cross-reactivity. The nature of this cross-reactivity varies among similar antigenic molecules and depends on the ability of the paratope to fit the epitope.

We have already seen that the paratopes of antibodies will bind to epitopes that are recognized either completely or partially. The immunoassayist must consider the possibility that the same or similar antigens may exist in a variety of infectious agents. For example, many cell-surface antigens are carbohydrate in nature and the same epitopes may be present on two cell types, one of which may be pathogenic whereas the other may be a commensal.

Similarly, some carbohydrates may be present in widely differing infectious disease agents (e.g., blood group like, ascarone). When polyclonal antibodies are produced in response to infection, antibodies to non–cross-reactive as well as cross-reactive epitopes will be produced and hence the problem of cross-reactivity can be minimized.

The problem of antigenic commonness becomes more obvious when using mAbs in diagnosis. In the developmental stage of an assay, the immunoassayist must consider which other antigens, including antigens from other infectious disease agents, might be involved in cross-reactions and develop the assay accordingly, bearing in mind the type of problems associated with such cross-reactions.

6. Other Techniques

The performance of good immunoassays also requires practical expertise in immunochemical techniques (or at least theoretical knowledge of when such techniques are to be used). The following list provides some techniques of use in the purification and characterization of antigens and antibodies:

1. Sucrose density gradient centrifugation
2. Polyacrylamide gel electrophoresis (PAGE)
3. PAGE followed by immunoblotting
4. Isoelectric focusing
5. Immunodiffusion in agar/agarose
6. Gel chromatography (DEAE, affinity, sephadex)
7. Salt fractionation of IgG
8. Enzyme conjugation methods

The nature and preparation of antibody fractions and their relevance in disease and assay should also be examined (i.e., whole molecule, Fc, Fab, $F[ab']_2$, IgM, IgA).

7. Units

Successful assays depend on a good knowledge of units of volume and weight. The concepts of accuracy in dilutions and the relevance of pipetting methods also fall within the necessary practice needed for assays.

Table 2
Relationship of volumes in microtiter assays

Volume	Symbol	Cubic centimeter	Microliters
Liter	L	1000	1,000,000
Milliliter	mL	1	1000
Microliter	μL	0.001	1

Table 3
Relationship of weights.

Unit	Relationship to gram
Gram	1
Milligram	10^{-3}
Microgram	10^{-6}
Nanogram	10^{-9}
Picogram	10^{-12}
Femtogram	10^{-15}
Attogram	10^{-18}

7.1. Volumes

The pipets used in microtiter plate assays are graduated in microliters (μL). The relationship of volumes is given in **Table 2**.

7.2. Weights

Note the relationship of weights as given in **Table 3**.

8. Dilutions

Difficulties are often encountered in the making of dilutions. It is essential that great care be taken in making the correct dilution and that there be no wasting of expensive reagents through making up convenient dilutions into an unneeded final volume. For example, we may need to make up a 1/1,200 dilution of a sample already at a 1/50 dilution in a final volume of 5.5 mL. Often operators attempt to round up volumes so that larger than necessary volumes are made, which is waste of reagents (e.g., conjugates).

Other problems such as making a 1/20,000 dilution in a final small volume such as 3-mL arise.

All problems of dilution are eased if all volumes in the calculation are converted to microliters (μL). The following examples illustrate this.

8.1. Making a 1/100 Dilution of Neat Sample at a Final Vol ume of 10 mL

Neat infers a sample is undiluted. Thus, we require a final volume of 10 mL. Convert the required volume to microliters:

$$10 \times 1{,}000\,\mu\text{L} = 10{,}000\,\mu\text{L}$$

The dilution required is 1/100. Divide this into the required final volume:

$$10{,}000/100{=}1/100$$

This is the volume of neat (undiluted sample) to be added into the required volume in microliters, which is therefore 100 μL.

In this example there would be little difficulty in using microliters. Thus, 10 mL/100 = 0.1 μL. We would therefore add 100 μL of the neat sample to 9,900 μL (9.9 mL) of diluent (final volume minus the volume of the added neat sample). The conversion of the 0.1 mL into the units of the micropipet would then have to be made, i.e., 0.1 mL = 100 μL.

A slightly more complex calculation illustrates the benefit of initial conversion to microliters of all the volumes.

5.8.2. Making a 1/200 Dilution of a Neat Sample in a Final Volume of 4 mL

Convert the required volume to microliters = 4 mL = 4,000 μL. The dilution factor is 200. Therefore, we need 4,000 μL/200 μL = 20 μL of neat sample. (A check on such calculations should always be made.) Thus, the dilution factor × volume of sample being diluted should equal the required volume. We therefore have 200 × 20 μL = 4,000 μL (4.0 mL). Note here by that using milliliters, we would have 4/200 = 0.02 mL. This becomes a little more difficult to relate to the microliter setting of the micropipets.

8.3. Calculating a Diluted Sample

When a sample is already diluted, we have to include this in the calculation. Thus, we have an already diluted sample at 1/50. We require a final dilution of 1/1,000 in a final volume of 20 mL.

This type of calculation causes most problems. Convert the required volume to microliters. The final volume required = 20 mL = 20,000 μL. The dilution factor required is 1,000.

Now, assume the sample was not already diluted. Then we would add 20,000/1,000 = 20 μL of neat sample. Therefore, since the sample is already diluted 1/50, we have to add more. The factor is determined by the known dilution factor (50); so we multiply the value for undiluted sample by this factor:

$$20\,\mu L \times 50 = 1{,}000\,\mu L$$

This may seem obvious, but taking a more complex dilution.

8.4. Dilution of a Final Volume

We require a 1/18,000 dilution in a final volume of 27 mL. We already have a dilution of the sample at 1/25. By converting to microliters we have a required final volume of 27,000 μL. Assume the sample was undiluted, then we would require 27,000/18,000 = 1.5 μL. Since it is already diluted, multiply 1.5 μL by the dilution factor:

$$1.5 \times 25 = 37.5\,\mu L$$

Check: 18,000 × 37.5/25 = 27,000 μL = 27 mL. When high dilutions are needed in small volumes, it may be necessary to make up a limited dilution series to avoid wasting reagents.

8.5. Requiring a High Dilution

Direct addition of the undiluted sample would require 5,000/100,000 = 0.05 μL. This volume is impossible to pipet. For most practical purposes, the pipetting of volumes < 5μL is not recommended. The high dilution just given can be achieved by two manipulations. There are alternatives, and these are governed by the availability of the reagent being diluted. If it is available in only small volumes, then the initial volume used to make the first dilution can be made small. Thus, a 1/100 dilution can be made into 1,000 μL by adding 10 μL of neat sample to 990 μL of diluent. Calculating the amount of this 1/100 dilution to be diluted as required in a final volume of 5 mL, we have 5,000/100,000 × 100 (the already produced dilution factor) = 5 μL. Thus, by adding an initial dilution into 1 mL of buffer, we can produce high dilutions using acceptable pipetting volumes.

8.6. Reviewing of Method for Dilution

Determine the final volume required and convert this to microliters.

1. Divide this by the dilution factor. This is the sample volume to be added to the final volume of diluent in microliters.
2. When there has been predilution of the sample, follow **steps 1** and **2**, and then multiply the predilution factor by the volume found in **step 2**.
3. When high dilutions are needed, make two or three dilutions of sample in small volumes.

8.7. Compensation of Volumes

Since we require a final volume (calculated in **stage 1** of **Subheading 8.6**), the addition of sample will obviously increase the final volume. As an extreme example, we may require a 1/10 dilution of a sample in 1 mL. This means adding 100 μL to a final volume of 1 mL. Following the procedures in **Subheadings 8.1– 8.6**, we would end up with a volume of 1,100 μL. Thus, this would not achieve an accurate 1/10 dilution – rather 1/11. The obvious course is to compensate for the addition of the sample volume by removing this from the final volume calculation. Thus, in the same example, the final volume required is 1,000 µL and the sample volume calculated is 100 µL. Therefore, we need to remove 100 µL of diluent to compensate for the extra 100 µL of sample added, and so we need 900 µL of diluent plus 100 µL of sample to achieve a perfect 1/10.

The accuracy then of the dilution depends on removing the sample volume from the final volume. However, this depends on the actual volume to be added. As an example, we may require a final dilution of 1/100 in 1 mL. Thus, we need a final volume of 1,000 µL and need to add 10 µL of sample. Here, we could compensate by removing 10 µL of diluent before adding the 10 µL of sample, but, in terms of accuracy, we can see that the difference between the dilutions with and without compensation are minimal. Hence, with compensation we have a dilution of 10/1,000 = 1/100, and without compensation, we have a dilution of 10/1,010 = 1/101. Effectively there is no practical difference.

8.7.1. When to Compensate

There can be no exact rule about when to compensate because there may be occasions in which the activity of a sample is affected by a very small difference in dilution. However, this is not usually true in ELISA, and as a strong guideline I suggest that when the volume of the sample being added is >2% of the required volume, compensation should always be used. Thus, to make a 1/200 dilution, 5 µL can be added to 1,000 µL (0.5%), 10 µL can be added to 1,000 µL (1%), 20 µL can be added to 1,000 µL (2%), 40 µL should be added to 960 µL.

9. Pipets

As in all assays, accurate pipetting is vitally important to obtain consistent results. Examine the multichannel pipet. It can be of fixed volume (dispensing a fixed specified volume) or of variable volume. For variable-volume pipets, the volume delivered can be adjusted by turning the knob at the top of the pipet so that the volume read on the side of the pipet handle is altered. These are digital pipets: The volume is shown as a number on the side in microliters.

Practice setting up different volumes. Remember to note where the comma (denoting the decimal point) is. Thus, 200 = 200 µL and 20.0 = 20 µL.

Some pipet volumes are altered using a vernier scale. Follow the instructions provided by the manufacturer. Generally these are not recommended because it is easier to make mistakes with them, and the scale tends to wear. Multichannel pipets are designed to deliver 4, 8, or 12 volume simultaneously, and therefore are ideal for microtiter plates. The pipets having 12 channels offer highest flexibility in that up to 12 channels can be utilized. Any number of the channels can be loaded with a tip (up to 12). This fact often confuses workers when they first encounter such pipets. Practice the pipetting action and putting on tips.

9.1. Pipg Action

Remember always to use the pipet whose maximum volume is nearest to the volume you require. All pipets should be calibrated on a routine basis (every month). Techniques for performing calibrations can be obtained from commercial companies supplying the pipets. Some companies also provide a calibration service. Special calibration tips with precise volumes marked on the outside allow routine examination of the volumes being dispensed. Pipets should also be checked for damage.

9.1.1. Picking Up Solutions

Press the button on top of the pipet to the first stop before you put tips in solution, and then place tips in solution. Release the button steadily. You will notice that a volume of liquid is taken up into each tip. Check that each tip has the same volume. If not, expel the liquid after noting which tip was "low" in volume. Press that tip on harder. Repeat the pipetting.

9.1.2. Dispensing Solutions

Put the points of the tips in the wells resting on the sides of the plastic, if possible. Press the knob to the first stop. Solution will be expelled; try to pull the tips out up the side of the wells. When you have finished, either pull the tips off by hand or press the tip ejector on the side of the pipet; this works with some tips but not others.

9.1.3. Single-Channel Pipets

Single-channel pipets are used to deliver single volumes of solution, particularly for small volumes. These can be the vernier or digital type, fixed or variable volumes.

9.1.4. Troughs

Reservoirs for liquid dispensing by multichannel pipets are used as reservoirs (containers) for the solutions in the ELISA for multichannel pipets. These can be homemade or commercial, and either single or multiple troughs. Some are only suitable for eight channels.

9.2. Pipetting Exercise

To get used to the pipets, perform some simple exercises in making dilution series in microtiter plates. The following materials are needed:

1. Multichannel pipet
2. Trough
3. Tips

4. Solution of dye (e.g., phenol red in water, trypan blue)
5. Water

Making a dilution series is highly important in immunoassay. In most cases, multiple dilution ranges can be made using the multichannel pipets. A dilution series is given next.

For a twofold dilution series, in 50-μL volume, add 50 μL of the substance to be diluted to 50 μL of diluent, mix, transfer 50 μL of this dilution to another 50 μL of diluent, and repeat to the required range.

In microtiter plates, the required volume of diluent is dispensed in the wells with the multichannel pipet. The substance being titrated is added either at the starting dilution (in the test volume) to the first well and to the second well as an equal volume of the starting dilution plus the volume of diluent in the well, or to the first row only in the test volume with the sample at twice the required initial concentration into the test volume of diluent. The solution in the first or second row is then mixed using the multichannel pipet, and the test volume is transferred to the next well containing the test volume of diluent, using the pipetting action of the multichannel pipet.

The process is repeated over all wells, each containing the test volume of diluent. In most cases, carryover of reagent can be ignored when the same tips are used for the dilution series. Thus any number of dilution series up to 12 rows (8 dilutions) or 8 rows (12 dilutions) can be prepared simply. Thus, for the exercise, the steps are as follows:

1. Add 50 μL of diluent (water) to each well of a plate.
2. Add 50 μL of dye solution to the first row (A–H) of the plate using a multichannel pipet.
3. Mix by pipetting action (first stop only used to avoid frothing).
4. Transfer 50 mL of diluted dye from row 2 to 3, and mix.
5. Transfer 50 μL from row 3 to 4, and mix.
6. Repeat to row 12.

We now have 8 rows (A–H) of the same dilution range of the dye. This is a twofold range (equal volumes transferred) from 1/2, 1/4, 1/8, and so on, to 1/4,096. You can make any fold dilution range provided the volumes you transfer are effectively large enough to be pipetted and mixed after transfer.

Examine the dilution range to ensure that the rows appear as if they have the same volume and that there is a logical dilution effect along the rows. Discard the first attempt, throw dye into sink, wash the plate under the tap, blot the plate dry, and repeat.

Try the following dilution ranges:

1. A threefold dilution range: 50-μL volume (25 μL carried over into 50 μL of diluent).
2. A fourfold dilution range: 50-μL volume (~17 μL carried over into 51 μL).
3. A fivefold dilution range: 60-μL volume (15 μL carried over into 60 μL).
4. A tenfold dilution range: 100-μL volume (11 μL carried over into 110 μL).
5. A fivefold dilution range: 100-μL volume (25 μL carried over into 100 μL).

9.2.1. Effect of Different Dilution Series

The choice of which dilution range to use depends on what activities are being titrated. Thus, if there is a large quantity of antibody in a serum, then a high dilution is necessary in order to assess this.

Preliminary experiments to assess ELISAs often involve the titration of reagents of unknown strengths. In such cases, the appropriate selection of dilution ranges is important. It is simple to make two-, three-, and fourfold dilution ranges, but what are the advantages? **Table 4** gives the effective dilutions of a sample using the different ranges over eight wells (eight dilution steps) and illustrates the ranges of dilutions covered by each.

This shows that a simple adjustment of diluting range markedly increases the dilution of samples. The three- or fourfold range is convenient in that the range titrates samples at relatively high concentration. Thus, low-titre samples might be observed but it is also useful in case samples have high titers. In the case of the twofold range a high-titer sample would show color across all the wells and no titer would be indicated. Preliminary experiments can be followed with the most suitable ranges according to the titer established as in **Table 4**.

Table 4
Dilutions obtained using different dilution series

	Dilutions Produced[a]							
Range	1	2	3	4	5	6	7	8
Twofold range	2	4	8	16	32	64	128	256
Threefold range	3	9	27	81	243	729	2,178	6,534
Fourfold range	4	16	64	256	1,024	4,096	16,384	65,536

[a]1-8 indicates the well number

10. Molarities

To make up a 1 M solution of a compound, we take the molecular weight of that compound in grams and dissolve this to 1 L (final volume) of liquid (usually distilled water).

Thus, the molecular weight of a particular compound must be calculated from the atomic formula or read off the reagent bottle. Take a simple example of sodium chloride (NaCl). The molecular weight is 58.5. Therefore, 58.5 g made up to 1 L in distilled water represents a 1 M solution. A 0.1 M solution would contain 58.5/10 = 5.85 g/L.

Often we do not require a large volume so that 100 mL of a 1 M solution of NaCl would contain 5.85 g of NaCl since 1 L of 1 M contains 58.5 g, and 100 mL = 1/10 L. Therefore, we require ten times less NaCl.

Another way to calculate this is to always calculate the amount of chemical needed to give the required molarity per milliliter. Thus, 1 M= 58.5 g/L = 0.0585 g/mL. If we require 50 mL at 1 M, we therefore require 50 × 0.0585 g made up to 50 mL. This helps calculation of more difficult molarities.

For example, we require a 0.125 M solution of NaCl in 35 mL. Calculate the number of grams per milliliters at the required molarity: 1 M= 58.5 g/L and 0.125 M= 58.5/8 (0.125 M/1 M) = 7.35 g/L = 0.0073 g/mL. We require a final volume of 35 mL. Therefore, 35 × 0.0073 = 0.256 g = 2.57 g (rounded up).

For 2 M solutions, we require twice the weight of that required for a 1 M solution, which is 117 g/L in the case of NaCl. If we require 17 mL of a 2 M solution of NaCl, 1 M NaCl = 58.5 g/L and 2 M NaCl = 117.0 g/L = 117/1,000 = 0.117 g/mL. We need 17 mL = 0.117 × 17 = 1.99 g.

Again, a fraction of a molarity is best calculated by assessing needs per mL; for example, we require a 0.15 M solution of NaCl in 25 mL. Therefore, 1 M NaCl = 58.5 g/L, 1.5 M= 1.5 × 58.5 g/L = 87.75 g/L, and 0.15 M = 87.5/10 = 8.75 g/L =.0088 g/mL. Hence, we need 25 mL = 25 × 0.0088 g = 0.22 g.

Sometimes molarities are expressed in millimolar quantities, e.g., 100, 10, 30 mM. One millimolar = 1/1,000 M. Thus, for NaCl, 58.5/1,000 = 0.0585 g/L = 1 mM.

Hence, a 10 mM solution contains 0.585 g/L, and a 100 mM solution contains 5.85 g/L.

References

1. Harlow, E., and Lane, D., eds. (1988) *Antibodies – A Laboratory Manual*, Cold Spring Harbor Laboratory Press, Cold Spring Harbor, NY.
2. Catty, D., ed. (1988) *Antibodies – A Practical Approach, Volume I*, IRL Press, Oxford, England.
3. Catty, D., ed. (1988) *Antibodies – A Practical Approach, Volume II*, IRL Press, Oxford, England.
4. Linscott, W.D.(1982)Linscott's Directory of Immunological and Biological Reagents, Linscott's Catalog, Mill Valley, CA.

Chapter 6

Practical Exercises

The aim of this chapter is to illustrate the principles of ELISA by *(1)* showing worked examples of each assay, including diagrams of plates and representational data from assays, *(2)* analyzing such data in terms of important rules that are learned at each stage, and *(3)* providing full working instructions for investigators to perform each assay so that they obtain their own data to be analyzed.

This chapter can be used in several ways. First, researchers without access to reagents will obtain a working knowledge of ELISA through the examples. Second, it can be used in training courses in which reagents may be provided (as indicated in the text). Third, the information will be useful for investigators who have already had some experience with the technique but may have had difficulties in obtaining and analyzing data.

Remember that it is the application of ELISA to specific problems, and not the methodology for its own sake, that is the most important reason the techniques should be mastered.

1. Test Schemes

You are already familiar with the concepts in ELISA, whereby an antigen binds to an antibody that can be labeled with an enzyme or, in turn can be detected with a species-specific antibody (enzyme labeled). All ELISAs described are variations on this theme. Inherent in the methods of ELISA is the attachment of one of the reagents to a solid phase, making the separation of bound (reacted) and unbound (nonreacted) reagents simple by a washing step. Before performing ELISA on disease agents, it is useful to train operators on how to use reagents of defined reactivity, which are easily available and which provide security problems. An ideal system is to use an immunoglobulin (Ig) –more particularly,

John R. Crowther, *Methods in Molecular Biology, The ELISA Guidebook, Vol. 516*

DOI: 10.1007/978-1-60327-254-4_6

an immunoglobulin G (IgG)–as an antigen. Do not get confused as you have learnt that the antibody population contains high levels of IgG acting as antibody. In the context of learning the principles, we are using IgG as an antigenic protein, because, *(1)* IgG from one animal species can be injected into another animal species so that a specific antiserum to that IgG is prepared; and, *(2)* such antibodies can be labeled with enzyme, or detected with a second species-specific antibody labeled with enzyme.

Such reagents are defined, easy to standardize, stable, and available commercially. The particular IgG system chosen in this chapter involves the guinea pig, but similar tests can be performed with IgG from other species using appropriate anti-species reagents. Systems described are analogous to the ones most commonly used to examine problems associated with diagnosis.

The schemes are described as symbols and as practical exercises in full as follows:

I= solid-phase microtiter plate well Ag = antigen Ag1, Ag2, etc. = particular antigens highlighted I-Ag = antigen passively attached to solid phase I-Ab, I-AB = particular antibodies passively coated to wells Ab = antibody AB = antibody from a different species to Ab Ab_X, Ab_Y = different antibodies identified by subscript letters Anti-Ab = anti-species specific antibody (species in which Ab was made) Anti-Ab*E = anti-species-specific antibody labeled with enzyme
W = washing step

+ = addition of reagents and incubation step

S= substrate/chromophore addition

R= reading the test in spectrophotometer.

Many of the practical steps are similar. The conjugates used are all horseradish peroxidase (HRP) and the substrate/chromophore is H_2O_2/*ortho*-phe-nylenediamine (OPD). The following practical details are helpful:

1. Substrate/chromophore. The easiest method is to use commercial tablets that are pre-weighed. Citrate/phosphate tablets can also be purchased (pH 5.0). Commercial preparations of this substrate/chromophore are available and require addition of only water. I recommend 30-mg tablets, which make 75 mL of solution in buffer. Unused OPD solution (without added hydrogen peroxide) can be stored at –20°C but should be examined closely for discoloration on thawing. Use the completely mixed solution as soon as possible. All liquids should be at optimal temperature. The hydrogen peroxide can be purchased as 3 or 6% solution and should be stored as instructed by the suppliers. Tablets of urea/peroxide can also be obtained and used to make up a stock of hydrogen peroxide of defined strength rather than purchasing liquid that has

certain transportation restrictions. Hydrogen peroxide should be added to the required concentration just before addition to wells; for example, add 5 μL of hydrogen peroxide (30% w/v) to every 10 mL of OPD solution (in citrate phosphate buffer pH 5.0) or 25 μL of 6% (w/v) hydrogen peroxide. It is imperative that the strength of the hydrogen peroxide be accurate.

2. The washing solution is phosphate-buffered saline (PBS) without addition of Tween-20. Washing requires addition and emptying of wells four times.
3. The blocking buffer is PBS containing a final concentration of 1% bovine serum albumin (BSA) and 0.05% Tween-20. This should be made in volumes necessary to complete tests as required, but can be stored at 4°C if contamination is avoided; it should always be warmed and inspected for contamination before use.
4. The stopping solution is 1 M sulfuric acid, and care should be taken in its preparation. It can be stored at room temperature.
5. Read implies using a multichannel spectrophotometer to assess the optical density (OD) values of plates and is in all cases in this chapter read at 492 nm. Plates should also be inspected by eye before reading, to determine whether there are gross errors and whether results are feasible.

1.1. Direct ELISA: Titration of Antigen and Antibody

1.1.1. Learning Principles

1. Measuring optimum concentration of antigen to coat wells.
2. Measuring optimum dilution of enzyme-linked antibody.
3. Using multichannel and single-channel micropipets.
4. Revising principles of dilution.
5. Making up and storing of buffers and solutions.
6. Learning to observe tests by eye and by using multichannel spectrophotometers.
7. Handling data.
8. Solving problems.

1.1.2. Reaction Scheme

$$\text{I-Ag}_{\text{W}} + \text{An*E}_{\text{W}} + \text{S} \text{ —READ}$$

where I = microplate wells (solid phase); Ag = guinea pig IgG adsorbed to wells; Ab*E = rabbit anti-guinea pig conjugated with HRP enzyme; S = H_2O_2 + OPD (chromophore); READ = observing by eye or reading with spectrophotometer (before or after stopping color development with H_2SO_4); + = addition of reagent and incubation at 37°C or room temperature for 1 h; and W = wash wells in PBS (four times).

1.1.3 Basis of Assay

The basis of this assay is to dilute the Ag across the plate one way in a buffer that allows passive adsorption, incubate the plate at 37°C or room temperature for 2 h, wash it and then dilute the conjugate across the plate, the opposite way to the Ag, obtaining a checkerboard titration (CBT) of Ag against Ab*. The Ab*E is diluted in a buffer to prevent nonspecific adsorption of the Ab*E to any free protein binding sites on the wells. After washing, all the wells receive a solution containing the substrate for the enzyme (H_2O_2) and a chromophore which can change color if the H_2O_2 is acted on by the enzyme. Thus, the color developing in each well depends on (1) the amount of antigen, and (2) the amount of conjugate that has bound to that antigen. The more conjugate, the more enzyme, and color.

1.1.4 Materials and Equipment

1. Ag: guinea-pig IgG in PBS at 1 mg/mL
2. Anti-guinea pig IgG prepared in rabbits conjugated to HRP
3. 96-well microplate for ELISA
4. 12-channel (tipped) micropipet (5–50 μL)
5. Single-channel micropipet (5–50 μL) plus tips and trough
6. 10- and 1-mL pipets
7. Carbonate/bicarbonate buffer, pH 9.5, 0.05 M
8. PBS containing 10% bovine serum albumin (BSA), 0.05% Tween-20
9. Solution of OPD in citrate buffer
10. Bottle of hydrogen peroxide (30% W/V, from 4°C)
11. Washing solution (PBS) reservoir
12. 1 M sulfuric acid in water
13. Paper towels or thin flat sponge
14. Small-volume bottles
15. Multichannel spectrophotometer
16. Clock
17. Graph paper

1.1.5. Practical Details

1. Examine a plate; note the position of letters A–H and the numbers 1–12. Place the plate with A at the top left-hand corner in front of you, as in **Fig. 1**. The 8 wells labeled with letters (A–H) are referred to as rows. The 12 wells labeled by numbers (1–12) are referred to as columns.
2. Use the 12-channel pipet with 12 tips to add 50 μL of carbonate buffer to each well of the plate. Use a trough to act as a reservoir for the buffer, and add 6 mL to give extra volume needed for the whole plate.

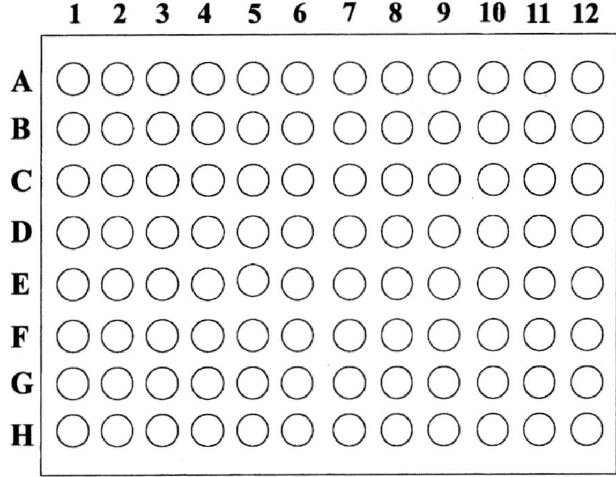

Fig. 1. Numbering and lettering on microtiter plate.

3. Dilute the antigen (1 mg/mL) to 10 µg/mL in carbonate buffer. Make up 1 mL of the antigen at this concentration; that is, add 1 mL of buffer to a small bottle. Pipet 10 µL of antigen into this. Mix well by manually rotating thebottle .(do not be over vigorous).
4. Set a single-channel micropipet to 50 µL. Add 50 µL of diluted antigen to all the wells of column 1. You should now have 100 µL of antigen in column 1.
5. Put tips into column 1, and mix the contents by pipetting up and down eight times, using the first stop of the pipet. Transfer 50 µL to column 2 (A–H), mix, and transfer 50 µL to column 3, and so on, to column 11. After the last mixing, discard the 50 µL left in the pipet. You should now have 50 µL of a dilution series in each row, ending with column 11. Check by eye the volumes are similar in all the wells (*see* **Fig. 2**).
6. Cover the plate with a lid and leave it on the bench (flat surface) for 2 h at room temperature, or at 37°C for 2 h or, if more convenient, leave it at 4°C overnight.
7. Wash the plate. The exact method depends on the equipment used. The principle is to discard the contents of the wells by "flicking" them into a sink (or suitable container bowl), then adding PBS and flicking this away four times. The major concern is that all the wells are filled at each stage.
8. Turn the plates onto absorbent paper (sponge), and remove most of the residual PBS by gently tapping the plates against the paper (picking the plate up to do this, well openings down).

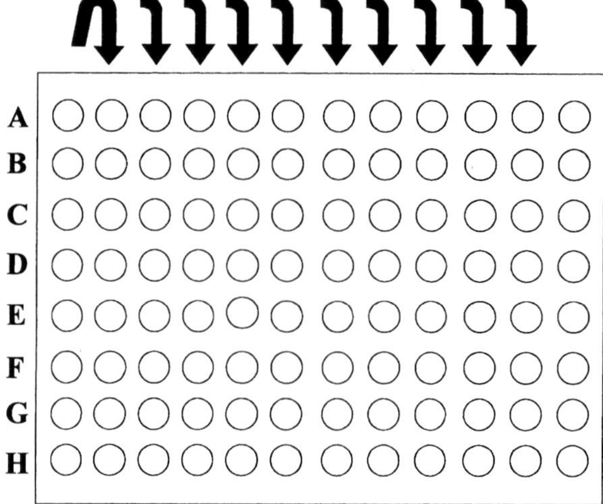

Fig. 2. Dilution of antigen across plate from columns 1 to 11.

9. To add the dilutions of conjugate, take the enzyme conjugate from the refrigerator. Check that it is rabbit anti-guinea pig IgG, conjugated to HRP (there may be variations in the particular species used to prepare the anti-guinea pig serum labeled; e.g., it could be sheep anti-guinea pig IgG). Make up 1 mL of a 1/200 dilution of the conjugate in a 5-mL bottle. Use the 5–50-μL single-channel pipet to add the conjugate: that is, add 5 μL of conjugate to 1 mL of blocking buffer. (**Note:** We do not wish to have any nonspecific adsorption of the conjugate to the plastic during the test.) Mix well by gentle swirling action; do not shake vigorously. Add 50 μL of blocking buffer to every well of the microplate using the multichannel pipet fitted with 12 tips. This is accomplished by adding about 6 mL of blocking buffer to a trough and pipetting from this. Wash the trough, after dispensing the blocking buffer, using tap water (or PBS). Dry the trough for use with conjugate with paper towel. Pour the conjugate dilution into a trough. Using the multichannel pipet with 12 tips attached, add 50 μL of the conjugate dilution into the first row (A, 1–12) of the plate. Thus, there is 100 μL of a 1/400 dilution of conjugate in this row. Mix using the multichannel pipet (eight times up and down). Transfer 50 μL of the conjugate from row A to B (1–12), and mix in row B (eight times). Transfer 50 μL to row C (1–12) and mix. Repeat the transfer of dilutions to the end of the plate (row H). There should now be 50 μL of conjugate dilutions in all wells, at a dilution range from 1/400 in row A to 1/51,200 in row H. This is diagrammatically shown in **Fig. 3**. Thus, a CBT has been performed relating to how the antigen and antibody have been diluted. Cover the plate and leave at room temperature for 1 h, or at 37°C for 1 h.

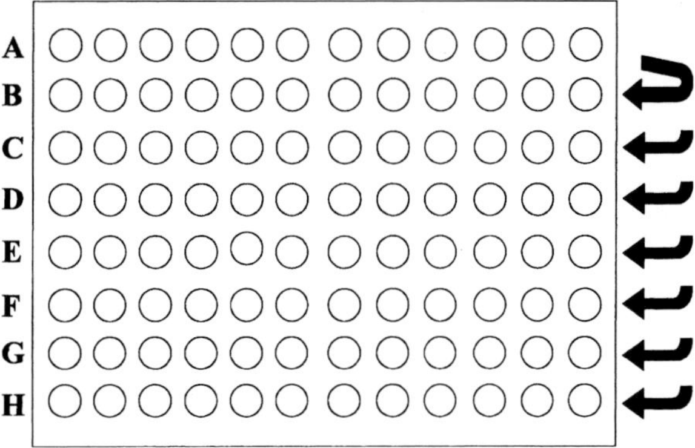

Fig. 3. Dilution of antibody from row A to H.

10. Wash the plate and flick free from excess washing solution (*see* **step** 7).
11. To add substrate/chromophore for color development, thaw 10 mL of citrate buffer containing OPD in a water bath or at room temperature (slower), or make up OPD solution from tablets. Ensure that the solution reaches an acceptable temperature, i.e., room temperature if this is fairly constant in your laboratory. It is a good idea to have a water bath at a temperature of 20°C and use this to equilibrate the OPD solution to achieve a standardized temperature, since this affects the rate of color development of the ELISA. Add 5 µL of hydrogen peroxide (30%)/10 mL of OPD. (Immediately, put this back in the refrigerator with a top screwed on tightly.) Mix gently. Pour the solution into a trough (must be washed and free of any previous reagents). Use a multichannel pipet to add 50 µL of solution to each well (8 or 12 tips used).
12. Leave the plate on the bench and examine color changes at ~1, 3, 5, 8, and 10 min after addition.
13. Add 50 µL of a 1 M solution of sulfuric acid in water (supplied) to each well after 10 min of color development (use a clean trough and multichannel pipets again) to stop color development.
14. Read the plate by eye and use a spectrophotometer.

1.1.6. Explanation of Data

Figure 4 is a diagrammatic representation of plates set up using the reagents as described, at different times before color development has been stopped. **Table 1** gives an assessment by eye of the development of color. **Table 2** presents the OD results for the plate stopped at 10 min. These results are analyzed graphically in **Fig. 5** and relate the color developing in the wells with different antigen-coating concentrations for different dilutions of anti-species conjugate.

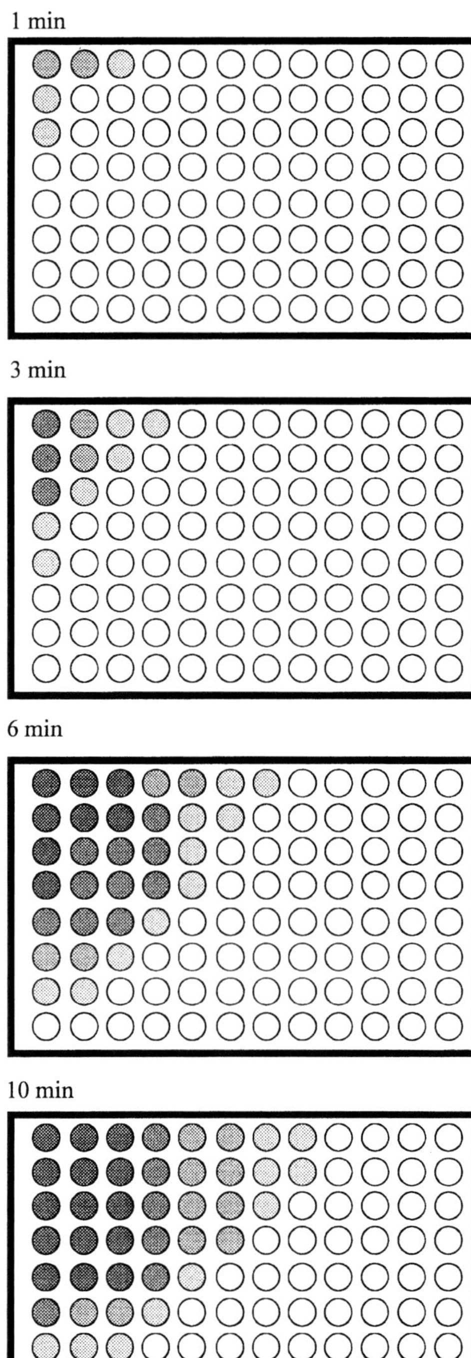

Fig. 4. Representation of color development at 1, 3, 6, and 10 min.

Table 1
Assessment of plates by eye

	1	2	3	4	5	6	7	8	9	10	11	12
Observed at 1 min												
A	+	+	–	–	–	–	–	–	–	–	–	–
B	+	+–	–	–	–	–	–	–	–	–	–	–
c	+	–	–	–	–	–	–	–	–	–	–	–
D	–	–	–	–	–	–	–	–	–	–	–	–
E	–	–	–	–	–	–	–	–	–	–	–	–
F	–	–	–	–	–	–	–	–	–	–	–	–
G	–	–	–	–	–	–	–	–	–	–	–	–
H	–	–	–	–	–	–	–	–	–	–	–	–
Observed at 3 min												
A	++	++	++	+	+	–	–	–	–	–	–	–
B	++	+	+	+	–	–	–	–	–	–	–	–
C	++	+	+	+–	–	–	–	–	–	–	–	–
D	+	+	+	+	–	–	–	–	–	–	–	–
E	+	+	+	–	–	–	–	–	–	–	–	–
F	+	–	–	–	–	–	–	–	–	–	–	–
G	–	–	–	–	–	–	–	–	–	–	–	–
H	–	–	–	–	–	–	–	–	–	–	–	–
Observed at 6 min												
A	++	++	++	++	++	++	+	+	+–	–	–	–
B	++	++	++	++	++	+	+–	–	–	–	–	–
C	++	++	++	++	++–	–	–	–	–	–	–	–
D	++	++	+–	–	–	–	–	–	–	–	–	–
E	+	+	–	–	–	–	–	–	–	–	–	–
F	+	+	–	–	–	–	–	–	–	–	–	–
G	–	–	–	–	–	–	–	–	–	–	–	–
H	–	–	–	–	–	–	–	–	–	–	–	–
Observed at 10 min												
A	++	++	++	++	++	++	++	++	+	+–	+–	–
B	++	++	++	++	++	++	+	+	–	–	–	–

(continued)

Table 1
(continued)

	1	2	3	4	5	6	7	8	9	10	11	12
C	++	++	++	++	++	+	+	–	–	–	–	–
D	++	++	++	++	+–	–	–	–	–	–	–	–
E	++	++	+	+	+–	–	–	–	–	–	–	–
F	+	+	+	–	–	–	–	–	–	–	–	–
G	+	+–	–	–	–	–	–	–	–	–	–	–
H	+	–	–	–	–	–	–	–	–	–	–	–

no detectable color; +– weak color; + definite color; ++ strong color

Table 2
OD results for plate stopped at 10 min

	1	2	3	4	5	6	7	8	9	10	11	12
A	1.89	1.88	1.67	1.34	1.10	0.97	0.86	0.57	0.44	0.32	0.31	0.31
B	1.87	1.86	1.63	1.29	1.04	0.93	0.84	0.53	0.35	0.24	0.23	0.21
C	1.68	1.45	1.32	1.14	0.96	0.86	0.64	0.45	0.29	0.19	0.17	0.16
D	1.14	1.03	0.94	0.83	0.57	0.45	0.38	0.29	0.19	0.18	0.15	0.16
E	0.99	0.91	0.74	0.54	0.46	0.36	0.29	0.19	0.18	0.15	0.13	0.14
F	0.66	0.44	0.39	0.33	0.24	0.21	0.19	0.15	0.18	0.16	0.14	0.12
G	0.34	0.20	0.16	0.18	0.16	0.18	0.15	0.16	0.14	0.12	0.14	0.13
H	0.21	0.22	0.15	0.18	0.17	0.15	0.13	0.14	0.15	0.13	0.12	0.12

Fig. 5 and **Table 2**, show the optimal dilution of conjugate that might be used in ELISA to detect guinea pig IgG. Also, the respective antigen concentration that might be used to detect antibodies (highly relevant in the indirect ELISA and explained fully in **Subheading 2**) can be observed. These figures provide individuals who have never seen an ELISA, an idea what to expect, and can be used as a comparison with their test results. They are also useful to those who obtain the text without access to reagents, in that it allows them to work through the examples without the need for setting-up an actual assay. Individuals who have performed an assay following the protocols in **Subheading 1.1**, can apply the observations on their plate to those demonstrated, and compare them critically.

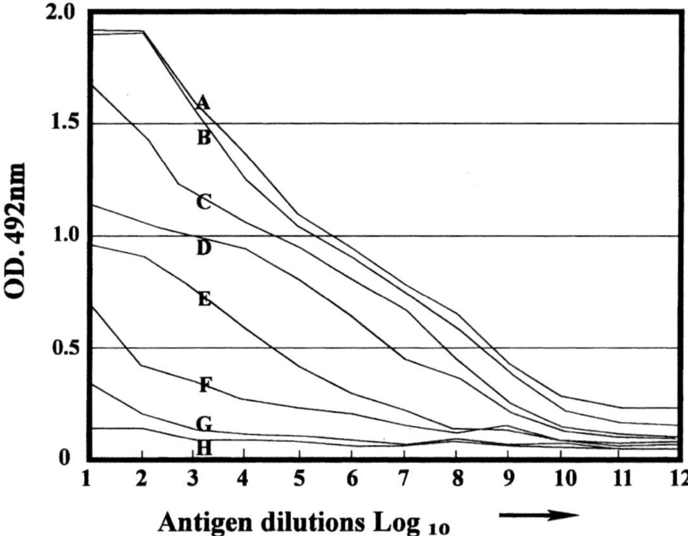

Fig. 5. Titration curves for conjugates against different dilutions of antigen (IgG) on columns 1–11 of plate.

1.1.7. Aspects of the Described Assay

Little happens during the first 30 s–1 min after the addition of substrate. Color then is detected in wells 1–3 of rows A and B and possibly C. The strongest color is detected in the wells containing the highest concentrations of antigen. By 3 min, the pattern should be confirmed, with detectable color in rows C–E. After 6 min, there is stronger color in rows A–D, all showing a gradual reduction in color as the antigen is diluted across the plate. The wells showing no color (no detectable antibody) for rows A, B, C, D, E, F, and G are 10, 9, 8, 6, 4, 3, and all rows, respectively.

At 10 min (the time for stopping color development), there is little change in the pattern, although intensity of the color may have increased. Note that there may be some color in the negative control well (12 at the strongest concentration of the conjugate). Also note the color change on addition of sulfuric acid (stopping).

1.1.8. Plate Reader Data

Now let us discuss the following factors:

1. Plateau height
2. Background, nonspecific adsorption of conjugate
3. Plate background

The color changes associated with each well have now been quantified, so that the exact situation can be assessed as shown in **Fig. 6**. Each line represents titration of a different dilution of conjugate against the same dilution range of antigen. Note that rows A and B are quite similar. Wells 1 and 2, have similar color, with no decrease in color when the antigen concentration is supposedly being decreased on the plate. This represents a plateau

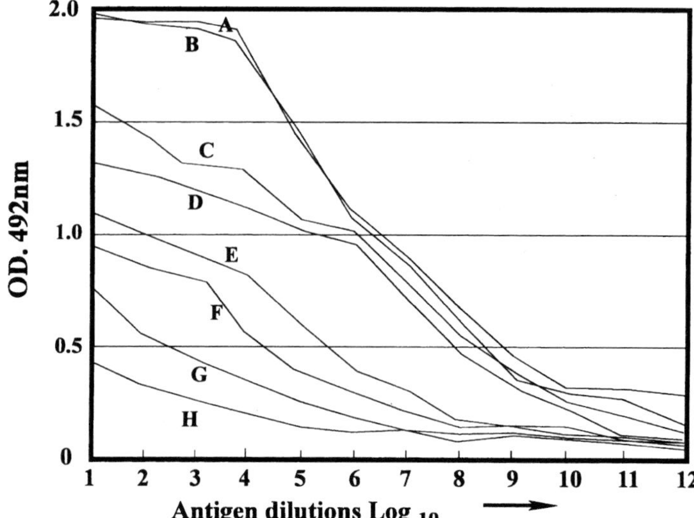

Fig. 6. Indirect ELISA: titration curves for anti-guinea pig serum dilutions (A–H) against different dilutions of antigen (IgG) on columns 1–11 of plate.

region (constant high color). Thus, the plate wells have similar amount of antigen as judged by the developing color which means that at antigen levels higher than those of well 2, no more antigen can attach to the plastic of the wells, due to the binding capacity of the plastic which may vary from protein to protein.

From well 3 in rows A and B, the color decreases, corresponding to the dilution of antigen on the wells. Note that A10–A12 show a similar color (around 0.31). This represents the end point of the titration at the respective conjugate dilutions of 1/400.

Although row B shows similar titration range, note that the color in rows 10–12 are similar to each other but lower than for row A. In particular, note well 12 for row B. This is the well that has no antigen, so the color developing in this row represents nonspecific adsorption of conjugate.

The color diminishes in column 12 as the conjugate is diluted (e.g., C12 = 0.16), and then stays at the same level. The conclusion here is that the 1/400 and 1/800 dilutions of conjugate cause some problems of nonspecific adsorption There is no further problem below these dilutions. The residual level of color, independent of the dilution of conjugate, is the plate background and is the result of change in color of the substrate independent of there being any enzymatic activity (oxidation owing to air and effect of light).

Row C shows good titration (high levels of color where there is antigen to low levels of color on antigen dilution) range of color. The end point of the titration is around well 9 (last dilution showing color above the plate background), which is similar to rows A and B (since their backgrounds are higher).

Row D also shows good titration of antigen, although the color is weaker, and the end-point is now around well 8. This indicates that some sensitivity is being lost in the titration of the antigen at this conjugate dilution. Wells E–G demonstrate loss in sensitivity on dilution of the conjugate, in particular well G, in which there is virtually no titration of the antigen.

1.1.9. Optimal Dilutions

We now may determine (1) the dilution of conjugate to be used in an ELISA to detect guinea pig IgG, and (2) what dilution of antigen (IgG) can be used on a plate in order to be used in other assays. Remember, this test is a demonstration of the principles to be used in specific antigen assays. The same test can be used for their standardization (more clearly demonstrated in **Subheading 2**).

Optimal Conjugate Dilution

The 1/400 and 1/800 dilutions give good titration with high backgrounds. The 1/1,600 gives a similar titration curve of similar end point to the 1/400 and 1/800 with a lower background. Thus, we could use this dilution without loss of sensitivity. The 1/3,200 also gives adequate titration of antigen, although there is some loss of sensitivity (ability to react with antigen), as judged by limiting of the end point. Thus, optimal dilution is somewhere between 1/1,600 and 1/3,200. In practice, dilution of 1/2,000 can be used for initial tests. This can be adjusted after later tests using particular antigens (e.g., if this assay was used to titrate anti-species conjugates which was then used in the Indirect ELISA).

Optimal Antigen Dilution

Optimal antigen dilution is relevant in other ELISAs in which specific antigens need to be titrated for use, e.g., in indirect assays. We might wish to use a constant dilution of IgG to detect antibodies against guinea pig IgG. The levels of IgG available on the wells after adsorption are reflected in the developing color. At high dilutions there is little color, and therefore little IgG is attached. In the plateau region (at plastic saturation level), there is an excess of IgG. The optimal amount to titrate antibody is arrived at when around 1–1.5 OD units of color are obtained using the optimal conjugate dilution. Therefore, the antigen dilutions in wells 3 and 4 are suitable for reaction with antibody. The exact value can be adjusted after actual assessments in specific assays.

1.2. Conclusion

Direct ELISA has been extensively described because it introduces the investigator to the ELISA. Many of the areas covered will need less explanation, so that protocols shown for ELISAs will have less detail. Direct ELISA is mainly used because ofits ability to titrate anti-species conjugates and thus avoid using preparations that are too strong or too weak. Some of the major principles of ELISA have been introduced–plateau height, end point, nonspecific reactions, backgrounds, and titration curves – and they will be constantly reviewed in all the assays described.

2. Indirect ELISA

This section describes the development of ELISA using nonpathogenic materials. Optimization of indirect ELISA is described, followed by an exercise in its use to titrate antibodies and later, the use of single dilutions to assess sera.

2.1. Learning Principles

1. Measuring optimal antigen concentration to coat wells
2. Titrating antisera
3. Using anti-species conjugates

2.2. Reaction Scheme

$$\text{I-Ag}_{\text{W}} + \text{Ab}_{\text{W}} + \text{Anti-Ab*E}_{\text{W}} + \text{S} \text{ —— READ}$$

where I = microplate wells; Ag = guinea pig IgG adsorbed to wells; Ab = rabbit anti-guinea pig serum; Anti-Ab*E = goat anti-rabbit serum conjugated with HRP; S = H_2O_2 + OPD; READ = observe by eye or read in spectrophotometer; + = addition and incubation at 37°C or room temperature for 1 h; and W = washing of wells with PBS.

2.3. Basis of Assay

The basis of this assay is to titrate antibodies that have reacted with an antigen by using an anti-species conjugate. The indirect aspect therefore refers to the fact that the specific antiserum against the antigen is not labeled with an enzyme, but a second antibody specific to the particular species in which the first antibody was produced is labeled. Such assays offer flexibility and form the bases of other ELISAs. In principle, optimization of reagents is similar to direct ELISA. However, three factors have to be considered:

1. Optimal dilution of antigen
2. Optimal dilutions of antisera
3. Optimal dilution of conjugate

The third factor was dealt with in direct ELISA. You should now be able to titrate the conjugate (anti-rabbit in this case). The main use of indirect ELISA is to titrate antibodies against specific antigens. In this case, constant amount of antigen is adsorbed to wells, and antisera are titrated against this as dilution ranges. Any reacting antibody is then detected by the addition of a constant amount of anti-species conjugate. Such assays can be evaluated fully from the diagnostic point of view in which numbers of field and experimental antisera (known history) are available.

Therefore, they can be used to assay single dilutions of antisera, and tests can be adequately controlled using standard positive and negative antisera. Thus, indirect ELISA has found many applications in epidemiological studies assessing disease status.

2.4. Materials and Reagents

1. Ag: guinea pig IgG at 1 mg/mL (1 g/L).
2. Ab: rabbit anti-guinea pig serum.
3. Anti-antibody*E: Sheep anti-rabbit serum linked to HRP (rabbit IgG needed if conjugate titration not done, as for titration of anti-guinea pig conjugate).
4. Microplates.
5. Multichannel and single-channel pipets.
6. 10-mL and 1-mL pipets.
7. Carbonate/bicarbonate buffer, pH 9.6, 0.05 M.
8. PBS containing 10% BSA and 0.05% Tween-20.
9. Solution of OPD in citrate buffer.
10. Bottle of hydrogen peroxide (30% w/v).
11. Washing solution (PBS) in a bottle or reservoir.
12. 1 M sulfuric acid in water.
13. Paper towels.
14. Small-volume bottles.
15. Multichannel spectrophotometer.
16. Clock.
17. Graph paper.

2.5. Protocol for Indirect ELISA

The first stage in this assay involves titration of the anti-species conjugate under conditions described for direct ELISA. Remember that the antigen used to titrate the conjugate must be appropriate; for example, if an anti-bovine conjugate is to be used, then use BSA as the antigen in the original CBT. If detection of an anti-bovine IgG is required, then use bovine IgG as the antigen in the direct ELISA CBT.

The anti-rabbit conjugate needs to be titrated so that we know the dilution to use in the indirect assay to detect any reacted rabbit serum (the optimal dilution of conjugate may be given in class if this procedure has not been carried out):

1. Titrate the anti-rabbit conjugate (optimal dilution may be given).
2. Take a microtiter plate with A1 at the top left-hand corner. Add 50 µL of carbon-ate/bicarbonate buffer to each well using a multichannel pipet.
3. Make a dilution range of the guinea pig IgG from 5 µg/mL from column 1 (eight wells) to 11. This is made exactly as

described for direct ELISA. Add 50 μL of the guinea pig IgG at 10 μg/mL (or 1/50 if the concentration is unknown) to column 1. Mix (pipet up and down eight times with a multichannel pipet), and then transfer 50 μL of dilution to column 2. Mix and continue transferring to column 11. Discard 50 μL remaining in tips after mixing in column 11. Thus, we have a twofold dilution range of IgG in each row A to H, excluding column 12 wells.

4. Incubate at room temperature or 37°C for 2 h.
5. Wash the wells in PBS (fill and empty the wells four times).
6. Blot the plates.
7. Dilute the rabbit anti-guinea pig serum to 1/50 in blocking buffer (PBS containing 1% BSA and 0.05% Tween-20). Make up 1 mL; therefore, add 20 μL–1 mL of buffer.
8. Add 50 μL of blocking buffer to all wells using a multichannel pipet.
9. Add 50 μL of the 1/50 anti-guinea pig serum to each well of row A. Mix and transfer 50 μL to row B, mix and transfer 50 μL to row C, and repeat this procedure to row H. We now have a twofold dilution series of antibody the opposite way to the IgG antigen.
10. Incubate the plate at room temperature or 37°C for 1 h.
11. Wash and blot the plate.
12. Make up the anti-species conjugate (kept at –20°C) to the optimal dilution found in direct ELISA (or as instructed) in the blocking buffer. Make up enough for all the wells of the plate plus 0.5 mL (~5.5 mL). This might appear wasteful but is convenient practice since it allows for minor errors in pipeting and avoids the need to make up a small volume of conjugate when one runs out on the last row (i.e., when the exact volume to fill the plate wells is made up). Add 50 μL of the dilution to each well using the multichannel pipet and a clean trough.
13. Incubate at room temperature or 37°C for 1 h.
14. Wash and blot the wells.
15. Thaw out the OPD (10 mL). Add 5 μL of H_2O_2 immediately before use. Mix well. Add 50 μL of this to each well, using a multichannel pipet and clean the troughs (make sure that the trough is not contaminated with conjugate from the previous addition to the plate).
16. Incubate for 10 min (note color changes).
17. Stop any color development by adding 50 μL of 1.0 M sulfuric acid to each well.

18. Read the plate by eye and with a multichannel spectrophotometer after titration of antigen (guinea pig IgG) and antibody (anti-guinea pig serum) as described above.

2.6 Results

Table 3 presents the microplate reader results. Note that the picture produced is similar to the direct ELISA results. Also, you should have observed that there is a similar development of color throughout the 10-min incubation after addition of the substrate solution. **Figure 7** shows the data graphically. Plots relating

Table 3
plate data from CBT of conjugate and antigen

	1	2	3	4	5	6	7	8	9	10	11	12
A	1.92	1.89	1.92	1.89	1.45	1.12	0.89	0.67	0.45	0.39	0.40	0.39
B	1.94	1.89	1.91	1.86	1.47	1.09	0.87	0.59	0.39	0.38	0.31	0.29
C	1.56	1.43	1.33	1.29	1.07	0.89	0.78	0.56	0.43	0.32	0.23	0.19
D	1.34	1.23	1.14	1.09	0.97	0.75	0.68	0.49	0.29	0.21	0.17	0.15
E	1.14	1.00	0.89	0.76	0.56	0.41	0.32	0.23	0.19	0.17	0.19	0.12
F	0.92	0.83	0.73	0.54	0.43	0.32	0.21	0.17	0.19	0.16	0.16	0.14
G	0.76	0.56	0.42	0.36	0.28	0.21	0.19	0.18	0.16	0.14	0.15	0.15
H	0.45	0.32	0.29	0.21	0.17	0.14	0.15	0.18	0.16	0.15	0.16	0.10

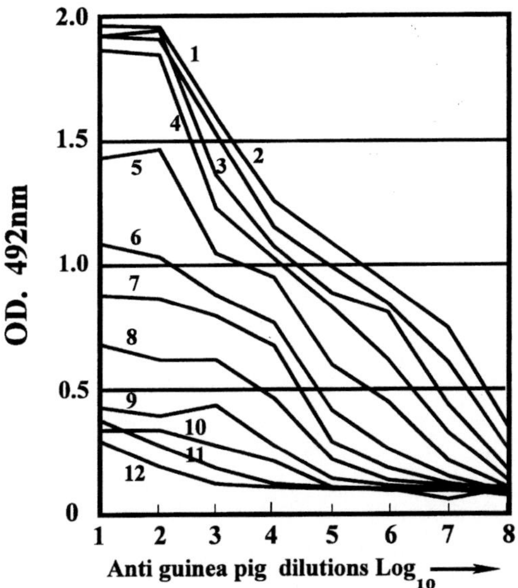

Fig. 7. Indirect ELISA: titration curves of anti-guinea pip serum (A–H) against constant antigen concentrations of IgG (columns 1–12)

concentration (or dilution) of the IgG (Ag) to the OD for different dilutions of rabbit anti-IgG are shown.

Plot the data relating to the IgG concentration on the plate as a $\log_{10}$ twofold series (micrograms/milliliter per well, or dilution if the actual concentration is unknown) against the OD for each dilution of antibody used. You should end up with eight lines on a single graph, one for each antiserum dilution. You have already observed similar results in the direct assay. Similar areas of reactivity can be identified on the indirect CBT.

1. Plateaus of similar high color are shown in rows A and B, wells 1–4.
2. Higher plate background values are seen in rows A and B (possibly C) than for more dilute serum.
3. The serum titration end points (where the OD value for a particular IgG concentration is the same as plate background) are similar for rows A–D. After this dilution of antiserum, there is loss in detection of IgG.
4. Loss of end point detection is matched by a loss in OD at high concentrations of IgG. For example, in rows F–H at 5 μg/mL of IgG, there is substantial and increasing loss in color, as compared to where maximal color (in antibody excess: row A) is observed. Note that row H barely titrates the IgG; very low color is obtained.

2.6.1. Optimization of Reagents

Rows A and B indicate that antibodies are in excess, and we have some problems of nonspecific attachment to the plate without antigen having been adsorbed (well 12). Note that in these rows, plateau regions extend to well

Thus, no more antigen (IgG) is able to absorb to the plate above the concentration in well 4. Rows C and D give optimal titrations of the IgG in that maximum values do not exceed 1.6 OD, and high end point titers are obtained. Below these dilutions, sensitivity for detection of IgG is lost. Thus, to detect the antigen optimally, and to use a single dilution of antiserum under the conditions of the ELISA described, use a dilution of about 1/400–1/800.

The optimum dilution of antigen that might be used as a single dilution to detect and maybe quantify antibodies is best assessed as the dilution (or concentration) that shows good binding across the whole range of antiserum dilutions. The best way to illustrate this is to draw a graph of the plate data, but this time, plot the dilutions of serum against the OD for the various antigen concentrations (or dilutions). This has been done in **Fig. 7.**

At the first four concentrations (dilutions) of antigen (IgG), there is little difference in the end-point detection, for the dilutions of antiserumarereduced. After this, the OD readings and end point detections are reduced. At the extreme, in column

10,barely no antibody is detectable, even where the serum is most concentrated.Higher values in rows A–C correspond to nonspecific binding to the wells seen in row 12. Thus, the dilution of antigen found in columns 3 and 4 is optimal to detect antibodies.

3. Use of Indirect ELISA to Titrate Antibodies

The optimized reagents in **Subheading 2.4** can be exploited to measure antibodies directed against the guinea pig IgG target.

3.1. Learning Principles

1. Titrating antibodies from positive sera using full-dilution ranges
2. Establishing ELISA-negative antibody levels for control of nonimmune sera
3. Duplicating samples tested

3.2. Reaction Scheme

$$\text{I-Ag}_{W} + \text{Ab}_{W} + \text{anti–Ab*E}_{W} + \text{S} \text{ —— READ}$$

where I = microplate; Ag = optimum concentration of antigen; Ab = test serum plus or minus in reaction for Ag; Anti-Ab*E = anti-species antibody linked to enzyme; S = substrate/color detection system; W = washing step; and + = addition and incubation of reactants.

In this exercise, the Ag and Anti-Ab*E are used at optimal dilution. The test or standard Abs is added as dilution ranges.

3.3. Basis of Assay

We are now able to titrate antibodies, as we know the antigen optimum and conjugate optimum dilutions for our given system. Thus, if sera are reacted with the antigen on the plate, and if they contain antibodies against the guinea pig IgG, they will be picked up by subsequent addition of the conjugate. The seropositive serum titration curves may then be compared with each other and to the seronegative curves, to establish antibody titers and examine the result of nonspecific reactions at various dilutions of the negative sera, within the system.

3.4. Materials and Reagents

1. Ag: guinea pig IgG, 1 mg/mL.
2. Ab: three rabbit serum samples after injection with guinea sera test bled at different times following inoculation with guinea pig IgG and three rabbit sera from antibody-negative animals (prebleeds).
3. Anti-Ab*E: sheep anti-rabbit serum linked to HRP.
4. Microplates.

5. Multichannel and single-channel pipets.
6. 10- and 1-mL pipets.
7. Carbonate/bicarbonate buffer, pH 9.6, 0.05 M.
8. PBS containing 1% BSA and 0.05% Tween-20.
9. OPD solution.
10. Hydrogen peroxide.
11. Washing solution (PBS).
12. 1 M sulfuric acid in water.
13. Paper towels.
14. Small-volume bottles/microdilution system.
15. Multichannel spectrophotometer.
16. Clock.
17. Graph paper.

3.5. Titration of the Antigen Dilution or Concentration for Use in Measuring Antibodies

Titration is performed as described earlier for the indirect assay (*see* **Subheadings 2.5** and **2.6**), in which we also titrated the optimum dilution of conjugate. Now we are concerned with the titration of antibodies against guinea pig IgG in rabbit sera. Therefore, we make the CBT of guinea pig IgG against the positive rabbit antiserum and use a constant dilution of anti-rabbit conjugate.

Note that while setting up an indirect ELISA, a positive serum against the particular antigen being detected is necessary . Such sera are often available as determined from other serological assays, from systems whereby specific antibodies are expected (e.g., from experimentally infected or vaccinated animals or from animals during the course of an outbreak). The exact conditions of the ELISA may therefore have to be altered during the developmental stages when many sera have been examined as compared to the originally used positive serum. For now, the original "optimal" conditions are determined using a defined (experimentally derived) positive serum.

3.6. Titration of Different Sera

1. Dilute guinea pig IgG (Ag) to optimum concentration in carbonate/bicarbonate buffer, pH 9.5, 0.05 M (as determined in **Subheading 2.1**).
2. Add 50 μL to each well of the plate using a multichannel pipet.
3. Incubate at 37°C for 2 h.
4. Wash and blot the plate.
5. Add 50 μL of blocking buffer to all the wells using a multichannel pipet and trough.
6. Take the six sera supplied. Label the three positive sera 1, 2, and 3. Label the three negative sera 4, 5, and 6. Dilute each

one to 1/20 in blocking buffer in small bottles, and make up a final volume of 0.5 mL of each (25 μL + 475 μL of blocking buffer).

7. Turn the plate with 50 μL of blocking buffer per well so that well H1 is on the left-hand top corner (*see* **Fig. 8**). Add 50 μL of serum 1 dilution to wells H1 and H2, add 50 μL of serum 2 dilution to wells H3 and H4, and add 50 μL of serum 3 dilution to wells H5 and H6. Repeat the process adding sera 4, 5, and 6 to wells H7 and H8, H9 and H10, and H11 and H12. We now have each of the sera diluted effectively to 1/40 in 100 μL of blocking buffer in the left-hand extreme row (H) of the plate (*see* **Fig. 9**).
8. Use the multichannel pipet with 12 tips attached to mix, and dilute the sera across wells G, F, E, D, C, B, and A, transferring 50 μL of each dilution. We now have twofold dilution range of the sera, in duplicate, that is, there are two dilution series of each of the sera (*see* **Fig. 9**).
9. Incubate at 37°C or room temperature for 1 h (the exact conditions you used in the indirect CBT are best).
10. Wash and blot the plate.
11. Add 50 μL of anti-rabbit conjugate per well (diluted in blocking buffer).
12. Incubate at 37°C (or room temperature) for 1 h (conditions as for 1-h incubation in CBT).
13. Wash and blot the plate.

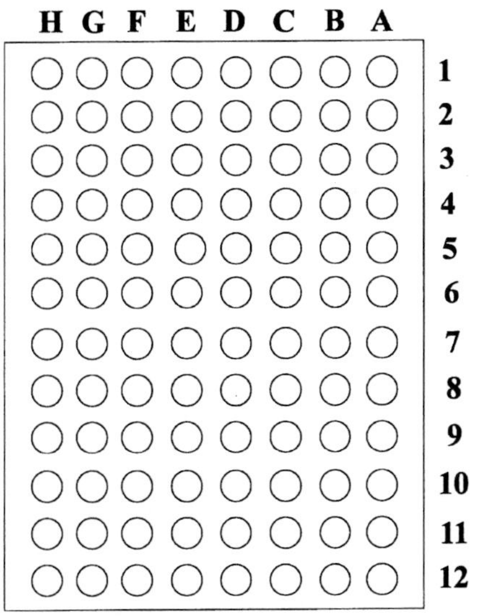

Fig. 8. Orientation of plate for dilutions of sera

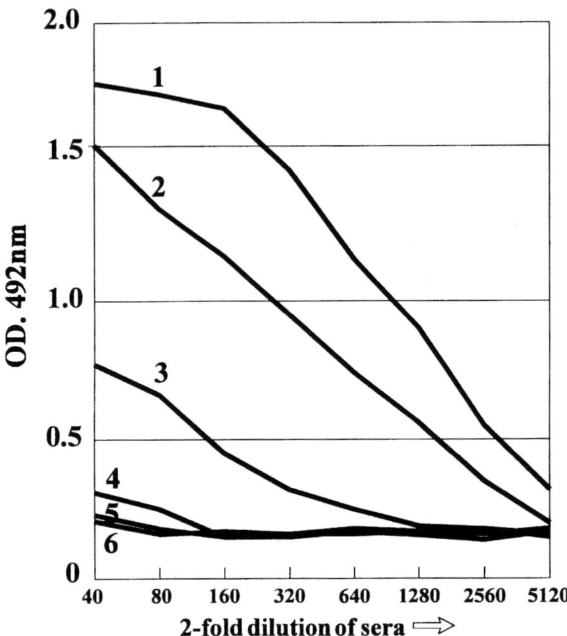

Fig. 9. Addition and dilution steps of sera to wells.

14. Add substrate and chromophore (50 μL).
15. Stop color development after 10 min.
16. Read the plate in a multichannel spectrophotometer. Remember to watch the plate as the color develops and make relevant notes.

3.7. Explanation of Data

Figure 10 gives typical results from this assay, and **Table 4** presents the OD readings.

1. Serum 1: The values of the duplicate samples are quite similar. The titration shows a plateau region where the values are the same (wells H1 and H2, and wells G1 and G2). Thus, there is a maximum color obtained up to 1/80; increasing the concentration of antibodies has no effect on the readings. This represents the region where the entire antigen is saturated with antibody. The value of the OD is dependent on the amount of antigen that has attached to the wells, which, in turn, is dependent on the adsorption characteristics of the plastic and concentration of antigen. On further dilution, the antibodies are no longer in excess, so they are titrated, as seen by a gradual decrease in the OD.
2. Serum 2: The OD levels even at 1/40 are not equal to those where antibody was in excess in serum 1. Thus, the antibodies are not saturating the antigen on the wells, and are

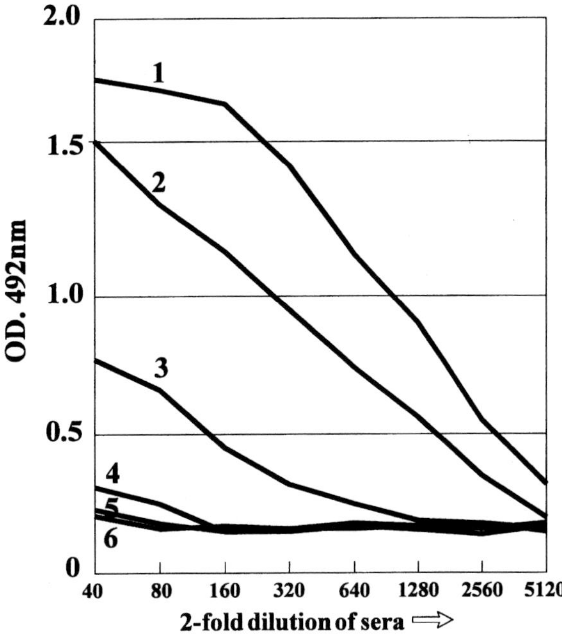

Fig. 10. Plots of data in **Table 4** showing titrations of six different serum samples diluted from 1/40 in a twofold series against constant antigen concentrations. Mean values for OD are used.

Table 4
Plate data

	Serum 1		Serum 2		Serum 3		Serum 4		Serum 5		Serum 6		
	1	2	3	4	5	6	7	8	9	10	11	12	Dilution
A	0.34	0.32	0.19	0.23	0.14	0.15	0.17	0.16	0.15	0.16	0.19	0.15	5.20
B	0.54	0.56	0.34	0.36	0.17	0.19	0.14	0.14	0.16	0.18	0.16	0.14	2.60
C	0.87	0.91	0.54	0.57	0.18	0.19	0.14	0.17	0.17	0.16	0.17	0.14	1.80
D	1.16	1.14	0.76	0.72	0.28	0.25	0.17	0.16	0.18	0.16	0.17	0.19	640
E	1.45	1.45	0.95	0.91	0.31	0.32	0.15	0.14	0.17	0.15	0.14	0.17	320
F	1.68	1.70	1.15	1.17	0.43	0.46	0.13	0.15	0.14	0.15	0.16	0.18	160
G	1.76	1.73	1.34	1.32	0.65	0.66	0.23	0.24	0.18	0.17	0.15	0.17	80
H	1.79	1.76	1.56	1.54	0.78	0.76	0.31	0.32	0.28	0.24	0.21	0.23	40

therefore not present in excess. The titration of the serum begins immediately on dilution. Note that the last dilutions give low OD values equivalent to the plate background, unlike serum 1.

3. Serum 3: Even at 1/40 OD values are low as compared to the serum samples 1 and 2. There are fewer antibodies in this serum than the other two! Again, the titration begins immediately on dilution and low OD (around 0.19) is attained at 1/1,280. Overall, these three positive sera have different reactivities in terms of quantity of antibody titrated. Thus, serum 1 has the highest titer, showing a plateau (is able to saturate the antigen). Serum 2 has the next highest amount of antibodies since it has an end point around 1/5,120 (point where OD equals the plate background). Serum 3 has the lowest amount of antibody, with an end point of around 1/1,280.
4. Serum 4: This is a negative serum (clinically). Therefore, by definition it should contain no antibodies. The color obtained reflects the nonspecific attachment of the serum to the antigen. Most nonspecific "sticking" might be expected in the least dilute sample as is the case here, with background levels at 1/40 and 1/80 serum dilutions. Note that the levels of nonspecific color are much lower than in the positive sera, but are distinct from the assumed plate background, which can be taken as the backgrounds observed for the negative sera at their highest dilution. Note that such wells (E, D, C, B, A) give similar results and no titration is observed on dilution.
5. Sera 5 and 6: These give results similar to serum 4, although there is a lower amount of color in the 1/80 wells, reflecting different amounts of nonspecific adsorption of serum proteins.

3.7.1. Curve Shapes

The plotted data, particularly for the positive sera, produces curves rather than straight lines. Generally, there is a region on the curve that contains three to five points that are more linear than the rest. Nonlinear regions occur at the top and bottom of a graph, and such sigmoidal curves are typical of serum titrations as shown in **Fig. 11**. End point determinations are difficult to assess exactly, because there is a pronounced "tail" at the low OD end of the results.

3.7.2. Comparison of Serum Titration Curves

The amount of specific antibody in each serum has been titrated over a dilution range. The serum containing the most antibodies will have a higher dilution end point (dilution where the OD is the same as the background OD). Thus, as already indicated, the end points may be compared as representing the titer of the sera. This can be assessed by eye as well as by machine reading.

A better estimate of the end point is made by drawing a straight line through the points on the curves that are nearly in a straight line. If this was done statistically, a regression analysis of the points would be made and the best line of fit would be given mathematically (*see* **Fig. 12**)., This may be approximated graphically to sufficient accuracy. Thus, the end points are assessed when

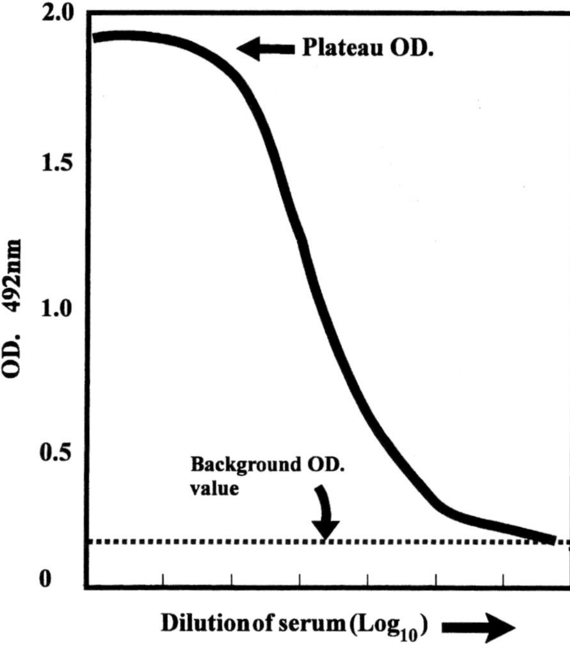

Fig. 11. Serum titration curves showing sigmoidal nature.

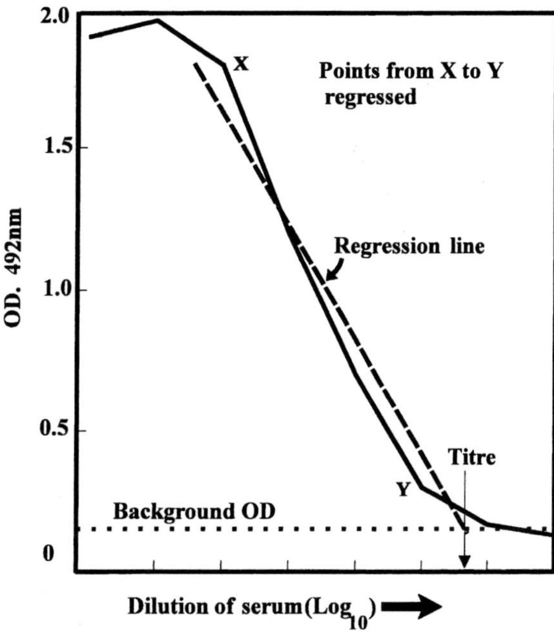

Fig. 12. Regression of points in serum titration curve to obtain a titer at the intersection of the background OD.

the regression lines (or graphically produced lines) cut the measured background OD line, assuming that the curves are of similar shape (the lines are then parallel). However, this may not always be the case, as different antibody populations may be responsible for the color of the ELISA. In this case, differences must be noted and taken into account when the implications of the titers found are considered. Note that the curves obtained for negative sera are very flat; even so, they have an end point. Sera may also show differences in maximum plateau heights and shape (**Fig. 13**).

Figure 14 attempts to explain why there are differences in plateau heights for different sera. Here, several sera are reacting maximally with the antigen as, there is no increase in color when their concentration is increased.. The plateau heights are different, however, showing that different weights of antibody have reacted with the same antigen for particular sera. This is a function of the number of reactive antigenic sites on the antigen and the quantities and specificities of antibody populations in the sera. Although this is uncommon when using polyclonal antibodies, it is common when using monoclonal antibodies (mAbs).

Where the curves are parallel, any point can be taken on them for comparison of samples. This is illustrated in **Fig. 15.** Analysis of as many sera as possible over full-dilution series and examination of the curves should be made to establish whether there is parallelism. This is important when spot tests are required so that a single dilution of test sample can be established.Dilution can be taken where samples give results in the parallel regions of curves.

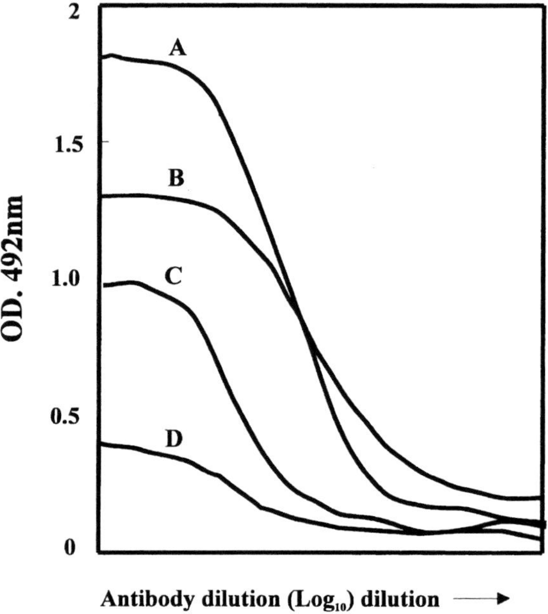

Fig. 13. Variation in sigmoid curves for serum titrations.

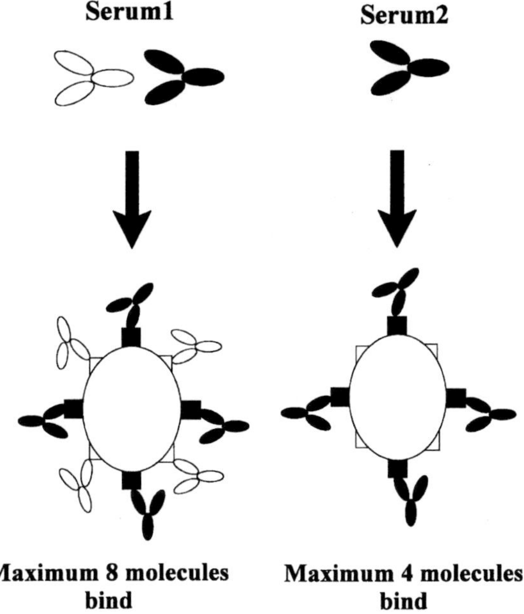

Fig. 14. Diagram representing maximum number of molecules of antibody that can bind to antigens. Differences in plateau height (maximum OD) can be attributed to different populations of antibodies in sera.

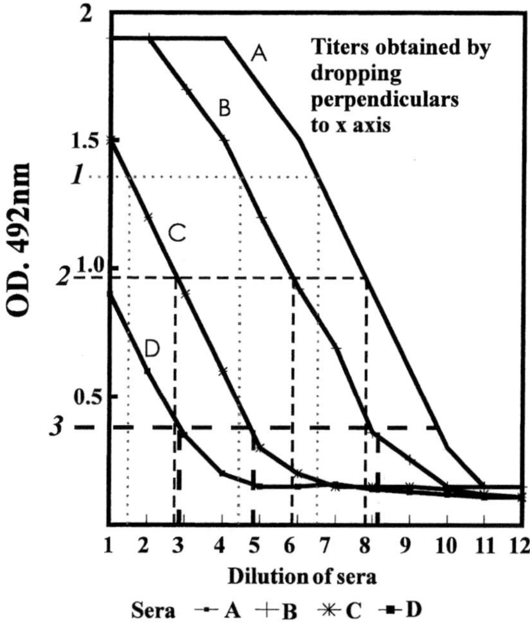

Fig. 15. Comparison of serum titration curves to standard serum titration at three points (OD values 1, 1, and 3) in parallel regions of curves. Titers can be read from the x-axis and related.

A line is drawn at a particular OD, and the dilution of serum giving this OD for all the sera is determined, thus giving relative titers. Such relative titers may be expressed compared to an accepted standard serum, which, in turn, can be given in any units. The actual activity of the standard serum may be known (e.g., number of micrograms/milliliter of specific antibody), so that all the sera compared to this can be expressed in the same units.

3.7.3. Negative Sera and Control Sera

The test undertaken involved only one control - that of negative sera. Ideally, a plate background should be included to measure the color in the wells with only the antigen and conjugate. This should correspond to the readings beyond the titration of the antibodies, observed when a low plateau is obtained even on dilution of the samples. Such backgrounds can be subtracted from the whole plate results before any processing of the data, or used to blank the spectrophotometer before reading. Treatment of the results of negative serum depends on what is known about the negativity in terms of other tests and clinical findings. For example, British cattle are ideal as negative sera when studying anti–foot-and-mouth disease virus (FMDV) antisera, because Britain is disease-free. This may not always be possible in countries where disease is endemic. Note also that control negative sera obtained from other countries may not reflect the same negative population of another country, since there are breed differences, complications owing to other infections, and so forth. This can affect the performance of kits in which standard negative sera are supplied to act as controls in the ELISA. Kits must be evaluated, wherever possible, in the country where they are to be used. The control value for the negative serum supplied may not reflect the mean value for negative sera.

3.7.4. Selection of a Single Serum Dilution to Perform a "Spot Test"

Examination of the serum titration curves for positive and negative sera can tell us which dilution may be suitable to use in the indirect ELISA so that antibodies may be assayed on single wells (or multiple wells using the same dilution). In **Fig. 10**, we thus observe that there is low nonspecific activity seen in the negative sera at 1/40 and 1/80. The positive sera still show high OD values at these dilutions so that the relative sensitivity of the assay (detection of specific antibodies) can be made at such dilutions. However, if dilutions greater than 1/80 are used, we can still measure antibody in the absence of nonspecific reactions. Sensitivity does drop, however. Remember that we are trying to balance sensitivity with low background in the presence of other serum proteins in the sample. If we had used the sera at 1/160, then we would have had values for the ELISA as shown in **Table 5.** Negative sera levels are therefore around 0.15, whereas all positive sera are above this value. The next exercise expands on this approach.

Table 5
Mean OD492 of anti-guinea pig sera at 1/60 dilution

Senim	OK
1	1.69
2	1.16
3	0.45
4	0.14
5	0.15
6	0.17

4. Use of Indirect ELISA to Determine the Positivity of Sera at Single Dilution

4.1. Learning Principles

1. Examining negative serum populations for establishing OD limits of negativity.
2. Examining antibody-positive serum populations.
3. Examining frequency of results in a population.

4.2. Reaction Scheme

$$\text{I-Ag}_W + \text{Ab}_W + \text{Anti-Ab}^*\text{E}_W + \text{S—READ}$$

where I = microplate; Ag = optimum concentration of antigen; Ab = test sera at single dilution; Anti-Ab*E = anti-species antibody linked to enzyme; and S = Substrate/color detection system.

In this exercise, we use Ag and Anti-Ab*E at optimal dilutions. The test sera are added at a constant dilution. Control positive antisera can be added at a constant dilution or as a dilution range, to produce a standard curve relating color to dilution or concentration of the antibodies added. Thus, the test sera can be related to the positive serum titration curve. The same can be done by including accepted negative control sera standards.

4.3. Materials and Reagents

1. Ag: guinea pig IgG (1 mg/mL) (or previously titrated)
2. Ab: 48 rabbit sera including high, moderate and low titer against guinea pig IgG (24) and negative sera (24)
3. Anti-Ab*E: sheep anti-rabbit serum linked to HRP
4. Microplates
5. Multichannel and single-channel pipets

6. 10- and 1-mL pipets
7. Carbonate/bicarbonate buffer
8. PBS containing 1% BSA and 0.05% Tween-20
9. OPD solution
10. Hydrogen peroxide
11. Washing solution
12. Paper towels
13. 1 M sulfuric acid in water
14. Small-volume bottles/microdilution equipment
15. Multichannel spectrophotometer
16. Clock
17. Graph paper
18. Calculator

4.4. Protocol for Spot Test

From the previous exercises, you should have assessed the dilution of test serum that can be used to discriminate between positive and negative nonspecific results, based on the difference noted between the selected positive and negative sera titrated over full-dilution ranges. We are now going to titrate all the sera at the dilution found as duplicates (two wells per serum dilution in the indirect ELISA).

1. Add the guinea pig IgG to the wells of a microtiter plate at optimum dilution (as in earlier exercises). Incubate at 37°C for 2 h (or under particular optimal conditions).
2. Wash and blot the plate.
3. Dilute the test serum samples appropriately, in blocking buffer. Sera may be diluted into small-volume bottles. However, this causes two problems: manipulation (capping and so on) is laborious, and transfer of serum dilutions must be made with a single channel pipet. The latter problem is important because it takes a long time to transfer all the sera to the different wells. Initially added samples will therefore receive a longer contact time with the antigen, which may affect the results. This can be avoided if the samples are transferred to other plates before dilution (e.g., plastic non-ELISA microtiter plates in volumes that need not be accurate). The plate can then be sampled using a multichannel pipet if the dilution factor for the sera is not too high. Initial dilution can be made directly into, say, 100 μL of blocking buffer in the non-ELISA plates. The transfer of the required volume of the diluted test sample can then be effected using a multichannel pipet. Thus, the samples are transferred at approximately the same time. Special systems have been developed for use with multichannel pipets. These are ideal for dilution and storage of test samples. Volumes of about 1 mL can be made up, making the accurate dilution of up to 1/200 (5 μL

of sample/mL) easy. The microtiter dilution system should be available for this exercise.

4. Add a volume of blocking buffer to the plastic tubes held in the tube holder. For example, if a dilution of 1/100 is required, add 0.5 mL of blocking buffer per tube, and then 5 μL of test sample. (*see* **Fig. 16** for a pattern of samples on a plate.) Incubate for 1 h, as in the previous exercise, and follow the same steps for washing and addition of reagents to the stopping stage. Read the OD values.

4.5. Example of Data

Table 6 gives typical results. Results obtained in your specific assay can be processed in the same way. **Figure 17** is a diagrammatic representation of a stopped plate.

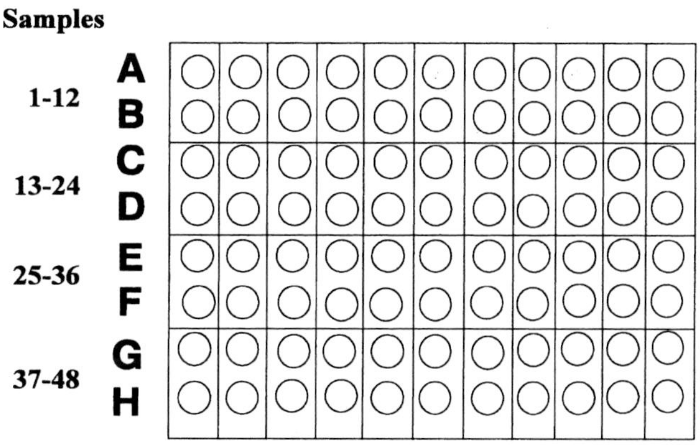

Samples

1-12 A B

13-24 C D

25-36 E F

37-48 G H

Fig. 16. Micronics system for dilution of samples, showing the order of samples.

Table 6
Plate data for example assay[a]

	1	2	3	4	5	6	7	8	9	10	11	12
A	1.21	1.09	0.78	0.32	0.12	0.66	*0.65*	0.17	0.67	0.34	1.34	1.11
B	1.19	1.03	0.69	0.31	0.16	0.64	*0.62*	0.16	0.64	0.37	1.28	1.17
C	1.00	0.23	0.45	0.56	0.78	0.13	0.19	0.45	0.56	0.78	1.00	0.56
D	0.97	0.27	0.49	0.54	0.72	0.16	0.20	0.44	0.53	0.75	1.01	0.55
E	0.13	0.14	0.18	0.09	0.07	0.12	0.14	0.09	0.08	0.12	0.16	0.14
F	0.12	0.13	0.16	0.09	0.08	0.11	0.13	0.10	0.09	0.11	0.13	0.15
G	0.15	0.18	0.13	0.14	0.10	0.15	0.13	0.12	0.13	0.13	0.12	0.08
H	0.13	0.16	0.13	0.15	0.12	0.13	0.12	0.14	0.15	0.12	0.11	0.09

[a]Duplicates of sample made are A1, B1; A2, B2; and so on. Suspect positive sera (24) are in rows A-D. Negative (prebleed Sera) are in rows E–H

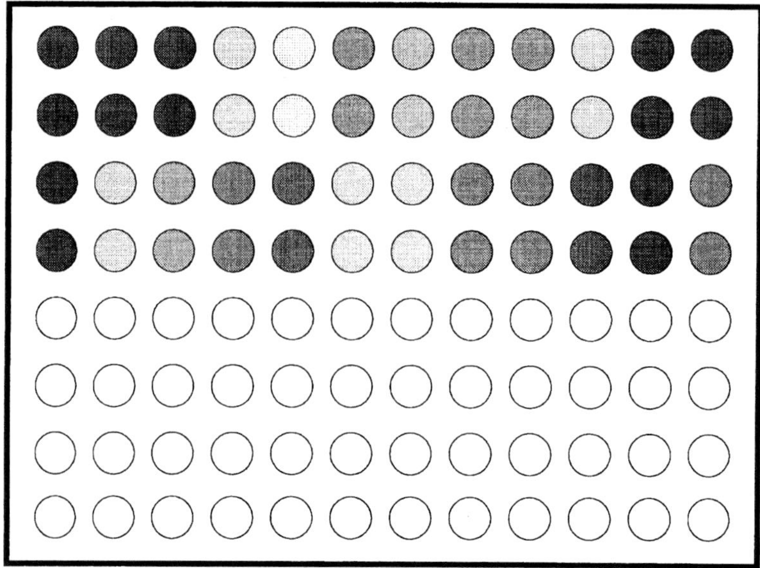

Fig. 17. Diagrammatic representation of a stopped plate.

As duplicates have been made, examine the variation between the values. This should not be high; i.e., there should be little difference between the ODs for both test wells of the same sample. Calculate the mean (average result) of the OD from both wells if the difference is not large. Variations in results are discussed later. Take the mean value to two decimal places.

4.5.1. Mean and Standard Deviation from Mean of Negative Serum Data

Take all the means of the negative sera and calculate the mean and standard deviation (SD) of the negative population using a calculator. (Note: Instruction should be given on the use of a calculator.) Non-course users of the manual should obtain a calculator and follow operating instructions to calculate same parameters.

4.5.2. Frequency Plots of Negative Serum OD Results

Plot the results for the negative sera as in **Fig. 18.** These relate the number of samples giving a particular OD..

A frequency distribution is obtained so that the distribution of negative results is got. Create a table of OD intervals and score the numbers of sera falling into the intervals. Add up the score, and plot this against the intervals. The mean of the data for the negative sera and the SD of the data can be found using a calculator. Thus, the population mean of a limited (in this case) negative population is found. If the population of negative ELISA readings is distributed normally (normal distribution statistics), then the upper limits of negativity can be ascribed with defined confidence limits, depending on the number of SDs from the mean that is used.

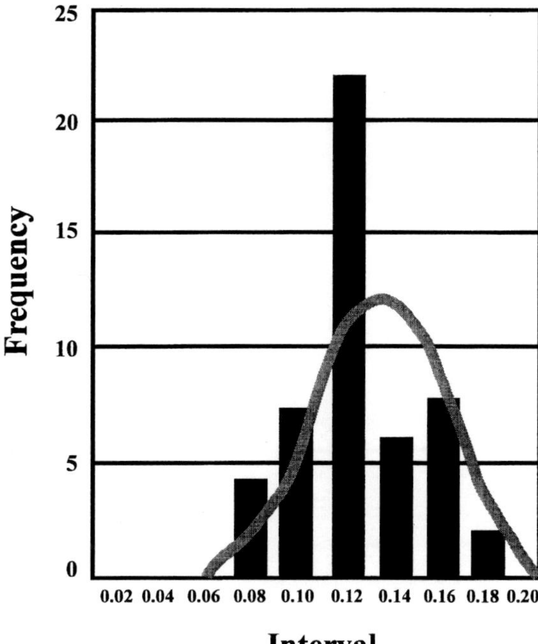

Fig. 18. Frequency plot relating number of sera giving particular OD values. Grey curve is the normal distribution plot.

The mean value in this case is 0.125, and the SD is 0.026. Thus, if we select 3× SD above this mean value (=0.084) and add this to the mean value (=0.209), values equal to or above this value are unlikely to be part of the measured negative population as defined by the fact that only ~0.1% of negative sera examined tended toward this value. Limits using 2× the SD above the measured negative population mean reduced confidence in the results for ascribing positivity (increase possible sensitivity but reduce specificity).

In practice, such distributions are skewed to the right-hand side, so that a tailing of results is seen at the higher ODs (*see* **Fig. 19**). To establish an OD reading that reflects the upper limit of negativity (as all negative sera have been studied), a statistical evaluation of the distribution is required. In general, since the distribution is skewed, a value of two times the mean OD for all the negative sera has been found to determine the upper limit of negativity (which corresponds to the lower limit of positivity) with a 95% confidence limit. Thus, we are 95% certain, that a sample giving an OD value equal to or greater than the value at two times the mean of the negative population OD results is positive. In practice, a confidence limit of 99% can be ascribed to results equal to or greater than two times the population mean.

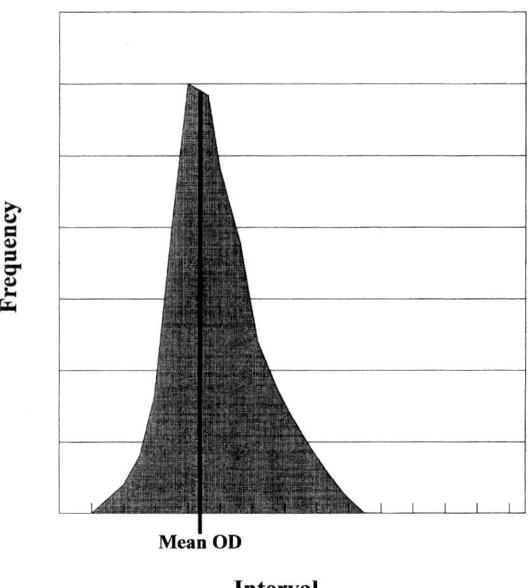

Fig. 19. Distribution skewed to the right.

4.5.3. Problems

When examining negative populations, we are assuming such sero-negativity, using one or more factors, such as other serological test results, knowledge of the clinical history of the animals, and epidemiological factors. Thus, it may be easy to identify seronegative animals in countries where a particular disease has never been recorded. However, this may not be true for countries that have endemic disease or where vaccination campaigns have been mounted at various times (with variable amounts of antibody against specific disease agents being elicited). In such conditions, the experimenter might make the best assessment of likely negative animals. In this case, after plotting the frequency curves, one of several distributions might be obtained:

1. **Figure 19:** One peak at the low OD end of distribution. The population is probably negative with all sera showing low OD.
2. **Figure 20:** Two peaks fairly well separated at the low OD and at the higher OD end of distribution. Distinct populations of animals that are positive and negative may reflect recent infection or vaccination.
3. **Figure 21:** Two peaks merged. There is no clear distinction between populations (the high and low ODs overlap greatly). These curves also illustrate what the picture looks like, after sampling total populations containing positive and negative animals. Thus, for the example in **Fig. 19**, there is no problem in ascribing an upper limit for negativity. Obviously the sera show the type of result expected of a totally negative population. However, in **Fig. 20** we have a percentage of

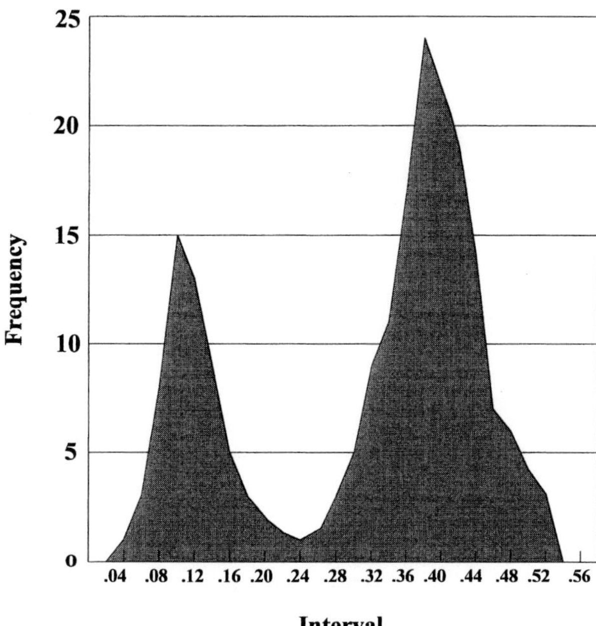

Fig. 20. Frequency plot of OD results from analysis of sera, with two peaks representing distinct populations

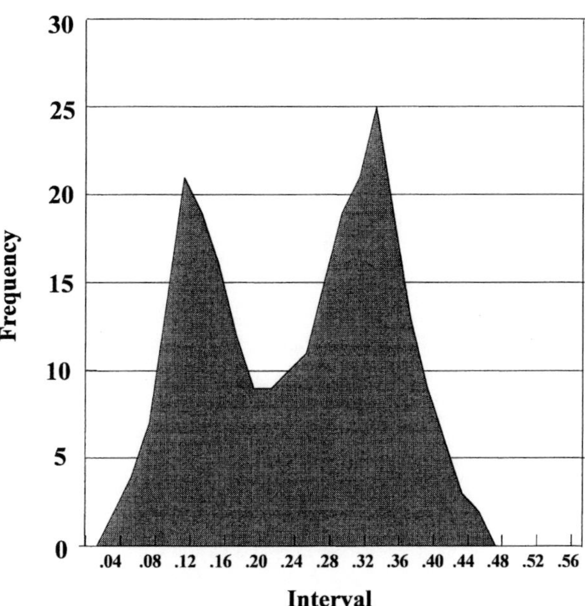

Fig. 21. Frequency plot of OD results from analysis of sera. No clear distinction is seen between populations.

high OD results. These probably represent positive animals, and we can use the clear difference in the two distributions obtained, to suggest strongly that the low OD results represent a negative population.

The distribution in **Fig. 21** demonstrates a situation in which there is a heterogeneous population of animals with respect to their levels of antibodies. Thus, it is probable, that the low OD range , shown by the situations in **Fig. 19** and **20**, represents negative animals. The merging of high and low results with high numbers of animals probably indicates that antibody levels have been reduced in the population after a past infection. Such a population can be studied, using a defined negative population (maybe from another source), but the negative distribution cannot be assessed from a study of this type of distribution alone. Hence, the experimenter might obtain serum samples from relevant species from countries where the disease they wish to study is absent. The negative value(s) obtained from such sera may not always be the same as that of the indigenous stock, but for most exercises it will suffice.

4.6. Establishment of Control Negative Sera

It is possible to use a limited number of negative sera, to act as controls, in any assay of antibodies. This can be done, only if a distribution of many negative serum OD levels has been made (~100 minimum). Thus, a serum typifying the mean of the population of negative sera can be used. If this is included as a single dilution in the indirect ELISA, the OD values obtained may represent the mean value for the negative serum population. The upper limit of negativity can then be calculated by multiplying this value by 2 ,as we know that this is a relevant value after studying the distribution. This approach is relevant when multi-channel spectrophotometers are to be used to read the color.

If assessment by eye is being done , control negative sera giving OD levels at the upper limit of negativity (around two times the mean) may be used. Color development in such assays should then be allowed until color is just detectable in the negative controls. The test should then be stopped. Therefore, any wells showing color more intense than the control wells would be positive for the antibody.

4.6.1. Data Analysis

You have calculated the mean OD of the negative population as well as the SD from the mean of the population. Now find a serum, which characterizes the mean of the population, as well as one that characterizes the upper limit (two times the mean), of the population.

4.7. Relating Single Test Dilutions to Standard Positive Antiserum Curves

If a characterized antiserum is available, it may be used as a standard in the indirect ELISA. In this case, a full-dilution range of the serum is made and titrated, under identical conditions, to the single dilutions of the test sera. A typical plate format is shown in **Fig. 22.** At the end of the test, a standard curve relating the OD to the dilution of standard positive serum is constructed. The titers of test samples can then be read from this curve so that a relative assessment of activity is obtained. This is demonstrated in **Fig. 23.** The standard serum may be given an

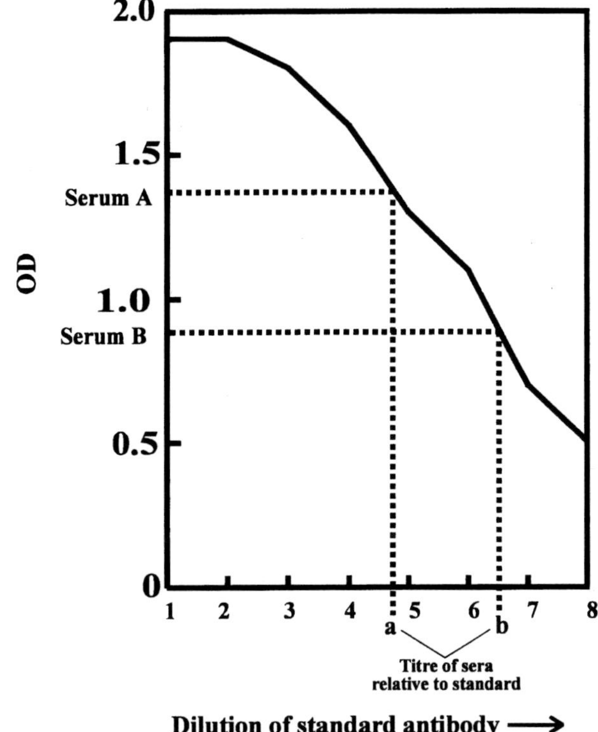

Fig. 22. Plate layout for comparison of test sera with standard serum titration.

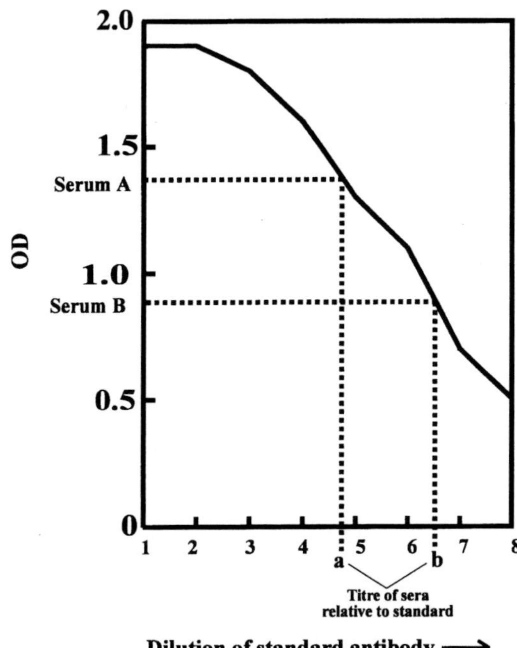

Fig. 23. Use of standard serum titration curve to assess titers of test sera. OD values obtained from serum A and B are read from the titration curve of the standard serum (a and b).

arbitrary activity (units) so that results may be expressed in those units. Such control positive sera may be useful when standardization between laboratories is required.

4.8. Complications of Actual Disease

Studies on many systems have shown that false positive results are obtained in a low percentage of animals, from a guaranteed non-infected population. It is difficult to determine why such reactions occur, but several reasons have been advanced, such as contamination of the serum with bacteria and fungi, dietary factors, and heating of the sera. The percentage can be of the order 1–2%; theseare easily read as very high ODs, as compared to the majority of samples, given the typical negative distributions already discussed. This nonspecificity can be eliminated, e.g., by using different antigenic preparations. However, the number of likely false positive results should be taken into account when diagnosing disease on a herd basis. Thus, if we know that 2 animals in 100 show this response and we find 20 animals in 100 show high responses, it is likely that disease is diagnosed. However, if only one to three animals are "positive," this finding could be due to identified nonspecific reactions.

5. Use of Antibodies on Solid Phase in Capture ELISA

This section examines sandwich ELISAs for measurement of antigens and antibodies.

5.1. Use of Capture ELISA to Detect and Titrate Antigen

1. Optimizing the amount of capture antibody attached to the wells
2. Optimizing amount of detecting antibody

5.1.1. Learning Principles

5.1.2. Reaction Scheme

$$(\text{I-AB}_X)_W + \text{Ag}_W + (\text{Ab}_Y)_W + \text{Anti-Ab*E}_W + \text{S—READ}$$

where I = microplate wells (solid phase); AB_X = capture antibody (species X) specific for Ag; Ag = antigen; Ab_Y = detecting antibody (species Y) specific for Ag; Anti-Ab*E = anti-species Y antibody linked to enzyme; S = Substrate/color detection system; W = washing step; and + = addition and incubation of reactants.

In this exercise, the capture antibody, the detecting antibody and the conjugate are used at optimal dilutions.

5.1.3. Basis of Assay

The following may happen to antigens: They may:

1. Attach poorly to plastics.
2. Be present in low quantity, e.g., in tissue culture fluids.
3. Be present as a low percentage of total protein in a "dirty" sample (e.g., in feces or epithelium samples).

4. Be unavailable for purification and concentration, as they are antigenically unstable when separated from other serum components.

In these cases, the indirect assay is unsuitable for handling the antigen, because it relies on the antigen attaching directly to the wells. The capture assay overcomes many of these problems, since the antigen is attached to the wells via specific antibodies. The test relies on the availability of two antisera from different species, so that the conjugate reacting with the second (detecting) anti-body does not react with the capture antibody. It is also essential that the antigen has at least two antigenic sites so that the antibody may bind to allow the sandwich (the antigen being the filling). Thus, when small antigens are being used (e.g., peptides), they may not react in such assays owing to their limited antigenic targets. The test offers an advantage over the indirect assay in the quantification of antigens, as direct attachment of proteins to wells is often nonlinear i.e., it is not proportional to the amount of protein in the sample. This is exaggerated if contaminating proteins are present with the antigen (e.g., serum components), because these compete for plastic sites in a nonlinear way. Because the capture antibody is specific, it binds antigen proportionally over a large range of protein concentrations. Thus, such assays give reproducible results when quantification is required. The assay is practically identical to the indirect assay except that an extra step (the capture antibody) is added. Thus, we have three parameters to optimize:

1. The capture antibody
2. The detecting antibody
3. The conjugate against the detecting antibody

5.1.4. Materials

1. Capture antibody (AB_X): = sheep anti-guinea pig Ig (an IgG preparation at ~5 mg/mL in PBS)
2. Ag: = guinea pig Ig at 1 mg/mL or as prepared by the worker
3. Detection antibody (Ab_Y): rabbit anti-guinea pig Ig serum (Ab)
4. Anti-Ab_Y*E: sheep anti-rabbit conjugate (HRP)
5. Microplates
6. Multichannel, single-channel, 10-mL and 1-mL pipets
7. Carbonate/bicarbonate buffer, pH 9.6
8. PBS 1% BSA/Tween-20 (0.05%)
9. Solution of OPD in citrate buffer
10. Hydrogen peroxide 30% (w/v)
11. Washing solution
12. 1 M sulfuric acid in water
13. Paper towels

14. Small-volume bottles
15. Multichannel spectrophotometer
16. Clock
17. Graph paper

5.1.5. Methods

Since you are now familiar with the indirect assay, steps in the optimization of the capture ELISA should be straightforward. The first essential step is to determine the amount of capture antibody to be attached to the wells. We have two situations in the laboratory, depending on the availability of specific reagents. We can use capture antibody as an IgG preparation, or if sufficiently high-titer serum is available, against the antigen, as whole serum. The easiest way to avoid serum effects is to prepare the IgG. Salt fractionation is usually adequate and does not affect antibody activity. Care must be taken to assess the effect of chemical preparation of IgG from mAbs.

Use of Ig Preparations

The advantage of using IG preparations is that the weight of Ig can be calculated, so that a defined quantity of reagent may be added to the plate. In general, a maximum amount of protein will attach to the wells. Because we know that a maximum possible binding of subsequently added antigen can be expected, we may add the Ig at "saturating" level. Thus, a good estimation of the activity of a capture antibody (the particular dilution/concentration to be used) can be assessed. As an example, if capture antibody is added at 5 μg/mL in 50-μL amounts, it represents the saturating amount of antibody protein that will attach to the wells. The ultimate activity will depend on the concentration of the specific Ig (against the Ag) in the capture antibody and spacing of the capture molecules.

Some assays perform better at lower than saturating levels of capture antibody so that a titration is needed. Generally, the amount of specific antibodies in a serum as a percentage of the total protein is about 1–5%. The preparation of Ig eliminates a large percentage of the serum proteins not involved in the assay (e.g., serum albumins). Therefore, the activity of the Ig protein (relative increase in the IgG fraction that will attach to each well) is effectively increased. In other words, there is a greater proportion of IgG sticking to the wells to act as trapping antibody if Ig preparations are used.

Use of Whole Serum

Dilutions of untreated serum can be used. However, as already indicated above, the proportion of specific IgG is low, and other serum proteins attach in a competitive manner. One cannot assume that putting on a low dilution of serum, will give a good level of capture antibody. The most usual event is that a bell-shaped curve of capture ability is obtained, with little activity at high concentrations of serum and a rise in activity as the serum is diluted. In general, serum has to be diluted to about 1/500 to 1/2,000. Thus, we must have fairly high titers to be able to use whole serum. **Figure 24**

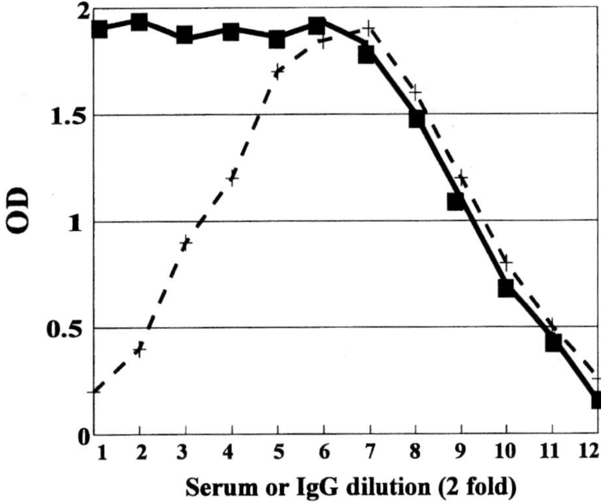

Fig. 24. Comparison of capture of IgG using whole serum or IgG as capture antibody. , IgG; +, serum

demonstrates the activity of whole and IgG capture antibodies as they are diluted down, to illustrate the bell-shaped curve.

Titration of Capture Antibody Using IgG

1. Dilute the sheep anti-guinea pig IgG preparation to 5 μg/mL in carbonate buffer. Add 50 μL to each well on the plate except column 12.
2. Add adsorption buffer alone to row 12. Incubate at 37°C for 2 h or overnight if more convenient (remember to put lids on the plates).
3. Wash the plates. (From now on we are performing a procedure similar to the indirect ELISA.)
4. Place the microtiter plate with well A1 at the top left-hand corner. Add 50 μL of blocking buffer to each well.
5. Make a dilution range of guinea pig IgG (the antigen of interest) from 5 μg/mL from column 1 (8 wells) to column 11 in blocking buffer. Add 50 μL of guinea pig IgG at 10 μg/mL to the first row 1 using a multichannel pipet. Mix and double dilute across the plate (you should be competent at this now). Remember to discard the last 50 μL in the tips so that each well contains 50 μL of fluid (check!).
6. Incubate the plates at room temperature or at 37°C for 1 h.
7. Wash the plates.
8. Add 50 μL of blocking buffer to each well.
9. Dilute rabbit anti-guinea pig serum to 1/100 in blocking buffer (make up 1.0 mL: add 10 μL of undiluted serum to 1.0 mL of buffer). Mix. Add 50 μL of the dilution to row A using a single-channel pipet. Dilute across rows A–H using a multichannel pipet. We now have a twofold dilution range from 1/200 (row A) to 1/25,600 (row H).

10. Incubate the plate at room temperature or at 37°C for 1 h.
11. Wash the plate.
12. Make up an optimum dilution of sheep anti-rabbit conjugate. Add 50 μL to each well using multichannel pipets.
13. Incubate for the standard time as used in the optimization of conjugate (1 h at 37°C or room temperature).
14. Wash the plate.
15. Add substrate and stop the color development at 10 min.

Data

Essentially we have produced a CBT of the antigen against the detecting antibody -as in the indirect assay. Thus, we have assumed that the capture antibody, put on the plate as an IgG, is at maximal reactivity. Results are therefore similar to those obtained in the indirect assay, and can be treated similarly. Each row from A–H has an identical dilution series of the antigen (guinea pig IgG) being captured by the same amount of antibody; thus the same amount of guinea pig IgG should be present, attached via antibody to the wells 1–11. The rabbit antibody against the antigen has been titrated at different dilutions, so that we can examine which dilution shows the best detection of IgG in rows A–H. The use of 5 μg/mL of capture IgG has been taken as that which from experience saturates the plastic sites available on the plate wells. Once the antigen and detecting serum optima have been established using this level of capture IgG, they can be altered to examine the effect on the assay. **Table 7** gives the spectrophotometric plate readings. A representation of the plate is also shown in **Fig. 25.**

Table 7
CBT of guinea pig IgG vs. rabbit anti-guinea pig IgG–constant capture antibody, constant conjugate

	1	2	3	4	5	6	7	8	9	10	11	12
A	1.67	1.67	1.68	1.65	1.54	1.34	1.09	0.89	0.67	0.54	0.34	0.23
B	1.68	1.68	1.65	1.56	1.51	1.31	1.04	0.84	0.59	0.51	0.32	0.17
C	1.56	1.54	1.52	1.43	1.34	1.23	0.99	0.76	0.52	0.43	0.23	0.09
D	1.12	1.09	1.00	0.94	0.87	0.78	0.67	0.56	0.45	0.34	0.19	0.08
E	1.00	0.97	0.89	0.78	0.67	0.56	0.43	0.34	0.23	0.21	0.17	0.08
F	0.78	0.74	0.71	0.56	0.51	0.43	0.32	0.21	0.19	0.14	0.09	0.10
G	0.54	0.51	0.51	0.42	0.36	0.32	0.21	0.16	0.14	0.09	0.08	0.09
H	0.34	0.34	0.32	0.21	0.18	0.15	0.16	0.09	0.08	0.07	0.08	0.09

Guinea pig IgG diluted 1–11; anti-guinea pig IgG diluted A–H

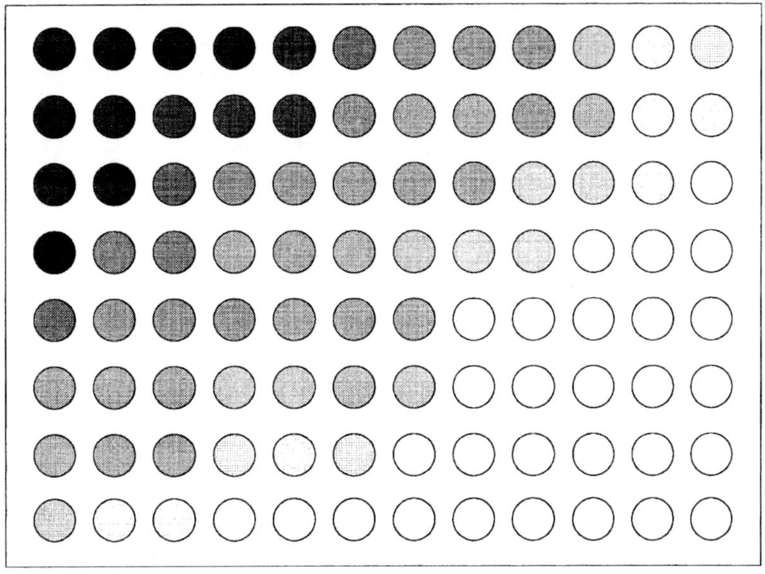

Fig. 25. Diagrammatic representation of plate showing results of CBT.

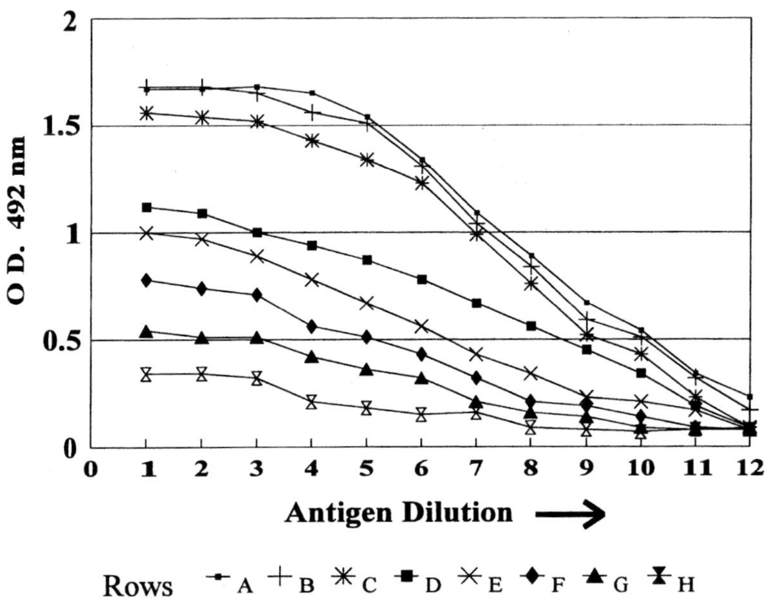

Fig. 26. Titration of guinea pig IgG using constant capture conditions. Each *line* represents titration of same dilution range of IgG using different concentration of rabbit anti-guinea pig IgG. The conjugate dilution is constant. Data from Table 7.

Plots of Data

Figure 26 shows data plotting the OD results obtained at different antigen dilutions for each dilution of rabbit anti-guinea pig serum.

Assessment of Data

Column 12 contained no antigen (guinea pig IgG), and therefore examination of the color here, gives a measure of the binding of the detection system to the plate or capture antibody. Thus, rows A and B show higher levels of color than the other rows. The value around 0.09 appears to be the plate background expected in the presence of the same dilution of conjugate. Thus, the end point detection of IgG is affected in rows A and B. Examination of the plateau heights indicates that the trapping system is saturated in columns 1–4, as we obtain similar OD values; e.g., we have around 1.67 for the first four wells using the 1/200 detecting antibody, although the actual plateau height value reduces on dilution of the detecting rabbit anti-guinea pig serum. **Fig. 26**, which relates the curves obtained for the detection of trapped Ig for different dilutions of the rabbit anti-guinea pig Ig, easily shows that the last dilution giving an optimal titration is in row C. After this dilution, the effect is to more markedly reduce the OD in the plateau region ,where the trapped Ig is in excess, and also to affect the sensitivity of detection of the Ig at higher dilutions, as indicated by a reduction in the end points where the test background is the same as the plate background.

Retitration of Capture IgG

The optimal dilutions chosen will depend on how the test is to be used. If an antigen is to be detected, then we might require high detection limits in the system, so that we can use a dilution of detecting antiserum to maximize this. We will see later, that capture assays are used in competitive situations, in which the amount of antigen to be captured needs to be reduced, so that a variation in reagent concentrations for that application may be necessary.

The established optima for the antigen and detecting serum can be reassessed using lower concentrations of capture IgG. Thus, a full CBT can be performed using 2.5, 1.25, and 0.625 μg/mL of the capture IgG. However, a simpler procedure is to coat plates with a dilution range of the capture IgG, and use constant antigen, detecting antiserum and pre-titrated conjugate dilutions; **Table 8** gives the results of a typical titration of this sort. Here plates were coated with capture anti-IgG at 5 μg/mL, in a two-fold range from row A to H, only columns 1–4; thus, quadruplicate samples were being examined. After incubation and washing, antigen (guinea pig IgG) at 0.625 μg/mL was added in blocking buffer. Following incubation and washing, the detecting antibody (rabbit anti-guinea pig IgG) was added at 1/400 diluted in blocking buffer. After incubation and washing, the anti-rabbit conjugate was added at the dilution used to optimize the reagents.

Table 8 shows that the capture IgG produces similar results at 5 and 2.5 μg/mL; thus, the l atter dilution can be used in an assay to capture antigen. Lower concentrations produce lower OD values, indicating not all the available antigen are being captured. The reduced ability to bind antigen (when in excess) is accompanied by a decreased ability to detect small amounts of antigen (the minimum detection limit is reduced).

Table 8
Titration of capture IgG against optimal antigen, detecting antibody, and conjugate

Capture IgG concentration (μg/ml)		1	2	3	4	Mean
5.0	A	1.50	1.48	1.49	1.51	1.50
2.5	B	1.49	1.47	1.51	1.46	1.48
1.25	C	1.25	1.21	1.24	1.27	1.24
0.63	D	0.95	0.94	0.96	0.93	0.95
0.32	E	0.67	0.69	0.69	0.66	0.68
0.16	F	0.36	0.37	0.40	0.37	0.38
0.08	G	0.14	0.12	0.15	0.12	0.13
0.08	H	0.05	0.04	0.04	0.03	0.04

Table 9
Assessment of constant capture system with different dilutions of conjugate

Conjugate dilution		1	2	3	4	Mean
200	A	1.95	1.87	1.87	1.95	1.92
400	B	1.84	1.82	1.84	1.82	1.83
800	C	1.45	1.41	1.44	1.47	1.44
1,600	D	0.95	0.94	0.96	0.93	0.95
3,200	E	0.77	0.79	0.79	0.76	0.78
6,400	F	0.36	0.37	0.40	0.37	0.38
12,800	G	0.15	0.14	0,15	0.14	0.15
None	H	0.05	0.04	0.04	O.03	0.04

Similar titrations of other reagents can be made, in which only one is diluted and others are kept constant. Thus, in the previous case, we have three conditions optimized under experimental conditions, with control sera and antigen. The capture IgG can be used at 2.5 μg/mL, the antigen can be used at 0.625 μg/mL, and the rabbit detector at 1/400, with the anti-rabbit conjugate at a constant dilution as assessed originally against the relevant IgG attached to a microplate.

We may wish to reassess the conjugate dilution under standardized conditions. Thus, using the capture IgG, antigen, and detecting antiserum optima just given, replicate wells can be used to titrate different dilutions of conjugate; an example is given in **Table 9**. Here, a dilution of 2–400 of conjugate gives similar results. Effectively, a dilution of 1/800 gives "optimal" results (OD value around 1.45), for an assay.

Titration of Capture Antibody When Used as Whole Serum

As already stated, whole serum can be used to coat plates and act as a capture reagent. However, this is not recommended as we cannot measure the protein Ig because it is contaminated with "blocking" serum proteins which compete for plastic binding sites preferentially over the IgG. The simplest method is to perform a CBT relating dilutions of capture serum to dilutions of detecting antibody and keep the antigen constant.

The diagram below illustrates this:

Reaction Scheme

$$\text{I-Ab}_{W} + \text{Ag}_{W} + \text{AB}_{W} + \text{Anti-AB}*\text{E}_{w} + \text{S} — \text{READ}$$

where I-Ab = dilution range of trapping antibody; Ag = constant dilution of antigen (high concentration); AB = dilution range of detecting antibody; Anti-AB*E = conjugated anti-species antibody; S = substrate/chromophore; andREAD = OD.

This assay is not described in detail. However, a description of the test is given with the relevant points highlighted. You should now have enough experience to be able to set up exact practical details, with help from the exercise titrating IgG as capture antibody.

Method

1. Dilute the serum containing capture antibody on plates in carbonate/bicarbonate buffer (begin at 1/100, twofold dilutions). Incubate and then wash the plates.
2. Add constant (excess) antigen diluted in blocking buffer. (It is difficult to specify here what excess might be for specific systems, for example, an undiluted tissue culture sample containing virus might be expected to have a high concentration of antigen.) Incubate for 1 h at standard conditions.
3. Wash and add dilutions of detecting antibodies in blocking buffer to obtain a CBT (dilute in opposite direction to the capture serum). Incubate and then wash the plates.
4. Add optimal conjugate, incubate, and wash.
5. Add substrate and then stop after at 10 min.

Data

Table 10 presents typical results. Data is plotted in **Fig. 27**. Rows A–H contain dilution ranges of the capture serum 1/100–1/51,200 and column 1 = 1/100, and column 12 = 1/51,200. Row A received the detecting antiserum at 1/200, row B at 1/400 and so on to row H at 1/12,800.

Table 10
Dilutions of capture serum 1/100 –1/51,200

	1	2	3	4	5	6	7	8	9	10	11	12
A	0.67	0.96	1.34	1.35	1.32	1.11	0.9S	0.76	0.56	0.45	0.23	0.12
B	0.66	0.99	1.42	1.37	1.29	1.09	0.89	0.75	0.54	0.36	0.22	0.11
C	0.65	0.98	1.36	1.34	1.15	0.99	0.87	0.72	0.52	0.31	0.17	0.09
D	0.56	0.88	1.23	1.19	1.01	0.88	0.74	0.65	0.43	0.26	0.14	0.09
E	0.45	0.67	1.00	1.09	0.98	0.78	0.56	0.45	0.34	0.21	0.12	0.07
F	0.23	0.43	0.78	0.76	0.56	0.45	0.40	0.33	0.23	0.16	0.12	0.08
G	0.15	0.23	0.34	0.35	0.21	0.15	0.16	0.09	0.08	0.07	0.09	0.09
H	0.15	0.19	0.18	0.17	0.16	0.10	0.09	0.08	0.09	0.07	0.07	0.09

Detecting serum deluted A–H 1/200 two fold.

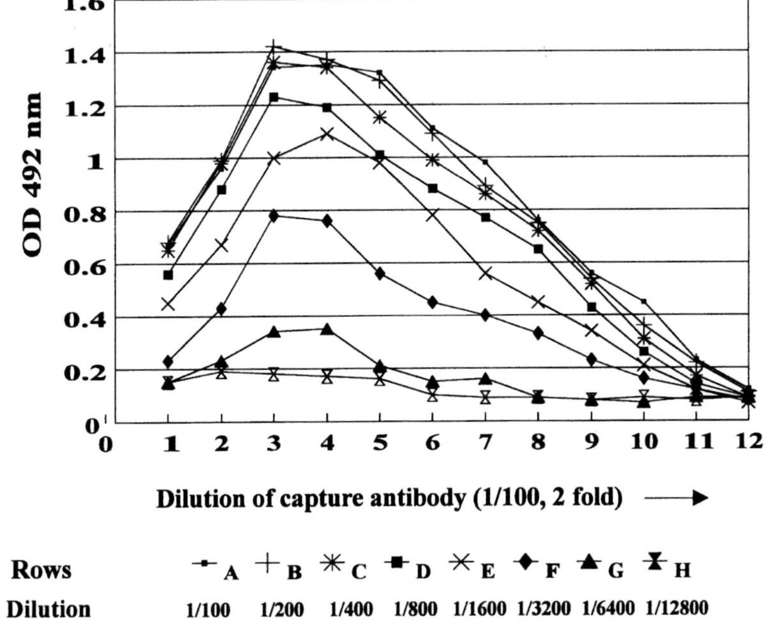

Fig. 27. Graph of data in Table 10. Columns 1–12 contain dilutions of capture antibody on wells. Rows A–H have different dilutions of detecting antibody.

Conclusion

1. The optimal dilution of capture serum is around row 5 -last row showing maximum OD.
2. The optimal dilution of detecting second antibody is around row C–D -last showing maximal titration curve of antigen.

3. Bell-shaped curves are obtained where low dilutions of capture serum give low OD values -columns 1 and 2.

Notes on Use of Capture ELISAs to Detect Antigens

Once the optimal conditions have been established, the capture assays can be used in several ways.

Diagnosis of Specific Disease Agents

$$\text{I-Ab}_W + \text{Ag}_W + \text{AB}_W + \text{Anti-AB} * \text{E}_w + \text{S} — \text{READ}$$

Here, a sample, possibly containing antigen, is added to a capture system (microtiter plate wells coated with an antiserum against a specific disease). Any bound antigen is then detected by another antibody from a different species. Such assays are important in serotyping in which the second antibody may further "divide" the disease agent into a serological grouping, such as is used routinely to serotype FMDV into one of seven distinct serotypes. The use of capture antibody means that relatively crude or contaminated samples can be used. Antigens may be quantified with reference to a standard antigen titration on the same plate.

Single dilutions of material containing Ag can then be titrated in the same system and the developing OD read against the standard titration. Again, the use of the capture antibody ensures an efficient and proportional uptake of the antigen on to the plate, which is unaffected by contaminating proteins.

5.2. Use of Capture ELISA to Detect and Titrate Antibodies

Essentially, the same parameters have to be standardized for antigen detection as for capture ELISA. However, the test is used to measure antibodies against a fixed amount of antigen captured on the plate. Thus, we must optimize the system, to have the correct amount of capture antibody and antigen, necessary to bind any test or control antisera. The test offers the ability to specifically capture antigen using a solid-phase antibody. Thus, relatively crude preparations can be used in cases in which the required antigen concentration may be low. Care must be taken to avoid reactions of the conjugate with components of the assay.

5.2.1. Learning Principles

1. Optimizing of capture antibodies
2. Optimizing of detecting antibody

5.2.2. Reaction Scheme

$$(\text{I-Ab}_X)_W + \text{Ag}_W + (\text{AB}_Y)_W + \text{Anti-Ab} * \text{E}_w + \text{S} — \text{READ}$$

where I = microplate; AB_X = trapping antibody (species X); Ag = antigen; Ab_Y = test or control sera (species Y); Anti-Ab*E = anti-species Y antibody conjugated with enzyme; S = substrate/color detection system; W = washing step; and + = addition and incubation of reagents.

5.2.3. Materials and Methods

1. Capture antibody (AB_X): sheep anti-guinea pig Ig at 5 mg/mL in PBS
2. Ag: guinea pig Ig at 1 mg/mL
3. Test antisera (Ab_Y: three rabbit anti-guinea pig Ig sera; also seronegative (Ab) rabbit sera
4. Anti-Ab_Y*E: rabbit antigoat Ig conjugated to HRP
5. Microplates
6. Multichannel, single-channel, 10-, and 1-mL pipets
7. Carbonate/bicarbonate buffer, pH 9.6, 0.05 M
8. PBS 1% BSA, 0.05% Tween-20
9. Solution of OPD in citrate buffer
10. Hydrogen peroxide
11. Washing solution
12. Paper towels
13. 1 M sulfuric acid in water
14. Small-volume bottles
15. Multichannel spectrophotometer
16. Clock
17. Graph paper

5.2.4. Optimization of Test

We need to know the following:

1. The dilution of capture antibody to use
2. The dilution of antigen to use
3. The dilution of conjugate to use

The aim is to have a constant system involving capture antibody (AB_X), antigen (Ag), and conjugate (Anti-Ab*E), which can then be used to titrate test sera (Ab_Y). We have already dealt with the use of capture antibody as whole serum or as IgG. For this exercise, we use sheep anti-guinea pig IgG (or the equivalent in an individual's systems). Thus, examination of the data in **Table 10** allows an estimation of the optimum capture IgG and antigen levels required to allow the detection of antibodies.

5.2.5. Data

Using titrations established in **Subheading 5.1**, we can obtain the optimal amount of antigen (guinea pig Ig in this case), that gives a high plateau OD , where the detecting antiserum is in excess. Turn to the data shown in **Table 7.** We can see that the plateau height is maintained to around column 4, showing that there is a maximum level of antigen to react with the antibodies in the positive serum. This concentration (or dilution) can be used in the capture assay, under the same conditions to titrate antibodies from any sera. We can therefore use the following quantities:

1. The capture antibody at 2.5 μg/mL if used as an Ig preparation or at the titrated level as found in **Subheading 5.1.5.4.** (**Table 8**).
2. The antigen at the concentration or dilution used in columns 4–5 (**Table 7**).
3. The conjugate as titrated initially as in Table 9.

5.3. Methods for Titration of Antibodies

We can examine sera for antibodies by using full dilution ranges or at a single dilution (spot test). This approach has already been described for the indirect ELISA (*see* **Subheadings 3.6** and **3.7.4**). Methodology for capture assays is similar, except that the antigen is presented to the test sera, after being captured by an antibody coating the microtiter wells. Optimum amounts of capture antibody and antigen are determined as in **Subheadings 5.1.5.1.–5.2.5**, The stages following this are very similar to the indirect ELISA, after plates have been prepared with an optimal amount of antigen. Set up the capture assay to present optimal amounts of guinea pig IgG. After washing the plates, use the same already examined in **Subheading 3.6** (rabbit anti-guinea pig sera) in a similar way, as described from stages 6–15 in **Subheading 3.6**. This entails making dilution ranges of sera, incubation, washing plates, addition, and incubation with anti-rabbit conjugate, washing, and addition if substrate/chromophore. Compare the data obtained with that in **Subheading 3.6**, **Table 4.**

Repeat the same procedure, but this time making spot dilutions of various rabbit sera as in **Subheading 4.3**. Compare the data with that in **Subheading 4.4**, and **Table 6.**

5.4. Problems in Using Capture Assays

1. Care must be taken to examine whether any of the reagents interact. Unexpected cross reactions can be found with immunological reagents. For example, the conjugated antibodies might react with different species other than which they were prepared. There are cross reactions between certain species ,so that conjugates against cow proteins will react with sheep and goat proteins. Thus, in such a system the use of sheep or goat Ig as a capture antibody precludes the use of anti-bovine conjugates to detect reaction of bovine antibodies with a particular antigen.
2. When relatively crude antigens are captured, contaminating proteins, which interfere with the assay, may also be trapped. For example, when purified FMDV is injected into an animal, there is a specific response against the virus, but also a response against contaminating bovine serum proteins present in extremely low amounts, which come from the tissue culture medium. Such sera used as capture reagent, will capture not only virus, but also bovine proteins. Thus, in typing exercises using tissue culture or bovine epithelial samples, a high quantity of bovine protein is captured. The use of anti-bovine

conjugates to detect bound bovine serum in a trapping assay therefore also binds to the trapped bovine protein giving high backgrounds. In the typing assay proper, guinea pig sera are prepared as the second typing detecting sera. These also bind bovine proteins and therefore detect bound bovine protein to the capture antiserum. Again specific typing is affected. However, the second antibody can be treated to remove cross- reactivity either by adding a high concentration of the cross-reactive protein to the reagent (in this case 1 mL of normal nonimmune bovine serum is added to 1 mL of typing guinea pig serum), or by using affinity reagents in which bovine serum is attached to a solid phase (e.g., agarose beads). This can be incubated with the serum so that cross-reactive antibodies are removed after incubation and separation of the beads is achieved by centrifugation. Or, as is most common, the test can be done using blocking buffers containing high levels (around 5%) of the cross-reactive protein.

6. Competitive ELISA

The direct, indirect, and capture ELISAs have now been examined. You should be able to optimize the conditions of the tests, and be able to use them, to measure antigen or antibody in a variety of formats. Competitive ELISAs include principles of all these types of assay.

Basically, they involve methods that measure the inhibition of a reactant for a pretitrated system. The degree of inhibition reflects the activity of the unknown. We can therefore measure antibody or antigen, and even compare small differences in the binding of antigens or antibodies so that antigenic subtyping may be performed by comparing the relative avidity of one antiserum for two antigens in the same system. As a reminder, let us consider the competitive assays based on the indirect test and the trapping test for the detection of antigens or antibodies in a diagrammatic way.

6.1. Indirect Assay: Antigen Detection by Competition

6.1.1. Reaction Scheme

$$\text{I-Ag1}_W + \text{AB}(+\text{Ag})_W + \text{Anti -Ab} * \text{E}_w + \text{S} \text{---} \text{READ}$$

A pretitrated indirect assay with optimal Ag1, AB, and conjugate, is competed for by Ag2, as a dilution range in the liquid phase. If Ag2 can bind AB, it will prevent AB binding that would normally react with Ag1 on the plate. The maximum expected OD for the pretitrated system without competitor (Ag2) is therefore reduced in the presence of the competitor Ag2. The degree of inhibition of the pre-titrated reaction is proportional to the relative amount of the competitor.

6.2. Indirect Assay: Antibody Detection by Competition

6.2.1. Reaction Scheme

$$(\mathrm{I\text{-}Ag})_W + \mathrm{AB}_W + \mathrm{Anti\text{-}AB}*\mathrm{E}_w + \mathrm{S} — \mathrm{READ}$$

A pretitrated system is challenged by a dilution range of Ab. The competing antibody is from a species that is not the same as that of the AB in the optimized system, and obviously the Anti-AB*E should not react with the Ab. The degree of inhibition of the pretitrated system depends on the concentration and interaction of the Ab competitor with the Ag - this time on the solid phase.

The direct assay could also be used for both these assays. Note that in the direct assay, any species of competing antibody can be used, since the AB is labeled with conjugate. Such assays are becoming increasingly relevant when mAbs are used.

6.3. Capture Assay: Antigen Detection by Competition

6.3.1. Reaction Scheme

$$\mathrm{I\text{-}AB}_W + \mathrm{I\text{-}Agl}\,(+\mathrm{Ag2})_W + \mathrm{Ab}_W + \mathrm{Anti\text{-}Ab}*\mathrm{E}_W + \mathrm{S} — \mathrm{READ}$$

The capture assay is optimized to detect the Ag1 trapped on the plates using Ab. Competition is achieved in which Ag2 is mixed with the Ab in the liquid phase. If this reacts, the amount of Ab available for reaction with the trapped Ag1 is reduced.

6.4. Capture Assay: Antibody Detection by Competition

6.4.1. Reaction Scheme

$$\mathrm{I\text{-}AB}_W + \mathrm{Ag}\,(+\mathrm{Ag2})_W + (\mathrm{Ab}_X)_W + \mathrm{Anti\text{-}Ab}*\mathrm{E}_W + \mathrm{S} — \mathrm{READ}$$

The capture antibody is optimized to bind Ag, which is detected by a constant amount of Ab_X (from animal species X). Competition involves the reaction of the Ag with antisera from species Y (which should not interact with the conjugate anti-Ab_X), in the liquid phase. The remaining Ag is then trapped and titrated with the Ab_X and the conjugate. A reduction in the expected OD for the system without any Ab_Y represents competition.

Next, we discuss the following assays:

1. Direct competition assay – antigen detection and quantification
2. Indirect assay – antigen competition
3. Indirect competition assay – antibody detection
   a. Full titration curves
   b. Spot test assessment of sera

7. Direct Competitive ELISA for Antigen Detection and Quantification

The direct assay for antigen detection and quantification has assumed an increased importance with the development of mAbs. A single mAb can be the one reagent that dominates a diagnostic assay, and therefore mAbs are worth labeling for use in an assay. The specificity of the assay is ensured and relatively crude antigenic preparations can be coated for use in a direct test format provided enough antigen attaches. This is also relevant to polyclonal antibodies. The demonstrated assays involve IgG/ anti-IgG systems.

7.1. Learning Principles

1. Optimizing of homologous system
2. Understanding competition curves

7.2. Reaction Scheme

$$\text{I-Agl}_{W} + \text{Ab}*\text{E}(\text{Ag2})_{W} + \text{S} \text{—READ}$$

where I-Agl = microplate with optimum concentration of antigen attached; Ag2 = competing antigen as a dilution range; Ab*E = conjugate specific for the Agl; S = substrate/color detection system; READ = spectrophotometric reading; + = addition and incubation steps; and W = washing step.

This exercise will most simply demonstrate the principles involved with competitive assays.

7.3. Materials and Reagents

1. Agl: guinea pig IgG at 1 mg/mL for attachment to solid phase
2. Ag2: Two samples: (a) guinea pig IgG (known concentration) and (b) rabbit IgG at 1 mg/mL
3. Ab*E: rabbit anti-guinea pig IgG conjugated to HRP
4. Microplates
5. Multichannel, single-channel 10- and 1-mL pipets
6. Carbonate/bicarbonate, pH 9.6, 0.05 M
7. PBS 1% BSA, 0.05% Tween-20
8. Solution of OPD in citrate buffer
9. Hydrogen peroxide
10. Washing solution
11. Paper towels
12. Small-volume bottles
13. 1 M sulfuric acid in water
14. Multichannel spectrophotometer
15. Clock
16. Graph paper
17. Calculator

7.4 .Practical Details

Repeat the exercise in **Subheading 1.1**, involving the CBT of antigen and enzyme-linked antibody. You should obtain a similar picture. Compare your results with those in **Table 11.**

The labeled conjugate dilutions are made from A to H, IgG is diluted 1–11, 12 has no antigen. **Figure 28** presents a

Table 11
Data from CBT of guinea pig IgG and anti-guinea pig enzyme conjugate in subheading 1.1

	1	2	3	4	5	6	7	8	9	10	11	12
A	1.89	1.88	1.67	1.33	1.10	0.97	0.86	0.57	0.44	0.32	0.31	0.31
B	1.87	1.86	1.63	1.29	1.04	0.93	0.84	0.53	0.34	0.24	0.23	0.21
C	1.68	1.45	1.32	1.14	0.96	0.86	0.64	0.45	0.29	0.19	0.17	0.16
D	1.14	1.03	0.94	0.83	0.57	0.45	0.38	0.29	0.19	0.18	0.15	0.16
E	0.99	0.91	0.74	0.54	0.46	0.36	0.29	0.19	0.18	0.15	0.13	0.14
F	0.66	0.44	0.39	0.33	0.24	0.21	0.19	0.15	0.18	0.16	0.14	0.12
G	0.34	0.20	0.16	0.18	0.16	0.18	0.15	0.16	0.14	0.12	0.14	0.13
H	0.30	0.J9	0.15	0.16	0.15	0.17	0.13	0.12	0.13	0.13	0.15	0.16

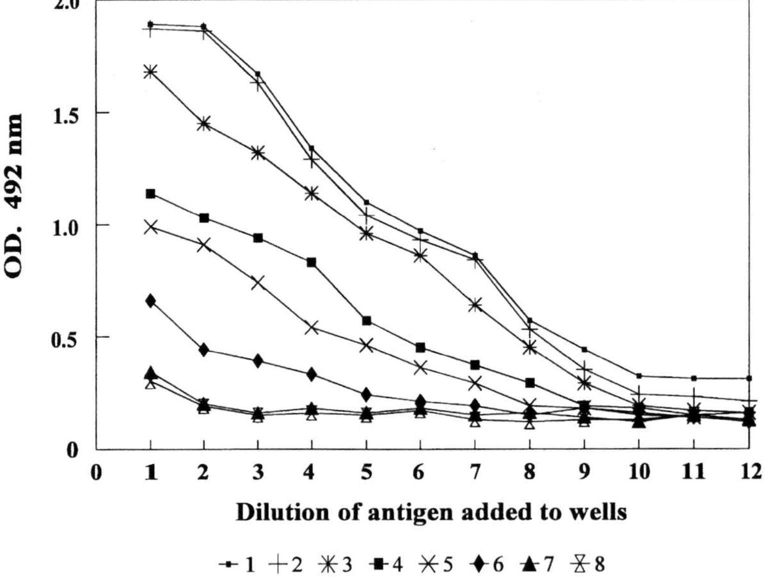

Fig. 28. Data from Table 11 relating antigen titrations at different concentrations of conjugate.

plot of a CBT of guinea pig IgG against rabbit anti-guinea pig conjugates.

7.4.1. Assessment of Data and Choice of Conditions for Competition

We are trying to make the same antigen (guinea pig IgG) and a different antigen (IgG from the rabbit), compete for a pretitrated homologous solid-phase reaction. The ultimate sensitivity of the assay depends on the exact relationship of the antibody and antigen attached to the solid phase. If we use too much antibody, so

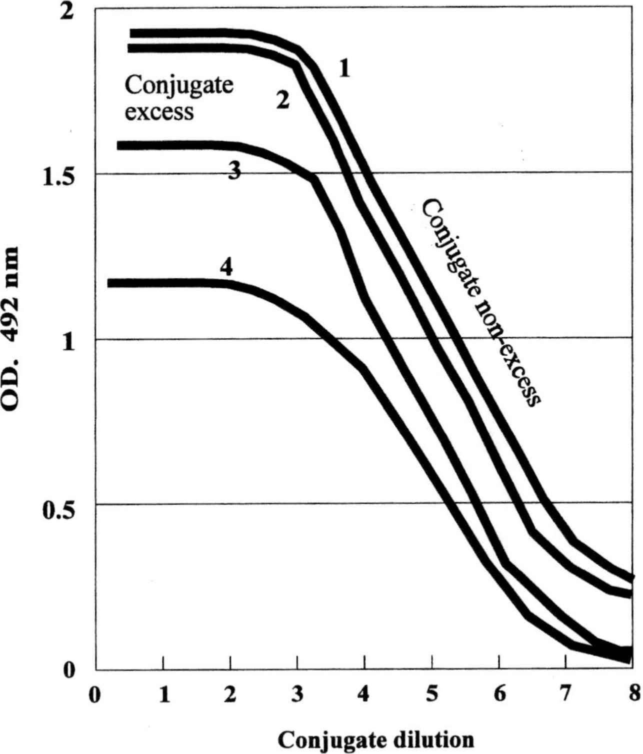

Fig. 29. Illustration of regions of conjugate excess and non excess, when titrating conjugate against constant concentration of antigen.

that it is in excess of that required to saturate the antigen, we will have a quantity of free antibody that may bind to the competitor, and there will still be an amount left to react with the solid-phase IgG. Thus, competition will only occur when extremely high concentrations of competitors are used.

This can be illustrated by an examination of the titration curves in **Fig. 29.** Note that the plateau region represents excess antibody for any given antigen concentration. The OD and extent of these plateau regions vary according to the exact amount of antigen attached to the solid phase. As we reduce the antigen, the plateau height values decrease. At the highest concentrations of antigen, titration curves are similar for different antibody concentrations, indicating that the antigen and antibody are behaving at maximum saturating levels. On dilution of the antigen, we see that the plateau height is reduced, even where we know that the antibody is available for higher OD values (curves 3 and 4). Here, the antigen is the limiting factor in color development. In the competition assay, a maximum plateau height dependent on the amount of antigen attached of around 1.0–1.5 OD should be selected. In other words, find out which dilution of antigen produces serum titration curves giving a maximum plateau of these values, e.g., curves 3 and 4. From this titration curve, we need to estimate the dilution of antibody yields about 70% of the maximum plateau OD. Using curve 1, we can illustrate this, as shown in **Fig. 30.**

7.4.2. Estimation of Antibody Dilution to Be Used in Competition Assay

The conditions are now set for competition. We have: (1) the antigen dilution as for curve, and (2) the antibody dilution estimated as shown in **Fig. 30.**

7.5. Competition Assay Proper

1. Prepare the optimum antigen coated with guinea pig IgG.
2. Wash the plates.
3. Dilute the guinea pig Ig (homologous competitor) and the rabbit Ig (heterologous competitor) to 40 μg/mL in blocking buffer.
4. Add 50 μL of blocking buffer to each well of the Ig-coated plate.

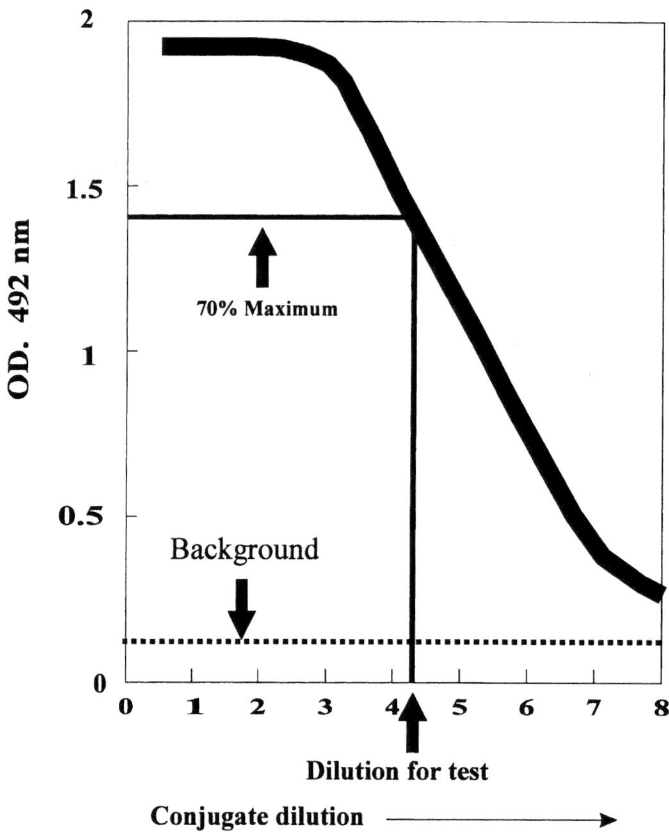

Fig. 30. Estimation of conjugate dilution for use in competition stage.

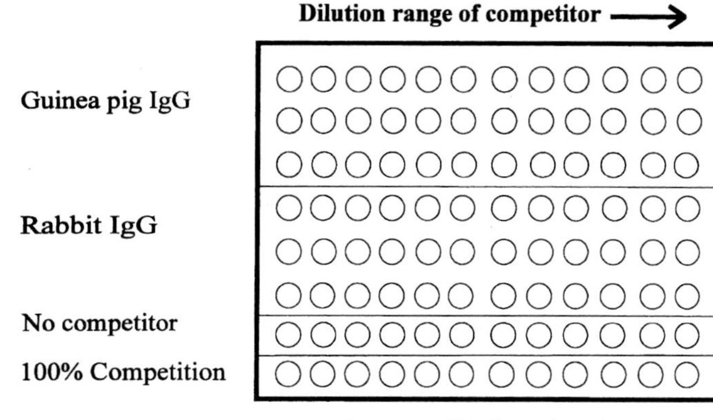

Fig. 31. Plate design for performance of competition assay.

5. See the plate design in **Fig. 31.** Make a twofold dilution range of the guinea pig and rabbit Ig by adding 50 μL of the Igs to the first row 1. Do this in triplicate (three rows for the guinea pig Ig – 1A, B, and C; and three rows for the rabbit Ig – 1D, E, and F).
6. Double dilute the IgGs across the plate (1–11).
7. Dilute the anti-guinea pig conjugate (pretitrated) in blocking buffer. Make up 6 mL.
8. Add 50 μL of the diluted conjugate to rows A–G. Do not add to row H. Mix the contents of the plates by gentle tapping. Add 50 μL of blocking buffer to row H.
9. Incubate for 1 h at room temperature (or under conditions you used to titrate the conjugate). Rotate the plate to mix reagents every 10 min.
10. Wash the plates.
11. Add OPD/H_2O_2 solution.
12. Stop the reaction after 10 min by addition of 50 μL of 1 M H_2SO_4.
13. Read the OD in spectrophotometer at 492 nm.

7.5.1. Data: Typical Results

Table 12 presents the results from the spectrophotometer readings of the plates. **Figure 32** relates the OD values to various concentrations of the competitors added. The results are processed initially as the mean OD for the triplicate estimations.

7.5.2. Further Processing of Data

1. Calculate the mean OD reading of row G. This represents the OD resulting from the reaction of the conjugate with only the solid-phase Ig and the conjugate. This value should be similar

Table 12
Plate data from the competition of samples of guinea pig and rabbit IgG for direct ELISA

	1	2	3	4	5	6	7	8	9	10	11	12
A	0.04	0.05	0.07	0.10	0.23	0.35	0.56	0.78	0.98	1.12	1.34	1.34
B	0.06	0.06	0.08	0.12	0.25	0.41	0.61	0.79	1.01	1.14	1.35	1.38
C	0.07	0.05	0.09	0.13	0.21	0.43	0.58	0.81	1.05	1.17	1.36	1.34
D	1.12	1.23	1.34	1.35	1.34	1.36	1.29	1.37	1.36	1.41	1.32	134
E	1.14	1.24	1.35	1.35	1.36	1.39	1.34	L36	1.33	1.34	1,32	1.38
F	1.13	1.25	1.34	1.38	1.38	1.41	1.42	1.35	1.33	1.38	1.34	1.32
G	1.35	134	1.41	1.35	1.36	1.32	1.29	1.34	1.37	1.39	1.32	1.45
H	0.05	0.06	0.05	0.07	0.08	0.04	0.07	0.05	0.04	0.07	0.08	0.04

A–C guinea pig IgG D–F rabbit IgG

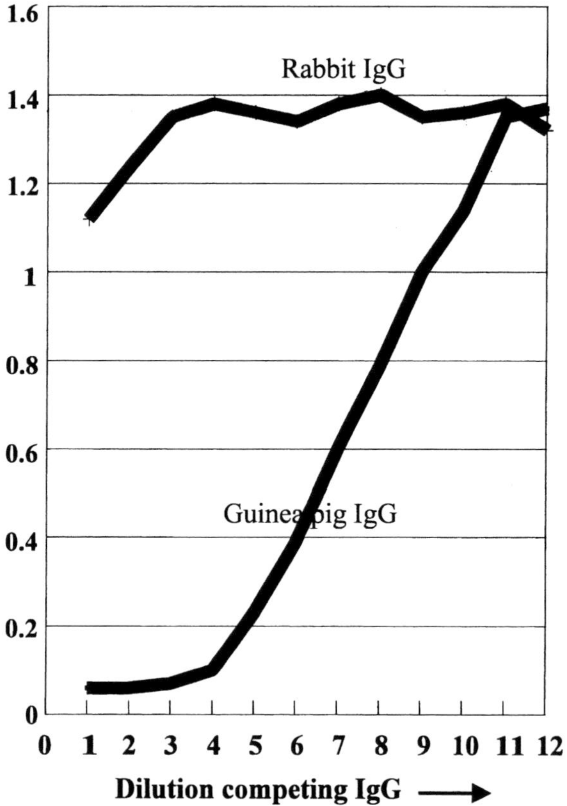

Fig. 32. Competition of guinea pig IgG and rabbit IgG for guinea pig system.

to that obtained when you titrated the conjugate. It represents the 0% competition OD, where most color is obtained.

2. Calculate the mean of the OD from row H. This represents the 100% competition level, i.e., where there is a total inhibition of the binding of antibody (not a strictly true 100% control since the conjugate was excluded from the test, but it approximates very well). Thus we have the 100% competition (degree of inhibition) and the 0% competition OD values.

3. Convert the OD values obtained for the wells that contained the two competitors into percentage of competition using the two values just calculated.

7.5.3. Example from the Data in Table 12

The mean of row G = 1.35, which is equivalent to 0% competition (a lot of color). The mean of row H = 0.07, which is equivalent to 100% competition (little color). Subtract the mean of row H from all the values obtained. If the value is minus then call it 0. This determines the 100–0% OD competition values (i.e., the range is from 0 to 1.29 OD). Using a simple formula, the percentage of competition of the samples can be calculated. **Table 13** presents the processed data with respect to subtraction of background for all data, using the following equation

Table 13
Mean values in table 12 for various dilutions of competing antigens[a]

	Mean ABC –row H guinea pig IgG	Mean DEF–row H rabbit IgG
I	0	1.17
2	0	1.18
3	0	1.29
4	0.01	1.35
5	0.16	1.28
6	0.33	1.27
7	0.51	1.27
S	0.73	1.29
9	0.93	1.28
10	1.10	1.29
11	1.28	1.26
32	1.29	1.27

[a]Mean row G – mean row H = 1.29 = the range.

$$\% \text{ competition} = 100 - \left\{ \frac{(\text{TestOD - backround})}{\text{Range}} \times 100 \right\}$$

As examples of further processing and estimation of competition, we have the guinea pig Ig competition experiment (backgrounds already taken off test results and range calculated):

Range = 1.29

Taking row 5 we have:

$$100–[(0.16/1.29) \times 100] = 87.7\%$$

Taking row 6 we have:

$$100–[(0.33/1.29) \times 100] = 75.0\%$$

Taking row 7 we have:

$$100–[(0.16/1.29) \times 100] = 60.0\%$$

Repeat this exercise for your data. Plot the data relating the percentage of competition against the concentration or dilution of the IgGs as in **Fig. 33.**

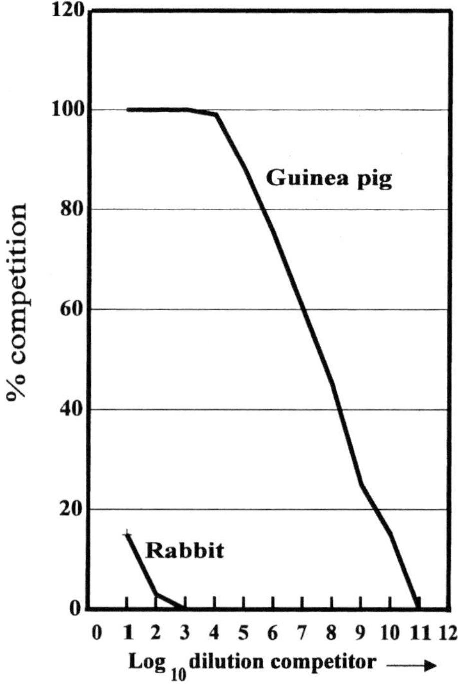

Fig. 33. Percentage of competition plots of guinea pig and rabbit IgG competing for the guinea pig system.

7.5.4. Analysis of Data

1. Note that as you dilute the homologous competitor (the guinea pig Ig), competition reduces.
2. Note that the plateau of 100% competition is where the competing Ig is in large excess over that on the plate.
3. Suggest what is happening at the 50% competition point.
4. Note that the competition curve is sigmoidal.
5. Note that the rabbit Ig hardly competes. Why?
6. Suggest how the sensitivity of the assay might be altered. A clue here is to examine what happens if we reduce (1) the amount of antigen on the solid phase and (2) the amount of conjugate in the test.

7.6. Indirect Assay: Antigen Competition

This exercise is similar to the direct competition assay for antigen except that the antigen is detected by an unlabeled antiserum (rabbit anti-guinea pig IgG), which in turn is detected using an anti-species conjugate. Here, the heterologous antigen is bovine IgG. Thus, the indirect assay is optimized as in **Subheading 2**. You can use the results of the CBT in this chapter (**Table 3**) to assess:

1. The best guinea pig concentration/dilution to adsorb to wells.
2. The optimum amount of antibody to give about 70% binding to the optimum amount of antigen found as shown in **Fig. 30.**

7.6.1. Materials

1. Ag1: guinea pig IgG at 1 mg/mL for attachment to solid phase
2. Ag2: samples of (a) guinea pig IgG standard solution (known concentration of 1 mg/mL, (b) three solutions of guinea pig IgG at unkown concentration, and (c) bovine IgG solution at 1 mg/mL
3. Ab: rabbit anti-guinea pig IgG
4. Ab*E: pig anti-rabbit pig IgG conjugated to HRP
5. Microplates
6. Multichannel and single-channel 10- and 1-mL pipets
7. Carbonate/bicarbonate, pH 9.6, 0.05 M
8. PBS 1% BSA, 0.05% Tween-20
9. Solution of OPD in citrate buffer
10. Hydrogen peroxide
11. Washing solution
12. Paper towels
13. Small volume bottles
14. 1 M sulfuric acid in water
15. Multichannel spectrophotometer
16. Clock

17. Graph paper
18. Calculator

These competition steps are identical to those of the direct assay and the data is processed in the same way. The extra step is to detect any reacted antibody with the anti-species conjugate.

7.6.2. Method

1. Coat the wells of a microplate with 50 µL of guinea pig Ig at optimum concentration found from CBT.
2. Wash the wells.
3. Dilute the homologous guinea pig IgG competitor of known concentration and the bovine Ig sample to 40 µg/mL in blocking buffer.
4. Take the three samples of unknown levels of guinea pig Ig and dilute 1/10 in blocking buffer.
5. Add 50 µL of blocking buffer to all the wells of the microplate coated with the optimum guinea pig Ig.
6. Make a twofold dilution range of all the diluted samples. Thus, add 50 µL of the initial dilution as shown in the plate plan in **Fig. 34.** Prepare duplicate columns of each for eight wells.
7. Add 50 µL of the pre-titrated antibody against the guinea pig Ig to columns 1–11. Add 50 µL of blocking buffer to column 12.
8. Incubate under conditions in which initial CBT were performed. Mix contents every 10 min (unless overnight incubation is being used).

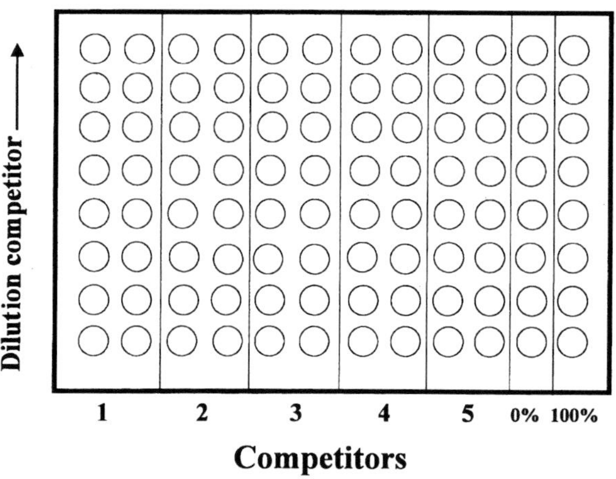

Fig. 34. Plate design for addition of competitors. 1, Guinea pig control; 2, bovine IgG; 3, sample A; 4, sample B; 5, sample C.

9. Wash the wells and blot.
10. Add 50 μL of the optimal dilution of the pig anti-guinea pig conjugate, per well and incubate at 37°C for 1 h. Wash the plates.
11. Add the OPD substrate/chromophore solution (50 μL per well), and stop the reaction by addition of 50 μL of 1 M H_2SO_4 after 10 min.
12. Read the OD using a spectrophotometer at 492 nm.

7.6.3. Data: Typical Results

Figure 35 represents appearance of the stopped plate. Plate data is as shown in **Table 14.**

7.6.4. Treatment of Data

1. Take the mean value of the OD from row 12 (0.08 in data from **Table 14**).
2. Subtract this from all the ODs of the rest of plate.
3. For each of the duplicate wells, find the mean OD for each competitor dilution. Thus, we have the values given in **Table 15.**
4. Take the mean result of column 11 in **Table 15** = 1.26. This is the 0% competition value. Use the following formula to calculate percentage of competition of each IgG dilution:

% competition = [(100 – OD in presence of competitor)/1.26 (range) × 100]

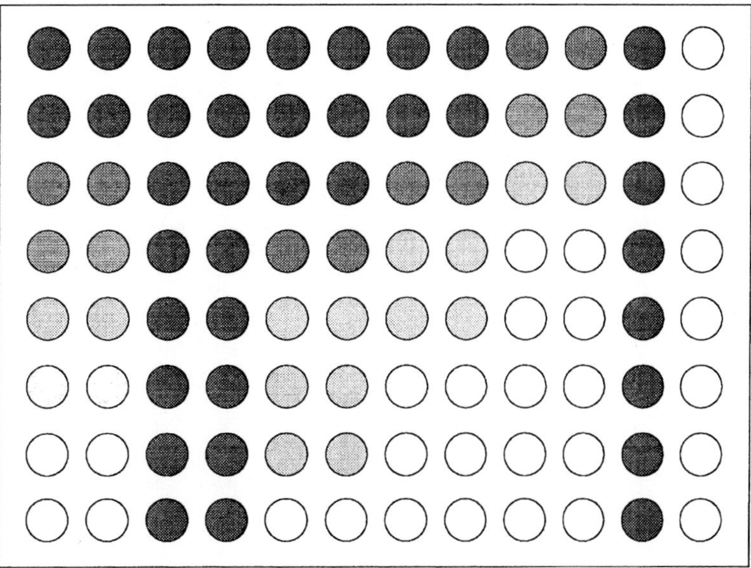

Fig. 35. Representation of place of competition assay. See data in Table 12.

Table 14
Plate data for indirect competitions ELISA to measure antigen

	Guinea pig test control		Bovine		Guinea pig 1		Guinea pig 2		Guinea pig 3		0%	100%
	1	2	3	4	5	6	7	8	9	10	11	12
A	1.31	1.30	1.31	1.33	1.32	1.32	1.26	1.34	2.12	1.10	1.34	0.06
B	1.12	1.14	1.32	1.34	1.28	1.29	1.21	1.18	0.88	0.83	1.32	0.08
C	0.79	0.77	1.29	1.28	1.09	1.10	1.00	0.98	0.68	0.66	1.34	0.09
D	0.57	0.54	1.27	1.19	0.85	0.79	0.76	0.74	0.44	0.43	1.32	0.06
E	0.33	0.36	1.25	1.24	0.67	0.69	0.47	0.48	0.22	0.23	1.29	0.08
F	0.18	0.15	1.25	1.26	0.41	0.45	0.26	0.27	0.09	0.09	1.34	0.09
G	0.09	0.10	1.21	1.22	0.30	0.29	0.16	0.17	0.08	0.09	1.33	0.08
H	0.08	0.07	1.15	1.18	0.13	0.15	0.09	0.07	0.07	0.06	1.35	0.06

Table 15
Mean values of plate data shown in table 14

	1 2	3 4	5 6	7 8	9 10	11
A	1.22	1.24	1.24	1.22	1.05	1.26
B	1.05	1.25	1.21	1.12	0.81	1.24
C	0.70	1.21	1.01	0.91	0.59	1.26
D	0.47	1.15	0.74	0.65	0.36	1.24
E	0.27	1.15	0.59	0.38	0.14	1.21
F	0.08	1.14	0.34	0.19	0.00	1.26
G	0.00	1.13	0.21	0.09	0.00	1.25
H	0.00	1.07	0.06	0.00	0.00	1.27

Thus, for data in **Table 15**, we have the processed data in **Table 16.** Plot the competition curves relating competition to $\log_{10}$ dilution or concentration as shown in **Fig. 36.**

7.6.5. Examination of Data

1. The bovine IgG competition is very low, and the slope of the curve is very different from those of homologous control guinea pig IgG.

Table 16
Competition percentage values from data shown in table 15

	% Competition				
	Guinea pig control 1–2	Bovine IgG 3–4	Guienea pig 1 IgG 5–6	Guienea pig 2 IgG 7–8	Guienea pig 3 IgG 9–10
A	6	5	5	7	20
B	20	5	7	12	36
C	35	9	20	28	53
D	67	10	42	49	71
E	79	10	53	70	100
F	93	11	75	87	100
G	100	15	87	100	100
H	100	20	95	100	100

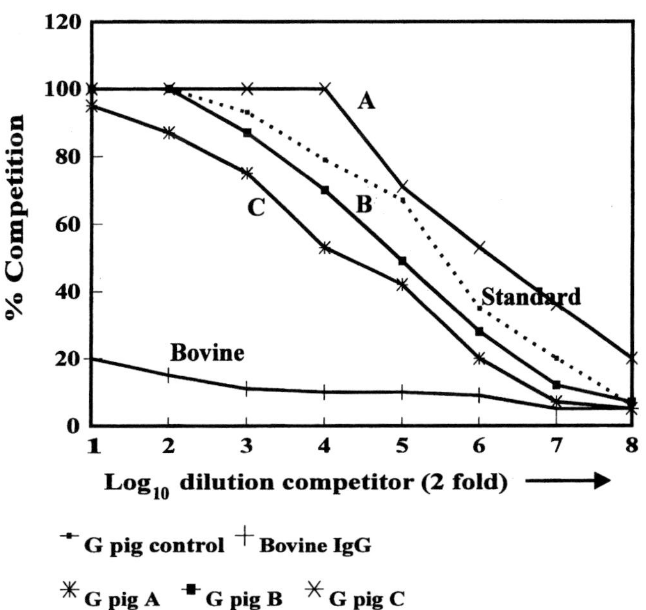

Fig. 36. Competition curves for various competitors. Data is shown in Table 12.

2. The curves for all guinea pig competitors are of similar shape.
3. The curves for test guinea pig IgG A, B, and C are displaced as compared to control IgG curve.

A standard curve relating concentration of guinea pig IgG competitor in the liquid phase to competition achieved, is shown by the control IgG. The concentration of IgG in the other samples can be determined with reference to this standard curve. Since the general slope of the curves is similar, we can compare the relative concentration at any point on the standard curve. Ideally, the best comparison point is at 50% competition. Therefore, draw a line across the 50% competition point on your graphs, as indicated in **Fig. 37.**

Read the dilution of the test IgGs that gives 50% competition, and then relate this to the known IgG concentration necessary to give 50% competition as determined from the standard curve at this point.

Thus, assuming a starting concentration of guinea pig IgG at 2 μg/mL, we have a standard IgG 50% competition = 1/64; a dilution for IgG A = 1/20; a dilution for IgG B = 1/40; and a dilution for IgG C = 1/140. Multiply the dilution factor by the 2 μg to get concentration/milliliters in the test IgG:

1. IgG C = 140/64 × 2 μg = 4.4 μg/mL
2. IgG B = 40/64 × 2 μg = 1.25 μg/mL
3. IgG A = 20/64 × 2 μg = 0.63 μg/mL

Remember that the dilution range is in $\log_{10}$ steps so that the antilog of the value has to be taken to obtain dilution factor at 50%.

7.6.6. Conclusions

1. We have used a standard curve relating a known concentration of homologous competitor to its competing ability, to measure unknown concentrations of the same IgG in samples. This

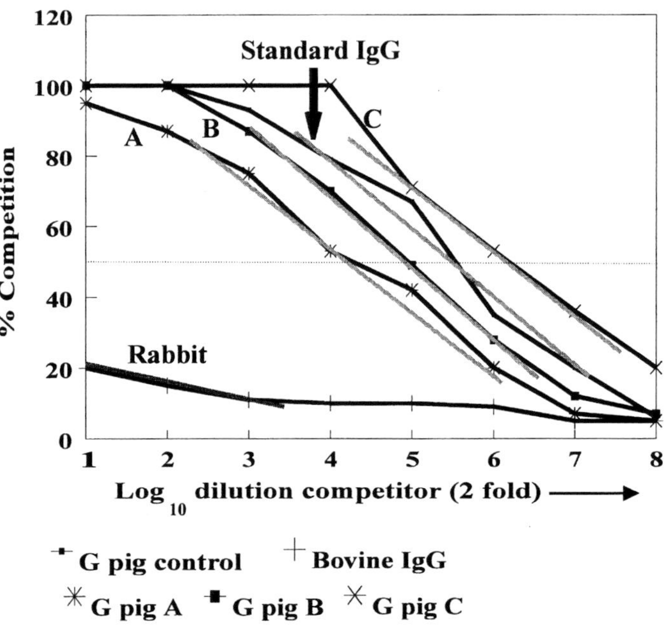

Fig. 37. Regression of competition curves for various competitors. Data from Table 14. Regression lines are gray.

has analogies to radioimmunoassay approaches used in quantification of hormones.

2. Note that if it is known that the substance for detection and quantification is the same immunologically (homologous) as the standard substance used to compute the standard curve, single dilutions of test could be used and their competing ability read from a standard curve.
3. Such competition assays can be used to determine the similarity of antigens in the same system competing for a single antiserum. The slopes of the competition lines can be compared to obtain a measure of antigenic relatedness.

7.7. Indirect Competition Assay for Antibody Detection

7.7.1 Reaction Scheme

$$\text{I-Ag}_W + \text{Ab} (+ \text{AB})_W + \text{anti-Ab*E}_W + \text{S—READ}$$

where I = microplate; Ag = antigen; Ab = pretitrated antibodies to Ag (species X); AB = competing antibody (from species different from Ab); Anti-Ab*E = conjugated anti-species in which Ab was produced; S = substrate and chromophore; W = washing step; + = addition and incubation of reagents; and READ = reading in a spectrophotometer.

In this exercise, the indirect assay is used to pretitrate the homologous antibody. The optimized system is then competed with a dilution range of antibodies from another species (the conjugate must not react with the competing antibodies). In this assay, the pretitration of the homologous serum is slightly different from the antigen competition indirect ELISA in that we need to add the amount of homologous antibodies which just saturate the antigen coated on the plate, as we do not wish to leave excess free antigenic sites that could react with the competing antibody and have little influence on the binding of the homologous antiserum. Note that this kind of assay can be made using the direct ELISA with a conjugated homologous serum, as for the direct antigen competition ELISA. Such assays are becoming more common with the advent of the use of mAb reagents.

7.7.2. Data

Figure 38 is a graph relating the antibody titration curves to the IgG concentrations on the wells. From these data we can do the following:

1. Assess the best antigen concentration for use in the competition assay, and select the IgG concentration that gives a plateau maximum (in antibody excess) of around 1–1.5 OD (curves 4 and 5).
2. Select the dilution of serum that just saturates this level of IgG (~1/100).

7.7.3. Increasing the Confidence of the Titration Curve Results

Since in the CBT we are using only a single-dilution range of antibody against the antigen, it is essential to titrate the antiserum in multiple rows against the antigen level found to be optimal.

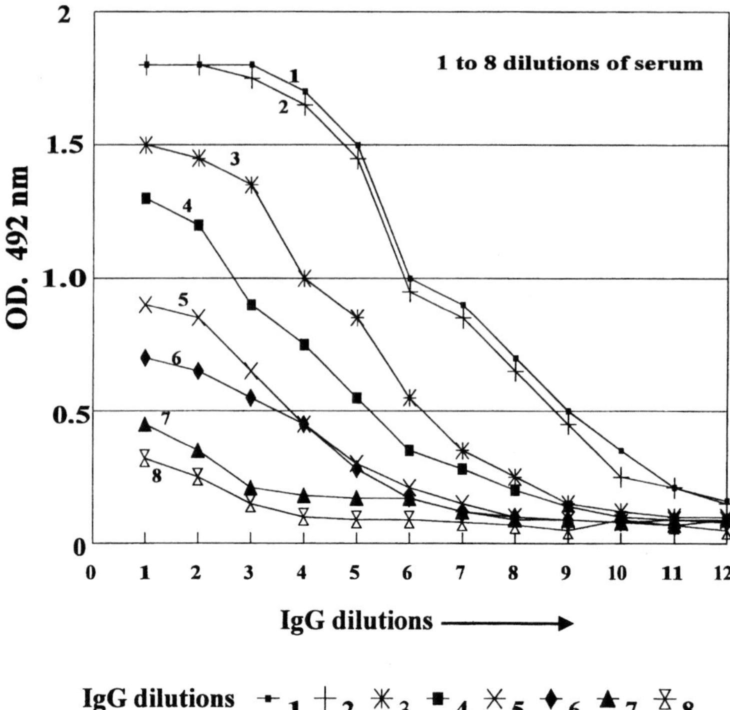

Fig. 38. Titration curves relating IgG dilutions on wells against different serum dilutions.

That is, we adsorb IgG at a level equivalent to the fourth or fifth dilution used in the preceding test, and titrate in quadruplicate a dilution series of serum against it. In this way, we can observe the variation in results and assess the confidence in the titer of antibody that just saturates the antigen used in the competition assay proper. This may be necessary when, e.g., one obtains poor competition in the test proper with low sensitivity, indicating that too high or much too low a concentration of antiserum was used.

7.7.4. Competition Assay Proper

1. Add 50 μL of guinea pig IgG to plates at optimal concentration found in stage 1, incubate, and wash the plates.
2. For the rabbit anti-guinea pig sera, label the standard antiserum 1, label the two unknown titer sera 2 and 3. Label the two sero-negative rabbit sera 4 and 5.
3. Dilute the rabbit sera to 1/50 in blocking buffer (make up 0.5 mL of each; i.e., add 10 μL of serum to 0.5 mL of buffer).
4. Add 50 μL of blocking buffer to all the antigen-coated plate wells.
5. Add 50 μL of rabbit serum 1 to wells H1 and H2. Add duplicate rows of other sera in row H (serum 2 in H3 and 4; serum 3 in H5 and 6; serum 4 in H7 and 8; serum 5 H in 9 and 10). Dilute the sera using a multichannel pipet, transferring and

mixing 50 μL for each step. We thus have a dilution range from 1/100 (row H) to 1/12,800 (row A) for each of the sera.

6. Incubate for 30 min at 37°C. Do not wash the plate.
7. Add 50 μL of the swine anti-guinea pig serum at the optimal dilution, found in stage 1, to each well from columns 1 to 11. Do not touch liquid in the wells when adding reagent. Add 50 μL of blocking buffer to column 12.
8. Incubate for 1 h at 37°C.
9. Wash the wells.
10. Add 50 μL of anti-swine conjugate to each well diluted in blocking buffer.
11. Incubate at 37°C for 1 h.
12. Add 50 μL well of substrate and OPD per well, and incubate for 10 min.
13. Stop the reaction by addition of 50 μL of 1 M H_2SO_4 to each well.

Typical Data

Figure 39 is a representation of the ELISA plate after stopping. **Table 17** presents the data.

7.7.5. Processing Data

Processing of the data is similar to the other competition assays performed:

1. Column 12 = 100% competition value, take the mean OD = 0.08
2. Subtract this from OD values of all wells.

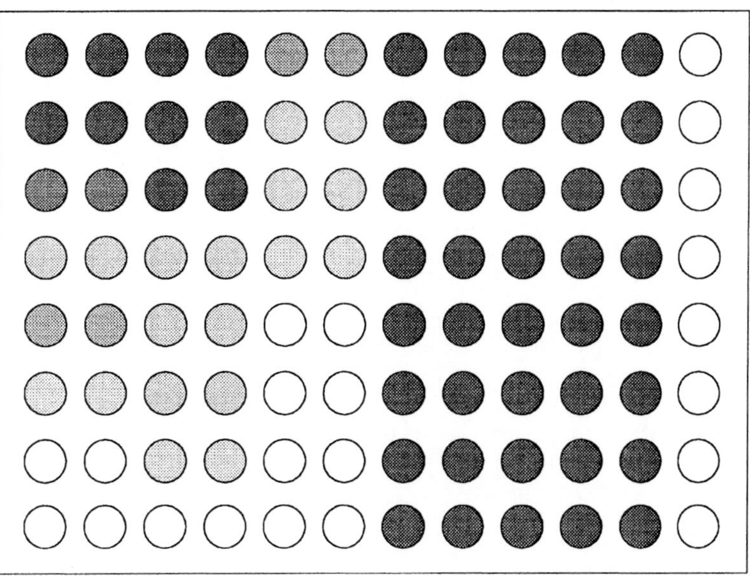

Fig. 39. Representation of plate showing competition assay. Data given in Table 17

Table 17
Plate data from exercise 7.7 in subheading 7.7.4 showing competition of indirect assay by antibodies

	Standard serum	1		2		3		4		100%		0%
	1	2	3	4	5	6	7	8	9	10	11	12
A	1.12	1.16	1.21	1.20	0.78	0.84	1.14	1.13	1.14	1.15	1.11	0.07
B	1.07	1.09	1.21	1 .19	0.56	0.58	1.15	1.12	1.16	1..4	1.15	0.09
C	0.89	0.91	1.10	1.09	0.34	0.32	1.13	1.09	1.15	1.12	1.17	0.07
D	0.63	0 61	0.87	0.89	0.21	0.19	1.10	100	1.13	1.15	1.16	0.06
E	0.42	0.41	0.63	0.65	0.09	0.08	1.16	1.09	1.14	1.13	1.15	0.08
F	0.23	0.26	0.43	0.45	0.08	0 07	1 13	1.14	1.14	1.16	1.15	0.07
G	0.13	0.12	0.23	0.25	0.07	0.08	1.15	1.12	1.16	1.15	1.17	0.06
H	0.08	0.09	0.12	0.10	0.08	0.07	1.14	1.16	1.14	1.15	1.15	0.07

Table 18
Mean values of data in table 17

	1–2	3–4	5–6	7–8	9–10	11
A	1.05	1.12	0.71	1.06	1.07	1.08
B	1.00	1.12	0.49	1.06	1.07	1.07
C	0.90	1.01	0.25	1.03	1.06	1.09
D	0.52	0.80	0.12	1.01	1.06	1.08
E	0.34	0.56	0.00	1.04	1.06	1.07
F	0.16	0.36	0.00	1.06	1.07	1.07
G	0.05	0.16	0.00	1.06	1.07	1.09
H	0.00	0.03	0.00	1.07	1.06	1.07

3. Take the mean OD of the duplicates for the competitors. This is shown in **Table 18.**
4. Plot the data, and relate the log 10 dilution of each antiserum to percentage of competition as illustrated in **Fig. 40.**

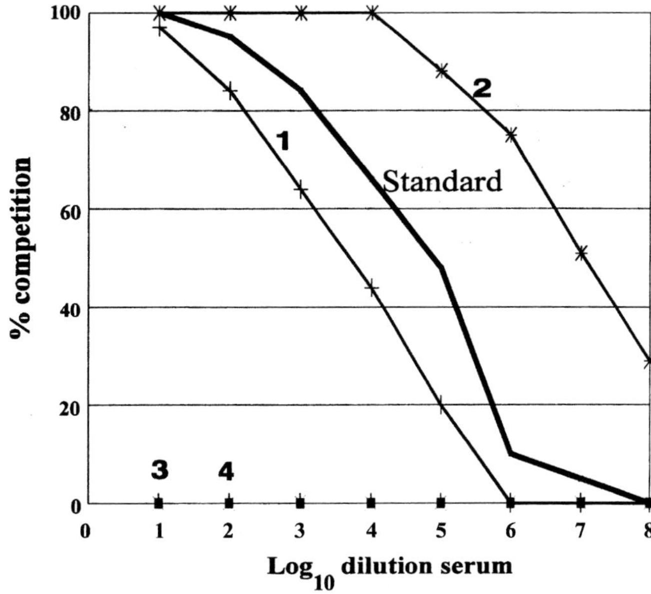

Fig. 40. Competition curves for various competing sera. Data from Table 18.

7.7.6. Analysis of Data

1. Note that the curves for the rabbit antisera are similar. All the samples compete. Sample 3 is a strong competitor as it gives high competition at higher dilutions than the standard (1). Sample 2 is a weaker competitor than the standard.
2. The negative sera give little or no competition even at low dilutions.
3. The activity of each of the two test sera can be compared to the standard competing antiserum (1). Arbitrary units can be ascribed to the standard serum so that serum titers could be expressed against this. As an example, let the titer of the standard serum at 50% competition be 1,000. The relative titers of the other two test sera can then be related to this. As the same dilution range was used for the samples, we have at 50% competition for serum 2, which is twice stronger than the standard. Therefore, we need twice as much antiserum to compete at the same level as the standard; hence the relative titer of the serum is 1/500. For serum 3 at 50%, we require five times less antiserum to produce the same result as the standard so the titer is 5,000. The difference in the dilution factors necessary to give 50% competition is easily assessed from the graphs in **Fig. 40.**
4. Note that this processing holds true only if the competition curves show similar characteristics (shape). Considerable variation in slopes indicates that there is a different population of

antibodies in the competing serum. As in all assays, the general picture of titration curves is best examined by the assay of as many sera as possible.

7.8. Indirect Assay Competition for Antibody Detection Using a Single Dilution of Test Serum

Here we use the standard competing rabbit serum as a full titration range in three rows of the plate. The rest of the plate contains a number of rabbit sera of high, medium and low titer against guinea pig IgG as used in **Subheading 7.6**. Not all the sera can be used in this exercise owing to the limited space on the plate. The assay is identical to that in **Subheading 7.6** except that duplicate samples of sera are assessed at a single dilution for their competing ability. The titer of the serum is then read from the standard curve obtained on full dilution of the standard serum. The test therefore has two stages: (1) the titration of the homologous antiserum and solid-phase antigen in a CBT indirect ELISA, and (2) the competition proper.

7.8.1. Materials and Reagents

As for **Subheading 7.7** except that rabbit sera are replaced by 32 rabbit sera including seronegative, low, medium, and high titers against guinea pig IgG.

7.8.2. Pretitration Stage

Repeat the first stage as in **Subheading 7.7**, or use this data to establish conditions. From the data the best antigen concentration, and dilution of swine antibody that just saturates the IgG, is determined.

7.8.3. Competition Assay Proper

1. Add 50 μL of guinea pig IgG to plates at optimal dilution Incubate and wash the plates.
2. Dilute the rabbit test sera to 1/50 in blocking buffer. Use micronics racks for dilutions so that the samples can be added using a multichannel pipet. Dilute the standard rabbit antiserum to 1/50.
3. Add 50 μL of blocking buffer to columns 1, 2, 11, and 12.
4. Add 50 μL of the diluted standard rabbit serum to H1 and H2. Make a twofold dilution range of the serum to A1 and A2.
5. Add the test samples to the wells as duplicates, as indicated in **Fig. 41.**
6. Incubate the plates for 30 min at 37°C.
7. Add 50 μL of the optimum dilution of swine anti-guinea pig serum in blocking buffer, incubate for 1 h at 37°C, and mix the contents of the plates every 10 min. Do not add this serum to column 12. Instead, add 50 μL of blocking buffer.
8. Wash the plates.
9. Add the anti-swine conjugate diluted in blocking buffer (optimum dilution). Incubate for 1 h at 37°C.
10. Wash the plate.

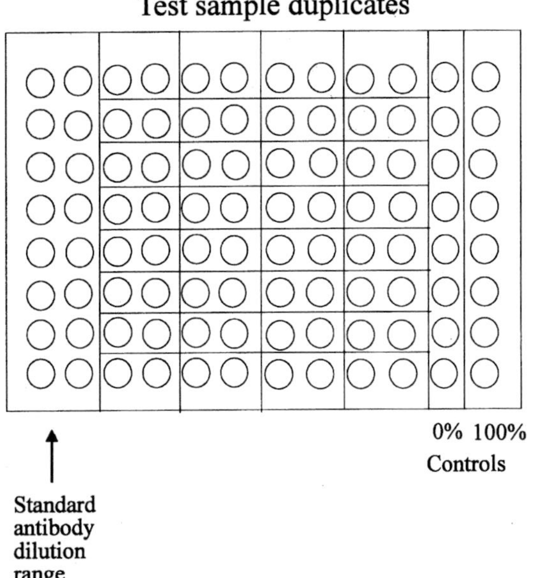

Fig. 41. Plate layout for spot testing in competition assay.

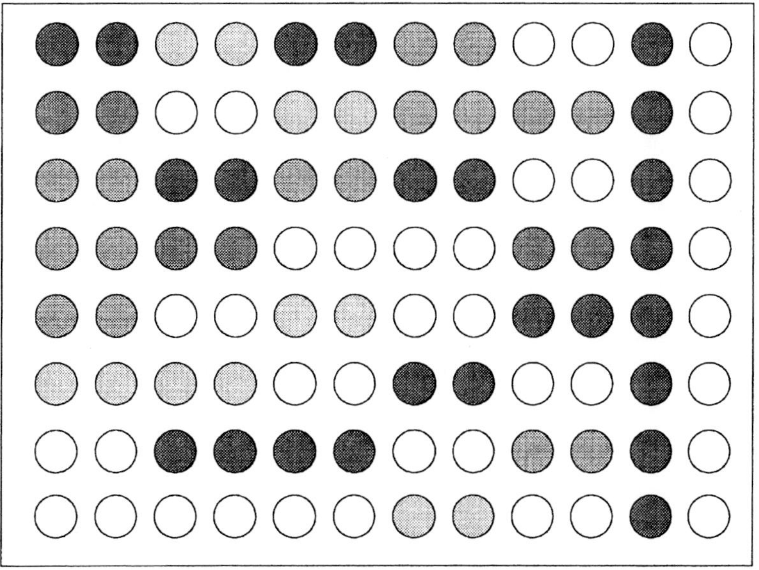

Fig. 42. Representation of a spot test competition assay. Data given in Table 19.

11. Add substrate/OPD, and incubate for 10 min.
12. Stop the reaction by addition of 50 μL of 1 M H_2SO_4 per well.
13. Read plate using spectrophotometer. (*see* **Fig. 42** for a representation of a stopped plate.)

7.8.4. Typical Data

Table 19 presents typical data for a spot test.

Table 19
Plate data from spot test

	1	2	3	4	5	6	7	8	9	10	11	12
A	1:31	1.30	1.31	1.33	1.32	1.32	1.26	1.34	1.12	1.10	1.34	0.06
A	1.21	1.24	0.34	0.32	1.23	1.21	1.12	1.12	0.09	0.09	1.23	0.07
B	1.03	1.05	0.19	0.18	0.43	0.45	0.56	0.58	0.78	0.78	1.21	0.09
C	0.91	0.90	1.13	1.15	0.67	0.69	1.11	1.13	0.12	0.14	1.24	0.08
D	0.76	0.73	0.98	0.96	0.13	0.12	0.16	0.13	0.78	0.80	1.24	0.09
E	0.53	0.54	0.06	0.04	0.34	0.36	0.16	0.18	1.23	1.21	1.23	0.08
F	0.31	0.34	0.34	0.36	0.14	0.16	1.17	1.19	0.08	0.10	1.21	0.07
G	0.12	0.13	1.21	1.23	1.14	1.11	0.09	0.07	0.67	0.69	1.26	0.05
H	0.06	0.08	0.06	0.09	0.15	0.12	0.23	0.27	0.10	0.12	1.23	0.06

7.8.5. Treatment of Data

For the other competition results, make the following calculations:

1. Calculate the mean of column 12, and subtract this from all results from the other wells.
2. Calculate the mean from column 11 (after subtraction in **step 1**).
3. Express the other ODs as a percentage of the range 0 to the mean column 11, i.e., from 0 to 1.16 in the example above.
4. Take the mean OD of the duplicate wells.
5. Use the following formula to calculate the percentage of competition in each well:

   $100 - [(\text{OD}/1.16 \times 100]$

   Plot the standard serum competition activity relating competition to $\log_{10}$ of the dilution.
6. Read the relative titers of the other competition results from the curve.
7. Another approach to evaluating spot testing is that in which, accepted negative sera are assessed as controls. Several sera can be included in a test so that their mean competition value and its variation can be assessed. Thus, sera giving higher values of competition under the same conditions (with prescribed confidence limits) can be assessed for positivity. Studies on a large number of negative sera give better population data as described for the other assays, so that chosen negative controls may be added from the defined population (*see* **Table 20**). In **Table 20**, the sera with asterisks can be the negative controls in order to test whether the system is ideal. The percentage

Table 20
Mean values of test sera from tale 19 processed as competition values

	Competition results (%)				
	1 2	3 4	5 6	7 8	9 10
A	0	73	2	16	99
B	16	90	68	57	39
C	28	7a	48	9	95
D	41	23	96	93	38
E	59	100	76	91	0
F	78	76	93	4[a]	98
G	100	100	95	84	97

[a]Sera could be used as negative controls.

value of their mean plus a defined interval as a percentage of this mean (as directed from large population studies) can be given. Here, we have mean = 3%. Assume that two times this mean is an acceptable upper limit for negative competition values. Therefore, sera can be ascribed as positive with competition values 6%.

7.8.6. Notes

We have used a dilution of 1/100 for the test sera in the example. This is based on preliminary studies establishing dilution as being optimal for distinguishing positive and negative values. This must be attempted in your laboratories for specific disease studies. The approach to examination of negative populations has already been discussed. In the case of competition assays, a lower dilution of test serum might be used (effectively increasing the sensitivity of the assay) since nonspecific factors detected in the indirect assay do not seem to affect competition assay results. Construction of full-scale serum titration competition curves of many negative and positive sera will indicate the best dilution (with definable confidence limits) of serum to be used. The sources of such sera have already been discussed.

Thus, for any particular dilution used in the competition assay, an upper limit of negativity should be definable (as a competition value) above which positivity of antibody will be detected. Once competition assays have been characterized in central laboratories, it is usually simple to read the assays by eye, with good levels of precision and sensitivity. In these cases, selection of appropriate negative controls that define upper limits of negativity as determined by eye is important.

7.8.7. Conclusions About Competition Assays

1. Competition assays provide a relatively simple method once the homologous systems have been titrated.
2. These assays can be read by eye, with some loss of sensitivity and reduction in confidence limits.
3. In all the examples given, we have used 50 μL of competitor and 50 μL of homologous serum as a mixture to compete for only 50 μL of antigen on the solid phase. You can alter the volumes to suit e.g.:
   a. 100 μL of antigen solid phase vs. 50 μL of homologous serum and 50 μL of competing antigen (or antibody). In this case, the pretitration would be with 100 μL of solid-phase antigen vs. 50 μL of serum dilutions + of 50 μL blocking buffer.
   b. 50 μL of solid-phase antigen vs. 25 μL of homologous serum + 25 μL competing antigen (or antibody). In this case the pretitration would be between 50 μL of solid-phase antigen and 25 μL of antibody dilutions + 25 μL of buffer.
   c. The competitor and homologous serum can be mixed together in another plate before addition to the solid-phase antigen plate. These types of assay can be termed inhibition assays since the reagents are not directly competing in the same system.
4. Differences in results can be observed by alteration of the sequence of reagents, i.e., when true competition and inhibition methods are used. In practice, the mixing of reagents in a true competition assay gives the most sensitive assays and best reflects avidity differences among reagents.

Chapter 7

Monoclonal Antibodies

The ability to produce and exploit monoclonal antibodies (mAbs) has revolutionized many areas of biological sciences. The unique property of an mAb is that it is a single species of immunoglobulin (IG) molecule. This means that the specificity of the interaction of the paratopes on the IG, with the epitopes on an antigenic target, is the same on every molecule. This property can be used to great benefit in immunoassays to provide tests of defined specificity and sensitivity, which improve the possibilities of standardization. The performance of assays can often be determined relating the actual weight of antibody (hence the number of molecules) to the activity. Often the production of an mAb against a specific epitope is the only way that biological entities can be differentiated. This chapter outlines the areas involving the development of assays based on mAbs. The problems involved addressinclude the physical aspects of mAbs and how they may affect assay design and also the implications of results based on monospecific reagents. Often these are not fully understood, leading to assays that are less than satisfactory, which does not justify the relatively high cost of preparing and screening of mAbs.

There are many textbooks and reviews dealing with the preparation of mAbs, the principles involved, and various purification and manipulative methods for the preparation of fragments and conjugation. There has been little general information attempting to summarize the best approaches to assay design using mAbs. Much time can be wasted through bad planning, and this is particularly relevant to mAbs. A proper understanding of some basic principles is essential. It is beyond the scope of this chapter to discuss all aspects, but major areas are highlighted.

1. Purpose of the Assay Involving the mAb

The fundamental question, "What is the purpose of the assay involving the mAb?" may never be properly considered in sufficient detail. The first considerations presented in the following

John R. Crowther, *Methods in Molecular Biology, The ELISA Guidebook, Vol. 516*

DOI: 10.1007/978-1-60327-254-4_7

list address the "state of knowledge" about a problem (disease organism, serology, antigenic structure, other tests) and available reagent base. These are in common with other test developments but are particularly relevant to mAbs:

1. How much knowledge do we have about other current assays?
2. How much information have do we have about the target antigen (organism)?
3. What information is there in the literature?
4. What time frame have we got for development of an assay?
5. What advantages and disadvantages will an mAb-based assay have over conventional techniques or polyclonal systems?
6. What polyclonal reagents do we have available from their use in other tests?

Analysis of this information should indicate whether mAbs are needed to provide the necessary properties of a test.

1.1. Availability of MmaAbs

mAbs are available from two sources. The first is from other laboratories. Such mAbs will have been subjected to various degrees of characterization, and it is vital that all data pertaining to the mAbs be are obtained. This will allow a better selection process for candidate mAbs for use in designing assays. The second source is to produce them either in-house where there are facilities, or through a contract with a specialist laboratory acting in a service capacity.

The cost of setting up and maintaining an mAb production facility is great, and usually resources are made available only where there is a need to produce a variety of mAbs against a number of agents. A typical laboratory making mAbs must consider carefully the logistical problems not only of tissue culture maintenance to a high standard but cloning, screening, amplification of mAb (increasing the amount of mAb produced), and storage of cell lines. In other words, careful planning with a full knowledge of the implications of mAb production is essential. Production methods have become easier as technologies surrounding the methods have improved, so it is feasible to set up production in a relatively small laboratory. The basics of production must include at least one dedicated worker responsible for maintaining the mAb production, animal facilities (with appropriate legal approvals), and enough financial support to have a sustainable work program.

A salutary truth is that there is no certainty of success when embarking on production. However, the first essential factor in planning is to decide exactly what the purpose of an mAb will be, so that the correct mAbs can be identified as quickly as possible and the work effort concentrated on these. It is far too tempting in practice to try to handle all the mAbs produced in a fusion.

1.2. Planning

Clear planning involves consideration of the immunization regime that might best give a range of mAbs most relevant to their intended task. Again, reference to developments in this field will give clues as to the best methods. Basically, mice (usually) have to be exposed to a specific antigen(s) and must stimulate antibody-producing cells. The approach can be "shotgun" in which a relatively complex and "crude" mixture of antigens is used as the immunizing agent, or it can involve administration of a pure, defined antigen. The first approach has implications when the antibody secreted from hybridomas (fused cells secreting antibodies) need to be screened for activity. Screening and selection of appropriate clones is are time-consuming, requires assay development, and should always have the aim of finding as quickly as possible the antibodies of direct relevance to the preconceived objectives of the required function. **Table 1** presents a typical scenario for the screening and eventual isolation and use of mAbs.

1.3. Screening mAbs after Fusion

Screening should be selective as early as possible. Thus, the appropriate antigen has to be used in screening to test for antibody binding. The ELISA systems are ideal for this and, often at this stage, rely on data from other polyclonal assays. As an example, the concentration of an antigen that gives a good level of coating and signal in a polyclonal serum-based assay might be known. This concentration can be used to screen for mAbs using an indirect ELISA.

The essential work in the early stages is to have actively growing hybridomas secreting IG, and to ensure that these stem from

Table 1
Scheme for prepration and characterization of mAbs using ELISA

1.	Growth of cells in microplates; secretion of immunoglobulin into maintenance medium	Spot test for levels; spot test for specific activity of mAbs
2.	Growth of selected hybridomas; stabilization; secretion of IG. into medium	Spot test for levels of IG; spot test for specific activity
3.	Larger-scale production in tissue culture, or ascites; secreted mAb or as ascites fluid.	Specific activity for each mAb determined using one or more antigen (epitope); isotyping
4.	Purification of mAbs; preparation of fragment?; conjugation; assay design	Specific activity of each mAb determined using different epitopes; quantification of IG; performance of mAbs as capture reagent; examination of conjugates
5.	Use of mAbs	Standardized reagents; differentiating reagents; specific diagnostic reagents; panels used to profile epitopes in epidemio logical studies; epitope characterization

single cells. Usually at the early stages of producing stable hybridomas, only a small amount of tissue culture fluid is available for testing, so that assays are made using a single dilution. This limits the possibilities of screening against a variety of antigens, which would allow some differential analysis of binding to be made at this stage. Therefore, it may be more useful to select an antigenic mixture at this stage. The specificity of the mAbs could then be determined when they are available in higher amounts.

The anti-mouse conjugate used must detect all isotypes of mouse IG equally well (these are commercially available). Mouse IGs have a number of specific isotypes and in order not to miss any possible binding, the conjugate must detect IgM, IgA, IgG_1, IgG_{2a}, IgG_{2b}, and IgG_3 isotypes.

There is a similarity in stages 2 and 3 in **Table 1**. This indicates that screening can be made quite early when it is reasonably certain that colonies of cells have been derived from single cells, depending on the methods used.

When single cells have been picked, there may be fewer clones to examine, but confidence in their clonality is high. Thus, screening here may be more relevant than for limit dilution methods. From a practical point of view, it might be useful to give a few figures for good and bad fusion results. An initial target of 200–500 clones (representing the handling of two- to four-microtiter plates) is reasonable. These reflect my experience and depend greatly on exactly which methods are used and the experience of the operators involved as well as the biological system being examined. They also depend on exactly how much work is put into the production. There must always be a realistic balance between achieving a target mAb and the maintenance of thousands of clones. Of these clones, many will turn out to be unproductive for various reasons, and hence useless. The maintenance and testing of 200–500 clones in the early stages is manageable by a single person. Increasing this number runs the risk of poor management. The essential target of this part of the operation is to produce colonies of cells that are secreting mAb. The testing of the mAb as early as possible will highlight candidate mAbs for further testing, stabilization, and use.

This scenario is further complicated if mAbs are being produced against several antigens are being produced by different operators. It is extremely difficult to control operations in which several runs are being made, each requiring operative procedures at different times.

The examination of whether colonies are secreting mouse IG might sometimes be useful, especially when there is little activity against target antigens in screening. Nonsecretors can also be discarded. This can be accomplished easily through developing a competitive assay. The competitive assay for determining mouse IgG is described next, for reference and to introduce techniques and terms that will be generally used.

2. Competitive Assay for Determination of Mouse IgG

2.1. Requirements

1. Mouse Igs isolated from whole mouse serum.
2. Anti-mouse enzyme-labeled conjugate (commercially available, reacting with all isotypes of mouse Igs).
3. Microtiter plates (96-well ELISA plates).
4. Micropipets (5- to 50-L variable volume), single and multichannel pipets (12 channel), and tips.
5. Reservoirs for reagents.
6. 5- to 20-mL bottles.
7. Relevant substrate/chromogen solution for enzyme conjugate.
8. Phosphate-buffered saline (PBS) (0.1 M, pH 7.4).
9. Blocking buffer: 5% skimmed milk powder in PBS.
10. Relevant agent/conditions for stopping reaction after addition of chro-mogen/substrate.
11. Multichannel spectrophotometer.
12. Samples for testing.
13. Washing solution (PBS, pH 7.4, 0.02–0.1 M).

2.2. Preparation of Mouse Ig

Preparation of mouse Ig requires a minimum of 2 mL of mouse serum. A relatively simple technique for the preparation of total mouse Ig from serum, and one that gives adequately pure Ig for this test, is to use ammonium sulfate precipitation. Once the Ig is obtained and dialyzed against, e.g., PBS as used in ELISA, the concentration can be assessed either by protein estimation using chemical kits or, more easily, by reading the absorbance at 280 nm in an ultraviolet (UV) spectrophotometer. The concentration of Ig can be related to the absorbance using the following formula:

Absorbance (280 nm) × 0.7 = mg/mL of Ig

However, the formula is only true for relatively pure IgG. Once this has been accomplished, a solution containing a known concentration of mouse Ig is available. It should be stored in small aliquots at –20°C. For the sake of this example, we can make the assumption that a sample with 1 mg/mL (i.e., 1,000 g/mL) has been obtained directly or has been diluted to this concentration.

This process should take a few hours to precipitate Ig followed by overnight dialysis allowing for changes in dialyzing solution.

2.3. Stage 1: Optimization of the Mouse/Anti-mouse System

The objective of this stage is to titrate the mouse Ig, when attached to the solid phase, against the anti-mouse conjugate. Optimal conditions specifying the dilution of mouse Ig (antigen) and conjugate will be determined. The system will then be challenged by the addition of known Ig concentrations to the conjugate on addition to the mouse Ig–coated wells. A standard curve relating the concentration of mouse Ig added and the degree of inhibition of pretitrated reaction between the mouse Ig antigen on the plate and the conjugate can be established. Readings of inhibition by samples possibly containing mouse Ig can then be used to estimate the concentration of mouse Ig. Although this may seem complicated, the test can be set up in 2 days. Such a system is also relevant for the determination of concentrations of Ig for any antiserum species. The prepared Ig will act as the standard solution for all competitive tests, so it needs has to be protected from contamination by storing at low temperature.

2.3.1. Practical Details of Stage 1: Chessboard Titration

1. Dilute the mouse Ig to 5 g/mL in PBS. Prepare a volume of 1 mL of this solution. For our example, we have 1,000 g/mL so we add 5 L of this to 1 mL (1000 L) of PBS. Mix well without causing frothing.
2. Add 50 L of PBS to columns 2–12 of a microtiter ELISA plate.
3. Add 50 L of Ig solution to columns A and B, using a 50-L pipet.
4. Place eight tips on a multichannel pipet, and set the volume to 50 L. Place the tips in column 2. Mix the contents (50 L of PBS and 50 L of Ig solution) by gentle pipeting action four times. Take up 50 L of mixed solution in column 2 and transfer to column 3. Repeat the mixing exercise in column 3. Transfer to column 4, repeat, and so on until column 11. Discard the last 50 L after final pipeting action in column 11. We now have the same dilution range of Ig in 50-L vol, added to rows A–H, beginning at 5 g/mL and diluted twofold to column 11.
5. Incubate the plates for 2 h at 37°°C.
6. Wash the plates by flooding and emptying wells 5 times in PBS. Then blot almost dry by tapping plates onto a sponge of paper towel.
7. Obtain conjugate and read the titer recommended by the commercial company. Make a dilution of approximately eight times that recommended; for example, if the recommended dilution is 1/400, make up 1/500. A final volume of 1 mL (1,000 μL) is needed in at this stage. Thus, add 2 L of conjugate to 1,000 μL of PBS. An examination of the appropriate pipet to use with small volumes is required. Where there is no pipet to deliver 2 μL accurately, then a 5-μL vol can be used into the appropriate volume; however, this does wastes conjugate. Mix the conjugate solution without undue force.

8. Add 50 L of blocking buffer to all the wells of the Ig-coated microplates using a multichannel pipet.
9. Add 50 μL of the diluted conjugate to each well of row A.
10. Using a multichannel pipet with 12 tips, mix the contents of row A. Transfer 50 μL to row B, mix, transfer to row C, and so on until row H. Discard the last 50 μL in the tips. We now have a dilution of conjugate in blocking buffer (50 μL per well) from 1/1,000 (since we added 50 μL at 1/500 to 50 μL of buffer) to 128,000.
11. Incubate the plates for 2 h at 37°°C.
12. Wash the plates, and blot.
13. Add the appropriate substrate/chromogen solution, leave for the prescribed time, and stop the reaction.
14. Read the OD values on a spectrophotometer.

2.3.2. Results

Table 2 gives typical results obtained with a horseradish peroxidase (HRP) conjugate/H_2O_2-*ortho*-phenylenediamine (OPD) system.

Chessboard titrations (CBTs) have already been considered in some detail (*see* **Chapter 4**). In **Table 2**, row E in this plate indicates that there is a good level of color development with the conjugate at 1/8,000. The plateau maximum value in the presence of excess antigen (mouse Ig) is acceptable, and the Ig is detected to column 11 (with respect to a plate background value of 0.1).

For the final competitive assay we require a single dilution of coating antigen. Ultimately, the sensitivity of the assay depends on the concentrations of conjugate and Ig, so that we are seeking a level of coating antigen Ig that does not saturate the wells, and a

Table 2
Data from CBT of Ig and conjugate

	1	2	3	4	5	6	7	8	9	10	11	12
A	2.2	2.3	2.2	2.1	2.0	2.0	1.9	1.6	1.5	1.3	0.8	0.6
B	2.2	2.0	1.9	2.0	1.9	1.8	1.7	1.5	1.3	0.8	0.5	0.3
C	2.1	2.0	1.9	1.9	1.8	1.7	1.6	1.5	1.2	0.7	0.5	0.3
D	1.9	1.9	1.7	1.8	1.5	1.2	1.0	0.7	0.5	0.3	0.2	0.1
E	1.8	1.8	1.7	1.5	1.3	1.1	0.8	0.6	0.5	0.3	0.2	0.1
F	1.3	1.3	1.2	1.2	1.1	0.8	0.6	0.5	0.3	0.2	0.1	0.1
G	0.7	0.7	0.7	0.6	0.6	0.5	0.3	0.2	0.1	0.1	0.1	0.1
H	0.4	0.3	0.3	0.3	0.2	0.2	0.2	0.1	0.1	0.1	0.1	0.1

[a]Conjugate diluted from A to H (e.g.,1/500 in above example). Mouse Ig is diluted from 1 to 11 (5 g/mL starting concentration in this example)

conjugate dilution that just reacts with all the coating Ig. The box in **Table 2** reflects the area where this is relevant. Stage 2 involves closer examination of the concentrations under competitive conditions to assess the best system in practice. This procedure takes only 1 day. The box in **Table 2** covers three antigen dilutions and two conjugate dilutions, which can be examined in stage 2.

2.4. Practical Details Stage 2: Competition Of of Standard IgG with Titrated Conjugate and Coating Ig

The materials needed are the same as those used in stage 10. Two microtiter plates are needed: plate 1 for the competition conditions, and plate 2 to set up controls for 100% competition values.

2.4.1. Materials

2.4.2. Method

The diagram in **Fig. 1** shows a template indicating the addition of reagents to plate 1.

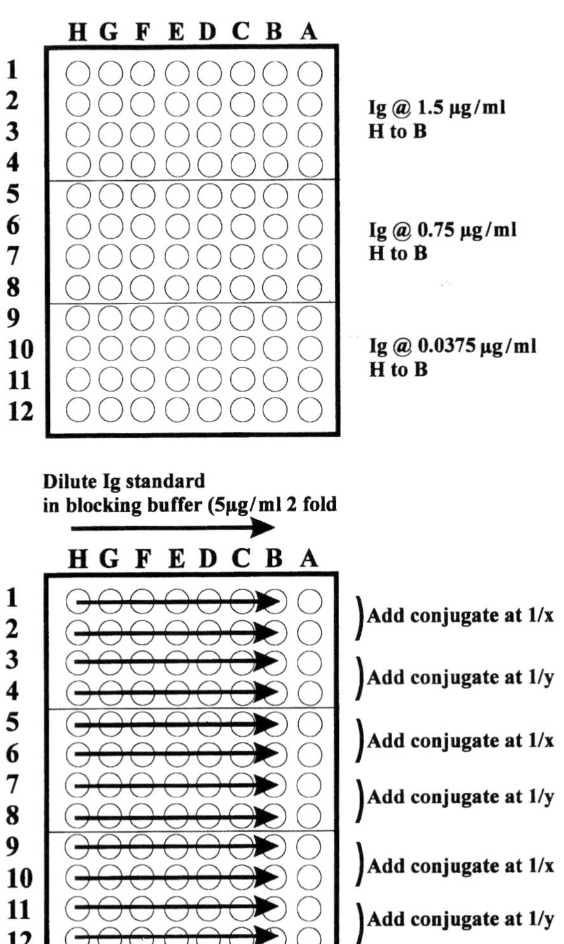

Fig. 1. Scheme for addition of reagents to assess optimal concentrations for competition assay.

1. Coat the wells of the plate (50 µL per well in PBS) with IgG at the three dilutions identified in stage 1. The microplate can be rotated so that the long edge is vertical and to the left of the operator (row H). Add the first dilution of IgG to wells 1–4, A–H. Add the second dilution to wells 5–8, A–H. Add the third dilution to wells 9–12, A–H. We have 1.5, 0.75, and 0.375 µg/mL for the three dilutions of Ig to coat the wells. The same conditions for coating concerning incubation and washing are as already described.
2. Wash the wells with PBS.
3. Add competing Ig as a dilution range from 5 µg/mL across seven wells. The Ig is diluted in blocking buffer to prevent it from coating the wells.
4. Add the conjugate (50 µL per well) as shown in Fig. 7.1. The dilutions *x* and *y* represent the dilutions identified in stage 1.
5. Incubate the plates for 2 h at 37°°C as in stage 1.
6. Wash the wells.
7. Add the appropriate substrate/chromogen, and stop the reaction.
8. Read the results on a spectrophotometer.

Plate 2

1. In place of the coating step with Ig, add 50 µL of coating buffer to wells H–A, 1–4. Incubate as for coating.
2. After washing, add PBS diluent (50 µL) to each well as a substitute for the competing Ig.
3. Add the two dilutions of conjugate used in plate 1 in 50-µL vol to the wells: 1/*x*dilution in blocking buffer from H–A, 1 and 2; 1/*y*dilution to wells H to A, 3 and 4. Incubate as for the competition stage in plate 1.
4. Wash and add substrate/chromogen, incubate, and stop the reaction as for plate 1. Read the results.

2.4.3. Results

Typical results are given in **Table 3**. The mean values for the replicates are shown in bold. In plate 1, the data show that the addition of Ig as a competitor for the labeled anti-mouse conjugate had the effect of reducing color when it was added at high concentrations, as indicated in the wells H, G, and F. As the competing Ig was reduced the effect was also reduced. Plate 2 results show that there is a low color representing the background.

To calculate the degree of competition, a calculation of the range of values with 100% and 0% competition is needed. The 100% competition values for both dilutions of conjugate used can be taken from mean values on plate 2. We have $1/x = 0.07$; and $1/y = 0/05$.

The 0% values for each of the conjugate dilutions and each of the IgG coating conditions are read for the respective concentrations in column A of plate 1. These are contained within the

Table 3
Plate 1 and 2 data

	H	G	F	E	D	C	B	A	Ig mg/mL
					Plate 2 data				
1	0.30	0.35	0.51	1.25	1.45	1.81	1.80	1.81	1.5
2	0.32	0.37	0.53	1.25	1.47	1.77	1.82	1.83	1.5
Mean	**0.31**	**0.36**	**0.52**	**1.25**	**1.46**	**1.79**	**1.81**	**1.82**	**1/x conjugate**
3	0.24	0.33	0.64	1.05	1.21	1.39	1.45	1.49	1.5
4	0.26	0.35	0.68	1.05	1.21	1.37	1.45	1.51	1.5
Mean	**0.25**	**0.34**	**0.66**	**1.05**	**1.21**	**1.38**	**1.45**	**1.50**	**1/y conjugate**
5	0.17	0.21	0.33	0.44	0.67	0.89	1.14	1.16	0.75
6	0.19	0.23	0.29	0.42	0.69	0.87	1.12	1.38	0.75
Mean	**0.18**	**0.22**	**0.31**	**0.43**	**0.68**	**0.88**	**1.13**	**1.17**	**1/x conjugate**
7	0.09	0.14	0.23	0.35	0.67	0.89	0.93	0.98	0.75
8	0.07	0.16	0.25	0.37	0.71	0.85	0.97	1.00	0.75
Mean	**0.08**	**0.15**	**0.24**	**0.36**	**0.69**	**0.87**	**0.95**	**0.99**	**1/y conjugate**
9	0.06	0.09	0.18	0.27	0.45	0.67	0.76	0.76	0.375
10	0.04	0.11	0.16	0.29	0.47	0.63	0.78	0.80	0.375
Mean	**0.05**	**0.10**	**0.17**	**0.28**	**0.46**	**0.65**	**0.77**	**0.79**	**1/x conjugate**
11	0.04	0.06	0.10	0.17	0.29	0.46	0.51	0.58	0.375
12	0.04	0.08	0,12	0.21	0.29	0.44	0.55	0.58	0.375
Mean	**0.04**	**0.06**	**0.11**	**0.19**	**0.29**	**0.45**	**0.53**	**0.58**	**1/y conjugate**
					Plate 2 data				
1	0.07	0.09	0.08	0.10	0.07	0.07	0.05	0.07	
2	0.06	0.04	0.08	0.05	0.05	0.06	0.05	0.08	
1/x mean of 16 wells = 0.07									
3	0.04	0.05	0.06	0.05	0.06	0.04	0.08	0.05	
4	0.06	0.08	0.05	0.4	0.05	0.03	0.04	0.05	
1/y mean of 16 wells = 0.05									

line drawn on the results of plate 1. These results show the color obtained for a particular coating concentration of Ig with the conjugates at different dilutions.

2.4.4. Calculations

The mean value of the conjugate control for both the dilutions of conjugate obtained in plate 2 is subtracted from the values

Table 4
Mean values in competition assa minus the background values for relevant conjugate dilution used

	0.31	0.36	0.52	1.25	1.46	1.79	1.81	1.82	
=	0.24	0.29	0.45	1.18	1.39	1.72	1.74	1.75	–1/x conjugate (0.07)
	0.25	0.34	0.66	1.05	1.21	1.38	1.45	1.50	
=	0.20	0.29	0.61	1.00	1.16	1.33	1.40	1.45	–1/y conjugate (0.05)
	0.18	0.22	0.31	0.43	0.68	0.88	1.13	1.17	
=	0.11	0.15	0.24	0.36	0.61	0.81	1.06	1.10	–1/x conjugate (0.07)
	0.08	0.15	0.24	0.36	0.69	0.87	0.95	0.99	
=	0.03	0.10	0.19	0.31	0.64	0.82	0.90	0.94	–1/y conjugate (0.05)
	0.05	0.10	0.17	0.28	0.46	0.65	0.77	0.79	
=	–0.02	0.03	0.10	0.21	0.39	0.58	0.70	0.72	–1/x conjugate (0.07)
	0.04	0.06	0.11	0.19	0.29	0.45	0.53	0.58	
=	–0.01	0.01	0.06	0.14	0.24	0.40	0.48	0.53	–l/y conjugate (0.05)

obtained in which that dilution of conjugate was used. This is shown in **Table 4.**

The values for the reaction between the conjugate and various concentrations of coating Ig without competition (0% competition) are shown in the gray boxes. This value is now used in the following formula to calculate the effect of adding the competing Ig:

$$\text{Competition} = 100 - [(\text{OD test}/\text{OD conjugate}) \times 100]$$

As an example: taking the first line of data we have the following values:

Value	
0.24	100 – [(0.24/1.75) × 100] = 100 – (0.14 × 100) = 100 – 14 = 86%
0.29	100 – [(0.29/1.75) × 100] = 100 – (0.17 × 100) = 100 – 17 = 83%
0.45	100 – [(0.45/1.75) × 100] = 100 – (0.26 × 100) = 100 – 26 = 74%
0.92	100 – [(1.18/1.75) × 100] = 100 – (0.67 × 100) = 100 – 67 = 33%
1.27	100 – [(1.39/1.75) × 100] = 100 – (0.79 × 100) = 100 – 79 = 21%
1.47	100 – [(1.72/1.75) × 100] = 100 – (0.98 × 100) = 100 – 98 = 2%
1.74	100 – [(1.74/1.75) × 100] = 100 – (0.99 × 100) = 100 – 99 = 1%

For the second row or results we have a different value for the % competition OD: 1.5 as follows:

Similar calculations can be made on all the other results. These are shown in **Table 5**, which lists all the data.

Value	
0.20	100 – [(0.20/1.45) × 100] = 100 – (0.13 × 100) = 100 – 13 = 87%
0.29	100 – [(0.29/1.45) × 100] = 100 – (0.19 × 100) = 100 – 19 = 81%
0.44	100 – [(0.66/1.45) × 100] = 100 – (0.46 × 100) = 100 – 46 = 54%
0.84	100 – [(1.05/1.45) × 100] = 100 – (0.72 × 100) = 100 – 72 = 28%
1.08	100 – [(1.21/1.45) × 100] = 100 – (0.83 × 100) = 100 – 83 = 17%
1.21	100 – [(1.38/1.45) × 100] = 100 – (0.95 × 100) = 100 – 95 = 5%
1.40	100 – [(1.40/1.45) × 100] = 100 – (0.97 × 100) = 100 – 97 = 3%

From these data we can determine optimal coating and conjugate dilutions to be used to test Ig in samples. Although it looks complicated, the whole procedure is accomplished in 2 days and is usually straightforward. Again, the calculations, seem problematic, but careful consideration will indicate that they are relatively simple.

In practice, examination of the data in the tabular form should be enough to set up optimal conditions. The optimal conditions can be assessed best if data are plotted. **Figure 2** illustrates features of the competition curves. All the curves illustrate that there is competition for the expected binding of the conjugates. The best combination of reagents to analyze samples is

Table 5
Percentage competition values

Conjugate	Competing antigen (μg/mL)							Coating Ig (μg/
Jilution	5	2.5	1.25	0.63	0.32	0.16	0.08	mL in 5μL)
1/x	86	83	74	33	16	2	1	1.5
1/y	87	81	54	28	17	5	3	
1/x	90	86	78	67	45	26	4	0.75
1/y	97	89	80	67	32	13	4	
1/x	101	96	86	71	46	19	3	0.375
1/y	101	98	89	74	63	25	15	

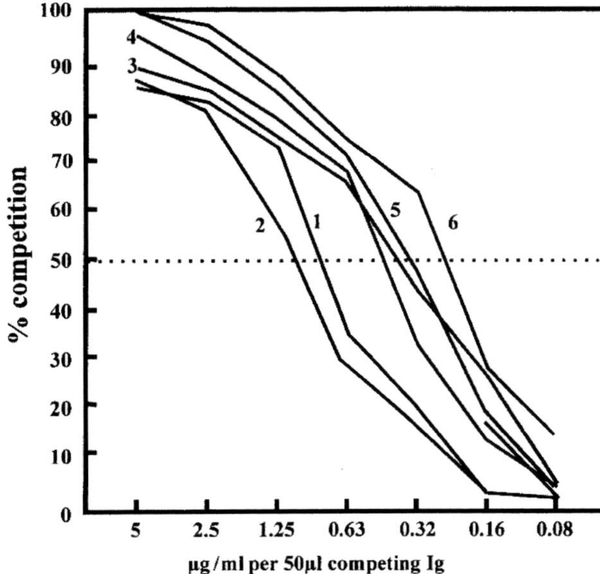

Fig. 2. The *six lines* show the competition data for the various combinations of coating concentrations and conjugate dilution. *Lines 1* and *2* show data for 1.5 µg/mL, 3 and 4 for 0.75 µg/mL, and 5 and 6 for 0.375 µg/mL coating. The conjugate dilution for 1, 3, and 5 was 1/*x*; for 2, 4, and 6, the conjugate dilution was 2/*y*. The 50% competition point is indicated by the *dashed line.*

obtained by considering the effective analytical sensitivity of each combination. The estimate of sensitivity is made by examining the weight of competing Ig at the 50% competition point. Thus, a line drawn across the 50% point is shown in **Fig. 2**. The weight of the Ig standard needed to give 50% inhibition of the conjugate binding for each combination can be measured as shown in **Fig. 3**, by plotting the perpendicular to the *x*-axis where the curve crosses the 50% competition line. Ideally, the weight of the competing Ig at the 50% competitive point should be the same as that added to coat the wells, assuming that all the Ig added was bound to the wells.

Note that it is much easier to plot the competition data on semilog graph paper. The competition is plotted on an arithmetic scale and related to $\log_{10}$ of the competing Ig concentration. In this way, the values for the various concentrations can be directly read from the scale. This approach also simplifies all other data plotting in which the *x*-axis is a scale of activity. **Figure 4** presents the same data plotted in this way. The values for the combination are shown in **Table 6.**

2.4.5. Conclusion

All conditions show that the conjugate was competed for on the addition of the known standard concentrations of Ig. A standard curve relating added Ig concentration to competition is obtained. The choice of best conditions is a balance between required

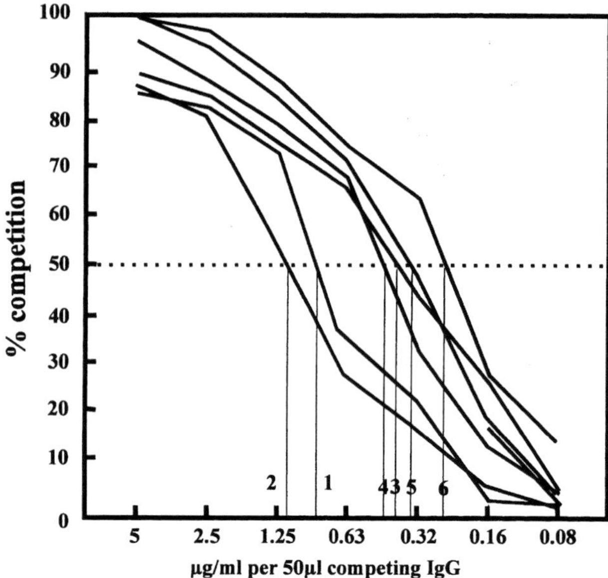

Fig. 3. The *six lines* show the competition data for the various combinations of coating concentrations and conjugate dilution. The competing Ig at 50% is indicated for each of the combinations 1–6.

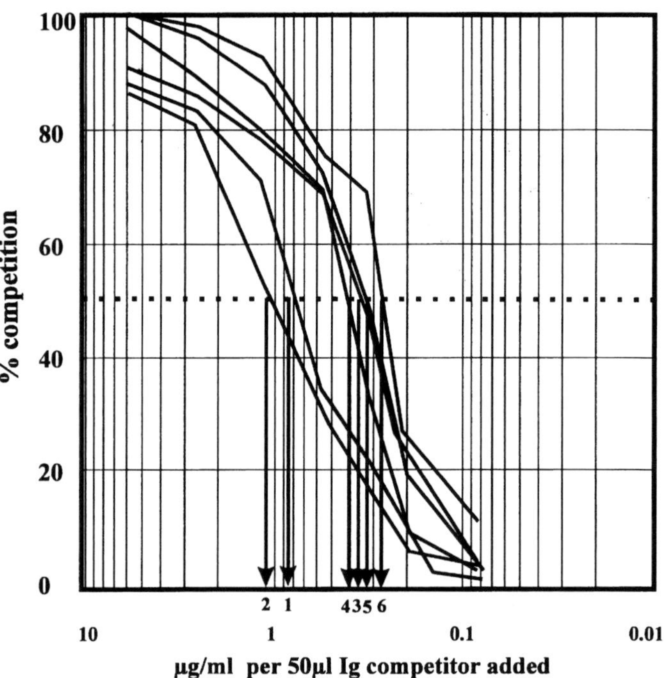

Fig. 4. Competition data plotted on long-semilog scale. The weight of competing Ig can be read directly from the *x*-axis. Combinations 1–6 are shown.

Table 6
Values for 50% compeition

Combinations of conjugate and coating IgG	Competing Ig giving 50% competition (μg/mL per 50/μL)	Plate concentration of Ig (μg/mL per 5Q(μL)
1	0.90	1.5
2	1.10	1.5
3	0.40	0.75
4	0.45	0.75
5	0.35	0.375
6	0.28	0.375

sensitivity and likely accuracy of the test. Screening for secretion of mouse Ig does not require high precision;, the results are relative within the standard system used with reference to the conjugate. The sensitivity is lowest when there are high levels of antigen Ig coating and higher levels of conjugate. In this case, there is more conjugate and antigenic target to be competed for. Reference to the OD values obtained for the 0% control indicates that this is rather high (OPD substrate system). The intermediate values of coating plates result in good titrations over the range of Ig added with OD values for 0% competition in a good area for this substrate. The sensitivity is increased here from about 1 μg/mL in 50 μL to about 0.4 μg/mL. The curves are also extended more into the area below which 50% competition is achieved. The third coating concentration gives a slightly higher sensitivity, but the OD values for control 0% competition can be regarded as too low. The variation in results increases with reaction in the colored product. An optimal dilution of coating Ig at about 0.75 μg/mL with a conjugate dilution equivalent to 1/*y* appears suitable for screening.

2.5. Use of Competition Assay to Assess Samples

The conditions established can now be used routinely for screening unknown samples for the presence of mouse Igs. The conditions for coating, washing, buffers, incubation, and so forth, are those described previsouly. A suitable template for addition of samples and controls (known Ig standards) should be developed. An example is shown in **Fig. 5.**

1. Wells should be coated with Ig at 0.75 μg/mL (50 μL per well). After incubation and washing, samples from mAb hybridoma studies can be added. A template as shown in **Fig. 5** is suitable.

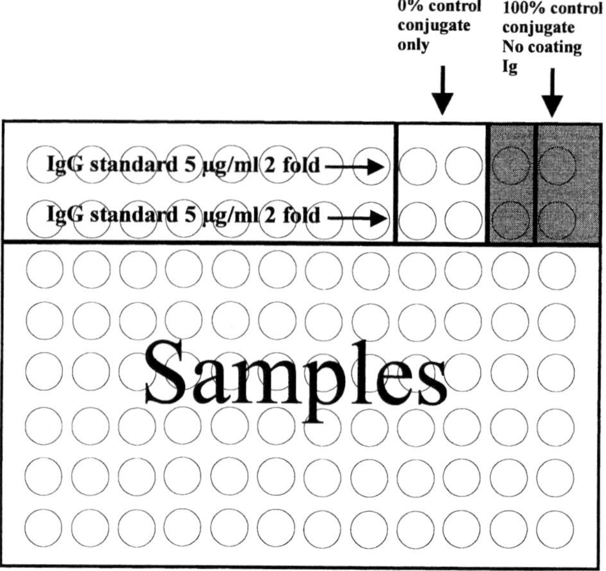

Fig. 5. Plate layout for measuring mouse Ig from samples. The gray box indicates no coating with IgG made. The standard dilution of Ig was make made as a duplicate two-fold dilution range. Zero percent control competition measures the reaction between coated wells and conjugate, and 100% competition is the reaction between conjugate and uncoated wells.

2. Add 25 µL of blocking buffer to each well except the control wells (*see* below). Add 25 µL of each mAb sample. Test mAb in duplicate if possible.
3. Add a dilution range of standard Ig preparation from 5 µg/mL by seven wells as in stage 2 (duplicate row).
4. Set up 0% controls (wells with blocking buffer added to Ig-coated wells).
5. Set up 100% competition controls.
6. Add conjugate to relevant wells (50 µL at 1/*y*) found in first stages.
7. Incubate, wash, add substrate, develop color, and stop.
8. Read the plates.

2.5.1. Results

Typical results are shown in **Table 7**. **Figure 5** shows the template used. Duplicate samples of mAb are titrated vertically.

For accurate treatment of data, the means of the results are calculated. The mean of the 100% competition data (A11 and 12 and B1 and 12) is subtracted from all means. The percentage competition is then calculated for the data using the same formula as in **Subheading 2.4.4.**

The standard curve can be plotted on semilog paper. The percentage values for the samples can be used to read off the

Table 7
Examination of samples

	1	2	3	4	5	6	7	8	9	10	11	12
A	0.05	0.13	0.22	0.37	0.68	0.89	0.99	1.07	1.09	1.08	0.05	0.05
B	0.06	0.15	0.20	0.35	0.66	0,91	0.97	1.09	1.08	1.07	0.04	0.06
C	0.04	1.08	0.56	0.43	0.04	0.91	0.89	0.67	0.56	0.05	1.07	1.04
D	0.06	1.06	0.58	0.47	0.06	0.89	0.91	0.65	0.60	0.07	1.09	1.02
E	1.08	1.10	1.12	1.00	1.12	0.98	0.67	0.32	0.43	1.09	1.07	1.06
F	1.10	1.06	1.08	0.98	1.10	0.98	0.65	0.28	0.41	1.07	1.05	1.06
G	0.56	0.45	0.32	1 07	1.06	0.76	0.45	3.04	1.09	1.21	0.12	0.13
H	0.58	0.51	0.30	3.11	1.10	0.78	0.43	1.10	1.03	1.09	0.10	0.11

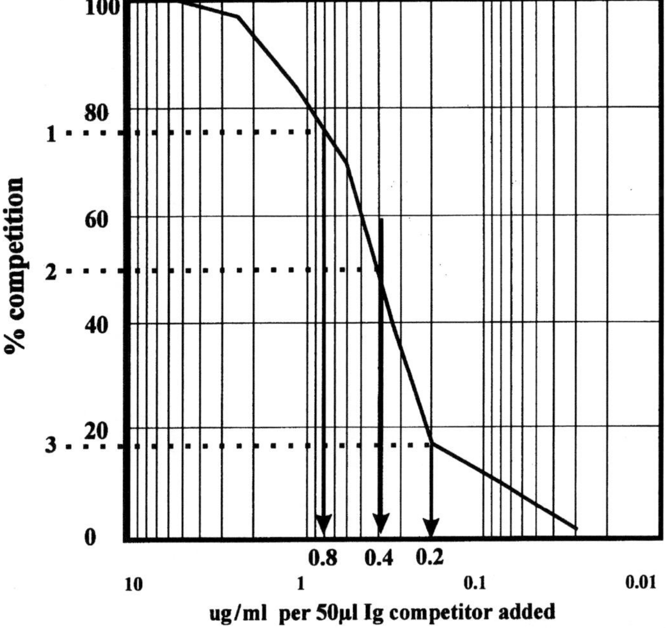

Fig. 6. Competition data for standards plotted on log-semilog scale. The weight of competing IgG in samples can be read directly from the *x*-axis. Three examples of test samples are shown, as indicated in the text. The estimated micrograms/milliliter values are shown for each sample below the *x*-axis.

relative activity as compared to the standard curve. This is illustrated in **Fig. 6**, in which only three samples are shown being read from the standard curve. When the sample values are equal to 100%, the effective concentration in the samples cannot be

Table 8
Competition data

1	2	3	4	5	6	7	8	9	10	11	12
0	0.04	0.16	0.31	0.62	0.85	0.93	1.03	1.03		100	
% 100*	**96**	**84**	**70**	**40**	**17**	**10**	**0**	**0**			
0	1.02	② 0.52	0.40	0	③ 0.85	0.85	0.61	0.53	0.01	1.03	0.98
% 100	**1**	**50**	**61**	**100**	**17**	**17**	**41**	**50**	**100**	**0**	**5**
1.04	1.03	1.05	0.94	1.06	0.93	0.61	① 0.25	0.97	1.03	1.01	1.01
% 0	**0**	**0**	**10**	**0**	**11**	**41**	**76**	**5**	**0**	**1**	**1**
0.52	0.43	0.26	1.04	1.03	0.72	0.39	1.02	1.01	1.11	0.06	0.07
% 50	**71**	**77**	**0**	**0**	**31**	**63**	**0**	**1**	**-7**	**94**	**93**

calculated. When they are lower, then effectively the concentration of Ig can be effectively assessed. Examination of the stopped plate by eye is useful and may be enough to indicate which wells or samples contain Ig. Thus, assessment as to wells which have no or very little color is enough to indicate Ig secretion. Similarly where wells have color equivalent to that in the 0% control wells, then they can be deemed "negative" with respect to Ig secretion to the limits of sensitivity as defined by the standard curve. The standard curve should also be examined in a "by eye assessment" and should indicate a gradual increase in color as expected by a decreasing level of competition.

Table 8 shows the data in **Table 7** and represents mean of replicates minus the mean value for the 100% competition controls, and the % competition values. The mean of replicates of 100% competition data is 0.05

3. Screening of mAbs for Specific Activity

A reminder is needed that the purpose of producing mAbs is to solve a particular problem. The screening of mAbs must reflect this purpose as early as possible. Reference to **Table 1** indicates when specific screening is best attempted. ELISAs measuring binding of fusion products to antigens are ideal for testing a high number of clones in a 96-well format. The screening does requires some pretesting of reagents to allow confidence that a system will detect mAb if produced. The usual source of developmental reagents comes from collecting serum from mice primed and vaccinated in the same way (or the actual mice used) as was used to prepare the mAbs. The polyclonal serum should contain antibodies that bind to a selected target antigen(s). This and preimmune serum can be used for developing an ELISA system for screening purposes.

A review of what is available in terms of likelihood, specificity, physical parameters, and availability is needed in order to assess the most suitable test. This also infers that there may be other reagents already exploited in ELISAs (e.g., polyclonal capture antibodies) that can be used. **Table 9** shows some considerations. The development of assays to detect bound mouse antibodies is no different from that for other assays. We need to be certain that a test will measure this binding and be reasonably assured that the test has good analytical sensitivity (can detect low levels of antibody).

The most obvious ELISA for general screening is the indirect system involving detection of bound mouse Ig using an anti-mouse conjugate. A commercial preparation reacting with all isotypes should be purchased. The antigenic target may well have been characterized in some other ELISA using polyclonal reagents so that the effective concentration can be assessed for use in detecting mAbs. Several scenarios will be described to indicate strategies.

These are probably available in laboratories equipped to produce mAbs because they have a research base. When reagents are unavailable (e.g., polyclonal antiserum raised against antigen[s]), then the mouse antibody detection system has to be worked up from basic principles. This is also illustrated. A key point in screening is that results are relative in the initial phases. One attempts

Table 9
Considerations of components of mAb screening

Question	Considerations
Is there an antigenic target?	Large antigenic complex, polypeptide, peptide, denaturable, single epitope expressed, multiple epitopes expressed
Is capture needed?	Is polyclonal available, species, concentration known?
Can it coat directly?	Concentration known?
What amount is available?	Examples: l/mL used at 1/10; 1/mL can be diluted l/2000, 5/mg used at 2g/mL
What is the degree of purity?	Amorphous mixture containing different antigens, purified product
Can it be used for vaccination?	With any of the above, assesses likelihood of spectrum of mAbs produced and complications using reagents specified

to identify mAb-producing cells as early as possible and to avoid maintenance of large numbers of cells in a blind fashion.

The factors considered in **Table 9** are relevant to the development of all ELISAs. Certain factors are more important when mAbs are to be exploited owing to the unique single specificity inherent in that reagent. This specificity can be both a great benefit and a problem, and care is needed to avoid unsuitable systems. The systematics of ELISA will be discussed after a few examples of how previous experience with the antigen helps in screening. These are meant only to illustrate principles and are not explored in great detail. The particular methods (e.g., CRTs, dilution ranges) are all examined in other sections.

3.1. Previous Experience in Helping to Develop an Indirect Assay

Our previous experience in developing an indirect assay involved antigen (Ag) coated directly to wells and a detecting serum in turn detected by an anti-species conjugate. In that case, the Ag concentration was known, and at this concentration, we know that a substantial amount of the antibodies bind, and that a good signal is seen on addition of the conjugate and substrate/chromogen. This concentration of antigen can be tested in the indirect ELISA; the mouse serum can be tested before and after the vaccination regime for producing the mAbs.

Assuming that the antigen in the indirect ELISA is the same as that used to prime and vaccinate mice, the polyclonal ELISA reagents can be used to assess antigen coating. The pre- and post-vaccinal mice sera can be titrated in a CBT against the anti-mouse conjugate. Some adjustment can then be made to the concentration of antigen and conjugate to allow optimization of all three components. The antigen is therefore controlled. There may be problems inherent in the presentation of the antigen to monospecific mAbs in screening, as compared to what is observed with polyclonal antibodies. This is explained in the **Subheading 9.**, dealing with the implications of mAbs in different assays.

3.1.1. Assay

1. A dilution (concentration) of antigen should be used on plates that gives a high OD in the presence of excess mouse positive serum. This will allow maximum binding of mAb from tissue culture preparations.
2. A volume of 25 μL of each mAb should be added in blocking buffer (as used in CBT of mouse serum). The mAbs can be added to wells already containing 25 μL of a solution of blocking buffer in which the blocking agent is at twice the normal concentration. This will compensate for the dilution of the mAb. A single dilution or, better, a duplicate sample should be used.
3. The mouse positive and negative sera should be added to some wells as controls to be indicators that the test is working. A dilution of positive serum that gives just gives the maximum

OD (plateau height maximum in the presence of excess mouse serum) can be added. A dilution of negative serum should be used to give an OD value that reflects background.

4. The incubation step to allow binding of mAb to antigen should be that used in the CBT. One hour at 37°°C while plates are being rotated is usually adequate.
5. After washing, the addition of anti-mouse conjugate (optimal concentration) and incubation are as in CBT.
6. Washing, substrate/chromogen addition, and stopping areas are as for the CBT.

3.1.2. Results

A typical plate might give results as shown in **Table 10.**

3.1.3. Conclusion

1. The control serum values indicate the test worked in that the wells were coated with antigen (gray box in **Table 11**).
2. High OD values are seen for certain mAb samples almost achieving plateau height seen with polyclonal serum (shown in boxes in **Table 11**). In G/H 5, a value greater than the polyclonal value is seen.
3. There are values with lower OD values but still high relative to others showing values around that of control negative wells (**Table 12**).

At this stage the concentration of the mAb is likely to be unknown, although the mAbs can be titrated in terms of mouse antibody, as explained earlier. Thus, the activities of the individual samples cannot be directly compared. A low OD may only mean that there is a small quantity of specific mAb, as compared to those that gave high ODs. The low OD values may have come from

Table 10
Tpical results from indirect ELISA screening of mAbs

	1	2	3	4	5	6	7	8	9	10	11	12
A	1.45	0.04	0.05	1.31	0.08	0.09	0.23	0.26	0.34	0.78	0.03	0.09
B	1.41	0.05	0.04	1.38	0.09	0.07	0.19	0.30	0.38	0.69	0.07	0.12
C	0.80	0.23	0.45	0.08	0.09	1.31	0.08	0.09	0.09	0.56	0.12	0.13
D	0.07	0.27	0.49	0.06	0.12	1.26	0.05	0.09	0.06	0.58	0.16	0.19
E	0.19	0.89	0.97	0.67	0.45	0.09	0.04	0.06	0.04	1.21	0.09	0.45
F	0.23	0.90	0.89	0.76	0.56	0.08	0.07	0.05	0.07	1.32	0.07	0.39
G	0 07	0.05	1.10	0.06	1.34	1.56	0.08	1.21	0.58	0.57	0.63	0.08
H	0.07	0.08	1.21	1.25	1.23	1.59	0.09	1.19	0.59	0.57	0.65	0.09

[a] AB 1 is positive serum control. CD 1 is negative serum control. Samples are as vertical duplicates.

Table 11
Higlighting strong positive samples in mAb screening

	1	2	3	4	5	6	7	8	9	10	11	12
A	1.45	0 04	0 05	1 31	0.08	0.09	0.23	0.26	0.34	0.78	0.03	0.09
B	1.41	0.05	0.04	1.38	0.09	0.07	0.19	0.30	0.38	0.69	0.07	0.12
C	0.80	0.23	0.45	0.08	0.09	1.31	0.08	0.09	0.09	0.56	0.12	0.13
D	0.07	0.27	0.49	0.06	0.12	1.26	0.05	0.09	0.06	0.58	0.16	0.19
E	0.19	0.89	0.97	0.67	0 45	0.09	0.04	0.06	0.04	1.21	0.09	0.45
F	0.23	0.90	0.89	0.76	0.56	0 .08	0.07	0.05	0.07	1.32	0.07	0.39
G	0.07	0 05	1.10	1.23	1.34	1.56	0.08	1. 21	0.58	0.57	0.63	0.08
H	0.07	0.08	1.21	1.25	1.23	1.59	0.09	1.19	0.59	0.57	0.65	0.09

[a] Gray box indicates positive control values. Open boxes show high OD readings

Table 12
Higlighting other clearl positive samples in mAb screening

	1	2	3	4	5	6	7	8	9	10	11	12
A	1.45	0.04	0.05	1.31	0.08	0.09	0.23	0.26	0.34	0.78	0.03	0.09
B	1.41	0.05	0.04	1.38	0.09	0.07	0.19	0.30	0.38	0.69	0.07	0.12
C	0.80	0.23	0.45	0.08	0.09	1.31	0.08	0.09	0.09	0.56	0.12	0.13
D	0.07	0.27	0.49	0.06	0.12	1.26	0.05	0.09	0.06	0.58	0.16	0.19
E	0.19	0.89	0.97	0.67	0.45	0.09	0.04	0.06	0.04	1.21	0.09	0.45
F	0.23	0.90	0.89	0.76	0.56	0.08	0.07	0.05	0.07	1.32	0.07	0.39
G	0.07	0.05	1.10	1.23	1.34	1.56	0.08	1.21	0.58	0.57	0.63	0.08
H	0.07	0.08	1.21	1.25	1.23	1.59	0.09	1.19	0.59	0.57	0.65	0.09

[a] Open boxes show values inclicating positive sampies. Gray boxes indicate low but probably still positive values

colonies with few cells. Therefore, all mAbs showing positivity at this stage have to be "grown on" to allow for more cells to be produced that secrete antibody.

The maximum OD of any mAb depends on the epitope density on the sample attached to the wells. The maximum OD for the polyclonal serum may well be greater than that for any mAb screened (unlike the example shown in **Table 10.**). This depends, to a large extent, on the number of different epitopes expressed on any solid phase "antigen" and the number of different polyclonal antibodies produced against it. When the single epitopes that mAbs identify are present in a low concentration, then the maximum binding of mAb as well as the maximum plateau will be low. This cannot be established in a single-dilution screening, but will be explained further below, when dealing with characterization of mAbs. Knowledge about the relative complexity of an antigen used in screening is very helpful in predicting the likely difference between polyclonal and mAb binding plateau maxima. As an example, at one extreme, in which a peptide is used with a single epitope, polyclonal sera will bind, giving maximum plateau similar to those of mAbs, and there will be a single saturating event in the presence of excess antibody from either source. Indeed, the mAbs may react better owing to their uniform structure.

Screening against more than one antigen may be relevant. It is possible that more than one antigen can be used at the first screening stage in order to establish some level of specificity of the mAbs at a very early stage. Thus, two specific antigens may be used and the relative binding of any secreting mAb determined. This can also serve to increase the likelihood of picking up mAbs that may not be detected because they have a low affinity against a particular antigenic preparation. If an operator is unsure as to the best antigen to use in a final assay, more than one can be tried. It must be emphasized that the objective in screening is to limit the number of clones to manageable proportions while successfully finding products for a defined purpose.

When the concentration of the mAbs is known, the activities can be compared with respect to the concentrations of Ig.

3.2. The Next Stage

Once you have identified mAbs that are secreting antibody, theyse can be selected for further growth, amplification of product, and complete characterization. This requires that supernatant fluids be retested to determine whether they are still secreting Ig. The same test is already described in **Subheading 3.1.1.** However, there is now a large increase in the volume of supernatant, which allows for additional testing. This stage may be the safest to begin accurate characterization. In this case, the more stabilized clones can be stored in liquid nitrogen to allow their restoration once characterization has identified the required mAbs.

A word of caution on screening using indirect ELISA is necessary. mAbs do show exquisite specificity, by definition. Solid-phase coating of antigens can affect certain epitopes in that they change their conformation. This prevents some mAbs from reacting (being dependent on conformation). Thus, in some cases, mAbs will be missed in the indirect ELISA.

3.3. Other ELISA Screening Systems

The exploitation of other ELISAs depends on the number of assays already developed and hence the reagents available. The antigen can be captured via polyclonal antibodies, allowing indirect sandwich ELISAs. Here again, the system can be worked out for a completely polyclonal set of conditions and the effective capture antibody concentration used to present antigen to the mAbs. There are some problems that depend on the nature of the antigen. As an example, when a small peptide is captured, the particular epitope targeted by an mAb may be already bound by the trapping serum. Thus, mAbs specific for that epitope would not be detectable. The presentation of more complex antigens with repeating identical epitopes will not affect screening. The capture of antigens also may protect the conformation of certain epitopes as compared to those directly coating wells.

Competitive assays may also be exploited. Thus, a fully validated polyclonally based assay can be used and challenged by samples containing mAbs. This is only successful with smaller, more limited antigenic targets, asince mAbs, by definition, will only compete for a single epitope with a single affinity. Polyclonal sera contain many antibodies directed at a variety of antigenic determinants. The antibodies themselves form complex interactions depending on the variable affinities of the individual molecules in the mixture (avidity). Thus, with more complex antigens, an mAb may completely compete off polyclonal antibodies from a single epitope, but, of course it fails to block reactions with all the other sites. The effect is that only a low maximum inhibition of binding is seen by mAbs. Owing to considerations as to the nature of the antigen (e.g., its physical state, the number of likely antigenic sites), its denaturability and size, will give a clue as to the best bet for screening.

4. Characterization of mAbs

Characterization of mAbs depends exactly entirely on the purpose of the mAb. The indirect ELISA with the detection of binding to a solid-phase antigen usually screens most mAbs of ultimate use, even when the mAbs are used in different systems. At this stage, there is the advantage that a larger volume of supernatant is available, so that more tests can be performed. We also now also have fewer concerns about sterility in sampling asince cells can be grown to allow supernatant production for testing alone.

5. Consideration of Use of mAbs

Table 13 lists some of the uses of mAbs and highlights their potential advantages and disadvantages. These stem from the single specificity of mAbs and the ability to standardize a product. The ultimate use must be considered to evaluate the need for sufficient quantities and the purity. Examples of these applications will be shown later.

6. Purification of mAbs

Purification of mAbs may be necessary to increase the concentration of Ig or to free the Ig from other proteins. The source of the mAb is important (how it is grown). **Table 14** presents some sources and typical concentrations of Igs in mAbs and polyclonal sera.

Table 13
Uses of mAbs in ELISA

1.	Differentiating closely related stains	Single, mAb or mAb panels 2 or more 100 s.All ELISAs
2.	Ability to capture defined antigen from mixture	Sandwich ELISA as capture andbody
3.	To specifically detect poiyclonally captured arttigen	Detecting mAb directly labeled or in indirect system (antifcouse conjugate)
4.	To use a reference standard	Activity defined by weight. Any ELJSAs
5.	To link sequence and structural data	Defining epitopes; mAb escape mutant studies. All ELISAs
6.	To define conformational and linear sitesh	Binding studies; All ELISAs
7.	To use a specific systems for quantification	mAbs used as capture and detecting reagents.
8.	To assess affinities against specific epitopes; compare epitopes and specific paratopes	Competitive ELISAs
9.	To use as isotype-specific assays	Use of anti-isotype conjugates to examine binding mixtures or single mAbs. Indirect and indirect sandwich ELISAs
10.	To use as multiple assays detecting different antigens	Mixture of mAbs; different labeled conjugates

Table 14
Sources of antibodies

Material	Serum	mAb tissue culture 10% calf serum	mAb serum free	mAb ascites in vivo
Antibody	Polyclonal	Monoclonal	Monoclonal	Monoclonal
Produced Total antibody Specific antibodies	5-10 mg/mL 1-5%	0.5-1 .0 mg/mL 5%	0.05 mg/mL 100%	1-15 mg/mL 80-90%
Contamination	Serum proteins antibodies	Calf serum/proteins antibodies	None	Mouse antibodies proteins
Purity specific antibody possible	10%	>95%	>95%	90%

Contaminants in mAbs depend largely on the method used to amplify the amount of Ig and the purification methods. These include non-antibody substances such as serum proteins, proteases, lipids, endotoxins, nucleic acids, and viruses. The actual purity of mAb depends on the ultimate use, and 95% is suitable for most assays. The purification procedure should be made as soon as possible. When this is not possible, mAb preparations can be stored. **Table 15** gives some conditions for storage.

Note again that mAbs are proteins and an excellent substrate for microbiological growth. Since mAbs are a single molecule, any physical or biological effect on one molecule will affect the entire antibody population. Care must be taken to store mAbs in buffered solutions and at suitable temperatures. Excessive freeze thawing should not be done. Ascites fluids are well buffered at the source, but purification procedures remove this buffer. Filter sterilization is recommended but possible losses must be taken into account.

Stabilization of mAbs is important if their reactivity is to be maintained. External factors such as excess of heat, pH, shaking, detergents, high salt, and chelating agents should obviously be avoided. Other chemical effects over longer times can also cause problems, such as, hydrolysis, crosslinking, and oxidation. However, these are less likely to induce problems in assays in which efficient use of controls and well-stored mAbs are maintained. Problems of aggregation and adsorption also reduce mAb activity. Approaches to stabilizing mAbs include freeze drying, addition of stabilizers in which proteins, sugars, amino acids, and fatty acids are present (1). Storage at a reduced temperature is still the most recommended procedure. mAbs are best stored in a neutral pH buffer solution containing ~0.1 M salt concentration.

Table 15
Storage conditions for mAbs

	Action	Storage	Stability
Celteulture supernaCants	Concentrated (10), filter sterilized	2-5°C	Few das
		-20°C	1 year
		-70°C	1-5 year
Ascites	Centrifuged, fat-free filter sterilized	2-5°C	Few days
		-20°C	1 year
		-70°C	1-5 year

Solutions should be relatively concentrated (~1 mg/mL), and higher if possible.

The addition of glycerol is recommended generally (1 vol glycerol to 1 vol mAb) with storage at –20 to –70°C.

The addition of preservatives is also recommended, e.g., merthiolate at a concentration of 1/10,000, or sodium azide (0.02–0.1%). Care is necessary in using both preservatives. Sodium azide also inhibits some ELISAs, and attention to its final concentration in any assay is necessary.

Lyophilization can provide a stable mAb preparation, particularly when supplied in kits, in which transportation and collection of reagents causes storage problems. Successful procedures for lyophilization are necessary to achieve a stable product.

6.1. Methods for Purification of mAbs

A wide variety of methods for purification are available. For most ELISA applications a purity approaching 95% may be sufficient to remove unwanted proteins. The method depends on the particular source material and its volume, and ultimately how much is needed. Techniques depend on fractional precipitation, electrophoretic, ion-exchange, ultracentrifugation, and affinity methods.

Generally, for immunoassays relatively small amounts (order of milligrams) are needed for developmental and applied work. Ultimately, the activity of any mAb can be associated with a defined weight of relatively pure product. Therefore, the available amount of mAb can be calculated with respect to any defined assay. This activity can be assumed on any subsequent preparation of mAb and the necessary steps taken to produce the required amount. As an example, a mAb is titrated for use in an ELISA at a dilution of 1/10,000 in a 50-μL vol. There is 1 mL of the preparation at 1 mg/L. This would allow 10,000 mL of reagent × 20 = 200,000 assay points. It can be determined whether this is enough to serve the needs in a given time. Note that the activity here can be related to the weight, i.e., 1/10,000 = 1 mg/mL. Preparation of the same mAb in the same way means that each milligram of mAb produced (and purified in the same way) should have a titer of 10,000. Such calculations based on mAbs are feasible as compared to polyclonal antibody considerations. Thus, when an mAb based test is envisaged for use in 20 laboratories all examining 10,000 samples per year for 5 years, the effective amount of mAb required can be calculated and production tailored to meet this need. This is an important consideration in all aspects of serology and avoids the embarrassment of validating particular sera for use (e.g., as standards in assays) only to find that, although a perfect serum is has been identified, only 1 mL usable at 1/800 is available. The distinct advantage of mAbs in this area is that an identical preparation can be produced on demand from the hybridomas.

6.1.1. Fractional Precipitation

Fractional precipitation methods can have damaging effects on certain mAbs. Pilot studies can examine this possibility. Methods classically involve the use of ammonium sulfate, sodium sulfate, caprylic acid, Rivanol, and polyethylene glycol. These separate mAb from the majority of other proteins in ascites. Following dialysis, this procedure may well be sufficient for use in ELISA.

6.1.2. Electrophoretic Separation

Electrophoretic separation techniques involve a good deal of instrumentation and also involve free-boundary electrophoresis, zone electrophoresis on celluloses acrylamide, and so forth, as well as isoelectric focusing techniques.

6.1.3. Ion-Exchange and Gel Filtration Chromatography

Anion and cation exchangers as well as gel filtration can be used to selectively purify mAbs – e.g., sephadex G series; sepharoses 2B, 4B, 6B, CVL; Sephacryl; as well as a variety of agarose or polyacrylamide beads.

6.1.4. Affinity Chromatography

Affinity chromatography offers efficient large and small-scale applications – e.g., the use of protein A, protein G, and protein A/G on a variety of matrices such as glass beads, avidin-biotin systems, antigen affinity columns to selectively purify mAb, and hydroxylapatite. There are many configurations exploiting affinity purification on the commercial market. Kits for small-scale purification and reagents to produce larger scale capacities can be purchased. Such techniques tend to favor the purification of specific Ig, and care must be taken to establish that particular mAbs are bound with sufficient affinity to the ligands. Recently kits have become available from Pharmacia (E-Z-SEP) that selectively precipitate Igs from heterogeneous mixtures by a volume exclusion technology through the use of nonionic linear polymers and special buffers. The kits are optimized for precipitation of globulins from ascites fluid, cell culture supernatants, bioreactor fluids, and animal sera. The isolation is independent of the species or subclass.

7. Characterizing mAbs by Isotype

The determination of the isotype of a particular mAb can be important in assessing its potential as a reagent, as well as allowing different possibilities of assay design. Early characterization of the isotype of an mAb may be important for a number of reasons. First, an isotype can determine the simplest method of purification. For example, IgG_{2a} and IgG_{2b} bind protein A, whereas IgG_1 mAbs do not bind protein A very well under standard conditions. Second, some isotypes are better suited to certain immunological techniques than others. For example, IgG_{2b} antibodies are the best isotype for complement-medi-ated killing of in vitro cells carrying the epitope. Third, isotype characterization also reveals the structure of the antibody, which may make it undesirable in some applications. For example, IgM exists as a pentamer composed of five 180-kDa subunits; therefore, IgM monoclonals are often too large for applications that require monomers. Fourth, an isotype determines the best method for preparing Fab fragments by proteolysis.

Several commercial kits are available to measure isotypes as well as specific anti-isotype reagents for mouse, rat, and human mAbs. The kits are expensive and care should be made to justify the need for isotype determination at any particular stage. Kits are based on various formats:

1. Agar gel immunodiffusion.
2. Coated latex particle strip assays, e.g., Boehringer Mannheim IsoStripTM, which is made simple by the kit's two components. Each development tube supplied with the kit contains colored latex beads bearing anti-mouse kκ and anti-mouse lλ antibodies, which will react with any mouse mAb regardless of its isotype. The isotyping strip bears immobilized bands of goat anti-mouse antibodies corresponding to each of the common mouse antibody isotypes (IgG_1, IgG_{2a}, IgG_{2b}, IgG_3, IgM, and IgA) and to the [kappa] and [lambda] light chains. Both sides of the strip also bear a positive control band. The diluted sample is added to the development tube, where the mouse mAb resuspends and forms a complex with the antibody-coated latex beads. When the isotyping strip is placed in the development tube, this complex flows up the strip (via capillary action) until it is bound by the immobilized goat anti-mouse antibody specific for the mAb's isotype and light chain. This takes ~5 min to perform.
3. Use of specific anti-isotype antibody measurement of mAbs in the ELISA format of choice, either directly with mAb after binding to a target antigen, e.g., Biomeda-Mouse Hybridoma IsoType Kit. The kit is designed to be used for determination

of the class and subclasses of mouse mAbs in mouse hybridoma supernatants or mouse ascites using enzyme immunoassay. The reagents in this package serve to detect primary antibodies of mouse isotypes IgA, IgG_1, IgG_{2a}, IgG_{2b}, IgG_3, and IgM origin, as well as to identify the kκ or lλ light chain antibodies in one simple, antigen-mediated immunoperoxidase assay. Purified antigen is absorbed to the microtiter plate wells. The remaining sites for protein binding on the microtiter plate are saturated with blocking protein solution. This complex is incubated with the antibody secreting hybridoma supernatants or diluted ascites. The mouse Igs bind to the antigen absorbed to the wells. Goat anti-mouse Ig isotype-specific antibodies are applied for isotype determination in the hybridoma supernatants. Signal is detected by incubation with HRP labeled rabbit anti-goat IgG. This step is followed by incubation with ready-to-use 3,3′,5,5′ tetramethylbenzidine chromogen.

Pierce offers ELISA-based mAb isotyping kits using HRP/2,2′-azino diethylbenzothiazoline sulfonic acid and Alkaline Phosphatase/*p*-nitro-phenylphosphate with two basic types of screening procedures. Antigen-dependent screening is as previously described above and involves coating the antigen on a microtiter plate. The hybridoma supernatant is then added, and the mAb is detected using an enzyme-conjugated anti-mouse antibody.

An antigen-independent screening method is also supplied when soluble antigens are difficult to obtain. ELISA plates are coated with an antibody to mouse immunoglobulin. This antibody then serves to capture the mAbs from the hybridoma supernatant. The presence of positive clones is provedn with enzyme-conjugated anti-mouse immunoglobulin.

8. Processing of mAbs

Applications involving the use of Ig fractions may offer advantages. The proteolytic cleavage and purification of products from mAbs (particularly of mouse origin) can be accomplished through the use of kits designed to give good yields. **Figure 7** gives the details of proteolytic cleavage of human IgG molecules. This illustrates the three major components of use and relevance in ELISA; the Fab_2 and Fab and Fc fractions. Care must be taken concerning with respect to the digestion of mouse IgG molecules since each isotype has a different degree of resistance to proteolytic cleavage. A good kit can be obtained from Pierce. These kits selectively cleave Ig molecules into Fab and $F(ab')_2$ fragments using papain, pepsin, ficin, and trypsin immobilized on

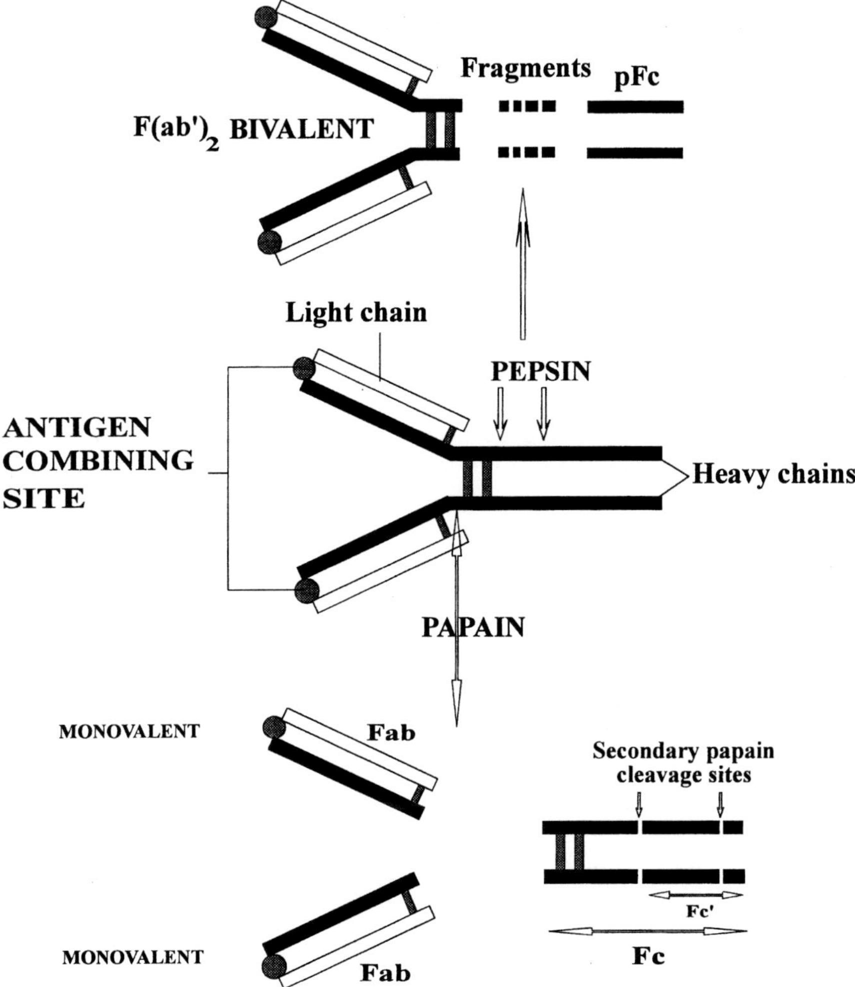

Fig. 7. Enzymatic cleavage of IgG. Pepsin cleaves the heavy chain to give F(Ab′) and pFc′ fragments. Further action results in greater fragmentation of the central protein to peptides. Papain splits the molecule in the hinge region to give two Fab fragments and the Fc fragment. Further action on the Fc can produce Fc'.

a crosslinked agarose support. Attaching the enzymes to a solid phase eliminates the problems often encountered with soluble enzymes to allow easy separation of enzyme from antibody fragments, no contamination with autodigestion products from the enzyme, and reproducible results.

9. Assay Formats Using mAbs

mAbs may be used in any assay format and they offer certain advantages over polyclonal reagents when used similarly. Care must be taken to assess the use in terms of the exact preparation

Table 16
Factors involved in assa design using mAbs

Valency	Example
Monovalent	Fab fragments
Bivalent	Whole $IgG_{1\text{-}3}$ Fab_2
Multivalent	IgM/IgA
Mixture	Not successfully cloned

(purity, isotype, fraction) of mAbs with due attention to the specificity of the interaction of the mAb and the epitope to which it binds and the nature of the antigen(s) that are involved in any assay. Certain formats used with mAbs can be used uniquely as compared to polyclonal sera. The valency of the mAb or mAb preparation can affect assays; **Table 16** outlines parameters.

Table 17 shows the direct, indirect, and sandwich systems using symbols for the reactants. Each system can be challenged with antigen or antibody and thus, be used to perform competitive or inhibition assays. Certain possible advantages and disadvantages of assays using mAB-based reagents as compared to polyclonal antibody reagents are shown.

The key features that can make mAbs potentially absolute reagents stem from their specificity. Therefore mAbs can be used effectively to measure only the epitopes against which they are directed and indirectly assess any other antibodies from other sources that bind with that epitope. The nature of the epitope (e.g., whether or not it is conformation dependent) and its overall expression are also important, and the antigen used in any assay has to be considered carefully. Factors affecting affinity are changes in antigen (alterations of epitopes by physical factors or differences among samples and their density of expression) and the valency of the mAb preparation. The epitope density also affects the binding according to the exact systems used. Such factors can be examined with reference to some of the assay systems described in **Table 17.**

9.1. Direct ELISA

The following list is a reminder of the systems as given in **Table 17**:

1. I = Ag + mAb*Enz.
2. I = Ag + Fab_2*Enz.
3. I = Ag + Fab*Enz.

Direct ELISA depends on being able to successfully bind antigen to a solid phase while maintaining a reaction with mAb. Binding of antigen can affect the availability and orientation of epitopes

Table 17
Use of mAb reagents in ELISA systems

Direct ELISA
I-Ag + mAb*Enz
I-Ag + Fab_2*Enz
I-Ag + Fab*Enz
Indirect ELISA
I-Ag + mAb + Antimouse*Enz
I-Ag + Fab_2 + Antimouse*Enz or Anti-Fab*Enz
I-Ag + Fab + AntimousE*Enz or Anti-Fab*Enz
Direct sandwich ELISA
I-mAbl + Ag + mAbl*Enz (same mAb detecting)
I-Fabj + Ag + mAb*Enz (same mAb detecting)
I-mAbl + Ag + mAb_2*Enz (different mAb detecting)
I-mAb + Ag + PC*Enz (poiyclonal antibody detector)
I-PC + Ag + mAb*Enz (polyclonal capture antibody)
Indirect sandwich ELISA
I-$mAb_{isotypel}$ + Ag + mAb $_{isotypel}$ + Antiiso2*Enz
I-Fab_3 + Ag + mAb + AntiFc*Enz
I-mAb + Ag + PC + AntiPC*Enz
I-Fab_2 + Ag + PC + AntiPC*Enz
I-PC + Ag + mAb C+Fabj or Fab)+Anti mAb*Enz (or Anti-Fab*Enz)

[a]I- = solid phase with attached reagent; mAb = whole mAb molecules; Fab_2 = bivalent mAb minus Fc; Fab - monovalent fraction; + = addition of reagent in sequence; Ag = antigen ; PC = polyclonal antibodies; *Enz = reagent conjugated to enzyme; Fc = Fc fraction of mAb Ig

(presentation to antibody) and also alter the antigenicity, particularly in which mAbs are directed against confor-mation-dependent epitopes. The mAb or fractionated mAb also has to be conjugated to the enzyme. Conjugation may affect the binding of mAbs. The specific activity of the mAb detector is related to the amount of enzyme. This type of assay is best suited for a competitive/inhibition format in which an mAb has been identified that provides useful information about a single property. Since

As the initial screening of mAbs probably involves the indirect ELISA, it is likely that mAbs that have been identified will bind to the coated-well antigen (if the same antigen preparation is used). The key is that several mAbs may have to be labeled until the best is identified. This is laborious and the use of the indirect ELISA, utilizing an anti-species conjugate, is recommended when many mAbs can be assessed in competition format.

9.2. Indirect ELISA

The following list is a reminder of the systems as given in **Table 17.**

1. I-Ag + mAb + Anti-mouse*Enz.
2. I-Ag + Fab_2 + Anti-mouse*Enz or anti-Fab*Enz.
3. I-Ag + Fab + Anti-mouse*Enz or anti-Fab*Enz.

mAbs screened already by indirect ELISA already should be suitable for this test. The main application is in competitive tests in which both antigen and antibodies can be assessed in samples. This involves pretitration of the system (Ag and mAb). Samples can then be added and mixed with the pretitrated concentration of mAb and incubated, or added simultaneously. The binding of Fab fractions may well show different characteristics to whole mAb since as bivalency of antibody molecules is lost. This affects the relative affinity of binding to the antigen. It may allow a greater density of binding of Fab molecules as compared to whole molecules. The use of Fab molecules in competition assays may reduce or enhance sensitivities depending on the exact distribution and effective relative affinities of binding to antigen.

9.3. Direct Sandwich ELISA

The following list is a reminder of the systems as shown in **Table 17**:

1. I-mAb1 + Ag + mAb1*Enz (same mAb detecting).
2. I-Fab_2 + Ag + mAb*Enz (same mAb detecting).
3. I-mAb1 + Ag + mAb2*Enz (different mAb detecting).
4. I-mAb + Ag + PC*Enz (polyclonal antibody detector).
5. I-PC + Ag + mAb*Enz (polyclonal capture antibody).

The advantage of this system is linked with the specificity of the mAb in possibly capturing only the targeted antigen. Bivalent mAbs usually capture well, but have to be tested individually for required performance.

The use of the same MmaAb for capture and detection (as in examples 1 and 2) can lead to problems in which there is a limited number or single (e.g., peptide) epitope being expressed, asince the capture antibody may effectively preclude any further reaction. However, the use of the same Ab can be exploited to achieve highly specific assays for the detection of particular complexes bearing an antigen, as is illustrated for specific detection of whole particles of foot-and-mouth disease virus (FMDV) from subunits. In this example, the key is that the initial capture by the mAb orientates the antigen complexes. The consideration of the effects of orientation is necessary in all tests involving mAb capture.

When more than one mAb is available, sandwich assays can be made by labeling mAbs and using them as detectors and can alleviate problems of orientation and limited epitopes. This can also lead to very specific assays.

Examples 4 and 5 show the use of a polyclonal serum to either capture or detect. As a capture serum, mAbs can be used to detect specific epitopes and increase the specificity of assays. Again, with antigens showing limited epitopes, the polyclonal capture may result in prevention of any more binding saturation of epitopes. When polyclonal antibodies are used as a general detector, they allow a number of mAbs to be screened for effective capture of antigens. The specificity of the initial capture depends on the mAb. Here, orientation effects are more limited (as shown in data, e.g., with foot-and-mouth disease virus (FMDV) in **Subheading 7.10.1**).

The assays developed (pretitrated) can all be used with competitive/inhibi-tion systems for the detection of antibodies. Examination of antigens is more difficult since as it must be ensured that the capture antibody is saturated with antigen because addition of competing antigen increases the effective concentration and free capture antibodies will bind to this. The same is applicable in indirect sandwich systems.

9.4. Sandwich ELISA – Indirect

The following list is a reminder of the systems given in **Table 17**:

1. I-$mAb_{isotype1}$ + Ag + $mAb_{isotype2}$ + Anti-iso2*Enz.
2. I-Fab_2 + Ag + mAb + Anti-Fc*Enz.
3. I-mAb + Ag + PC + Anti-PC*Enz.
4. I-Fab_2 + Ag + PC + Anti-PC*Enz.
5. I-PC + Ag + mAb(+Fab_2 or Fab) + Anti mAb*Enz (or Anti-Fab*Enz).

In cases in which mAbs are available in pairs and their isotype is known, mAbs with different isotypes can be used to capture and detect antigens, as shown in example 1. This is made possible by the use of an anti-mouse isotype specific conjugate, which allows a higher level of screening of mAbs provided that the enzyme conjugates are affordable. When the bivalent Fab_2 is prepared, the whole molecule mAb or different mAbs can be used. These are detected using an anti-Fc specific conjugate (example 2). Thus, a large number of mAbs can be screened using a single successful capture reagent.

The use of polyclonal antibodies and mAbs is shown in examples 1–3. Examples in 3 and 4 show the benefit of screening mAbs for capture activity using a general detecting reagent and anti-species conjugate, and example 3 is probably the most widely used application.

When polyclonal antibodies are used to capture antigens, the screening of mAbs is relatively easy, and whole mAb or fractions can be used with appropriate anti-species conjugates (example 5).

The preparation of polyclonal reagents in experimental animals or characterization from field sera is important in the development of assays. Such sera can be used directly as components of assays and also as reagents defining mAb reactivity. This is particularly important in research areas. Often the best assays involve the use of polyclonal and mAb reagents, one allowing generalized reactivity and the other high specificity.

The systems can all be used in competition/inhibition ELISA for examination of antibodies. The target antigen can be captured first and then competition performed for the detecting antibody.

In summary, the use of mAbs and mAb-polyclonal systems offers a large number of possibilities. The particular advantage of any one has to be determined in the feasibility stages of the development of assays. The production of polyclonal reagents is recommended, to allow greater flexibility and possibly avoid too great a specificity of reaction at the various phases of the ELISAs; for example, polyclonal reagents may serve as a general capture reagent for a polyvalent antigen and the specificity of the mAb detector for a particular epitope exploited. Assays can be evolved with limited reagents, e.g., the use of mAb combinations using isotype-specific conjugates. Care must be taken to examine the use of mAbs in combination with respect to the orientation of antigens and subsequent elimination of binding of the detector. Some knowledge of the antigen(s) should be sought (molecular weight, density) to aid the designing of the assays.

10. Examples of the Use of mAbs

Examples of the use of mAbs are now given in detail and involve studies on FMDV:

1. The quantification of whole virus particles in the presence of subunits bearing the same epitope using the same mAb as capture and detector (direct sandwich ELISA).
2. The use of panels of mAbs at a single dilution to differentiate antigenic differences among many virus isolates, involving polyclonal capture sera, mAb detectors and anti-mouse conjugate (indirect sandwich).

3. The use of mAb-based competition assay for detection of antibodies against rinderpest virus and the development of kits.

The methods illustrate the interface of different technologies and disciplines needed to produce a successful ELISA for a specific purpose. This typifies the interaction of research facilities necessary to develop assays and a thorough understanding of the biological entities being examined.

10.1. Quantification of Whole Virus Particles of FMDV in the Presence of Virus Subunits, Using mAbs in a Sandwich ELISA

10.1.1. Background

The immunogenicity (ability to elicit protective antibodies in animals) of FMDV vaccines depends, to a large extent, on the production of whole virions (146S particles, so named because of their sedimentation characteristics in sucrose density gradients) in tissue culture and the stability of these particles after virus inactivation procedures and formulation into vaccines. The immunogenicity of subunits (12S particles) is very poor, weight for weight, compared to the 146S particles. Both whole and subunit particles are produced in the infectious process during the manufacture of vaccines. The specific quantification of 146S particles is made using physical methods using such as either $CsCl_2$ or linear sucrose density centrifugation methods. Both these methods are laborious, take a relatively long time, are subject to standardization problems, require expensive equipment, and do not assess whether the virus has been affected by proteolytic enzymes.

Serological methods for estimating the specific weight of 146S are complicated asince whole particles and subunits share most of the same epitopes. Thus, polyclonal sera produced against purified 146S particles cross react with subunits and, therefore, cannot be used directly to assess the weight of whole particles specifically.

Virus-neutralizing mAbs offer serological systems that can overcome the problems of crossreactivity. Neutralizing mAbs against most serotypes of FMDVs have been prepared and characterized in many laboratories worldwide. Such reagents have been used to compare virus isolates antigenically, to prepare and characterize mAb escape mutants allowing the identification of epitopes at the amino acid level, and as reagents in assays to measure antibodies. From such studies, the antigenic makeup of the surface of FMDVs is becoming more clearer, particularly when studied in conjunction with X-ray crystallographic data.

One strategy for the specific detection of 146S would be to select an mAb that bound only to the whole virion and not to the subunit particle. This has been proved possible, but such mAbs are not commonly isolated. Another strategy is to use the same mAb as capture and detector. This strategy has another advantage when commonly produced mAbs of a particular specificity have been defined. The use of centrifugation methods involves the sedimentation of virus and its assessment by reading the absorbance of fractions at 259 nm in a spectrophotometer. This measures the RNA content of the fraction, which is then used to calculate the protein weight using a formula. The association of protein to RNA of the correct sedimentation value indicates that virions are being quantified; however, it does not indicate whether the proteins in the virion are cleaved. Cleavage of protein VP1 in the virion capsid can dramatically alter the immunogenicity of the vaccine. If cleavage is to be estimated, then the peak fractions measured from the gradient have to be analyzed by polyacrylamide gel electrophoresis (PAGE), which is a laborious and limiting procedure. The complete procedure of centrifugation and analysis on PAGE, which gives full confidence in the vaccine, does not allow the prospect of on-line testing for virus as it is being produced during the vaccine run. The use of mAbs similar to those identified in this chapter will not only quantify 146S specifically but will identify whether the VP1 protein has been cleaved. The system could also be adapted to the on-line continuous testing for 146S virus, which would allow a greater control of the manufacturing process so that the virus could be harvested at the time of maximum production.

10.1.2. Materials and Methods

Viruses

Type O1 Kaufbeuren FMDV was grown in BHK-21 cells in the absence of bovine serum. Infected tissue culture fluid was clarified by low-speed centrifugation and the protein precipitated by the addition of an equal volume of saturated ammonium sulfate (pH 7.4, controlled by the addition of NaOH). After 1 h at room temperature, the precipitated protein was collected by centrifugation (~6,000 *g*; Mistral 6L centrifuge). The sediment was resuspended in a minimum volume of PBS and clarified by centrifugation at 10,000 *g*. The supernatant was then centrifuged at 100,000 *g* for 2.5 h to pellet the virus. One milliliter of PBS was added to cover the pellet, which was then left overnight at 4°C to allow the pellet to rehydrate. The pellets were then resuspended by agitation with a pipet and brief sonication in a water bath sonicator. Purification was made on linear 15–45% sucrose density gradients after the addition of sodium dodecyl sulfate (SDS) to a final concentration of 0.1%. The concentration of purified virus (146S) was established by examination of the RNA adsorption at 259 nm. Peak samples were stored at –70°C without further additions.

Preparation of 12s Subunit Particles

One milliliter of purified virus containing 200 mg of virus was acidified by the addition of 2 mL of 0.1 M NaH_2PO_4. Phenol red indicator solution was added (0.05 mL), and the mixture was left at room temperature for 10 min, after which the pH was adjusted to 7.4 by the addition of 0.1 M NaOH.

Preparation of Trypsin-Treated Virus

To 200 mg of purified virus in 1.0 mL of sucrose was added to 50 mL of trypsin solution (2 mg/mL in 0.1 M phosphate buffer, pH 7.4). The mixture was incubated at 37°C for 15 min. The virus was then diluted to the assay concentrations in the relevant buffer with no further treatment.

Preparation of Denatured Virus

To 1 mL of purified virus containing 200 mg was added 10 mg of SDS (giving a final concentration of 1%) and 20 mL of mercaptoethanol (to a final concentration of 2%). The mixture was heated for 3 min in a boiling water bath. The virus preparation was dialyzed against PBS, and the volume after dialysis was noted to allow an accurate determination of concentration of the protein relative to the starting material.

Antisera

Guinea pig and rabbit polyclonal antisera against type O and SAT 2 FMDVs were prepared after multi-vaccination of animals with purified inactivated virus containing antibodies with a wide spectrum of activity against all FMDVs components.

Monoclonal Antibodies

mAbs were prepared as described in **ref.** *2*. Acites fluids were prepared by ip inoculation of the hybridoma cells into mice previously sensitized with Freunds' Complete Adjuvant (FCA). Ascites fluids were clarified by centrifugation and stored at –20°C. The anti–type O mAbs B2, C8, C9, and D9 have been extensively characterized using serological tests and mAb escape mutant studies (*3–5*).

Enzyme Conjugation of mAbs

Ascites fluids were labeled with HRP using the method described in **ref. *6***.

10.2. ELISAs

10.2.1. Titration of mAbs as Capture Antibodies

The ascites and the polyclonal rabbit serum were diluted in 0.05 M carbon-ate/bicarbonate buffer, pH 9.5, in 50-µL vol into wells of a microtiter ELISA plate (Nunc7 Maxisorb). Twofold dilution series from 1/20 were made across 11 wells, in quadruplicate. The plates were incubated at 4°C overnight or at 37°C for 2 h. Plates were then washed by flooding and emptying the wells four times with PBS. Plates were blotted almost dry and 50 µL of the respective purified FMDV, 12S, trypsin-treated virus (TTV), or denatured virus (DNV) were added to each well at 2 µg/mL, diluted in PBS containing 5% bovine skimmed milk powder (Marvel) and 0.1% Tween-20 (blocking buffer to prevent nonspecific attachment of protein). The plates were incubated at 37°C for 1 h while being rotated. Plates were then washed and 50 µL of the relevant type of specific polyclonal guinea pig anti-FMDV serum was added at optimal dilution to each well, diluted in the blocking buffer just described. Plates were then incubated at 37°C for 1 h while being rotated. Anti-guinea pig whole IgG HRP conjugate was then added, 50 µL per well diluted in blocking buffer, and the plates were incubated for 1 h at 37°C while being rotated. Plates were then washed and 50 µL per well of OPD/H_2O_2 chromogen/substrate was added. Color was allowed to develop for 10 min, and then the reaction was stopped by the addition of 50 µL of 1 M H_2SO_4. The results were quantified by reading the plates on a multichannel spectrophotometer. Data relating the activity of each mAb dilution to capture virus as detected by the polyclonal system were plotted. Optimal dilutions of each mAb were measured to allow a single dilution to be assessed in virus quantification studies. The effect of using different concentrations of mAbs as capture reagents was also examined when assessing the various antigen preparations.

10.2.2. Titration of Enzyme-Labeled mAbs

Plates were coated with 50 μL per well of an optimal dilution of the relevant rabbit anti-FMDV serum in carbonate/bicarbonate buffer (1/5,000). After incubation overnight at 4°C or at 37°C for 2 h, the plates were washed. Purified 146S and 12S (50 μL) were then added at 2 μg/mL in blocking buffer and incubated for 1 h at 37°C while being rotated. Each of the conjugated mAbs was tested on the relevant virus capture plates by titration in twofold dilution series from 1 to 10 across 11 wells. The conjugates were diluted in 50 μL of blocking buffer as just described and incubated for 1 h at 37°C while being rotated. Plates were then washed and the chromogen/substrate steps followed as in **Subheading 10.2.1.** Data were obtained relating the activity of the conjugates on dilution to estimate the optimal dilution to be used in the virus quantification studies.

10.2.3. Titration of Virus Using Dilutions of mAb as Capture and Detecting Reagents

Optimal dilutions of each of the mAbs, as assessed under **Subheadings 10.2.1.** and **10.2.2.**, were used to coat wells under the same conditions. After washing, known concentrations of 146S, 12S, TTV or DNV were added as twofold dilution series in 50 μL of blocking buffer (beginning at 5 μg/mL). Plates were incubated at 37°C for 1 h. Labeled mAbs were then added at optimal dilutions in 50 μL of blocking buffer. After 1 h of incubation at 37°C, the plates were washed and substrate/chromogen was added, followed by stopping and reading in a spectrophotometer. Different combinations of mAbs were used as capture and detecting reagents. Virus and virus preparations were also captured using the rabbit serum and then detected with the mAb reagents. Guinea pig serum was also used to quantify the antigens when mAbs and rabbit serum had been used as capture reagents.

10.2.4. Titration of 146S in the Presence of 12S

The effect of adding high concentrations of 12S to a constant amount of 146S was examined using different concentrations of mAb capture reagents. The same systems were also examined using guinea pig polyclonal detecting serum.

10.2.5. Standardization of 146S Titrations

A standard preparation of known concentration was established using purified 146S virus quantified by UV spectrophotometry. This standard was stored in small volumes at –70°C, and samples were thawed and used once in the assays. The standard was diluted in quadruplicate in 50 μL of blocking buffer to produce a standard curve relating the weight of 146S to OD, and the variation at each point was calculated. For the assay of virus contained in tissue culture samples, four different infected tissue culture supernatants were diluted 1/2, 1/4, 1/8 and 1/16 in blocking buffer and then assayed in quadruplicate in 50-μL vol. The weight of the virus in the samples was then calculated for the different dilutions by referring to the curve obtained for the standard 146S titration. The standard 146S acted as a control for each test plate, and examination of the cumulative data from all the test plates allowed the variation of the assay to be determined.

Determinations of the concentrations of the virus from three of the tissue culture samples were made over ten tests on ten separate days.

10.3. Results

Figure 8 shows the titration curves obtained using different dilutions of mAbs and the polyclonal rabbit serum as capture reagents for constant amounts of the various antigens. Captured antigens

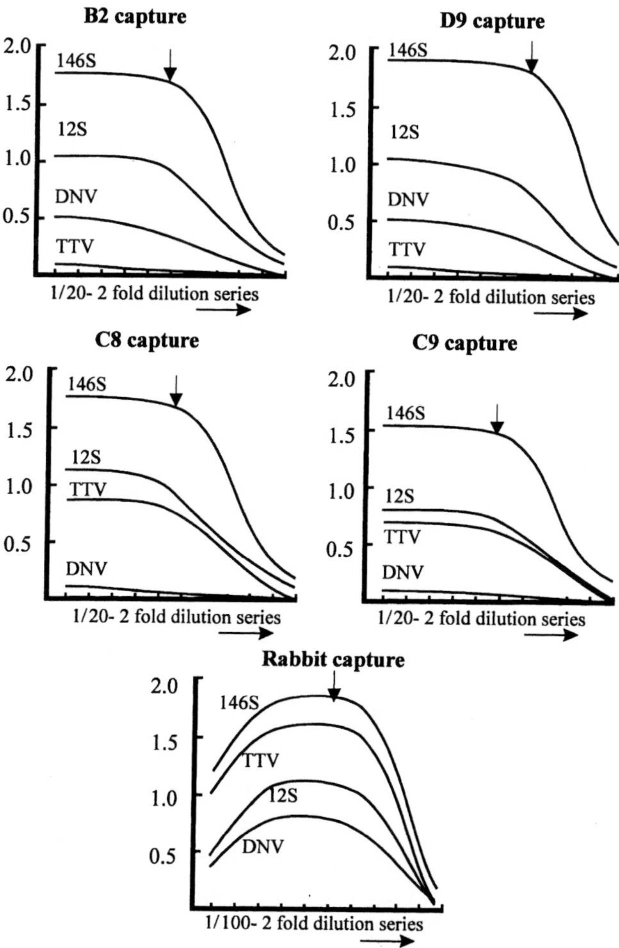

Fig. 8. Use of mAbs and rabit sera on solid phase to capture various antigenic preparations of FMDV. *Downward arrow*↓ = optimal dilution of capture reagents.

were detected using polyclonal guinea pig serum/anti-guinea pig conjugate. All the mAbs captured both 146S and 12S, although the plateau maximum OD for 12S was significantly lower than that for 146S, particularly for mAbs B2 and D9. This was also true for the rabbit capture/guinea pig detector system. Neither TTV nor DNV was detected when the B2 and D9 mAbs were used as capture reagents, whereas mAbs C8 and C9 were capable of presenting TTV to the detecting antibody. The polyclonal system detected all antigens, although dilution of the serum was needed to achieve optimal capture. The optimal dilution for each of the mAbs and the polyclonal sera for the capture of 146S are arrowed.

Figure 9 shows the titration curves for each of the mAb-enzyme conjugates where constant amounts of 146S and 12S were captured by the optimal dilution of polyclonal rabbit serum indicated in **Fig. 1**. All the mAb conjugates were capable of detecting both antigens, the plateau height differences between 12S and 146S resulted from the limiting factors of the polyclonal rabbit serum to capture 12S as explained diagrammatically in **Fig. 10**. The reduction in plateau height for the titration of the

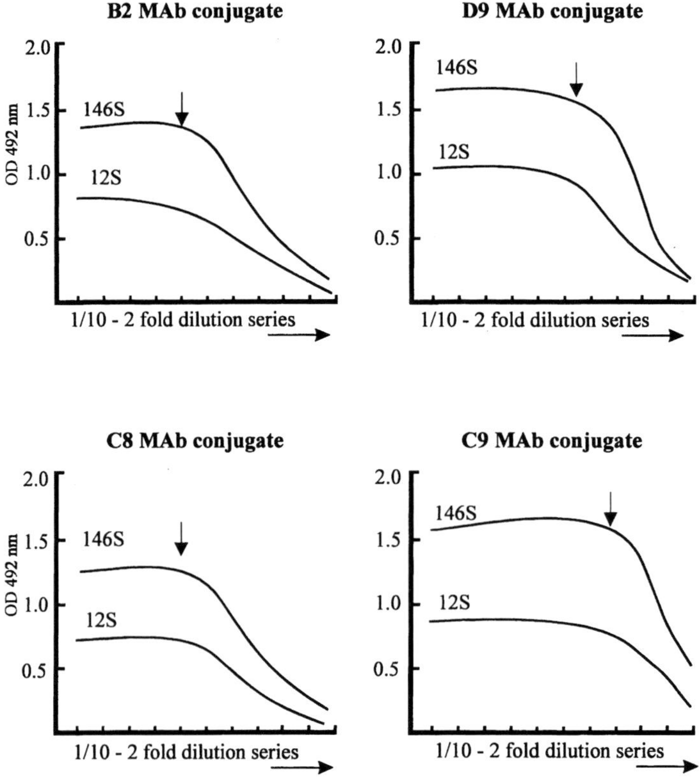

Fig. 7.9. Titration of mAb enzyme conugates against 146S and 12S captured by rabbit serum. *Downward arrow*, Optimal dilution to detect maximum amount of 146S virus.

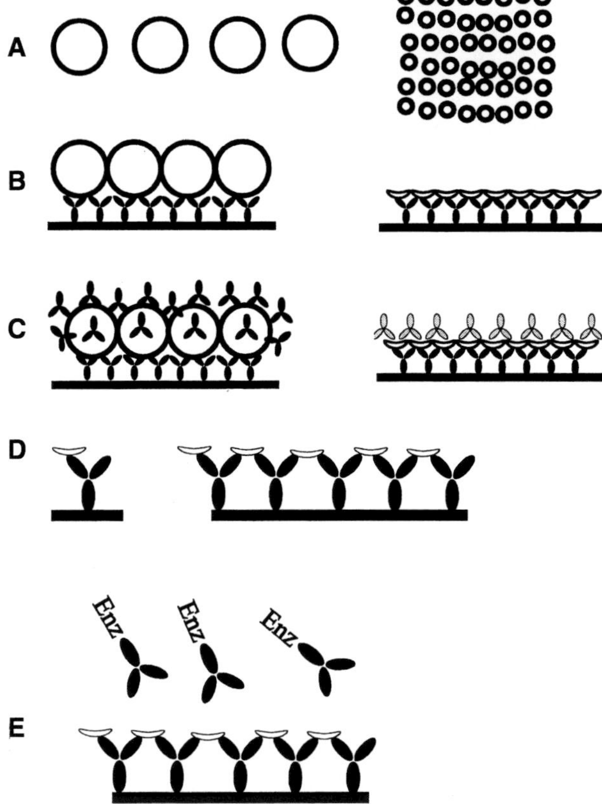

Fig. 10. Consequences of binding virus and subunits via mAbs or polyclonal sera. **(A)** Relative subunit number to four virus particles. **(B, C)** Capture of 146S virus particles and subsequent detection presents more antigenic sites that than with optimal capture of subunits generated from the same number of particles, thus affecting plateau height maxima. **(D)** mAbs orientate subunits to present internal epitopes, unlike presentation of captured 146S particles. **(E)** Detection of mAb captured subunits with the same mAb as used to capture does not work, as relevant epitopes are already bound, unlike detection of epitopes on whole particles in the same system.

same weight of 12S was also shown in the polyclonal capture/ detection system.

Figure 11 shows the titrations of various antigens using optimal dilutions of the same mAbs as both capture and detecting reagents. The rabbit capture/ guinea pig detection system is also included for the same materials assessed. This shows that B2 and D9 detected 146S but not 12S, TTV or DNV; whereas C8 and C9 detected 12S and TTV. The polyclonal system demonstrated that all the antigens were present in the samples and that there were marked effects on the maximum OD obtainable for 12S and DNV, with a small effect on TTV.

Figure 12 shows the effect of measuring two different concentrations of 146S in the presence of a dilution series of 12S.

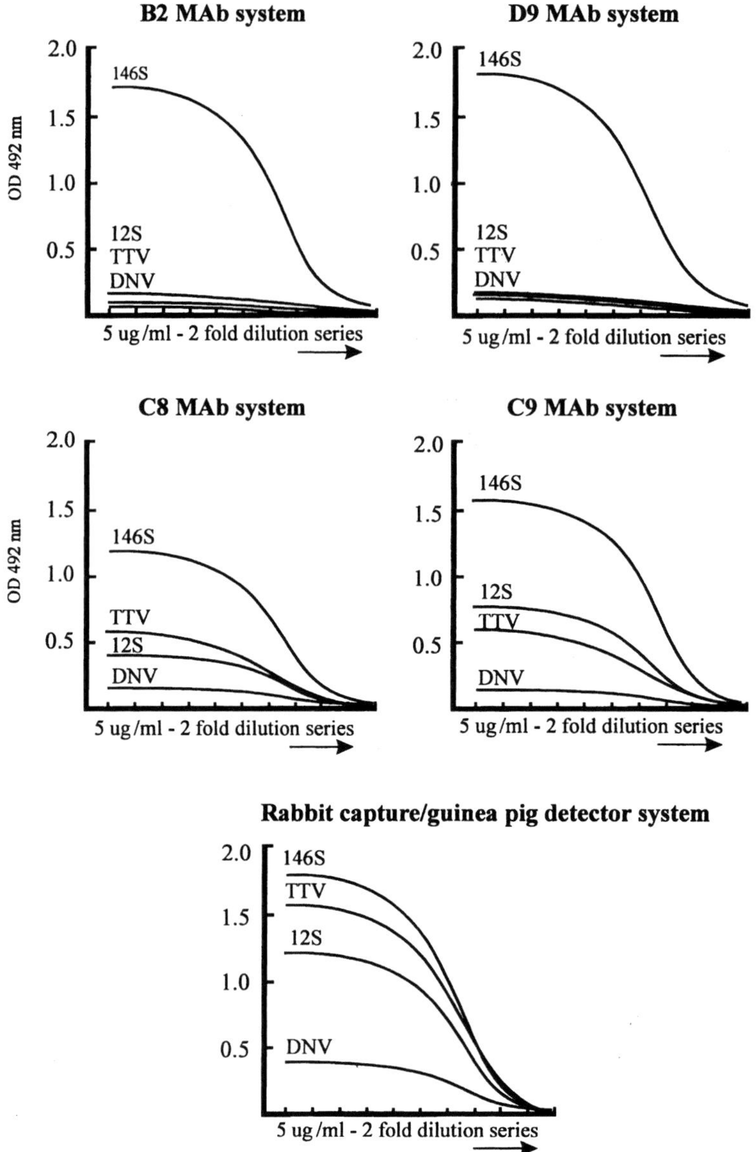

Fig. 11. Titration of mAbs as capture and detection systems against dilutions of 146S, 12S, TTV, and DNV.

The rabbit/guinea pig system demonstrated that the 12S was titratable. There was no significant effect on the detection of the constant amount of each of the 146S samples in any of the mAb capture/detector systems. Error bars representing 2 × *SD* from the mean OD of each sample are shown.

Figure 13 shows the results of titrating 146S in the presence of a relatively high concentration of 12S. The rabbit/guinea pig system indicates that the level of reaction owing to the 12S

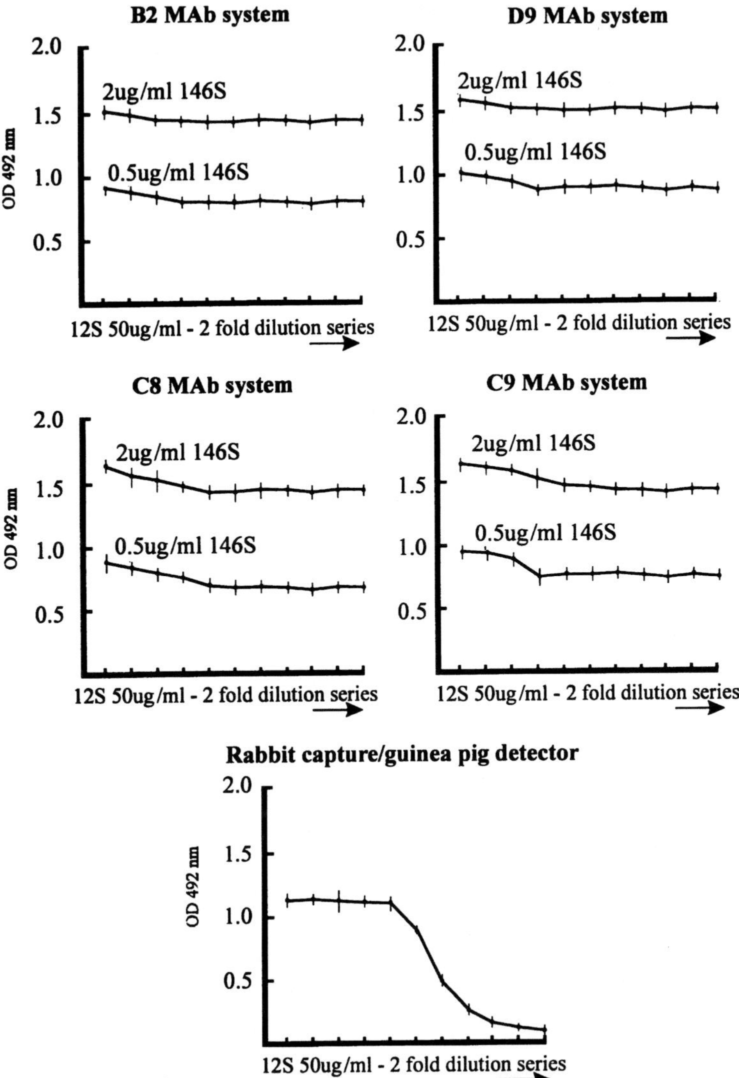

Fig. 12. Measurement of 146S in the presence of a dilution series of 12S using mAb capture and detection system.

observed after the 146S is diluted to a level below that of the 12S. No such plateau is observed in the mAb systems.

Figure 14 shows a curve of cumulative data obtained on 10 estimations of the standard 146S performed on different plates over 2 wks using the B2 and D9 mAb systems. The variation in results is shown as bars (1 × *SD* mean) for each of the titrations (quadruplicate estimates). A line has been drawn through 1.0 OD to highlight the mean and upper and lower limits of the

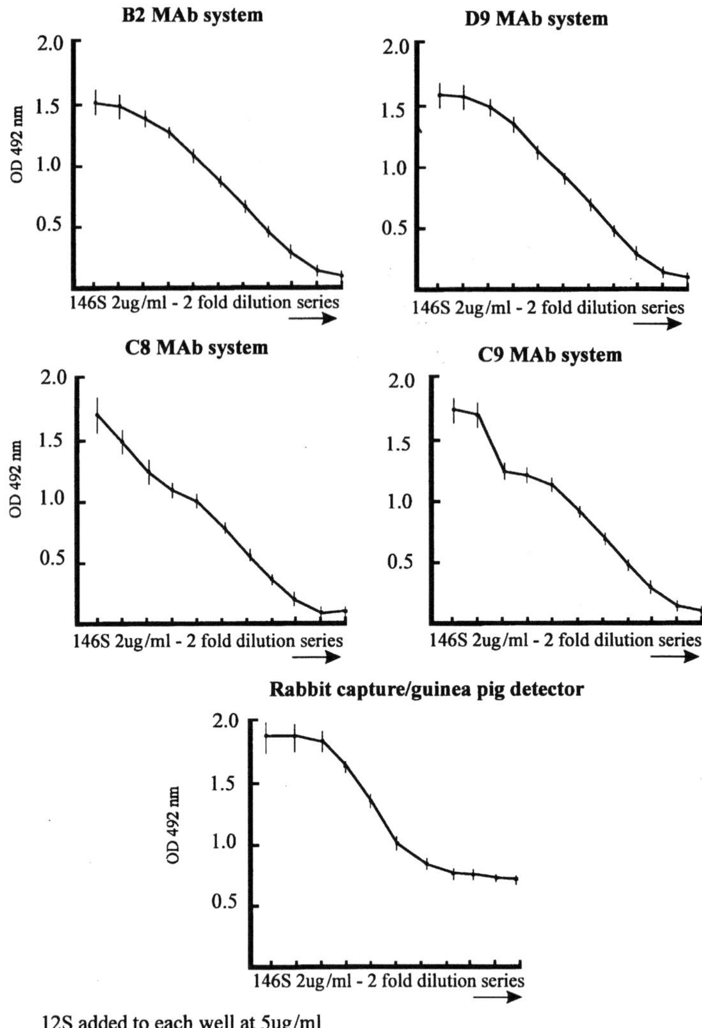

Fig. 13. Titration of 146S in the presence of a constant amount of 12S using mAb capture and detection systems.

data for each mAb. This represents the most precise area on the standard curve.

The concentration of virus in unknown samples was best estimated when OD values of 0.6–1.3 were obtained, corresponding to a range of ~0.03–0.5 μg/mL of virus on the standard curve. **Table 18** shows the results for the determinations of the 146S in four infected tissue culture samples. **Table 19** shows data for three of the samples assessed at a single dilution over 10 tests.

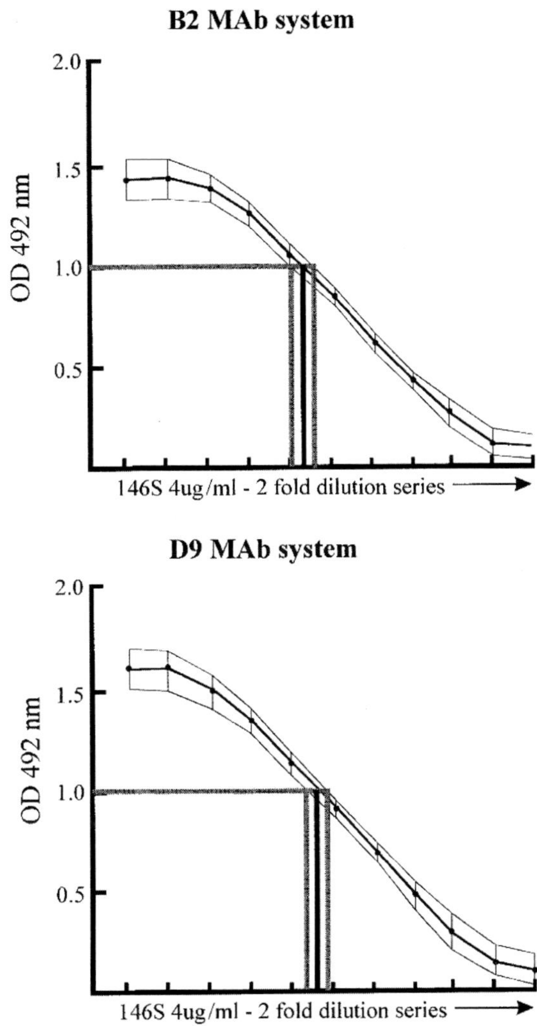

Fig. 14. Cumulative data for titration of 146S using mAb capture and detection systems.

Figure 15 is a diagrammatic representation illustrating the relationship B) to 12S subunits derived from those particles (**Fig. 15C**). The relative sizes of the particles are drawn to scale along with an IgG molecule. A side view of the 12S pentamer (**Fig. 15D**) illustrates that epitopes are contained internally as well as externally (in common with 146S external sites). The consequences of mAb or polyclonal antibody capture/detection is are examined in **Fig. 15E** and **F**.

Note in **Fig. 10**. **Figure 10a–c** that for the same antigenic mass (illustrated as four virus particles), a higher number of subunits are available for capture. However, the ability of the capture

Table 18
Quantification of 146S virus from four tissue cktre samples at different dilutions

				Weight from mean value read from standard curve (μg/mL)[a]		Concentration in original (μg/mL)[a]	
Sample		OD	so	Mean	*SD*	Mean	± *SD*
A	3/2	1.51	0.09	>4	–	>4	–
	1/4	1.45	0.09	1.71	0.10	6.84	6.44–7.24
	1/8	1.30	0.06	0.83	0.07	6.64	6.08–7.20
B	1/2	1.35	0.07	1.01	0.12	2.02	1.78–2.26
	1/4	1.29	0.05	0.81	0.05	3.24	3.04–3.44
	1/8	1.10	0.04	0.37	0.03	2.96	2.72–3.20
C	1/2	1.12	0.04	0.39	0.02	0.78	0.74–0.82
	1/4	0.89	0.03	0.20	0.01	0.80	0.76–0.84
	1/8	0.76	0.02	0.11	0.01	0.88	0.80–0.96
D	1/2	0.11	0.01	0.008	0.004	0.016	0.008–0.024
	1/4	0.10	0.01	0.007	0.004	0.028	0.012–0.044

[a]Weights measured using mean value from sample. The variation of standard curve at this OD was used to establish the standard deviation (SS) for the test sample

[b]Obtained by multiplying the weighjs of virus obtained for the mean and±SD by dilution factor

Table 19
Assessment of 146S virus from three tissue culture samples

Sample	Dilution	Weight (μg/mL)	SD (μg/mL)	CV%
A	1/16	7.1	0.51	7.1
B	1/8	3.1	0.19	6.3
C	1/8	0.8	0.05	6.1

[a]Coefficient of variation (%)

system to bind all the units released on producing 12S is more limited. This affects the number of antibodies binding as compared to the antigens exposed on virions. **Figure 10d** illustrates that the binding of capture mAbs to external 12S epitopes in common with 146S has the effect of preventing the same mAb binding, thus allowing differentiation of 12S and 146S particles, even though they share the same epitope.

10.4. Discussion

A novel method is described for the detection and quantification of whole 146S particles of FMDV using mAbs as capture and detecting reagents. The key to the success of the system relies on the fact that, although the epitopes identified by the mAbs are common to 12S and 146S, they are on the outer capsid surface. The subsequent presentation of the mAb-bound 146S and 12S to the same mAb allows detection of only 146S asince the cross-reactive epitopes on the 12S particles are orientated toward the plate by interaction with the capture mAb.

The capture of 12S by the mAbs and polyclonal serum was shown through its detection using the polyclonal guinea pig antiserum detector in **Fig. 7.9**. Note the different reaction for the same weights of 146S and 12S by all the systems. In polyclonal capture/detection systems in the sandwich ELISA, there is always a reduction in the plateau height (a constant maximum OD observed for a range of concentrations in which the detecting serum is in excess), asince there is both a reduction in the number of 12S particles (antigenic mass) that can be captured from the equivalent weight of 146S owing to physical reasons, and an orientation factor for 12S (similar to that described for the mAb) depending on the exact nature of the polyclonal antibodies and the extent that the capture and detecting antibodies react with internal and external epitopes. The sandwich ELISA has been used successfully as an analytical method for the estimation of total degradation of the 146S using a defined polyclonal system in the analysis of the pH stability of 146S and 75S particles.

All the mAbs examined were capable of detecting 146S and 12S when used as detecting reagents, as shown in **Fig. 7.9**. The reduction in plateau height was again observed. However, mAbs used in combination did not detect 12S even at high concentration, but were capable of specifically measuring 146S. **Figure 7.12** illustrates this and also shows that mAbs B2 and D9 did not detect TTV or DNV, although both these mAbs have been shown to react with continuous epitopes (linear determinants) on the VP1 loop of type O FMDV in the indirect ELISA. However, the sandwich conditions presumably inhibit any second antibody binding asince denaturation and disruption of the virus produces small polypeptides and peptides containing the linear epitopes that bind exclusively to the capture antibodies.

The use of such virus-neutralizing mAbs reacting with linear epitopes on VP1 on the outside of the capsid that are sensitive to proteolytic cleavage allows not only the quantification of virus but also a qualitative assessment of the antigen. This is vital in preparing vaccines that show poor immunogenicity when cleavage of VP1 has occurred. mAbs that react with similar epitopes have been characterized, so it is envisaged that there will be little difficulty in identifying reagents suitable for this assay for the assessment of vaccines. The prerequisite is that the mAb can bind to the vaccine strain of interest.

Titration of 146S in the presence of large excesses of 12S could interfere with the specific quantification of 146S. This could occur asince the capture mAbs bind 12S, which may affect the capture potential for 146S. The results in **Figs. 12 and 13** confirm that this was not a problem. There was a slight increase in the expected OD values for the 146S, when 12S was added at 100 and 50 times the weight of 146S, particularly using the C8 and C9 systems. Such ratios are not expected to be present in infectious tissue culture samples prepared during the manufacture of vaccine.

The use of standard curves for calculation of virus weight should be successful if precautions are taken to avoid thermal and chemical effects on standard preparations. Thus, once a purified virus has been assessed spectrophotometrically and stored in small aliquots at ~–70°C or in liquid nitrogen, and when used as single batches, it should be possible to standardize assays precisely. This was shown by titration of the same virus on 10 different days where the best range for the estimation for virus was when OD values were from ~1.2 to 0.4, corresponding to 0.5 and 0.03 μg/mL of virus/mL. The data in **Tables 18** and **19** indicate that reproducibility of the assay is acceptable for the purpose of assessing of 146S in vaccines.

11. Use of mAbs T to Examine Antigenic Variation in Type A FMDV

11.1. Background

Any mAbs produced against members of serotype A FMDVs can be been used to examine antigenic differences. The mAbs used in this study were obtained from various laboratories in Europe and South America. A microtiter plate sandwich ELISA was used to measure the binding of the mAbs with virus field isolates, vaccine strains, and mAb escape mutants relative to binding with homologous virus. Different amounts of serological and biochemical data were available as to the characterization of the mAbs, particularly for the identification of the critical amino acid sequences bound by individual mAbs. The use of a relatively high number of viruses allowed mAbs of similar reactivities to be compared and grouped using multivariate statistics. The antigenic relationships between the viruses were also evaluated in the same way, and the relevance of results to the epidemiology of strains was examined. The study has allowed the frequency of different epitopes on type A viruses to be examined and the consideration of the epidemiological significance of the findings. Recommendations are made for the use of a limited number of mAbs to act as a standard panel to allow rapid antigenic analysis of isolates.

mAbs against most serotypes of FMDVs have been prepared and characterized in many laboratories worldwide. Such reagents offer the potential for rapid antigenic characterization of virus isolates in simple binding assays such as ELISA. Antigenic variation of FMD viruses is important in many areas involving the control of diseases, such as assessing field strains for their potential threat to animals vaccinated with vaccine strains, comparing vaccine strains among producers, monitoring the vaccine strain throughout production, examination of challenge strains used to evaluate vaccine efficacy which are produced by passage in animals, and examining of persistent viruses (carrier state).

This study shows how mAbs produced against serotypes A5, A10, A22, and A24 viruses, from different laboratories, can be used to group viruses according to their similar properties; examine the distribution and variation of the epitopes; recommend an assay for the rapid comparison of epitopes on type A viruses; and to define a limited panel of type A mAbs that might be useful in comparing type A field, vaccine, and challenge strains.

11.2. Materials and Methods

11.2.1. Viruses

The viruses were obtained from the World Reference Laboratory (WRL), at Pirbright, UK. Certain isolates were selected as representatives of vaccine strains. The isolates were amplified by growth in tissue culture usually through bovine thyroid (BTY) primary cells, then passaged in continuous monolayer cultures of baby hamster kidney (BHK-21). Some of the viruses also were passaged in continuous renal swine cells (RS). The passage history of most of the isolates is indicated by the number following the cell line. Most of the samples for use in the ELISA were obtained by a further passage of seed stock virus in BHK cells, but the last manipulation of the virus is shown by the last cell line indicated. When monolayers were totally disrupted, the mixture was centrifuged (2000*g* for 10 min) to remove debris, and the supernatant was stored at –70 or –20°C after the addition of an equal volume of sterile glycerol.

11.2.2. Antisera

Rabbit and guinea pig polyclonal antisera against type A5, A22, and A24 viruses were prepared as described in **ref.** *2*. These sera, used as capture antibodies and detecting antibodies, respectively, in ELISAs were produced after multivaccination of animals with purified inactivated virus, containing antibodies with a wide spectrum of activity against all FMDVs components.

11.2.3. Monoclonal Antibodies

The mAbs used in this study came from the IAH, Pirbright, UK, and from various laboratories in Europe and South America. These were obtained as ascites fluids or tissue culture preparations.

11.2.4. Data Obtained For for mAbs

Different methods were used to characterize the various mAbs, including use of various ELISAs with various antigenic preparations of the viruses. The data were also used to evaluate the findings of the sandwich ELISA.

11.3. Sandwich ELISA to Compare Binding of mAbs to FMDVs: Antigenic Profiling

The sandwich ELISA was conducted as described in **ref.** *7*. Briefly, microtiter plate wells were coated with a pooled mixture of rabbit antibodies produced against type-purified isolates characterizing A24, A22, and A5 FMD virus subtypes. Such a mixture has been shown to be effective in capturing most of the type A FMDV isolates examined in the WRL at Pirbright. The rabbit antiserum was added in 50-μL vol to the wells and diluted in 0.05 M carbonate/bicarbonate buffer, pH 9.6. Plates were incubated overnight at 4°C or 1 h at 37°C. Plates were then washed with PBS, and the various virus preparations were added in duplicate in 50-μL vol, (as shown in **Fig. 16**) diluted in 50 μL of blocking buffer (PBS containing 3% bovine serum albumin, 0.1% Tween-20, and 5% nonimmune [normal] bovine serum). The homologous virus was always included on row A of each plate to demonstrate the maximal interaction of the mAbs so that relative assessments of binding could be examined, as discussed next.

Plates were washed and mAbs were added as shown in **Fig. 17**. The mAbs were diluted in blocking buffer as described for the virus dilution. The dilution of mAb used was determined from the studies on mAb binding to homologous virus using indirect and sandwich ELISAs; an excess of mAb was always used. The last two columns of the plates received guinea pig serotype-specific serum at a pretitrated dilution in blocking buffer. This serum was broadly reactive (produced in a way similar to the rabbit capture antibodies), and has been tested to react with all viruses within a serotype. The values in these columns served to estimate the amount of each virus captured. The last row received no virus but the respective column mAb. This acted as the background control for any mAb interaction. Plates were incubated at 37°C for 1 h while being rotated. Plates were washed, and then each well that had mAb added received anti-mouse IgG enzyme conjugate

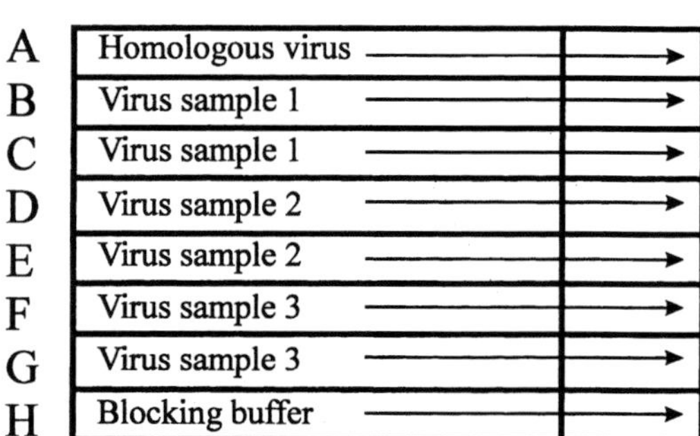

Fig. 16. Sandwich ELISA for mAb profiling. All wells of the plates are coated with polyclonal anti-FMDV-type specific serum. A mixture of rabbit antibodies against A5, A22, and A24 serotypes is used. After incubation and washing, a single dilution of different virus suspensions is added (in blocking buffer) as shown, in duplicate rows for test samples (B, C; D, E; and F, G). Row A contains the virus responsible for eliciting the mAbs used, and row H receives only blocking buffer.

at a pretitrated optimal dilution in blocking buffer. The last two columns received anti-–guinea pig conjugate as described for the virus titrations. The plates were incubated at 37°C for 1 h with rotation and then the OPD substrate solution was added. The color development was stopped after 10 min and the color quantified by a multichannel spectrophotometer.

The dilution of each virus was usually determined by previous titration in a sandwich ELISA in which plates were coated and viruses diluted in triplicate as twofold series, in blocking buffer. After incubation with rotation, the plates were washed and a pretitrated anti-serotype-specific guinea pig serum was added diluted in blocking buffer. The plate was then incubated as for the virus stage and washed, and then each well received a dilution (in blocking buffer) of anti-guinea pig HRP conjugate. After incubation as before, H_2O_2/OPD substrate was added. Color development was stopped at 10 min. The plates were read in a multichannel spectrophotometer (492 nm). The devel-

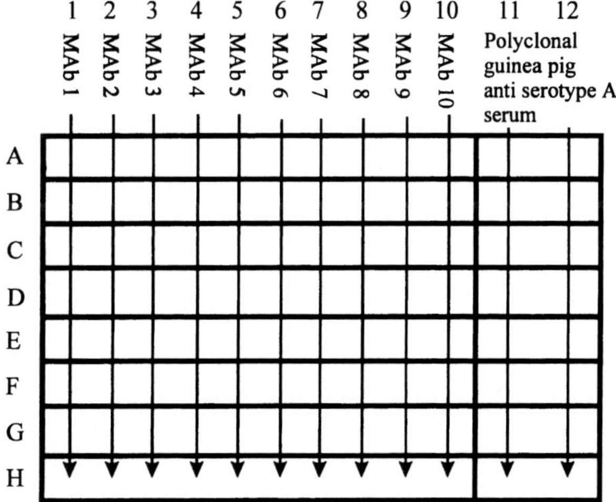

Fig. 17. Addition of mAbs to profiling plates. mAbs 1–10 are added in columns 1–10 at a single dilution in blocking buffer. Polyclonal anti-–type A serum is added in columns 11 and 12. Plates are incubated and washed, after which anti-mouse enzyme conjugate is added to columns 1–10 and anti-–guinea pig enzyme conjugate to columns 11 and 12. After incubation and washing, substrate chromophore is added and color development stopped. The OD values are read and the relative binding of mAbs to viruses is determined with reference to the reactions of the mAbs with the homologous virus. The OD values in row H are subtracted from each OD value in the respective column. The OD values for each duplicate mAb reaction are then averaged. This mean OD value is then expressed as a percentage of the mean value obtained for the virus/ guinea pig binding for each respective virus. Finally, this percentage value is expressed as a percentage of the value obtained for the homologous virus. Thus, the relative weights of each virus are taken into consideration by with reference to the examination of the guinea pig polyclonal readings, and results are therefore comparing a comparison of the relative binding of the same mAbs to different viruses as compared to the homologous virus.

oped color was related to the dilution, and the dilution giving 1.2– to 1.5 OD was used in the antigenic profiling ELISA described in **Subheading 11.3.1.** The plates were incubated for 1 h at 37°C while being rotated at approximately three revolutions per second. In practice, it was found that most tissue culture preparations contained high levels of virus and that dilutions of 1/3 to 1/16 could be used to provide excess virus for the trapping rabbit serum. Therefore, the amount of rabbit serum was limiting in this step.

11.3.1. Processing of Data

Processing of the data is described in **ref.** *7*. Briefly, the OD values in the last row (mAb negative antigen control) were subtracted from each column. The OD values for each duplicate were then averaged. This mean value was then expressed as a percentage of the mean value obtained for the virus/guinea pig binding for each respective virus. Finally, this percentage value was expressed as a percentage of the value obtained for the homologous virus. Thus, the relative weights of each virus were taken into consideration by reference to the examination of the guinea pig polyclonal readings. Results are therefore compare ing the relative binding of the same mAbs to different viruses as compared to the homologous virus. This is illustrated in Tables 7.20 with simplified results.

The criteria for assessing the results and statistical considerations were examined in **ref.** *7*. The data were analyzed with a computer-based package using multivariate statistics to perform hierarchical analysis (block method, complete linkage). The mAbs

Table 20
Stlized data and methods for calculation

(i) Untreated sylized OD data (duplicates made the same)

	1	2	3	4	5	6	7	8	9	10	11	12
A	1.1	1.5	1.3	1.0	1.0	0.8	0.9	1.I	1.2	1.3	1.6	1.6
B	0.1	1.4	1.1	1 I	0.1	0.1	0.7	1.1	0.1	0.1	1.5	1.5
C	0.1	1.4	1.1	1.1	0.1	0.1	0.7	1.1	0.1	0.1	1.5	1.5
D	1.1	1.4	1.2	0.1	0.1	0.1	0.1	1.2	1.0	1.0	1.5	1.5
E	1.1	1.4	0.2	0.1	0.1	0.1	0 1	1.2	1.0	1.0	1.5	1.5
F	0.5	1.1	1.3	0.1	0.5	0.8	0.9	1.1	0.1	0.1	1.2	1.2
G	0.5	1.1	1.3	0.1	0.5	0.8	OP	1.1	0.1	0.1	1.2	1.2

(continued)

Table 20 (continued)

(i) Untreated sylized OD data (duplicates made the same)

	1	2	3	4	5	6	7	8	9	10	11	12
H	0.1	0.2	0.3	0.1	0.1	0.1	0.1	0.1	0.1	0.1	0.2	0.2
(ii) OD minus row H value in each column												
	1	2	3	4	5	6	7	8	9	10	11/12	
A	1.0	1.3	1.0	1.5	0.9	0.7	0.8	1.0	1.1	1.2	1 4	
B	0	1.2	1.0	1.0	0	0.1	0.6	1.0	0	0	1.3	
C	0	1.2	1.0	1.0	0	0.1	0.6	1.0	0	0	1.3	
D	1.0	1.2	0.9	0	0	0.1	0	1.1	0.9	0.9	1.3	
E	1.0	1.2	0.9	0	0	0.1	0	1.1	0.9	0.9	1.3	
F	0.4	0.9	1.0	0	0.4	0.7	0.8	1.0	0	0	1.0	
G	0.4	0.9	1.0	0	0.4	0.7	0.8	1.0	0	0	1.0	
(iii) Means of OD values after subtraction												
	1	2	3	4	5	6	7	8	9	10	11/12	
A	1.0	1.3	1.0	1.5	0.9	0.7	0.8	1.0	1.1	1.2	1.4	
B/C	0	1.2	1.0	1.0	0	0.1	0.6	1.0	0	0	1.3	
D/E	1.0	1.2	0.9	0	0	0.1	0	1.1	0.9	0.9	1.3	
F/G	0.4	0.9	1.0	0	0.4	0.7	0.8	1.0	0	0	1.0	
(iv) Percentage value of OD mAb/OD value polyclonal, for that virus in 11/12												
	1	2	3	4	5	6	7	8	9	10	11/12	
A	71	93	71	107	64	50	57	71	79	86	100	
B/C	0	92	77	77	0	8	46	77	0	0	100	
D/E	77	92	70	0	0	8	0	84	70	70	100	
F/G	40	90	100	0	40	70	80	100	0	0	100	
(v) mAb percentage in each column as percentage of homologous virus value												
	1	2	3	4	5	6	7	8	9	10		
A	100	100	100	100	100	100	100	100	100	100		
B/C	0	99	108	72	0	16	80	108	0	0		
D/E	108	99	99	0	0	16	0	118	89	81		
F/G	56	97	140	0	61	140	158	140	0	0		

were then assessed according to their reactions with the viruses, and the viruses were related according to their reactions with the mAbs. Cluster analyses were made grouping the reactions of the mAbs and viruses, respectively. The reactions were related to obtain dendrograms of the mAb and the virus groups.

11.3.2. Results

All the mAbs were examined initially for their binding characteristics against 20 selected field strains, using the antigenic profiling sandwich ELISA. From all data, 30 of the mAbs were selected for use in larger-scale antigenic profiling studies, in which a higher number of virus isolates wereas examined. The conclusive final relationships for the mAbs and the antigenic relationships of the viruses were based on the use of these 30 mAbs and 60 viruses. The data in the dendrograms in **Fig. 18** show the cluster analysis for the mAbs. Ten clusters were selected as being distinct; these are indicated in **Fig. 19** (in which the origin of the mAbs is also indicated). That the mAbs in these clusters reacted with different epitopes was further confirmed through the examination of other available data. In **Fig. 19**, mAb L13 is boxed in because it reacts with a conformational epitope, whereas the other mAbs bind to a linear epitope.

The relationship of the viruses as elucidated from the binding pattern with the mAbs is shown as a dendrogram in **Fig. 20**. The distance at which the viruses within a cluster are assessed as being very similar but different to from another cluster has been put at 5.0.

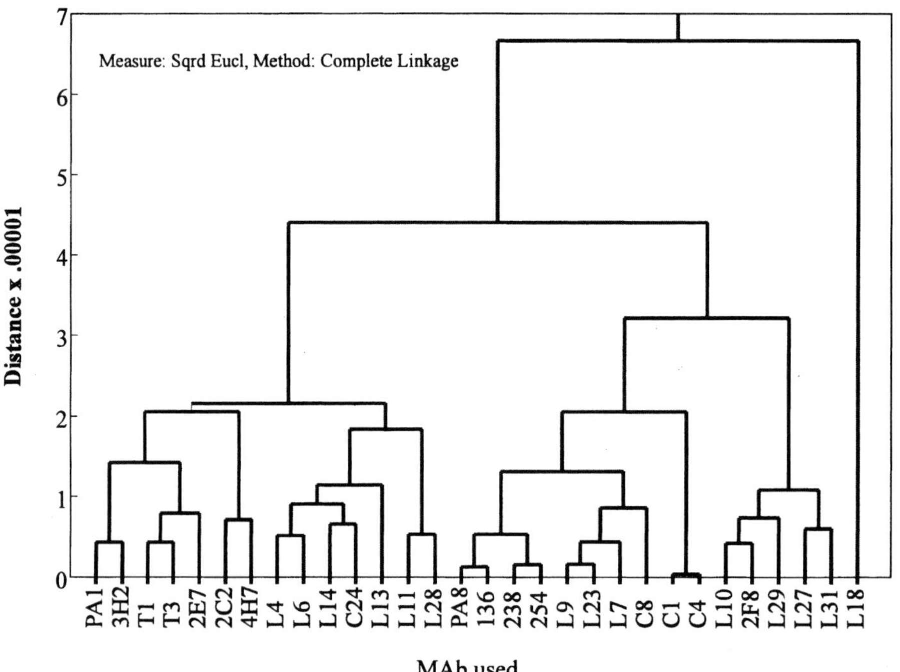

Fig. 18. Grouping of mAbs according to reaction patterns against viruses. Analysis was by multivariate statistics.

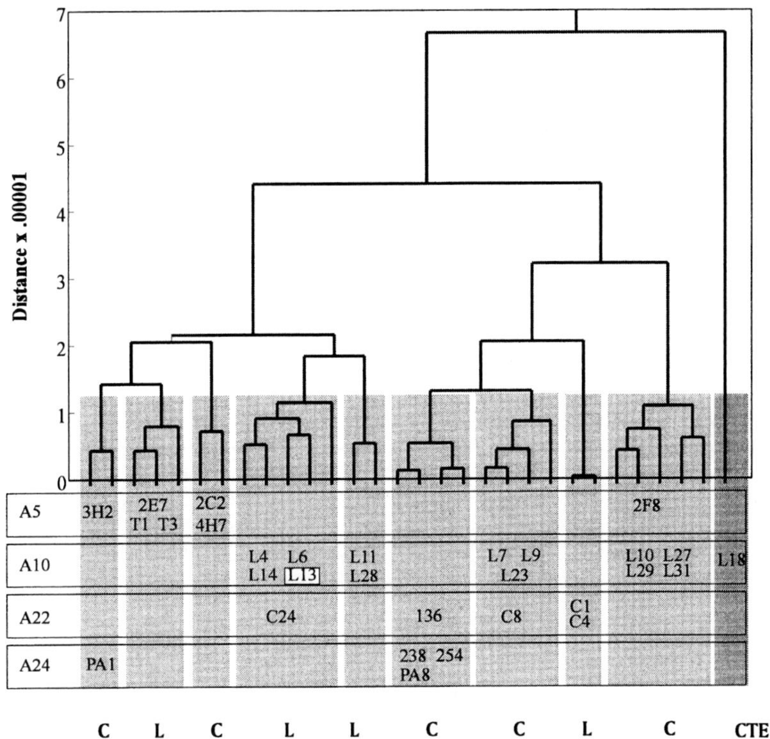

Fig. 19. Grouping of mAbs according to reaction patterns against viruses. Analysis was by multivariate statistics. There was clustering of mAbs with similar reactivities. Data were examined in the light of the origin of mAb and known reactions from other tests. Serotypes used to generate mAbs are shown as A5, A22, A24, and A10. C, mAbs binding to conformation-dependent epitopes; L, mAbs binding to conformation-independent epitopes (*linear*); CTERM, mAbs demonstrated to react with the C-terminus of structural protein VP1.

This is demonstrated by the line drawn across the dendrogram in **Fig. 20**. This value is based on assessing the relevance of the observed clusters to existing epidemiological knowledge of virus isolates. Sixteen clusters are produced, as shown in **Fig. 21**. The virus profiling data showed two major clusters separating A22-like viruses from the A24-like and A5/A10-like viruses;, the latter two clusters were more closely related. The first cluster group indicates closely related South American A24 Cruzerio isolates. The profiling confirms the identity of two vaccine and challenge strains produced after passage in cattle and indicates their similarity to the A24 Cruz reference strain. Viruses from Peru in 1971 and 1972 appear to be similar to each other and to the reference strain. The second cluster within the A24-like viruses comprises two virus isolates from Brazil in 1979 and A24 Venceslau in 1970. Both these clusters have a similar relationship to clusters 3 and 4. These clusters contain South American viruses expected to be A24-like (A Col/Sab/85 and A Col/Boy/89); however, viruses of African origin (A Egypt 1/77, A Cam 5/75, and A Sau 1/76) are also included. Cluster 5 has more similarity to the A5/A10 viruses and again contains both South American (A Bra/68, A27 Col/ 67) and African (A Libya 3/79, A Alg 5/75) viruses. This cluster is similar to clusters 6 and 7, which contain early European (A5 West/51, A Greece 1/76), Middle Eastern (A Sau 23/68) and African (A Ken 1/76) viruses. Cluster 8 is more distinct than clusters 1–7 and comprises the A10 Holl/42, A10 Arg/61 (known to be related), and A5 Spa/73 virus. In turn, this group is strongly related to A5 viruses from Italy and France.

A representative mAb profile from some of the clusters is shown in **Fig. 22a–d**. Such profiles relating to binding of mAbs are typically produced. Their evalua-tion is more difficult. Comparison by eye estimation is not valid; this section has attempted to introduce statistical methods for the easy comparison of data.

11.3.3. Discussion

The method used for the rapid analysis of virus isolates relied on the specificity of mAbs. In this study, a relatively large panel was used, the mAbs of which were prepared against several classical

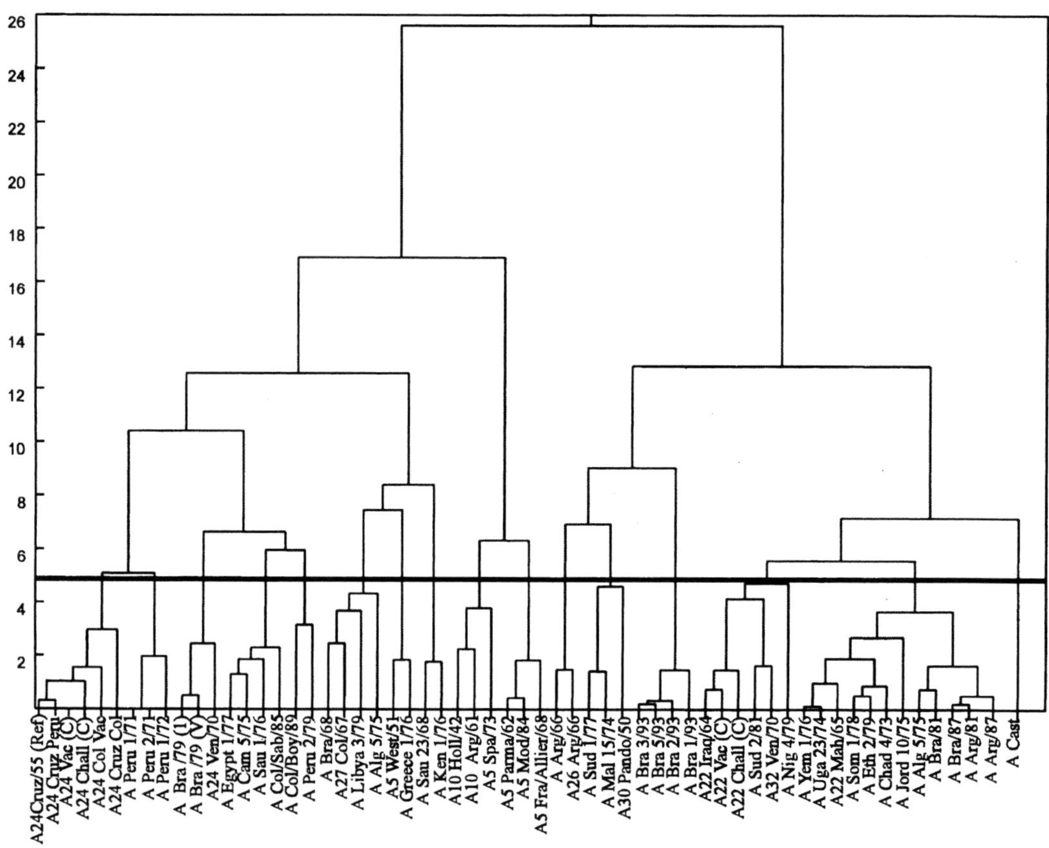

Fig. 20. Grouping of viruses according to the their similarity of their binding profiles with mAbs.

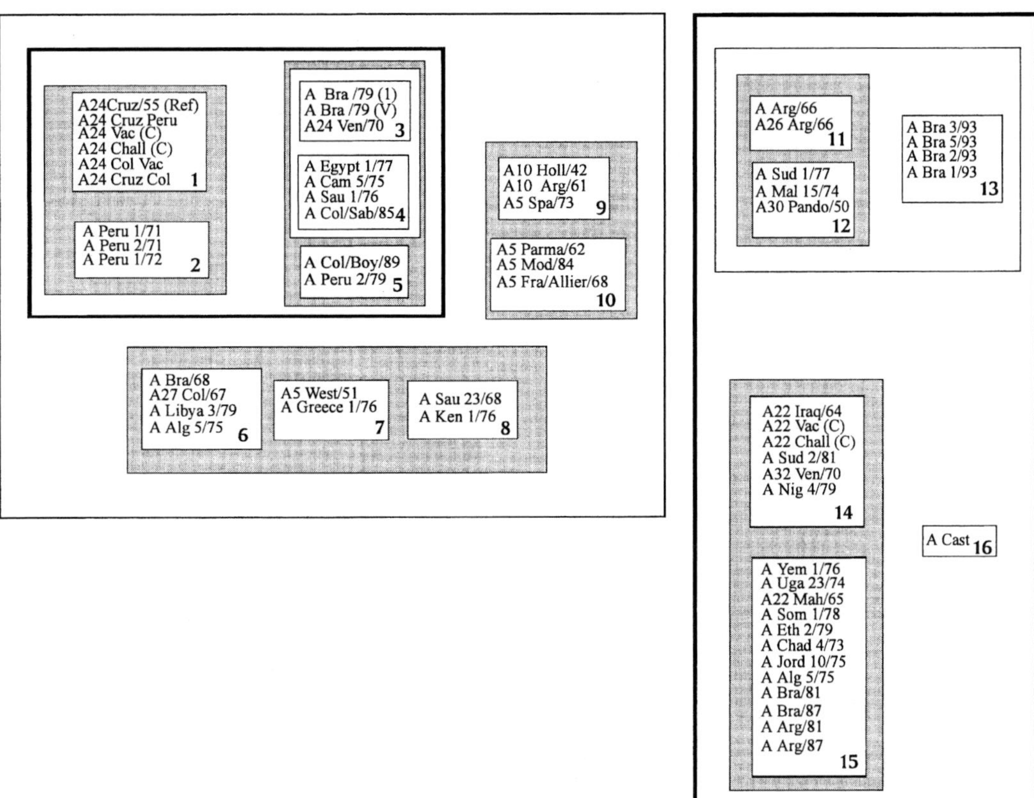

Fig. 21. Virus clusters (1–16) taken from data in Fig. 7.21. The closeness of relationships is indicated by boxes.

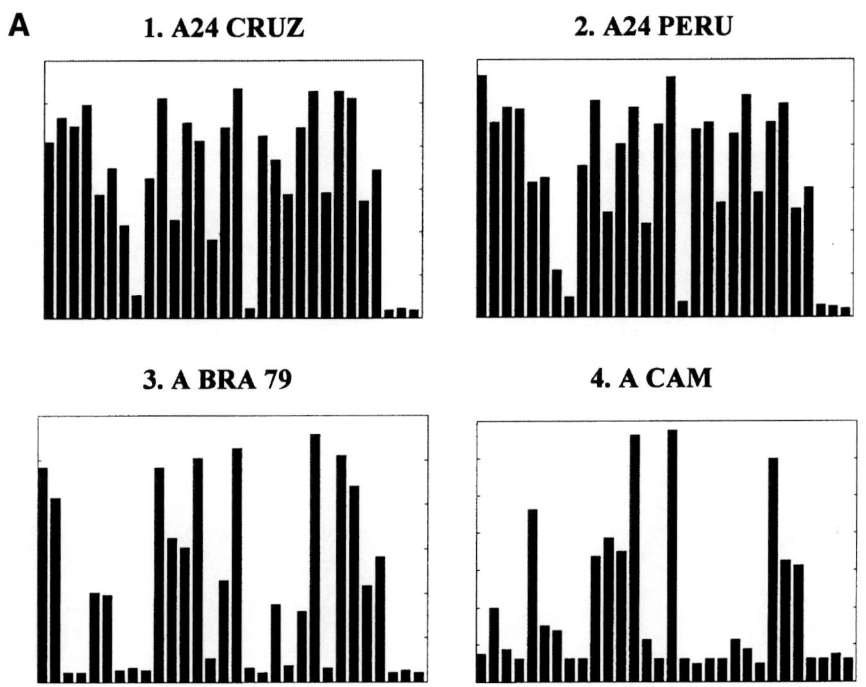

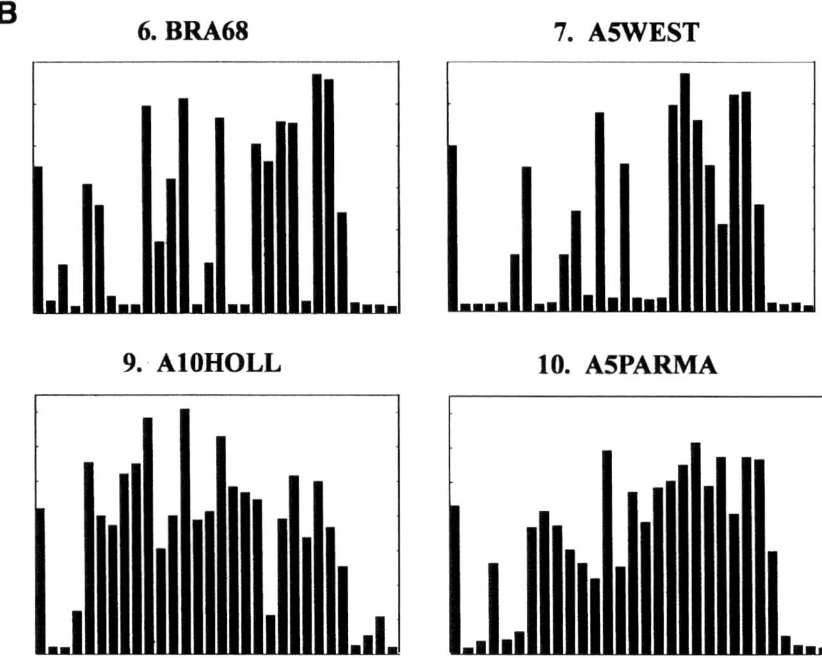
B
6. BRA68
7. A5WEST
9. A10HOLL
10. A5PARMA

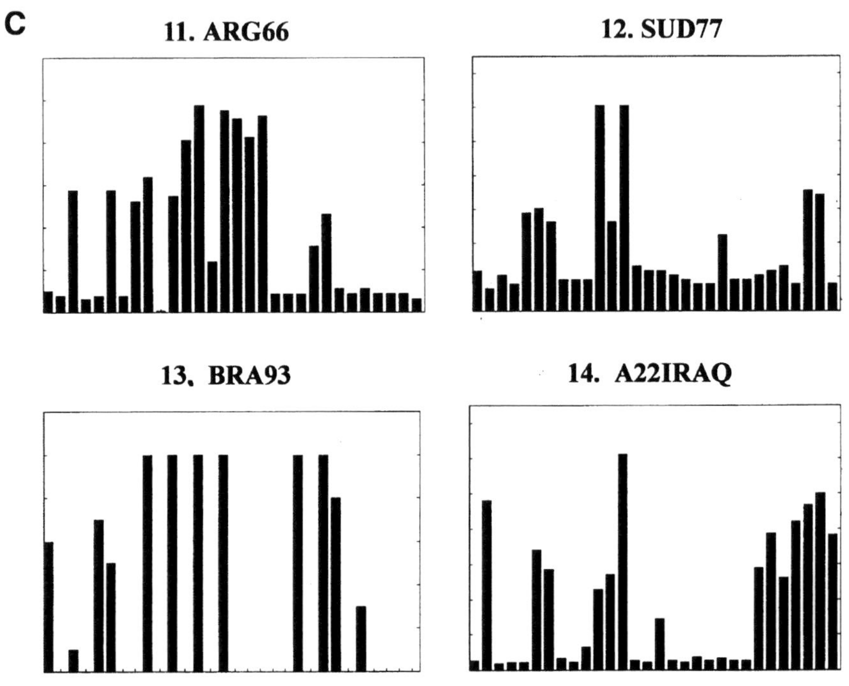
C
11. ARG66
12. SUD77
13. BRA93
14. A22IRAQ

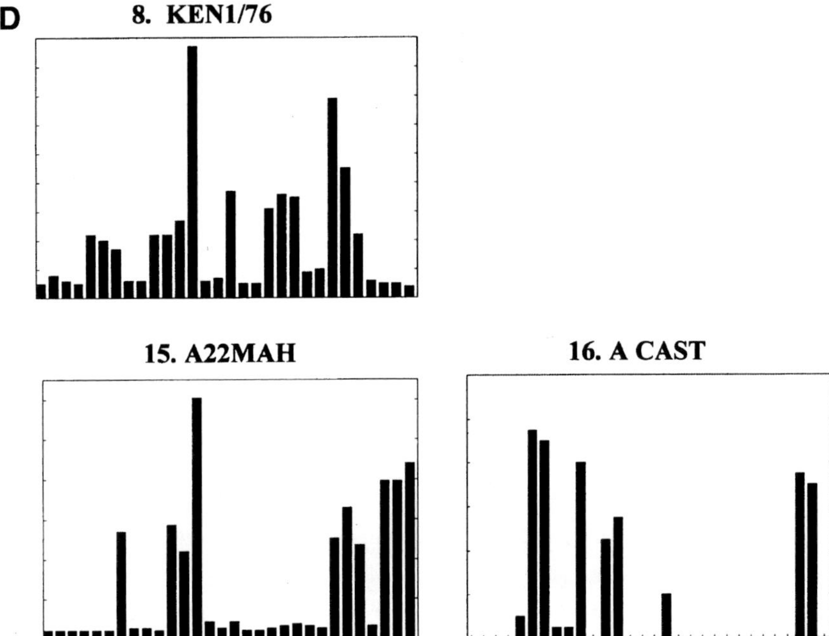

Fig. 22. **(A)** Profiles showing individual mAb reactions with particular viruses. 1–4, members of those cluster groups specified in Fig. 22. **(B)** Profiles showing individual mAb reactions with particular viruses. 6, 7, 9, and 10: members of those cluster groups specified in Fig. 22. **(C)** Profiles showing individual mAb reactions with particular viruses. 11–14: Members of those cluster groups specified in Fig. 22. **(D)** Profiles showing individual mAb reactions with particular viruses. 8, 15, and 16: Members of those cluster groups specified in Fig. 22. Scale (y-axis) is from 0–120% binding with respect to homologous binding of mAb to parental strain.

type A viruses representing epidemiologically important groups. Thus, one aspect of the study allows an examination of the distribution of epitopes identified by the mAbs. The characterization of the specific mAbs in terms of, e.g., reaction with conformational and linear sites, amino acid sequences important to binding, and trypsin sensitivity, allows various antigenic properties to be ascribed to the viruses where binding of antibody is observed. Such properties can be used to directly compare possible biological properties of isolates and thus predict problems in vaccine formulation, identify specific changes to viruses during the manufacture of vaccine and examine viruses and virus proteins produced and expressed using molecular biological techniques. The data collected for the mAbs is included to allow a comprehensive list of properties to be available to other researchers.

The use of a large number of virus isolates also allowed the rapid comparison of all the mAbs. Thus, the variation in antigenic properties of the isolates allowed identification of patterns of reaction of the mAbs, thereby producing groups (clusters) of identically or similarly reactive mAbs and distinguishing them from other clusters. This approach is only possible where a large number of epidemiologically distinct isolates is are available (as is true of the WRL), and a limitation of the variation in antigenic makeup of the isolates would have an effect on the patterns of reaction of the mAbs. Thus, if only two strains were used in this study, it would be likely that only two to three groups of mAbs would be observed. The clusters observed for the mAbs through examination of many isolates are verified with reference to data from this and previous studies on mAb escape mutants as well as reference to the binding characteristics of the mAbs.

This exercise also allows a limited panel to be designated whereby the relationships between isolates can be made with a low number of mAbs, which greatly simplifies assays. Confidence that limited panels reflect true antigenic differences comes only through a thorough examination of mAbs against a large number of viruses. Such an approach is also quite useful to workers in laboratories without access to a large number of isolates because the mAbs they produced can be compared to others by standardization laboratories. The mAbs can be identified as fitting into particular clusters (already defined), and properties common to those clusters can be ascribed.

The method used to examine the virus/mAb binding used mAb in excess (i.e., at a high concentration). This can have a distinct effect on the binding profiles observed. The relative affinity of each of the mAbs depends on the exact differences between the epitopes presented on the heterologous viruses as compared to the homologous virus. The assay used is essentially a binding assay, and small differences in affinity constants among isolates are not reflected by differences in binding in which there is a large excess of antibody molecules. Thus, any differences noted in this study reflect relatively large differences in affinity (a significant difference in epitope). Such differences also fit in with the examination of the virus-neutralizing capacity of the mAb for homologous and heterologous viruses. Not all mAbs that bind 100% to heterologous isolates will neutralize that virus (results not shown). This is a result of the differences in the conditions in the virus neutralization test (VNT). In the VNT, the amount of virus used represents about 100 TCID50 (~10^5 virus particles assuming 1 TCID50 is equivalent to 10^3 noninfectious particles). In the ELISA, ~0.05 μg is present to bind with mAb (~8×10^9 virus particles). The same concentration of mAb is used in both assays; thus, by the Law of Mass Action, the ELISA tends to effect reaction owing to the high concentration of virus (~× 80,000 times that in the VNT). Therefore, mAbs with reduced affinity tend to have the reaction driven in the ELISA but not in the VNT.

Differences in affinity for strongly binding mAbs can be assessed easily using competitive assays in which a homologous system involving pretitrated virus and homologous mAb (submaximal binding concentration) is challenged by the addition of heterologous virus. Here, the relationship of competition slopes comparing homologous and heterologous viruses reflects the relative affinity of the mAb for the two isolates (data not shown).

12. Conclusion

Figure 23 shows the features of mAbs relevant to the ELISA. Although the mAb is, by definition, a specific reagent with respect to the binding to epitopes, the physical state of the mAb, its density, and the distribution of epitopes all affect assay performance.

Let us review the diagrams in **Fig. 23**:

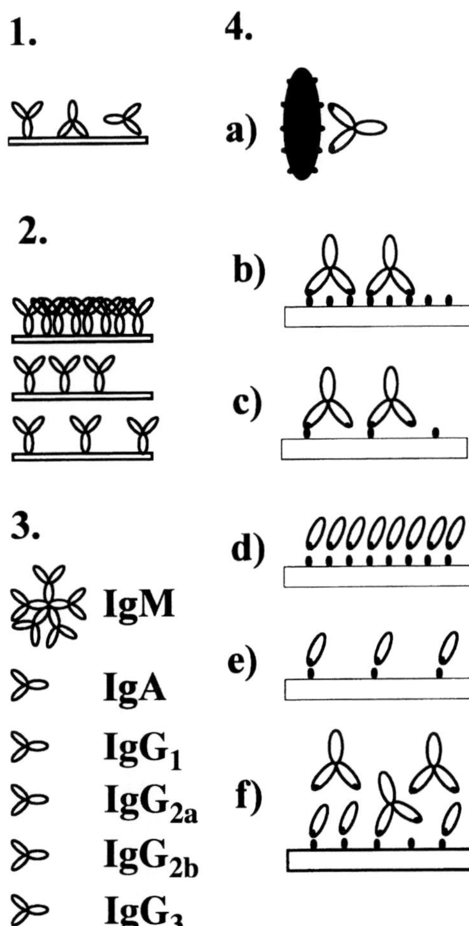

Fig. 23. Properties of mAbs relevant to performance of ELISA. (1), The orientation of molecules affects capture properties; **(2)**, density of molecules affects performance through interference. The correct spacing of mAbs also is important with reference to epitope spacing and density; **(3)**, the isotype of mAbs can be important; **(4a)**, optimal binding of bivalent mAb needs spacing of epitopes on multivalent antigen target; **(4b)**, spacing of small molecules is important to maximal bivalent binding; **(4c)**, where the distance between FAB fragments is too large, only monovalent binding takes place; **(4d–4e)**, Fab fragments are free to bind and the reaction is limited only by concentration of epitopes; **(4f)**, the most common mixture of bivalent and Fab molecules used in assays

1. Diagram 1: This indicates that the orientation of the mAb on the plastic surface can affect subsequent binding to antigens (e.g., in capture ELISA). Since As the mAb is a single population of molecules with identical chemical structure, any tendency for such orientations (depending on the exact nature of plastics used and the solutions used to bind the mAb), will be translated to all molecules. This means that a variety of plates and solutions of different ionic strengths and pHs can be used in cases in which an mAb apparently does not perform well as a capture reagent.
2. Diagram 2: This indicates that the density of mAb can affect binding, even when the orientation is correct and Fab molecules are present. Full-dilution ranges of mAbs should be performed to allow an assessment of binding properties, since as it is possible that lower concentrations of mAb are better spaced to allow capture. This is also dependent on the nature of the antigen.
3. Diagram 3: This reminds us that the isotype of an mAb can be important. Generally, IgM molecules are poor capture reagents. The use of mAbs of different isotypes can be exploited through the use of specific anti-mouse isotype reagents.
4. Diagram 4a: When bivalent molecules of mAb are reacting with epitopes on a complex, the spacing of the epitopes has a profound effect on the actual affinity of the mAb. When epitopes are spaced too far to allow bivalent binding, effectively a single Fab interaction takes place. The orientation of the epitopes is also important.
5. Diagram 4b: When small molecules (e.g., polypeptides) are coated, mAb may also have optimal bivalent binding in which the spacing (and presentation/orien-tation) is optimal.
6. Diagram 4c: Here, the spacing is too large to allow bivalent binding and hence the effective affinity is reduced as compared to diagram 4a.
7. Diagram 4d: The deliberate processing of mAbs to Fab fragments affects the affinity. Here, the spacing of the molecules is not as important as in diagrams 4a and 4b, since as the Fab fragments are free to interact in solution.
8. Diagram 4f: This probably reflects the most common situation in which mAbs are used as a relatively impurified unpurified mixture of bivalent and monovalent molecules. Here, the binding of Fab fragments and bivalent molecules can be regarded as competitive. Assays developed with such reagents may suffer asince the distribution of Fab to bivalent molecules is different from batch to batch and owing to physical changes on storage. When a purified product is used, the results may be different. This is also relevant when considering mAbs as capture reagents (as in diagram 1).

References

1. Grandic, P. (1994) Monoclonal antibody purification guide Part 3. . *Am. Biotechnol. Lab.* 12(8), 16, 18.
2. Butcher, R. N., Obi, T. U., and McCullough, K. C. (1991) Rapid isolation of monoclonal hybridoma cultures by a fusion-cloning method: the requirement for aminopterin. *Biologicals* 19, 171–175.
3. McCullough, K. C., Crowther, J. R., Butcher, R. N., Carpenter, W. C., Brocchi, E., Capucci, L., and De Simone, F. (1986) Immune protection against foot-and-mouth disease virus studied using virus neutralising and nonneutralising concentrations of monoclonal antibodies. *Immunology* 58, 421–429.
4. McCahon, D., Crowther, J. R., Belsham, G. J., Kitson, J. D. A., Duchesne, M., Have, P., Meleon, R. H., Morgan, D. O., and De Simone, F. (1989) Evidence for at least four antigenic sites on type O foot-and-mouth disease virus involved in neutralisation: identification by single and multiple site monoclonal antibody resistant mutants. *J. Gen. Virol.* 70, 639–664.
5. McCullough, K. C., Crowther, J. R., Carpenter, W. C., Brocchi, E., Capucci, L., De Simone, F., Xie, Q., and McCahon, D. (1987) Epitopes on foot-and-mouth disease virus particles. I. Topology. *Virology* 157, 516–525.
6. Nakane, P. K. and Kawaoi, A. (1974) Peroxidase-labelled antibody: a new method of conjugation. *J. Histochem. Cytochem.* 22, 1084–1091.
7. Samuels, A. R., Knowles, N. J., Samuel, G. D., and Crowther, J. R. (1991) Evaluation of a trapping ELISA for the differentiation of foot-and-mouth disease virus strains using monoclonal antibodies. *Biologicals* 19, 229–310.

Chapter 8

Validation of Diagnostic Tests for Infectious Diseases

1. Validation

Validation involves all processes that determine the performance of an assay to achieve a defined set of objectives. Only when the actual data have been obtained can test parameters be assessed and confidence in results be assigned in a statistical sense. Validation is a continuous process, in which increasing knowledge about an assay is gained each time it is run. The continuous process also involves data obtained when the test is performed in hitherto untried scenarios. Because most assays begin in the research arena, the use of validated assays in the form of kits by a large number of scientists, varying widely in expertise, equipment, and climatic conditions can cause problems. The objective in validation is to be able to define an assay in terms of statistically quantifiable parameters with measured confidence. The designation of "validated assay" is only merited when it has been defined in terms of its capacity to classify samples with regard to the presence or absence of a particular analyte. Validation relies on the examination of as many factors as possible. At any stage, quantifiable parameters must be defined, describing the test and mechanisms to reevaluate and be put into place.

A validated assay, therefore, depends on the characteristics of the assay design that ensure the results. This leads to a robust assay (not easily affected by physical factors, operators, or geographical location where used or where samples came from). Such assays generate data that can be compared directly, irrespective of which laboratory uses it, and to what population of animals it is applied.

John R. Crowther, *Methods in Molecular Biology, The ELISA Guidebook, Vol. 516*

DOI: 10.1007/978-1-60327-254-4_8

In the context of the ELISA, the development and validation of an assay is usually made using a limited number of tests, on samples from a selected group(s) of animals or patients, and made over a short time frame. The data defines the performance of the assay, and the characteristics of these performances are published, and possibly certified by governing authorities. In this case, what constitutes a validated assay obviously depends directly on the experiences limited to the samples analyzed. The conditions established during this validation phase can also be modified based on experience with the assay's capacity to correctly classify the infection status of animals from various populations over a longer time period. Such a situation is unavoidable as a single laboratory cannot have access to all samples at all times. However, the validation methods followed must be clearly described so that at least variations from the accepted criteria can be determined and possibly accounted for.

1.1. Definition of a Validated Assay

The concept of a validated assay has many shades of meaning among laboratory diagnosticians and veterinary clinicians. For this chapter, a validated assay is described in terms of its use as an assay that provides results that consistently identify animals as being positive or negative for the presence of a specific analyte (antibody or antigen), and by inference, accurately predict the infection status of animals with a known (measurable) degree of statistical certainty. The principles underlying the development and maintenance of such validated assays are examined here.

1.2. Components of Assay Validation

The development and validation of an assay is a multicomponent operation consisting of at least three general areas:

1. Feasibility of the method including choice and optimization of reagents and protocols.
2. Determination of the assay's performance characteristics.
3. Continuous monitoring of assay performance during routine use.

The third component may not be immediately considered as part of assay validation, but it is included because a test can be considered valid only when the data is generated and their interpretations are, respectively, accurate and meaningful and updated. The development of an indirect ELISA for antibody detection can be used to illustrate points 1–3. This is a test format that can be difficult to validate as there is signal amplification owing to both specific and nonspecific components.

1.3. Feasibility Studies

In our ELISA example, feasibility studies are first made to examine whether the selected reagents have the capacity to distinguish between a range of antibody concentrations and the infectious agent in question, while providing minimal background activity.

This can be a rapid process (a few weeks) and uses a minimum of samples. It establishes whether the test is feasible for further examination.

1.3.1. Samples for Feasibility Studies: Serum Controls (Standards)

Developments in ELISA rely on the availability of some reagents of relevance to the problem at hand. Thus, other tests can provide information, e.g., about antibodies measured in a serum, which allows them to be used in ELISA development. In the case of the indirect assay, we are trying to estimate antibodies against a specific agent through their binding to that agent (on a plate), and subsequent detection with an anti-species conjugate. We are also trying to produce an assay that can differentiate between samples containing (positive) and not containing (negative) antibodies.

The availability and selection of four or five samples (positive sera in our example) that range from high to low levels of antibodies against the infection/infectious agent in question is quick and useful. The availability of such samples relies on a continuity of work at a given institution or their preparation in animals with specific disease agents. In addition, a sample(s) containing no antibody is required. Such control positive and negative samples should be taken, wherever possible, from known infected or uninfected samples from a representative population of animals for which the eventually validated assay will be applied (target population). Preferably, the samples should have given expected results in one or more serological techniques other than the one being validated. These same samples are used to optimize reagents throughout the feasibility studies. The samples are preferably taken from individual animals but they may represent pools of samples from several animals. A good practice is to prepare or obtain a significant volume (e.g., 10 mL) of each sample and divide it into 0.1-mL vol, to be stored at –20°C. One volume of each is thawed, used for experiments, and stored at 4°C between experiments until depleted. Then, another aliquot may be thawed for further experimentation.

This procedure aims to provide the same sample source of sera, in which the same number of freeze/thaw cycles is maintained for all experiments. This precaution is a strong element in reducing any variation that may be introduced, since freeze thawing can denature protein and hence antibodies. Excess shaking of samples is also to be avoided as the shearing action in vigorous mixing also denatures protein. Shaking also causes frothing (excess bubbles), which produces partitions of proteins so that the antibody may be enriched in the bubbles (hence, depleted in the main volume of liquid).

Care is necessary to ensure that samples taken from the freezer are mixed thoroughly, because freezing causes the protein content of the serum to separate at the bottom of the tubes. Basically, samples (including test samples) should be treated gently.

Note that the qualitative nature of antibodies making up a serum may be altered greatly even though the quantity of antibody measured appears, by some tests, to stay the same. As an example, shaking may destroy a high-affinity IgM population of a serum, allowing a more stable but lower-affinity IgG population to react with a target antigen. The net result (titer) may not alter in a specific assay, but the overall avidity of the serum may.

Conversely, other test systems may detect the drop in IgM, or increase in IgG, and hence show great alterations in respective titers. Note also that the problems with physical handling are more acutely important when levels of antibodies are low since there is a low level of positive antibody (protein), and small amounts of denaturation can turn a weak positive control into a negative one.

The approach of using the same sera has the added advantage of generating a data trail for the repeatedly-run samples. After the assay is validated, one or more of the samples can become the serum control(s) that may be the basis for data expression and repeatability assessments both within and between runs. They may also serve as serum standards if their activity has been predetermined by other accepted methods; such standards provide assurance that runs of the assay are producing accurate data.

1.3.2. Expression of Data

The method use to normalize and express data should be decided preferably no later than at the end of the feasibility studies. Comparisons of results from day to day and among laboratories are most accurate when done using normalized data. For example, in ELISA systems, optical density (OD) values are absolute measurements that are influenced by ambient temperatures, test parameters, and photometric instrumentation. Therefore, results need to be calculated and expressed as a function of the reactivity of one or more serum control samples that are included in each run of the assay.

Classically, normalization of data is accomplished in indirect ELISA by expressing OD values in one of the several ways – e.g., by expressing the OD values as a percentage of a single high-positive serum control that is included on each plate. This method is adequate for most applications.

More rigor can be brought to the normalization procedure by calculating results from a standard curve generated by several serum standards. This requires a more sophisticated algorithm such as linear regression or log-logit analysis to calculate the normalized value for each test sample. These approaches are more satisfactory because they do not rely on only one high-positive control sample for data normalization, but, rather, utilize several serum controls to plot a standard curve from which the sample value is extrapolated. This allows for some experimental error correction; for example, if one of the control samples was omitted or gave a high variation from the expected value, then the test may be accepted provided the other controls were acceptable.

Whatever the type of assay, it is essential to include additional controls for any reagent that may introduce variability and thus undermine attempts to achieve a validated assay.

1.3.3. Repeatability: Preliminary Estimates

Evidence that an assay is repeatable is necessary for further development. This is accomplished by calculating the intra- and inter-plate variation using the same samples run in different plates and on different days (and with different operators). Ideally, such tests should be run on at least 10 plates on 10 separate occasions. Coefficients (CVs) of variation (standard deviation [SD] of replicates, of mean of replicates, of equal to or less than 15% for the raw OD values indicate adequate repeatability at this stage of assay development. Such data obtained on a number of different plates and days also allows confidence limits to be ascribed to the variation observed (comparison of different means with their respective variations). However, if there is evidence of excessive variation (>20%) within and/or between runs of the assay, more preliminary studies should be made. This either will confirm that stabilization of the assay is possible or will determine ultimately whether the test format should be abandoned. This is extremely important because an assay that is inherently variable has a high probability of not withstanding the rigors of day-to-day testing on samples from the targeted population of animals.

1.3.4. Choice of Optimal Assay Parameters

Optimal concentrations/dilutions of the antigen adsorbed to the plate, serum, enzyme-antibody conjugate, and substrate solution are determined through chessboard titrations (CBTs) of each reagent against all other reagents after confirming the best choice of reaction vessels (usually evaluation of two or three types of microtiter plates, each of which has different binding characteristics).

Additional experiments determine the optimal temporal, chemical, and physical variables in the protocol, including incubation temperatures and durations; the type, pH, and molarity of diluent, washing, and blocking buffers; and equipment used in each step of the assay (e.g., pipettors and washers that give the best reproducibility). There are numerous publications detailing the reagents and protocols available for assay development. Often these, publications give examples of assays dealing with similar antigens and species of sera being examined.

1.3.5. Analytical Sensitivity and Specificity

Experiments to establish the analytical sensitivity of the assay (the smallest detectable amount of the analyte in question) and the analytical specificity (the degree to which the test does not cross-react with analytes associated with other infections) are needed. Note that sensitivity and specificity here are not strictly the same as when being considered in a purely immunological way, but are an attempt to quantify the "detection" level of any assay (sensitivity) that is affected by unwanted crossreactivity (specificity considerations).

Analytical sensitivity can be assessed by end point dilution analysis, which measures the dilution of serum at which point antibodies are no longer detectable. Analytical specificity is best assessed by examining test performances using a panel of sera derived from animals that have experienced related infections that may stimulate the crossreactive antibody. If, e.g., the assay does not detect the antibody in limiting dilutions of serum with the same efficiency as other assays, or crossreactivity is common when sera from animals with closely related infections are tested, the reagents need to be recalibrated or replaced, or the assay abandoned.

1.4. Determining Assay Performance Characteristics

When feasibility studies indicate that an assay has potential for field application, the next step is to characterize the assay's performance characteristics. Estimates are needed of diagnostic sensitivity (D-SN) and diagnostic specificity (D-SP).

D-SN is the proportion of known infected reference animals that test positive in the assay; infected animals that test negative are deemed false negative results. D-SP is the proportion of uninfected reference animals that test negative in the assay; uninfected animals that test positive are deemed false positive results. The number and source of reference samples used to derive D-SN and D-SP are thus of paramount importance if the assay is ever to be properly validated for use in the general population of animals targeted by that assay.

These are primary parameters obtained during validation of an assay. They are the basis for calculation of other parameters from which inferences are made about test results. It is important that estimates of D-SN and D-SP are as accurate as possible. Ideally, they are derived from testing a series of reference samples from reference animals of known infection status, relative to the disease or infection in question.

1.4.1. Intended Use of the Assay

It must be determined how many reference samples should be tested to achieve statistically significant estimates of D-SN and D-SP with an acceptable error. This depends on the intended use of the assay. When a screening test is needed for application to a highly pathogenic disease, the threshold that separates seropositive from seronegative animals can be set at a low level, so that it is unlikely that any infected animals will be misclassified as uninfected. However, a consequence of the low threshold is that uninfected animals showing nonspecific activity will be misclassified as infected. This will directly contribute to a lowering of assay specificity.

Alternatively, if the test is for a highly endemic but less pathogenic disease, generally the threshold can be set relatively high because it is important that the test not classify an animal as infected when in fact it is uninfected. Because of its high specificity, such a test is often used as a confirmatory test. Having determined whether high sensitivity or high specificity is the primary requirement for the assay, it is theoretically possible to calculate the number of samples required to establish valid estimates of D-SN and D-SP.

8.Serum Panel Required for Calculations of D-SN and D-SP

The optimal way to determine D-SN and D-SP of any assay is to test a large panel of reference sera that represents two groups of animals. One group should be proved to be infected with the agent in question. The second group should be known to be free of infection. In theory, the number of infected animals tested to achieve the desired diagnostic sensitivity of the test (± allowable error) can be approximated by the following formula:

$$n=\{[4 \times ds \times (1 - ds)]/e2\}$$

in which n = the number of animals that need to be tested in the new assay; ds = the diagnostic sensitivity that is sought (i.e., the expected proportion of infected animals that will test positive); and e = the amount of error allowed in the estimate of diagnostic sensitivity.

For instance, if a 95% diagnostic sensitivity is desired with ±5% error allowed in that estimate, the theoretical number of animals that is needed in the test validation = $\{[4 \times 0.95 \times (1–0.95)]/0.052\}$, which is 76 infected animals. If one wishes to increase the diagnostic sensitivity to 99% ± 2%, then the theoretical number of animals required is only 99.

These estimates of sample size may be misleading because they assume that the reference animals represent the same and a normal frequency distribution in the total population. This is unlikely as the latter population is influenced by many unquantifiable biological and environmental variables. Factors such as breed, age, sex, stage of infection, differing responses of individuals to infectious agents, differing host responses in chronic versus peracute infections, and the effect of diet and environment are but a few examples. All may have an impact on antibody production. Additionally, an antibody to closely related infectious agents may cause crossreactions in the assay, and if this combination of agents is found only in one portion of the total population targeted by the assay, but is not represented in the panel of reference sera, then obviously the estimates of D-SN and D-SP derived from the reference panel will be wrong. It is therefore impossible to represent fully all variables found in a target population of, say, 25 million animals, using a sample of 100 animals.

The way to reduce the error in any statistical estimate is to increase the sample size (the larger the sample size, the more confident one can be about the estimate of the population). The experience of people validating assays indicates that it is necessary to evaluate sera from several hundred known infected animals to account for many of the variables in a large population. As the number of variables is indeterminate, we recommend that at least 500–1,000 samples be selected randomly from throughout the target population in which the assay will eventually be used. Such an exercise serves to define a population and may be further refined if distinct environmental regions can be regarded as having similarly influenced animals. In this way defined populations can be compared as to their distribution statistics. The extension of assays through active use in the evaluation of different populations and comparative testing against other methods also serves to allow a reestimation of the sensitivity and specificity of ELISAs.

The calculated number of uninfected reference animals required to establish diagnostic specificity of the assay is even greater. To validate an antibody detection test that will be 99% specific (only one false positive per 100 uninfected animals), an extremely large population of uninfected animals must be tested, representing as many biological and environmental variables as possible. This will allow an estimate of confidence in the test specificity. Again, the assumptions in the statistical calculations are a major concern; therefore, one should think in terms of at least 1,000, and preferably upward of 5,000 samples from animals that are known to be uninfected and not vaccinated with the agent in question, to establish a reasonable estimate of specificity.

1.4.3. The Gold Standard for Classifying Animals as Uninfected

The term *gold standard* refers to the method or composite of methods giving results that are regarded as unequivocally classifying animals as infected or not infected. The results obtained from the new method are compared to those obtained using the gold standard during the validation process. In statistical terms, the gold standard results are regarded as the independent variable whereas the result from the new assay is the dependent variable. The results of the new assay are deemed correct or incorrect relative to the gold standard.

Classifying a population of animals as unequivocally uninfected with the agent in question using culture or isolation techniques or serology is not possible. One cannot rule out the possibility of false negative results, but it is possible to combine several sources of information to determine the probability that reference animals have never experienced an infection with the agent.

Accordingly, reference animals selected to represent the uninfected group in the assessment of assay specificity need to be selected as follows:

1. From geographical areas where the disease has not been endemic for at least 3 years.
2. From herds from those areas that have not had clinical signs of the disease during the past 3 years, nor herds that have been vaccinated against the agent in question.
3. From herds that are closed to importation of animals from endemic areas and do not have infected neighboring herds.
4. From areas where there is no evidence of antibody to the agent in question based on repeated testing over the past 2–3 years.

If all of these criteria are met, one can be reasonably certain that these animals have not been in contact with the agent in question. Sera from such animals could then be used as the reference sera for the uninfected reference animal group.

1.4.4. Gold Standard for Classifying Animals as Infected

Several standards have been described that can be used with varying success to characterize the animals that serve as a source of reference sera:

1. Verification of infection: an absolute gold standard. The only true gold standard for classifying an animal as infected is the isolation of infectious agents or unequivocal histopathological criteria. Sera from such animals are used to establish analytical and diagnostic sensitivity of a new assay designed to detect antibody to that agent.
2. Comparative serology: a relative standard of comparison. It may be impractical, technically difficult, or impossible to obtain definitive proof of infection via culture or isolation techniques. In the absence of such a gold standard, less exacting methods must serve as the standard of comparison with the new assay. If the other tests have already established assay performance characteristics (e.g., the Rose Bengal screening test followed by the complement fixation confirmatory test for detection of antibody to *Brucella bovis*), their results taken together provide a useful composite-based standard by which the new assay may be compared.

When the new test is evaluated by comparison with another serological test or combination of tests, the estimates of D-SN and D-SP for the new test are called *relative diagnostic sensitivity* and *relative diagnostic specificity*. These standards of comparison, however, have their own established levels of false positivity and false negativity that are sources of error carried over into the new assay. Therefore, the relative D-SN and D-SP for the new test will be underestimated. It follows that the greater the amount of false positivity and false negativity in the test that is used as the standard of comparison, the more the new assay's performance characteristics will be undermined. In other words, care must be taken when the "new" test in fact shows a better diagnostic capability than those previously accepted.

1.4.5. Experimental Infection or Vaccination: an Adjunct Standard of Comparison

Another standard for assessment of antibody response is sera taken sequentially, over several months, from experimentally infected or vaccinated animals. The strength of this standard is that it measures the ability of the assay to detect early antibody production and to follow the kinetics of antibody production to the agent in question. This also can be relative to preintervention treatment through the taking of samples before treatment. If it is evident that animals become infected, shed organisms in low numbers, but have no detectable antibody during the first 2–3 months using the new assay, the analytical sensitivity of the assay may be inadequate, and estimates of diagnostic sensitivity will be low. Alternatively, if the antibody appears quickly after inoculation of the infectious agent, and earlier than in the conventional assays used as standards of comparison, the new assay may have greater analytical sensitivity (and associated increased diagnostic sensitivity) than the conventional assay.

The interpretation of experimentally derived infected/vaccinated antibody response must be done carefully. The particular strain of organism, route of exposure, and dose are just a few variables that may stimulate an antibody response that is quantitatively and qualitatively atypical of natural infection in the target population. The same is true of vaccination. Therefore, it is essential that experimentally induced antibody responses are relevant to those occurring in natural outbreaks of the disease caused by the same infectious agent, otherwise the estimates of relative D-SN and D-SP may be in error. Because of the difficulty of equivalence in the responses of naturally infected and experimentally infected/vaccinated animals, the relative D-SN and D-SP data derived from such animals should be considered as an adjunct criterion and should not be used alone to determine a new assay's relative D-SN and D-SP.

1.5. Random Testing of Samples from a Population Endemic for Disease: No Standard of Comparison

Validation of assays can be made in the absence of a standard. The validation then relies on statistical tools such as cluster or mixture analysis. Assuming that a few sera of known status are available to establish the feasibility of the assay system, it is possible to obtain a rough estimate of the assay's performance characteristics. Then, several thousands of animals in the target population can be tested in the absence of known infection status data other than possibly scattered clinical observations. If a clear bimodal frequency distribution becomes evident with a large peak consisting of many animals at the low end of the antibody scale, and a second peak extended over a wide range of higher antibody responses, it may be possible to estimate a cutoff in antibody response that separates presumed uninfected from presumed infected animals. Since in this scheme there is no proof of the infection status of the animals, this approach should be done as a last resort with later confirmation after definitive standard(s) of comparison become available. This process also is inherent in the cumulative analysis of data from the field on the continuous use of a kit.

1.6. Repeatability and Reproducibility: Calculations

During feasibility studies, preliminary estimates of repeatability should be obtained. Selected sera from a bank of reference sera used to determine the assay's D-SN and D-SP can be tested using a series of runs of the assay within the same laboratory. It is useful to have several operators of the assay system do this exercise independently. This will provide an indication of assay repeatability that addresses the robustness of the assay.

Similarly, reproducibility of the assay (agreement among results of samples tested in different laboratories) needs to be established by testing the same sera in several other laboratories. The evaluation of both repeatability and reproducibility should be made on normalized data. For repeatability data, CVs for replicates should not exceed 10%, and regression analysis of normalized reproducibility data among laboratories generally should not give significant differences at the 95% confidence level.

1.7. Selection of the Positive/Negative Threshold (Cutoff)

After all the reference sera are tested, frequency distributions of results from infected and uninfected populations can be established. Both distributions are plotted on the same graph with the vertical axis representing the number of animals having test results that fall within each of 20 or so intervals of result values plotted on the horizontal axis.

For instance, when the data are expressed as a percentage of the value for the high-positive control sample (PP), 20 intervals of five units each (0–4%, 5–9%, 10–14%, and so on) could represent the horizontal axis. There is usually an overlap in these frequency distributions. The selection of a cutoff value for the new test will fall somewhere within this overlapping region.

The extent of the overlap may vary considerably from one assay to another. If only a small percentage (e.g., 2%) of the results from infected and uninfected animals are overlapping, and the cutoff selected is at the midpoint of the overlapping region, then the D-SN and the D-SP will both be 99%.

Alternatively, if the overlap involves a greater percentage of animals (e.g., 10%), then the cutoff chosen may be shifted to the left to minimize the false negative results (favoring greater D-SN), or to the right to minimize the false positive results (favoring greater D-SP), depending on the intended application of the assay. Once selected, the cutoff will determine the D-SN and D-SP, which, in turn, are the bases for calculating predictive values for positive and negative test results.

1.7.1. Details

When giving further consideration to cutoff values one needs to recognize that there is invariably an overlap (as already stated) between populations containing negative and positive test results. Thus, the estimation of a perfect discriminatory cutoff is not possible. **Figure 1** presents a hypothetical (but typical) overlap of positive and negative distributions of ELISA. The cutoff value is the point set on the test scale that determines whether the response is positive or negative. The observed overlap reduces confidence in such statements for certain samples. The importance of false negative or false positive results depends on the required levels of diagnostic sensitivity against specificity. As already indicated, setting a cutoff of two or three times the SD of the negative control group is the accepted practice. This assumes that there is a normal distribution statistic in both types of population and that a representative sampling procedure for the whole population is being measured. The rationale here is that ~95% of normally distributed observations are expected to fall within a range of mean 2 × SD, and would test negative. However, as already indicated, the normal distribution is not always realized, and the distribution of positives (particularly) is neglected. This may be, and often is, biased. The major flaw in this method is that it deals with the specificity of the assay results but not the sensitivity.

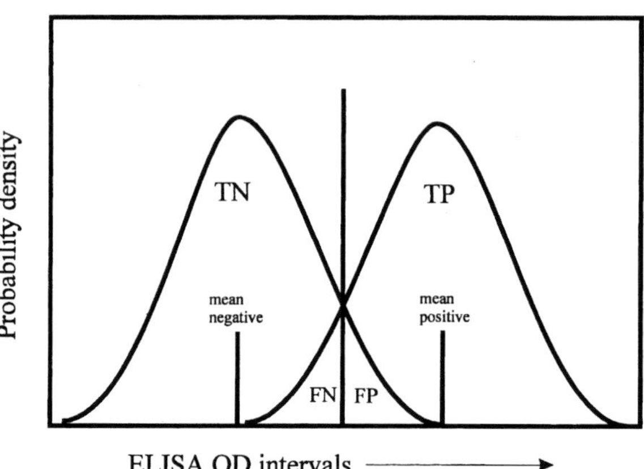

Fig. 1. Hypothetical distribution density of ELISA results of populations of noninfected (*left-hand curve*) and infected (*right-hand curve*) individuals. The FN and FP area is referred to as "*gray area*," and results falling here must be regarded as suspect. The importance of retesting depends on how important the result is to classification of the test unit. The setting up of cutoff values depends on knowledge of such overlaps and the variability of the test used. FN, False negative; FP, false positive; TN, true negative; TP, true positive.

The value can be regarded as a good reference value. The continuous validation of assays, with reference to evaluating a wider number of epidemiological niches using the same reagents, often modifies the cutoff value using this criterion. The relationship between sensitivity and specificity cannot be forgotten in any consideration. Raising the cutoff value increases specificity, and reducing it increases diagnostic sensitivity (reduces specificity). Whether this matters, depends on the problem being tackled, and the types of results that can be accepted. For example, false positive results may be unacceptable. This is true in, say, the diagnosis of AIDS. However, it is important that none should be missed either. False negative results may be acceptable in cases in which another test can be used in parallel. The first screening of samples could be with an ELISA set to have low sensitivity, but would be specific and reduce the number of clear positives, to relieve the burden on another more sensitive assay (e.g., polymerase chain reaction [PCR]).

Borderline or intermediate results require cautious interpretation. Statistically this gray zone defines a range of cutoff values that would result in a sensitivity or specificity less than a predefined level. Although there are techniques to attempt to compensate for unknown factors, the best approach is to assimilate as much data from all sources. This allows explanation and then manipulation (selection) of data to help eliminate bias. The flexibility in altering the cutoff value is data dependent and a continuous process in test validation.

1.8. Calculation of D-SN and D-SP: Predictive Value of Diagnostic Tests

The inferences from test results rather than observed test values are of interest to the diagnostician. Thus, the use of the assay rather than the technology itself is the key. Measurement of disease state, level of protective antibody, and transition of disease status are all objectives. Rarely is there a perfect correlation between disease status and any test result. Thus, there is always some degree of false positivity or negativity. The establishment of the correlation is regarded as diagnostic evaluation. The standard for presenting such results is in **Table 1**, which relates true positive (TP), true negative (TN), false positive (FP), and false negative (FN) results represented as frequencies of the four possible decisions. These can be shown in a 2 × 2 (*see* **Table 1**).

D-SN and D-SP can be estimated from test results on a panel of reference sera chosen early in the validation process. Calculations of D-SN and D-SP, therefore, only apply to the reference sera and can be extrapolated to the general population of animals only insofar as the reference sera fully represent all variables in that targeted population. The paramount importance of the proper selection of reference sera is thus self-evident.

Other terms based on these values can be defined as follows.

Table 1
Relationships of disease status and test results[a]

	True disease state	
Test	D+	D−
T+	TP	FP
T−	FN	TN

[a]Diagnostic (clinical) sensitivity = [TP/(TP + FN)] × 100. Diagnostic (clinical) specificrty is [TN/ (TN + FP)] X 100

1.8.1. Prevalence of Disease (P)

Prevalence of disease denotes the probability of a subject as having a disease:

$$\text{General probability } (P) = \Pr(D+)$$

$$P = (TP + FN)/N$$

P is an unbiased estimator of the prevalence in a target population if animals can be randomly selected and subjected to both the reference test (to establish D) and the new test (T).

1.8.2. Apparent Prevalence

Apparent prevalence (AP) denotes the probability of a subject to have a positive test result:

$$AP = \Pr(T+)$$

1.8.3. Predictive Value

The predictive value of a positive test gives the percentage of subjects suffering from disease correctly classified as positive by the test, and defined as follows:

$$[TP/(TP + FP)] \times 100$$

The predictive value of a negative test gives the percentage of healthy subjects correctly classified as negative by the test, and defined as follows:

$$[TN/(TN + FN)] \times 100$$

1.8.4. Components of Diagnostic Accuracy

Accuracy is the ability of a test to give correct results (diagnostic sensitivity). As already indicated, this can be estimated by the observed agreement of the new and reference test. There are two components.

Sensitivity

Sensitivity (Se) is the probability of a positive result (T+) given that the disease is present (D+):

$$Se = TP/(TP + FN)$$

Specificity

Specificity (Sp) is the probability of a negative results (T–) given that the disease is not present (D–):

$$Sp = TN/(TN + FP)$$

1.9. Combined Measures of Diagnostic Accuracy

1.10. Efficiency

The overall efficiency (Ef) of a diagnostic test, defined as the percentage of subjects correctly classified as diseased or healthy, with a given prevalence of P, is estimated using the following relationship:

$$Ef = [(TP + TN)/(TP + FP + TN + FN)] \times 100$$

1.10.1. Youden's Index

Youden's Index (J) is the measure of the probability of correct classifications that is invariant to prevalence. In terms of Se and Sp we have:

$$J = Se + Sp - 1$$

1.10.2. Likelihood Ratios

Likelihood ratios (LRs) are important measures of accuracy that link estimations of pre- and posttest accuracy. They express the change in the likelihood of a disease based on information gathered before and after making tests. The degree of change given a positive result (LR+) and given a negative result (LR–) depends on the SDe and Sp of the test.

Likelihood Ratio of a Positive Test Result

The likelihood ratio (LR) of a positive test result is the ratio of the probability of disease to the probability of nondisease given a positive test result, divided by the odds of the underlying prevalence [odds (P) = (P/1–P)]:

$$LR + = Se/(1 - Sp)$$

Likelihood Ratio of a Negative Test Result

The likelihood ratio of a negative test result is the ratio of the probability of disease to the probability of nondisease given a negative test result, divided by the odds of the underlying prevalence:

$$LR - = (1 - Se)/Sp$$

Odds Ratios

Odds ratios (ORs) combine results from studies:

$$OR = (TP \times TN)/(FP \times FN)$$

1.11. Examples Relating Analytical and Diagnostic Evaluation

In a new ELISA, 250 sera have been examined from nonexposed animals and 92 infected animals. **Table 2** presents the results.

The following data reflect some of the features already discussed:

Table 2
Relationship of disease status and test results

	Infection status	
Test	D+	D−
T+	76	0
T−	16	250

1. Sensitivity (Se) = 76/92 = 0.826
2. Specificity (Sp) = 250/250 = 1.000
3. Efficiency (Ef) = 326/342 = 0.953
4. Youden Index (J) = 0.826 + 1–1 = 0.826
5. Likelihood ratio (LR+) = 0.826/0 = cannot be defined
6. Likelihood ratio (LR–) = 0.174/1. 000 = 0.174

As already stated, the perfect test would exhibit 100% sensitivity, specificity, and efficiency. This is not possible in practice. Thus, the values of each depend on the decision level or point chosen (cutoff values, reference values, and so forth). The setting of the criteria for decisions is not solely based on statistics since there are ethical, medical, and financial implications, particularly in the human testing fields. The relationship of sensitivity to specificity has to be considered. A high cutoff favoring specificity reduces diagnostic sensitivity. Increasing sensitivity leads to false positive results. Different tests can be performed on samples in which there is to be increased confidence such that results are false positives, for example, the use of PCR may provide a higher degree of specificity. This pairing of sensitivity and specificity is inherent in all assays. The two parameters can be evaluated in terms of receiver operating characteristics (ROC) curves.

1.12. ROC Analysis

ROC analysis was developed in the early 1950s and extended into medical sciences in the 1960s. It is now a standard tool for the evaluation of clinical tests. The underlying assumption in ROC analysis is that the diagnostic variable is to be used as the discriminator of two defined groups of responses (e.g., test values from diseased/nondiseased animals, or infected/noninfected animals). ROC analysis assesses the performance of the system in terms of Se and 1–Sp for each observed value of the discriminator variable assumed as a decision threshold, e.g., cutoff value to differentiate between two groups of responses. For ELISA, which produces continuous results, the cutoff value can be shifted over a range of observed values, and Se and 1–Sp are established for each of these. Setting this as *k* pairs, the resulting *k* pairs ([1–Sp] Se) are displayed as an ROC plot. The connection of the points leads to a trace that originates in the upper right corner and ends in the lower left corner of the unit square. The plot characterizes the given test by the trace in the unit square, irrespective of the original unit and range of the measurement. Therefore, ROC plots can be used to compare all tests, even when the tests have quite different cutoff values and units of measurement. ROC plots for diagnostic assays with perfect discrimination between negative and positive reference samples pass through coordinates (0; *1)*, which is equivalent to Se = Sp = 100%. Thus, the area under such ROC plots would be 1. 0, and the study of the area under the curve (AUC), which evaluates the probabilities of (1–Sp) and Se, is the most important statistical feature of such curves.

8.1.12.1. Area under the ROC Curve

The theoretical exponential function underlying the ROC plot is estimated on the assumption that data from two groups are distributed normally (bimodally). The ROC function is then characterized by parameter *A* (standardized mean difference of the responses of two groups) and the parameter *B* (ratio of SDs). Thus, for a set of data for a positive and negative reference group with means of x_0 and x_1, in which $x_0 < x_1$ and the SDs are s_0 and s_1, respectively,

$$A = (x_1 - x_0)/S_1$$

$$B = S_0/S_1$$

The AUC can be estimated making assumptions about the distribution of test results. Therefore, a nonparametric test is based on the fact that the AUC is related to the test statistic *U* of the Mann-Whitney rank sum test:

$$\text{AUC1} = U/n_1 n_0$$

With $U = n_1 n_0 + n_0 (n_0 + 1)/2 - R$, R = rank sum of squares. A parametric approach can be taken. Here,

$$\text{AUC}_2 = \theta[A/(1 + B^2)^{0.5}]$$

Here we can see that for AUC = 0.5, then $A = 0$. Equal values for negative and positive reference populations indicate a noninformative diagnostic test. Theoretically, AUC < 0.5 if A is negative. In practice, such situations are not encountered, or the decision rule is converted to obtain positive values for *A*.

The bimodal distribution may not be justified for a given set of data, and other methods have been developed based on maximum likelihood estimates of the ROC function and the AUC.

8.1.12.2. Optimization of Cutoff Value Using ROC Curves

The optimal pair for sensitivity and specificity is the point with the greatest distance in a Northwest direction, from the diagonal line Se = (1–Sp) (*see* **Figs. 2** and **3**).

8.1.12.3. Example of ROC Analysis

The principle of ROC analysis is to generate plots using a spreadsheet (e.g., EXCEL) in which:

1. A grid of possible cutoff values is generated.

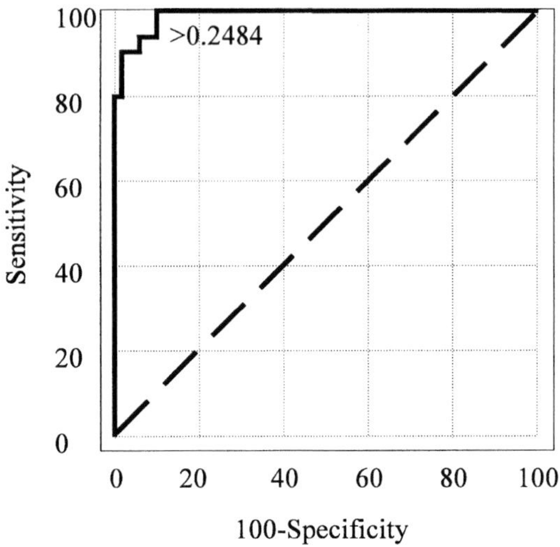

Fig. 8.2. ROC plot for T3 data (T1 assumed as reference test, n = 100). Area under plot = 0.993; standard error (SE) = 0.012; 95% confidence interval (CI) = 0.950–0.998.

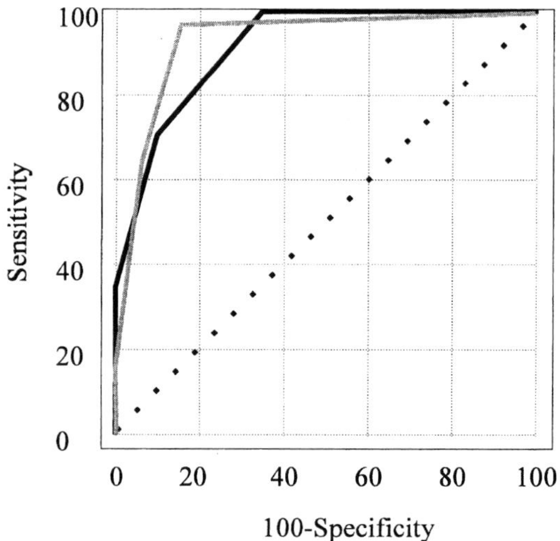

Fig. 8.3. ROC plot for data T7 and T10 (T1 assumed as reference test, n = 100). T7 area under plot = 0.920; SE = 0.039; 95% CI = 0.848–0.965. T10 area under plot = 0.957; SE = 0.029; 95% CI = 0.896–0.987. Difference between areas = 0.037; SE = 0.029; 95% CI = –0.046 to 0.130. Significance level = 0.437. The difference between the areas is not significant.

2. For each cutoff value, the resulting sensitivity (Se) and 1–Sp are calculated.

3. The values of Se are plotted against 1–Sp for all grid points. Many statistical packages can be used to construct ROC plots and shareware is available in the public domain. In this example (taken from **ref. *1***), the AUC is estimated for an ELISA for T3 using a test reference (T1), given the mean values of 1.04 and 0.11; the SDs 0.47 and 0.13; and the sample sizes 25 (positive subpopulation) and 75 (negative subpopulation). The rank sum and the *U* statistic are as follows:

$$A = (1.04 - 0.11)/0.47 = 1.97$$

$$B = 0.13/0.47 = 0.276$$

$$R = 2864$$

$$U = 2575 + 75\ (75 + 1)/2 - R = 1861$$

$$\text{AUC1} = 1861/1875 = 0.9935$$

$$\text{AUC}_2 = \theta\ [1.97/(1 + 0.13^2)^{0.5}] = \theta\ (1.953) = 0.9745$$

Thus, the nonparametric test and parametric estimates of the AUC for T3 data are 0.9935 and 0.9745, respectively. **Figures 2** and **3** show examples of ROC plots.

1.13. Monitoring of Assay Performance During Routine Use

If we accept the proposition that a validated assay implies provision of valid test results during routine diagnostic testing, it follows that assay validation must be an ongoing process consistent with the principles of internal quality control (IQC). Continuous evaluation of repeatability and reproducibility are thus essential for helping to ensure that the assay is generating valid test results.

Repeatability between runs of an assay within a laboratory should be monitored by plotting results of the control samples to determine whether the assay is operating within acceptable limits. It is useful to maintain a running plot of the serum control values from the last 40 runs of the assay and to assess them after each run of the assay to determine whether they remain within 95% CI. If results fall outside of the CIs or are showing signs of an upward or downward trend, there may be a problem with repeatability and/or precision that needs attention. Similarly, when several laboratories assess samples for inter-laboratory variation, reproducibility of the assay is monitored. The assay should also be subjected to tests for accuracy. This may be done by including samples of known activity in each run of the assay or by periodic testing of such samples. In addition, it would be desirable to enroll in an external quality assurance program in which a panel of samples, supplied by a third party, are tested blind to determine proficiency of the assay. Inclusion of such QC schemes in routine use of an assay that was validated at one point in time, ensures that the assay maintains that level of validity when put into routine use.

1.14. Updating Validation Criteria

We have stressed that an assay is valid only if the results of selected sera from reference animals represent the entire targeted population. Because of the extraordinary set of variables that may affect the performance of an assay, it is highly desirable to expand the bank of gold standard reference sera whenever possible. This follows the principle that variability is reduced with increasing sample size; therefore, increases in the size of the reference serum pool should lead to better estimates of D-SN and D-SP for the population targeted by the assay. Furthermore, when the assay is to be transferred to a completely different geographic region (e.g., from the Northern to Southern Hemisphere), it is essential to revalidate the assay by subjecting it to populations of animals that reside under local conditions. This is the only way to ensure that the assay is valid for that situation.

1.15. Assay Validation and Interpretation of Test Results

It is wrong to assume that a test result from a validated assay correctly classifies animals as infected or uninfected based solely on the assay's D-SN and D-SP. The calculations of D-SN and D-SP are based on testing the panel of reference sera and are calculated at one point in time. This is unlike the ability of a positive or negative test result to predict the infection status of an animal because this is a function of the prevalence of infection in the population being tested. Prevalence of disease in the target population, coupled with the previously calculated estimates of D-SN and D-SP, is used to calculate the predictive values of positive and negative test results.

For instance, assume a prevalence of disease in the population targeted by the assay of only 1 infected animal per 1,000 animals, and a false positive rate of the test of 1 per 100 animals (99% D-SP). Of 1,000 tests run on that population, 10 will be false positive and only 1 will be true positive. Therefore, when the prevalence of disease is this low, positive test results will be an accurate predictor of the infection status of the animal in only about 9% of the cases. Thus, if assay validation is concerned with accuracy in test results *and their inferences*, then proper interpretation of test results is an integral part of providing valid test results. It is beyond the scope of this chapter to discuss the many ramifications of proper interpretation of test results generated by a validated assay.

1.16. Validation of Assays Other than ELISA

Although the example we have used was an indirect ELISA test, the same principles apply in the validation of any other types of diagnostic assay. Feasibility studies, assay performance characteristics, the size and composition of the animal populations that provide reference sera, and the continuing assessment and updating of the performance characteristics of the validated assay are all essential if the assay is to be considered thoroughly and continuously validated.

2. More Principles of Validation

This section reexamines the process of validation in a slightly different way. Other terms are introduced and explained. The initial steps in assessing the performance of an assay are really a technical evaluation. Various experimental procedures can be used to assess aspects affecting the performance of assays. These examine the following areas:

1. Precision (reproducibility).
2. Sensitivity.
3. Accuracy.
4. Specificity.

These factors help cover potential sources of error in assays that may be:

1. Systematic: errors that consistently affect repeated measurements of the same sample.
2. Random: errors affecting individual measurements randomly causing a scatter.

2.1. Precision

Precision can be regarded also as reproducibility and is a statistical measure of the variation in samples on repeat determinations of the same sample either within the same run or from day to day, or operator to operator in time. This is always examined first in any assay development because an assay with great imprecision in the early stages is not likely to be of any routine use, despite later attempts to improve this factor. Precision testing involves testing samples many times to accumulate data for analysis within and between runs. Different samples, reflecting the target population in which the test is to find practical use, should be examined.

The statistics involves *(1)* the mean (X), *(2)* standard deviation (SD), and *(3)* coefficient of variation (CV), which is expressed as follows:

$$CV = \%CV = (SD/X) \times 100$$

The performance of an assay can be examined through profiling the precision measured for different sample (analyte) concentrations and conditions. Such assessment at any stage can be regarded as a precision profile.

2.1.1. Precision Profile

Precision profiles are obtained by plotting the values of %CV against the concentration of measured analyte. To construct such curves, between 10 and 20 replicates of each standard concentration (dilution) should be run. At least three dilutions should be examined representing high medium and low signal in the ELISA. These should include samples representing ~80, 50, and 20% of maximal activity measured. This can give useful information about reproducibility for different concentrations. The minimum acceptable precision can be defined, and estimates of about a maximum of 10% should be accepted. Differences in reproducibility are evident in assays at different concentrations of reagents used in development as well as for different concentrations of analyte being detected. **Figure 4** shows an example of %CV plots against concentration of analyte detected. Usually nonuniform error is seen across the concentration range used as illustrated. The acceptable precision is drawn on the graph, and this would define a "working" range within which there were acceptable limits for the variation in the assay. On further validation extending development into a kit format, this degree of variation can be measured and limits acceptable to the kit imposed.

Precision should be estimated not only within runs but also between runs from day to day. Usually there is more variation day to day (and operator to operator), but the continuous exercise of precision analysis allows limits to be determined statistically that define the test. The variation measured during development is the sum of all the errors that affect the test.

2.2. Sensitivity

Sensitivity is the assay's capacity to measure the smallest amount of target analyte under the standard conditions defined. For a full treatment of the approaches to determining the theoretical sensitivity of assays, *see* **ref.** *1*. This explains the Yalow and

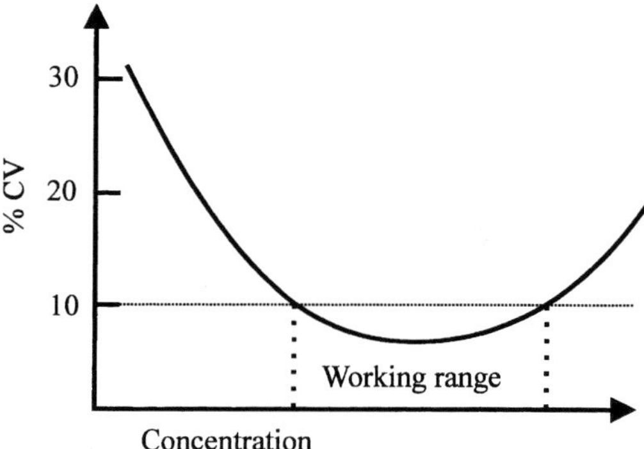

Fig. 4. The precision profile of an assay showing nonuniform error. The CV is plotted against the analyte concentration. The working range of the assay can be defined as the range where imprecision is below a preset level such as 10%, as shown.

Berson and Ekin models defining antigen and antibody interactions and points to the features inherent in assays that affect the sensitivity. The required sensitivity is a consideration here and practically depends on the balance between obtaining maximal sensitivity and the precision of the results compared to suboptimal conditions of sensitivity conditions. It may be advantageous to reduce the sensitivity for certain assays to improve both accuracy and specificity. Thus, conditions can be assessed that reflect the likely concentration of the analyte being determined. The factors involve the examination of the concentration of reagents, the time for incubation, the effects of temperature, the mixing of reagents, the sequence in which reagents are added, and, to improve precision, the number of replicates run.

2.3. Accuracy

Accuracy is the concept of being able to measure the true value of the analyte. The use of control standards, which, by definition indicate the true value, can give a measure of accuracy and evaluate any bias in the functional aspects of the use of an ELISA.

The bias may be proportional when the results indicate a constant percentage higher (positive bias) or lower (negative bias). The assay may involve both types of bias, depending on the range of standards assessed. **Figure 5** shows the relationship of precision, accuracy and bias.

Accuracy can be affected by all components of an assay. Generally, accuracy has to be determined by comparing results to a reference method. However, in most cases, only an indirect assessment is possible, and several methods are used, including calibration standards, recovery studies and parallelism.

2.3.1. Calibration Standards

The provision of standards for ELISA is not as simple as for other assays involving more physical methods (e.g., in which a defined substance can be measured by weight or wavelength, and in which it is known that test samples contain the same substance known to be identical in structure). Even in these cases, methods used to extract the sample or other physical treatments may alter the measurements in a test to increase imprecision. In the ELISA we rely on measuring activity through many steps and assessing the activity of reagents such as antisera, which show variability in their own right. The inability to supply standards in biological fields, which can reflect all activities of similar reactants, is a drawback to using calibration studies. Some areas have better chances of assessing accuracy with respect to standards, e.g., monoclonal antibodies (mAbs), which can be defined exactly in terms of epitope recognition and physical structure. In this case, a standard preparation can be classified through considerations of weight to activity measured.

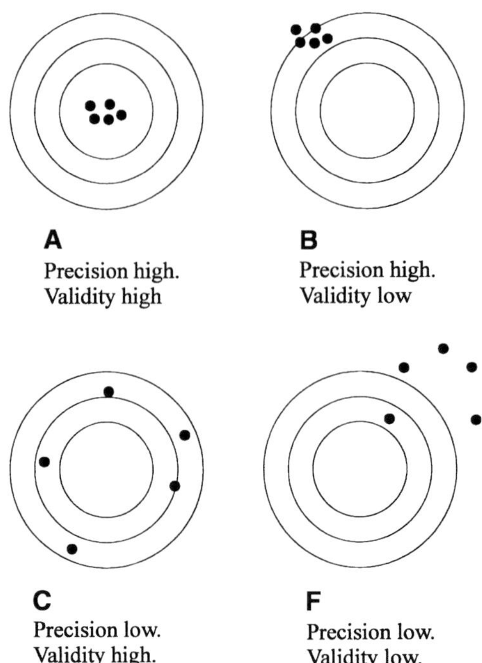

Fig. 5. Representations of precision (reproducibility) and validity (accuracy). The target for accuracy of a test result is represented by the central disc. For example, this is the correct mean for a sample analyzed by ELISA. Results from five tests are shown as *black dots*. **a** Data are grouped tightly (reproducible) and all are in the correct result disc (accurate). **b** Although the data are precise (all showing similar results), they all are inaccurate and biased toward the *upper left*. **c** This shows a wide dispersion of data (not reproducible), but the average result of the data predicts the accurate result; confidence in these data is low. **d** This shows both irreproducible results in which the control mean is not reflected by the average of all the results; the test is inaccurate and variable.

2.3.2. Recovery Studies

A recovery study determines the ability of a test to measure a known incremental amount of standard analyte from a sample matrix. Thus, in practice, a known amount of analyte (A) is added to base (B) and the recovery (C) is calculated as a concentration after performing the assay. The percentage of recovery is as follows:

$$(C - B)/A \times 100$$

This system is applicable to standards which can be highly defined and whose purity can be a guarantee, e.g., drugs, steroids, peptides. Again this method suffers in typical uses of ELISA for diagnosis where purity and heterogeneity of samples are the norm.

2.3.3. Parallelism

Parallelism relies on dilutions of standards and testing these in an assay. Correction of the measurements for samples, with respect to the dilution factors, should show that there is equivalent "activity." The easiest way to treat results is to simply multiply the found concentration by the dilution factor. The results can be plotted against dilution, and a parallel response is inferred from an observed horizontal line. Statistics can be used to examine the significance of the correlation of activity to dilution.

In assays of antibody, both the concentration and avidity of the serum have to be considered. Parallelism will only be demonstrated when the avidity of the test antibodies corresponds exactly to those in the assay calibrators. Thus, samples with high-affinity antibodies will show over-recovery on dilution whereas those with low-affinity antibodies will show under-recovery. Hence, the serial monitoring of antisera and the consequential nonlinearity of the antibody titers can give rise to clinical interpretation. One method of minimizing this is to use reference preparations that best reflect the average avidity (sum of all affinities of antibodies in a sample). In this way samples dilute correctly on "average" in which approximately half will show apparent under-recovery and half over-recovery. In simple terms, standards are "sought" from a population that best reflect the average avidity of sera in a population. Diluents affect such considerations, and the dilution matrix should be maintained throughout the range chosen.

2.4. Specificity

The accuracy of an assay ultimately relies on its specificity. Thus, the ability for accuracy relies on the assay determining only the required parameter, probably when mixed with other components. With polyclonal antibodies, the specificity is complicated owing to the heterogeneity of the antibodies, which have varying affinities even against the same epitope. mAbs offer better reagents because they are, by definition, reactive as a single population of antibody with a single affinity. However, even in this case, minor variations in the same epitope affect the binding of a mAb and hence the specificity. The existence of cross reactivities and the variation in a specific response against a required single antigenic site of choice, complicate the measurement of a specific activity. Such factors include the existence of endogenous molecules that are structurally similar to the principle analyte, the in vivo production of metabolites of the principle analyte with common crossreactive epitopes, and the possible administration of similar analytes as vaccines or medications (*see* **ref.** *2*).

2.5. Testing of Ruggedness (Robustness of Test)

The entire process of developing assays and their validation involves determining the effect of all operational parameters and the tolerances for their control. This includes all the systematic factors, assay temperatures, times for incubation, volumes, separation procedures for samples, order of addition of reagent, and signal detection. In short, all the factors that can be examined and the effect of changes in conditions should be understood. The examination of the tolerance of the assay to changes is a measure of the ability of the test to resist changes and maintain its test results within tolerable limits. The tolerances can be measured against different conditions depending on the intended environment of the assay. A robust assay might be viewed as one whose reagents are stable at high temperatures, which might be more suitable for use in countries where the environment is hot and where laboratory temperature control is not available. The suitability of an ELISA may in fact be dominated by its intended end user, and the relevant factors should be examined to allow the best chance of a successful assay. The development of kits to be used worldwide should consider the robustness or ruggedness carefully. Some factors for consideration are examined in the next section. Often, validation requires that a set of reagents and a defined protocol be field tested to allow an estimation of robustness. Indeed, it may not be possible to test all factors in a central laboratory to account for the types of challenge to the assay experienced through its dispersion. Often changes have to be made to assay components, systems, methods of sending materials, and so forth, according to the feedback from extended validation.

3. Kits

The definition of what comprises a kit rests on considerations on test validation, the perceived objective of the kit, the market or end users who are to exploit the kit, and, the factors involved in sustainability. The last area is perhaps the most important and needs examination in the light of commercial interests and international bodies supplying help through technology transfer to developing countries. Thus, the equation for a kit is complex, involving technical performance, supply and profit motives, and continuity. Kits, at best, also have to be accepted by international bodies to fulfill their ultimate role of standardization of a given approach and allow harmonization with other tests measuring the same or similar factors. It would be useful here to examine some generalized ideas about kits in all fields of human and veterinary applications. The separation of developments in humans and animals is also relevant and is examined subsequently.

Where do kits stem from? It could be assumed that kits always supply a need identified by careful assessment of existing problems and the current solutions, and thus that there is a direct route from need to development to the end product. This is not generally true. Rarely is there such a clean scenario. Rather, some developments in research are harnessed to prove feasibility of an approach, which then leads to a relatively moderate amount of validation followed by exploitation. Who exploits the reagents and in what form usually determines the success of the kit and its long-term prospects and, more important, its actual benefit. This area has to take into account the profit motive as well as technical aspects. The possibilities for profit are great in the human medical sphere and concentrated on relatively few diseases, whereas the veterinary market is fragmented, centered more on application in developing countries, and hence lacks appeal to the commercial sphere.

Having indicated that kits can be relatively poorly thought-out entities, it is probably incumbent that I define the ultimate kit. Such a definition or statements may then be examined against kits being used by readers or used to help design better kits. Having said this, there is no perfect kit that deals with biological systems. The section on validation of assays strongly indicates that the process is continuous and that data derived from the use of kits constantly redefines the particular test. The gathering of information from kits and the modification of reagents/conditions/protocols is necessary to account for the many variables that cannot be assessed at a single time point or in a single laboratory. The validation also involves changes in the biological systems examined, such as alteration in the antigenicity of agents examined, which necessitates action.

3.1. A Definition of a Perfect Kit

1. A kit should contain everything needed to allow testing including software packages for storage, processing, demonstration, and reporting of data.
2. The reagents should be absolutely stable under a wide range of conditions of temperature (rugged, robust).
3. The manual describing the use of the kit should be foolproof.
4. The kit should be validated in the field as well as in research laboratories.
5. All containers for reagents should be leakproof.
6. IQC samples should be included.
7. External quality assessment should be included in the kit package.
8. Data on the relationship of kit results to those from other assays should be included.
9. Attention should be made to ensuring that all equipment used in the kit is calibrated (spectrophotometers, pipets).
10. Training courses should be organized in the use of kits.
11. Information exchange should be set up to allow rapid online help and evaluation of results when there are perceived problems.
12. The internationally sanctioned supply and control of standards used in kits should be maintained.

3.2. Other Considerations for Kits

Allied to validation and ruggedness testing, the implication for a kit is that the reagents can be supplied over an extended time. This can mean that different batches or lots of materials are produced at different times. It is essential that there be monitoring of reagents to ensure consistency. The degree of inaccuracy owing to great variation is ultimately determined by the manufacturer (the tolerance limits). Typical tolerance limit could be of 2–10% or 1–2 SDs of the difference among lots. Examples of lot changes include all materials in an ELISA such as changing the anti-species conjugate. This can have a profound effect on an assay and care should be taken to retitrate conjugates to equivalent activities. In fact, all aspects are relevant from the solid phase, control antisera, buffers, substrates, and so on. The control of this element of kits was originally the supplier's responsibility. QC is essential and measurement of the new errors with respect to those of the previously established lots. Changes in lots should also be reported to users, who may encounter problems owing to local conditions. If these are reported to the supplier, the supplier may indicate that changes are made. Microtiter plates can be a problem, and it should not be assumed that different batches supplied from manufacturers are the same for any specific assay, since the tests used to establish batch-to-batch variation by plastics manufacturers are not the same as those for any particular assay. Thus, a statistically valid number of plates should be tested when they are from a different batch number.

3.3. Quality Assurance/Quality Control

Some consideration of Quality Assurance (QA) and QC is relevant. It is also considered with reference to controlling a single assay. IQC should be designed to ensure that results are within acceptable (given) limits of accuracy and precision. Thus, all aspects that might influence assay performance should be monitored, such as routine assessment of equipment performance, reagent stability, technique, assay conditions, and sample handling. QC samples should be included in every assay at regular intervals (if not every time, and such samples should reflect the concentration range where "clinical" decisions can be made with regard to samples from a "population." The QC samples therefore control retrospectively the within assay, between assay, bias, drift, and shift in results.

The most common method of presenting of data and the statistical analyzes is through Shewhart or Levy-Jennings control charts *(3)*. These charts require the estimation of the mean and SD for each control used.

3.4. External Quality Assurance Schemes

External Quality Assurance (EQA) schemes attempt to provide an independent assessment of a laboratory's performance usually with respect to a defined assay. Such schemes complement (and use) ICQ. The basis of the schemes is that an organizer sends the same control samples to all participating laboratories for testing at regular intervals. The samples are tested in the routine cycle of the laboratory and the results are transmitted back to the organizer.

Successful schemes need not require many samples (e.g., five). The transmission of IQC data and a questionnaire also add a great deal to the EQA (*see* **refs.** *4–7* for reviews on IQC and EQA).

3.5. Standards

An ELISA can be developed to measure a substance that has not been previously examined. Thus, a reference preparation may not exist. Generally, the substance may not be characterized by a single chemical structure. A well-defined compound of high quality, purity, and stability, can be adequate as a standard. However, in the ELISA, many biologically active substances are only available in crude forms. Three types of reference preparations are commonly used for standardization of immunoassay kits.

3.5.1. International Standards

An international standard (IS) or international reference standard (IRS) must be used to calibrate a new method for biological analytes. As examples, materials for such standards are collected, tested, and stored by the World Health Organization International Laboratory for Biological Standards. An international unit for activity is assigned to these preparations, and collaborative efforts among several laboratories maintain these as reliable reference preparations. The IRS status is reserved to designate preparations that do not meet the very demanding criteria for an IS. The ISs are available in limited quantity for a small charge for calibration purposes of national or reference preparations. They are not available in sufficient quantities to serve as routine standards.

3.5.2. Reference Materials

Reference materials are not as extensively tested as ISs, but they do have certain potency and purity of data. Such preparations are useful in cases in which substances cannot be completely characterized by physical means alone.

3.5.3. In-House Reference Preparations

In-house reference preparations are produced by the laboratory that develop the assay or are those that have been acquired without reliable potency estimates. Frequently, these materials are calibrated against an IS.

3.5.4. Working Standards

Working standards are very important forms of standards and are prepared in the laboratory in relatively large volumes. The extensive testing and validation required for the introduction of reference standard is not normally necessary, but the donor laboratory must assume responsibility for maintaining appropriate quality. This form of standard is common in animal disease diagnosis.

4. Shelf Life and Reagent Considerations

QC relies on the source and accurate preparation of reagents. The quality of reagents for certain stages can be more critical than others. With in-house assays, new reagents must be thoroughly characterized, and once this is done the controls can be restricted to those used for monitoring assay performance. Regular checks are needed to examine deterioration in reagents. Assays based on kit material also require attention even though reagents are provided, because often producers do not provide complete test formats of individual reagent batches. A major problem is that test kit reagents have to be transported, and this can affect reagents (factors of robustness have already been mentioned). Each kit delivered must be checked. Kit overlapping is important, in which the new kit is evaluated against the old by testing the same samples. Reagents from the old kit can be substituted in order that the activity of new reagents can be determined. Instructions for the kits must be followed exactly, e.g., the reconstitution of freeze-dried reagents. These must be opened very carefully, because powdered material can easily be lost owing to the difference in pressure (lower) in the vial. There are manufacturing guidelines concerning reagents *(8)*. These can be summarized as follows:

1. Liquid and freeze-dried reagents should be stored at 2–8°C.
2. Reagents transported in dry ice should be stored at –20°C.
3. After reconstitution, freeze-dried reagents should be stored at 2–8°C for short times, or as samples at –20°C.
4. Thawed reagents should not be refrozen.

4.1. Liquids

Water quality plays a critical role for some reagents. Untreated water can contain inorganics, organics, dissolved gases, suspended solids, colloids, microorganisms, and pyrogens. Deionization and reverse osmosis are used to prepare water for laboratory use. Cation and anion-exchange resins are used to remove all dissolved ionizable substances and provide a primary water source. When coupled to specific ion-exchange resins or activated carbon resins, all organic or colloidal matter can be removed. Reverse osmosis uses a semipermeable membrane to separate substances from the water.

Most immunoassays can be performed with a water quality of 5/cm at 25°C with an organic content of <2 ppm. Thus, use of deionization controlled by a conductivity meter is adequate to obtain water for the assay and washing use in ELISA.

Water quality can be a major problem in some countries. Attention has been focused on devising special units suitable for developing countries.

4.1.1. Aqueous Protein Solutionsa

Proteins can be relatively fragile in aqueous solution so that enzymes and antibodies need to be handled with care. High temperatures, and acid or alkaline solutions should be avoided. Temperatures above 40°C cause denaturation of proteins. Solutions of proteins that are stirred vigorously are denatured by shearing action. The shelf life of proteins is prolonged by cold storage but attention should be focused on the state of the protein. For most enzymes in a dry phase, storage at 2–8°C is good. Other enzymes may be unstable even dry and should be stored at −20°C. Repeated thawing is disastrous. Organic solvents should be avoided with enzymes except at concentrations of <3%. Enzyme labels can be supplied as liquids but need addition of cryoprotectants such as glycerol and polyethylene glycols, (~40% final concentration).

4.1.2. Preservatives

Common preservatives in diagnostic reagents are as follows:

1. Thimerosal (0.01%): This is expensive, difficult to dispose of (mercuric compound), and can affect assays.
2. Sodium azide (0.02–0.1%): This is biostatic, difficult to dispose of, and can inhibit enzyme reactions.

Although both are used for various reagents in ELISA, they do pose problems of safety and disposal. A commercial product, ProClin™, from Rohm and Haas, Spring House, PA, is recommended in **ref.** ***8***. It is reported to be a broad-spectrum biocide, having good compatibility and stability and low toxicity at in-use levels. It eradicates bacteria, fungi, and yeast cells at very low concentration, does not interfere with enzyme reactions, and can be disposed of without restrictions.

4.2. Shelf Life Evaluation

Evaluation of shelf life is related to the ruggedness of a test. The shelf life is a measure of the time within which the performance characteristics of a test are maintained under specified handling conditions. The change in quality is a function of factors such as storage temperature, humidity, package protection, and formulation. These are the key factors in kits, which have to be dispatched and which may not be collected or used under the predetermined optimal conditions. This is particularly important in some developing countries, so that kit formulations must be tested for performance under a wider set of variables. There is an attempt to measure product expiration times with commercial kits through practical determination of stability. This is also tied up with governmental regulations. For example, the Food and Drug Administration requires written testing programs designed to examine the stability of products based on these factors:

1. The sample size and the test intervals for each attribute measured.
2. Reliable, specific, and meaningful tests to assess quality.
3. The conditions under which held-back samples are stored.
4. Testing to be conducted under the same conditions as in the intended market.
5. Tests to be conducted at the time of dispensing, as well as after reconstitution of reagents.

4.2.1. Types of Stability

Physical, bacteriostatic, and functional stabilities are important. Physical appearance such as discoloration and precipitation is undesirable. Most products contain bacteriocidal or bacteriostatic compounds to prevent deterioration through microbial growth. Thus, on storage, the active component must remain at a sufficiently high level to work. Functional changes are damaging to the assay's performance (can reduce analytical and diagnostic sensitivity and specificity). These can involve functional changes owing to antibody degradation, as well as chemical changes affecting function, e.g., in chromophore quality owing to oxidation or reduction.

4.2.2. Criteria for Shelf Life

A typical quality criterion for shelf life is that the product must retain at least 90% of its original value throughout its life. This performance is often applied to assessing the results of stability testing. Reagents used in ELISA, and diagnostic kits in general, must have a long shelf life. Most reagents are stable when unopened. It is desirable to have single lots of reagents, which can be used over a long period in many laboratories. Stability involves factors of degradation. The rates of degradation for given reagents are defined by the laws of chemistry and physics. The dominating factor for a given pH, ionic strength, composition, and so on, is temperature. Thus, degradation of any product can be monitored at high temperatures and the information extrapolated to the anticipated storage temperature, to determine the usable shelf life.

4.3. Real-Time Stability Testinga

The testing of products in real time has to be regarded as the gold standard for determination of expiry dates. However, this is not practical in most cases. Products must be left to allow a degradation to be observed. Methods to measure at least a 1% degradation, as distinct from interassay variation, must be available.

The reliability can be increased if a single lot reference is included with each test point. Sample recovery among samples can be normalized to this reference to minimize the impact of systematic drift and imprecision. The reference materials themselves should be sufficiently stable so that a single lot provides unchanging performance throughout stability testing. In brief, the real-time data collection is complicated by drift or changes in the testing method used over a period of time.

4.4. Accelerated Stability Testing

Accelerated stability testing is often used when developing clinical reagents, to provide an early indication of shelf life. The method involves subjecting products to several high temperatures. The amount of heat input needed to cause product failure is determined. An efficient system requires at least four "stress" temperatures *(9)*. Temperatures that cause denaturation should not be used. This is particularly true for labile proteinaceous reagents, such as antibodies and enzymes. One advantage is that samples can be subjected to elevated temperatures, stored at low temperature, and then assayed at the same time as unstressed controls. There are several approaches to analysis, involving different mathematical methods.

4.4.1. Protocol for Accelerated Stability Testing

Four parameters for accelerated stability testing must be considered *(10)*:

1. Preparation of samples: The samples must be as close to, if not identical to those to be used in assays. This includes containers.
2. Storage conditions: Four temperatures for storage should be examined. The highest temperature is determined by the type of substance being examined (e.g., to avoid denaturation of proteins, and by the length of time available to devote to the assays). Lower temperatures may be needed when the containers themselves are affected.
3. Analytical procedures: The analytical method used must be meaningful for the active reagent of the product. Chemical assays are reliable up to 2°C but biological assays only to 5°C. It is vital that the initial assay be titrated extremely accurately in multiple replicates to allow the determination of degradation.
4. Analysis and interpretation of data: Methods are reviewed in **ref.** ***8*****, Chapter 10**. These exploit the Arrhenius relationship, which states that the functional relationship between time and stability of a product stored under constant conditions is dependent on the order of reaction and the rate constant that determines the speed of reaction. A general guideline is shown in **ref.** ***8*****, Chapter 10** which delineates the steps as follows:

a. Select four temperatures. Define degradation, e.g., loss of total function or clinical parameter (enzyme concentration, percentage of binding of a reference material to an antibody at a predetermined concentration, and so on). Place the reagents in incubators at the predefined temperatures. If degradation is not observed within a reasonable time (e.g., 1–2 mo), then select higher temperatures. There must be degradation for determination of shelf life.

b. Place a sufficient amount of reagent in the final containers, at the selected temperatures, for specified time periods. This will depend on the estimated rate of degradation. The volume/amount will depend on test method requirements, but there should be enough to allow testing to run duplicate assays for each point of a minimum three-point assay curve. Higher temperatures should be sampled more frequently than lower. The following protocols are suggested: 37°C once every 5 days; 45°C once every 4 days; 50°C once every 3 days; 60°C once every 2 days; and, 80°C once every day.

c. Samples should be cooled on removal from elevated temperatures and analyzed promptly.

d. Measurements can be made on any critical components.

e. Data plotted against day number should give an approximate straight line using semilog graph paper. Conventionally, the slope is measured. However, the measure of the length of time for activity (potency) to drop by 90% of the original value, or any other appropriate criterion, can be selected and determined from the graph. The real situation requires an estimation of the maximum allowable drop in activity that would not affect the functioning of the product and thus the assay performance.

f. From such a set of data, one can predict the time required to reach 90% potency at the desired temperature. The logarithms of the t_{90} values are related linearly to the reciprocal of the absolute temperature.

g. A semilog plot of t_{90} values (ordinate) and $1/T$ in Kelvins (abscissa) should give a straight line. From this, the predicted shelf life at the desired storage temperature can be calculated.

Based on the experiences of the author in **ref.** *8*, here are some guidelines to approximate the shelf life of a product at a desired temperature.

1. One month at 50°C is equivalent to 1 year at room temperature.
2. Two months at 50°C is equivalent to 2 years at room temperature.

3. Three months at 37°C is equivalent to 1 year at room temperature.
4. Six months at 37°C is equivalent to 2 years at room temperature.
5. Seven days at 37°C is equivalent to 1 year at 4°C.
6. Three days at 37°C is equivalent to 3–6 months at 4°C.

5. Literature

Further information on the various aspects of validation can be obtained in **refs.** *9* and *11*. In addition, an excellent review of advanced methods for test validation and interpretation in veterinary medicine is available in **ref.** *12*.

6. Statistics

This section reviews some statistical terms and principles. The purpose of ELISA is to measure quantities or compare antigens or antibodies through measuring the level of binding or inhibition of binding of some labeled material. Statistical analyzes are applicable to both the assay itself, through examination of the variation inherent under different conditions and to the data generated and its relevance to the problem investigated. Thus, statistical analysis is inherent in ELISA development, for continuous use (monitoring performance), and to analyze the results for specific samples (e.g., whether a sample falls into a positive or negative population). Statistics also assess results in terms of confidence in the values obtained.

It is vital to understand that statistical examination should never be regarded as the last thing to do when faced with data. Consideration of what statistical methods are to be used must be made during the planning stages, so that the data can be immediately assessed, particularly since computer software is often used. A key is to ask, How can anyone prove anything associated with an assay? The proof statistically is, by definition, a measure of the probability of an event. The stronger the measure of the statistical probability, the more true the measure is.

8.6.1. Populations

A major use of ELISA is to obtain data from sample analysis and assess whether a particular sample is positive (contains a particular analyte) or negative (does not contain analyte). This requires both the examination of the specific assay parameters (assessing sensitivity and specificity) and the defining of a specific population in terms of data obtained and with reference to other data from other tests. The establishment of a population statistic requires that the data be obtained and analyzed. The analysis determines the type of distribution of data, and hence any sample value can be assessed with reference to all data in that population. The amount of data obtained to establish a population affects the certainty of any result, as does where the samples were taken from to establish the population (sampling/survey statistics).

6.2. Basic Terms

These are a few basic terms:

1. The *mean* is the arithmetic mean of a set of data.
2. The *median* defines a value or interval range of values in the middle of a set of values in a population.
3. The *mode* defines the value or interval range that is most frequent in any population.

These are illustrated in **Fig. 8.6** as a plot of the data is shown in **Table 8.3**. These are OD results from the analysis of a supposedly negative population of samples. The interval has been selected as 0.02 OD units represented on the *x*-axis, and the numbers of samples in any defined interval are plotted on the *y*-axis.

Figure 8.6 represents actual data for 77 results taken from a population of samples. We can see that there is a peak where most of the data are placed from intervals about 0.08–0.16. Lower numbers are observed on either side of this. The mean, median and mode can be described for this data as shown in **Fig. 8.7**. The

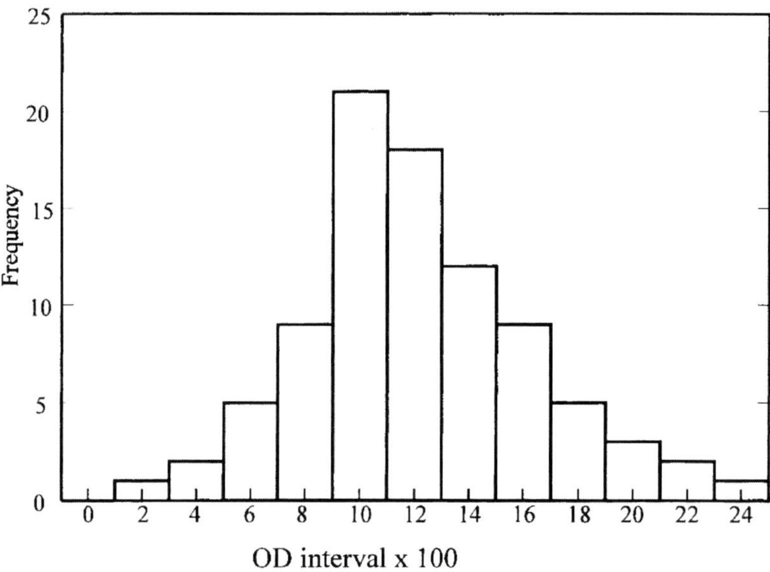

Fig. 6. Frequency histogram of data in **Table 8.3**.

Table 3
Data from analysis of samples

OD interval	Number (frequency)
0.00–0.02	1
0.02–0.04	2
0.04–0.06	5
0.06–0.08	9
0.08–0.10	21
0.10–0.12	18
0.12–0.14	12
0.14–0.16	9
0.16–0.18	7
0.18–0.20	4
0.20–0.22	2
0.22–0.24	2
0.24–0.26	0

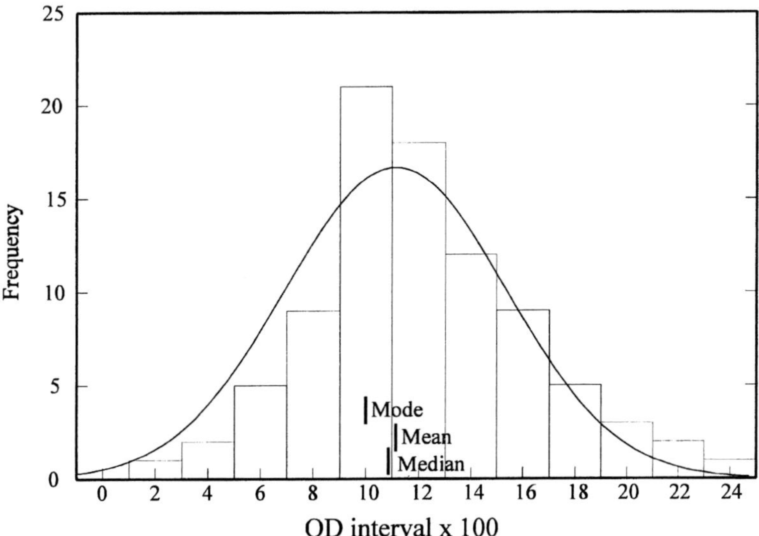

Fig. 7. Frequency histogram of data in **Table 8.3** with normal distribution plotted and the mean, median, and mode highlighted.

data is shown as a distribution curve and these can be defined mathematically according to the distribution they fit in. Some distribution curves are shown in Fig. 8. The statistics involving normal distribution curves are illustrated in Fig. 9.

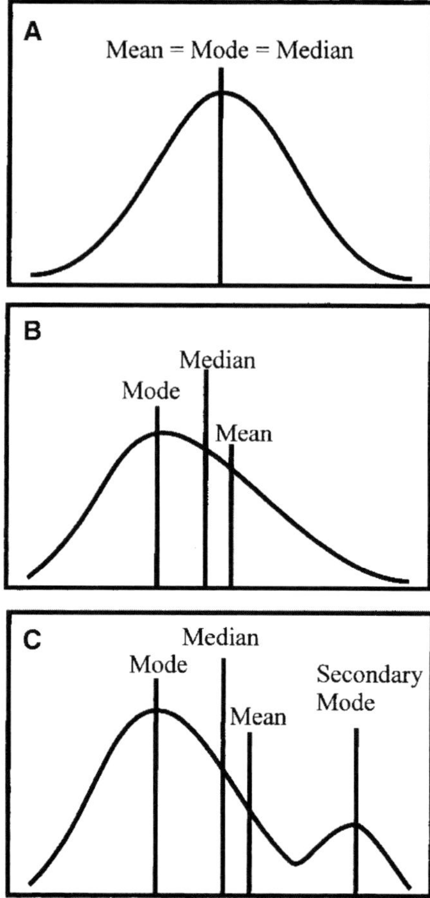

Fig. 8. Population distributions. **a** Gaussian or "normal" distribution. This is symmetrical about the mean and the values of the mean, median, and mode are the same. **b** A long "tail" of higher values, this represents a nonsymmetrical distribution in which there are different values for the mean, median, and mode (**c**)

6.2.1. Normal Distribution

When the distribution is symmetrical, it is referred to statistically as a Gaussian or normal distribution. In a perfect case, the mean, median, and mode are identical. Although this perfect situation is never achieved in practice, most situations for ELISA regard distributions as normal. The normal distribution can be described in mathematical terms with regard to the mean (X) and the SD of the observed values. The use of sampling techniques and the examination of distribution in samples attempts to determine the true mean (u) and variance (S^2) of the entire population from which the samples are taken. The breakdown in the statistical considerations of a normal distribution are shown in **Fig. 9.** The

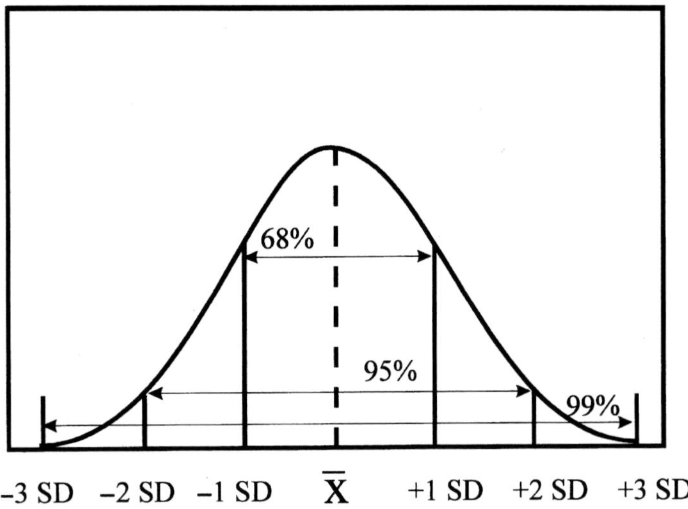

Fig. 9. Probability distribution for a population defined by Guassian curve. Mean *X*, and plus or minus 1, 2, 3 × SD encompases the percentages indicated. Thus, e.g., 95% of all results in a population would be distributed about the mean between +2 and −2 × SD.

key here is that whatever the measured values, a certain percentage of the sample is always contained within the SD values. One SD on either side of the mean contains 68% of all values under the curve of that distribution. In the same way, 1.96 × SD on either side of the mean contains 95% of the entire population. The 99% limits fall 2.58 SDs to either side of the mean.

The methods involved in calculating the mean, median, mode, and SD are usually made through the use of a statistical package, and the theory of their calculation can be examined in any fundamental book on statistics.

The confidence in results is important in the examination of distributions. This is considered in the calculation of the distribution statistics *per se*, but generally the greater the number of samples analyzed to calculate a distribution, the greater the confidence one can have in evaluating any result with respect to that distribution. The confidence value for any sample can be measured and used to ascribe confidence in a result with regard to the distribution statistic, although this is not common.

6.2.2. Nonnormal Distributions

The analysis of nonnormal distributions requires more complex mathematical considerations. Differences among mean, median, and mode alert the operator to nonsymetrical distributions.

6.3. Variation in Practice

The mean (X), SD, and %CV are used as indicators of the variation on data. The formula for X is as follows:

$$X = X_i / N$$

in which X is an individual component and N is the sample size. The formula for SD and %CV are as follows:

$$\mathrm{SD} = (X_i - X)^2 / (N - 1)$$

$$\%\ \mathrm{CV} = (\mathrm{SD}/X) \times 100$$

Worked examples of the use of statistics is most worthwhile.

6.3.1. Example Data

A number of supposedly negative samples (n = 421) have been analyzed by an indirect ELISA for the detection of antibodies. A single dilution was measured for each sample and the data were collected as OD values and based on a validated assay. Note that one concept in validation is the examination of populations to establish what we think of as a negative result. The distribution of data from a selected "negative" population will help describe any other test result as falling into or out of that population. Whether the population is actually negative with respect, e.g., to detecting a specific antibody is important and not always easy to ascertain. Examination of a large data set will indicate possible problems in determining whether there is wider dispersion (range) of results than might be expected. What is expected in a negative population is that all results will be low (OD) with a low variation. This can be examined, and any results with very high ODs can be reexamined. The object here is to plot the data as a frequency distribution and then calculate the mean and SD of that population. The selection of a negative population is easier from countries where there has never been a particular disease, but this does not rule out nonspecific results nor that the parameters measured, say, in cattle from England are the same as those in the Sudan.

Data

Figure 10 shows all the data plotted as a frequency distribution. Since we have taken a relatively large population, this might be reasonably expected to represent the distribution inherent in the whole population. However, the sample must be regarded with respect to the estimated total number of animals in a population and the possible geographical variations.

Note that the calculated mean, median, and mode are similar, indicating a normal distribution. We can therefore use statistics to set various limits as to values with respect to the mean and SD. Thus, from the data shown in **Fig. 10**, we see that the mean is 13.18 and that the SD is 5.76. Hence, 95% of all results lay between plus and minus 2 × SD of the mean. Therefore, the mean plus 2 × SD = 24.7, and the mean minus 2 × SD = 1.68. Any values outside the upper value of 24.7 would be more unusual in the population of negatives, and above 3 × SD very unusual. The population examined appeared to give results that were normally distributed. The mean value of this population and the SD can be used to determine the positivity of samples.

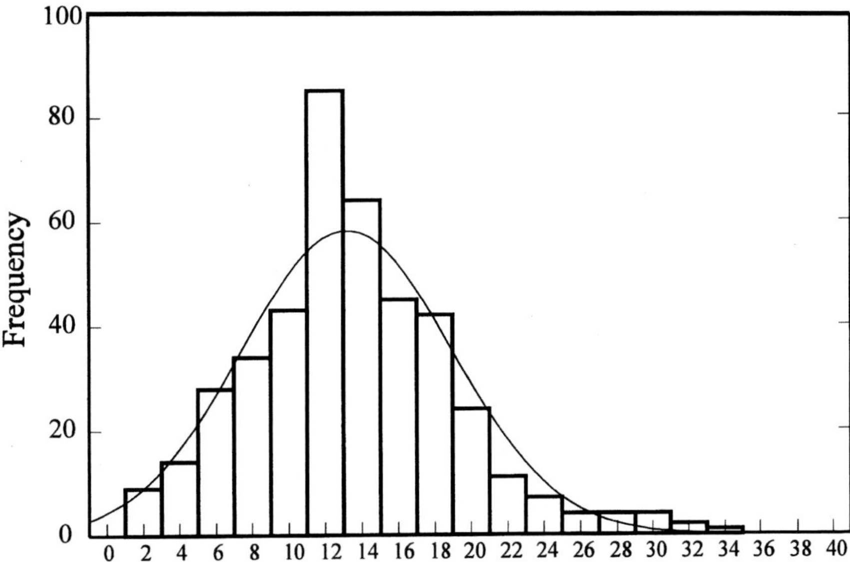

Fig. 8.10. Distribution plot of 421 samples. Data were analyzed in a statistical program and showed the following: mean = 13.18; mode = 11.68; median = 12.00; lower quartile = 10; upper quartile = 16; interquartile range = 6; standard error of mean (SEM) – 0.28; variance = 33.20; SD = 5.76; CV = 0.44.

The confidence we can have in any datum point (sample) can be determined with respect to the calculations based on the negative population examined. This requires the consideration of some statistical terms.

6.4. Confidence Interval

The CI for a mean essentially describes where the population mean (u) lies with respect to the sample mean X with a given probability. If several means are available from different groups of measurements of the same sample, the individual means will also be distributed normally around the grand mean. The random variation in a population of means is described by the SEM:

$$S_X = \mathrm{SD}/N$$

By using the SE of the experimentally determined mean one can give a CI that has a known probability of including the true population mean. This depends on the number of measurements (N), the SD and the level of confidence desired:

$$\mu = X \pm (t\mathrm{SD}/N)$$

or

$$\mu = X \pm (tS_X)$$

The value of t is taken from a table and depends on the level of confidence required or the level of probability (p) that u is outside the CI because of chance alone and the number of degrees of freedom (v, which is one less than the sample size) associated with the estimation of SD. Thus, values such as $p = 0.05$ indicate a 95% confidence limit [100 (1–p)%], that the interval includes the true mean. Basically, this means that we examine the variation in the result for a single sample (its mean and variation as error), and see where this fits in the distribution (with its internal variation).

The t values also fit a normal distribution. Here, one is making an assumption that the true population mean and SD are known, and because the CI is being made to include the true mean, the 0.5 probability that μ is beyond the calculated limits a is spread over both ends of the distribution (both tails). Here a two-sided interval, $p = 0.5$ t value, is used. The uses in which a single tail (above or below the mean) is considered, a one-sided t value ($p = 0.025$ is used (equivalent to the two-sided $p = 0.05$). The object then is (1) to have a defined total population statistic and (2) to examine where and with what confidence a sample value fits into this population. Some points need to be made concerning confidence limits.

1. No error can be calculated in which a single sample alone is measured. One element during the development of an assay is that the random error can be measured for many samples. This generally tends to be a compound of the internal variations of all aspects of sample analysis, and thus an overall generalized error can be calculated and "imposed" on all samples.
2. The SD of the population mean (S_X) is smaller than the sample SD. The SD decreases as the square root of the number of samples is averaged; thus, obviously, the mean of the population is a better approximation of the true mean (u) than any single sample. As the number of samples increases, the CI for the mean increasingly decreases, because of the decreasing SD of the mean and of the decreasing value of t.
3. The defining of confidence limits requires the analyst to make a subjective choice of a level of confidence. The higher the level of confidence, the wider the limits.

As indicated already, the calculation of confidence limits does depend on the random errors following a Gaussian distribution, and this can be tested by χ^2 squared or Kolmogorov-Smirnov testing, but in the main immunoassay, data follow the Gaussian statistic, which can often be proved throughout assay validation through repeat testing of samples.

7. Optimization of ELISA Procedures: New Approach

Recently, a method for optimizing ELISA procedures has been demonstrated *(13)*. This method attempts to compare the net effects of different conditions using an experimental design called the Taguchi method. The method attempts to reduce the effects of the interactions of optimized variables, making it possible to access the optimal conditions even in cases in which there are large interactions among variables. The proposed scheme is said to allow calculation of the biochemical parameters of the ELISA. Thus, the calibration curve and the intra- and the interassay variability can be calculated in one step. This compares with the step-by-step approach of CBTs. The method is exemplified using an ELISA required to be optimal for the detection of the single-chain fragment of variable phages. The calculations are made through a spreadsheet program. This procedure is worth examining when considering the optimization of ELISAs and is one of the few designs intended to allow optimization based on a simple statistical evaluation. The design is based on that used to optimize the PCR *(14, 15)*.

References

1. Deshpande, S. S. (1996) in *Enzyme Immunoassays from Concept to Product Development*, Chapter 9, Chapman and Hall, International Thomson Publishing, New York.
2. Miller, J. J. and Valdes, R. (1991) Approaches to minimizing interference by cross-reactive molecules in immunoassays. *Clin. Chem.* 37, 144–153.
3. Westgard, J. O., Barry, P. L., and Hunt, M. R. (1981) A multi-rule Shewhart chart for quality control in clinical chemistry. *Clin. Chem.* 27, 493–501.
4. Blockx, P. and Martin, M. (1994) Laboratory quality assurance, in *The Immunoassay Handbook* (Wild, D., ed.), Stockton Press, New York, pp. 263–276.
5. Seth, J. (1991) Standardization and quality assurance, in *Principles and Practice of Immunoassays* (Price, C. P. and Newman, D. J., eds.), Stockton Press, New York, pp. 154–189.
6. Perlstein, M. T. (1987) Immunoassays. Quality control and troubleshooting, in *Immunoassay: A practical Guide* (Chan, D. W. and Perlstein, M. T., eds.), Academic, Orlando, FL, pp. 149–163.
7. Gosling, J. P. and Basso, L. V. (1994). Quality assurance, in *Immunoassay: Laboratory Analysis and Clinical Applications*, (Gosling, J. P. and Basso, L. V., eds.), Butterworth-Heinemann, London, pp. 69–81.
8. Deshpand, S. S. (1996) *Enzyme Immunoassays from Concept to Product Development.* Chapman and Hall, International Thomson Publishing, New York.
9. Jacobson, R. H. (1998) Validation of serological assays for diagnosis of infectious diseases. *Rev. Sci. Tech. OIE.* **17**, 469–486.
10. Anderson, G. and Scott, M. (1991) Determination of product shelf life and activation energy required for five drugs of abuse. *Clin. Chem.* 37, 398–402.
11. Office International des Epizooties (1998) Principles of validation of diagnostic assays for infectious diseases, in *Manual of Standards for Diagnostic Tests and Vaccines,* Office International des Epizooties (OIE), Paris, pp. 8–15.
12. Gardner, I. A. and Greiner, M. (1999) *Advanced Methods for Test Validation and*

Interpretation in Veterinary Medicine. Freee University, Berlin and University of California, Davis, CA (report).

13. Jeney, C., Dobay, O., Lengyel, A., Adam, E., and Nasz, I. (1999) Tagushi optimisation of ELISA procedures. *J. Immunol. Methods* 223, 137–146.
14. Cobb, B. B. and Clarkson, J. M. (1994) A simple procedure for optimizing the polymerase chain reaction (PCR) using modified Taguchi methods. *Nucleic Acids Res.* **18**, 3801–3805.
15. Burch, G. J., Ferguson, C. H., Cartwright, G., and Kwong, F. Y. (1995) Application of Taguchi experimental design to the optimization of a baculo expression system. *Biochem. Soc. Trans.* 23(1), 107S.

Chapter 9

Charting Methods for Internal Quality Control for Competition ELISA

This chapter deals with relatively simple ways to use control charts to monitor the performance of ELISAs. A rinderpest competition ELISA, for the estimation of antibodies in serum samples, is used to demonstrate the methods. This assay is available in a kit form. Constant evaluation of the use of the kit is part of what is called internal quality control (IQC). **Figure 1** shows an overview of the ELISA scheme described in this chapter. The details of the procedure, which involves plotting the data graphically (charting methods), are explained herein. The objectives of charting data are as follows:

1. To keep a constant record of all data.
2. To monitor the assay from plate to plate in any one day's testing.
3. To monitor the tests made from day to day, week to week, year to year.
4. To allow rapid identification of unacceptable results.
5. To allow recognition of reagent problems.
6. To identify trends in results (increasingly poor performance).
7. To identify when a new set of kit reagents is necessary.
8. To allow identification of differences among operators of the assay.
9. To fulfill various criteria for good laboratory practice.
10. To fulfill necessary requirements for external recognition to prove that tests are being performed at an acceptable level (increasingly important when results are used for international trading purposes).

John R. Crowther, *Methods in Molecular Biology, The ELISA Guidebook, Vol. 516*

DOI: 10.1007/978-1-60327-254-4_9

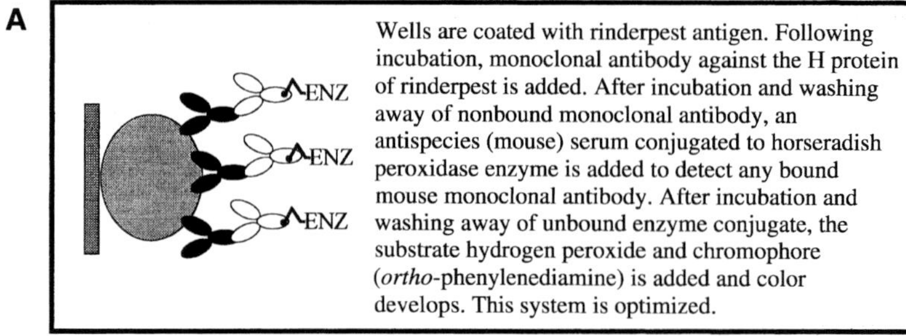

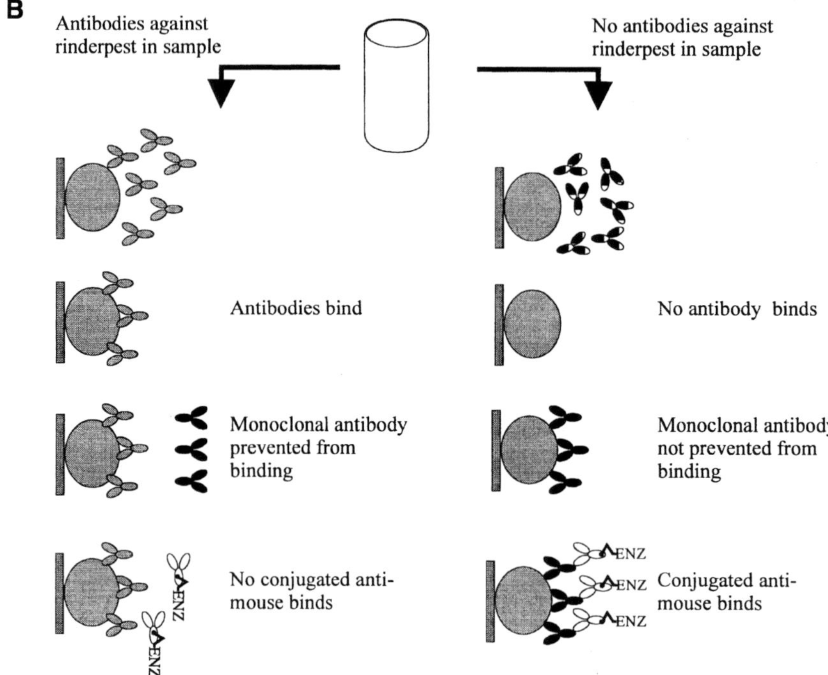

Fig. 1. Principles of competitive ELISA for measuring antibodies against rinderpest virus: (**A**) pretitration of indirect ELISA; (**B**) blocking of ELISA to detect anti-rinderpest antibodies in serum samples.

1. Good Practice of IQC

IQC methods allow test operators as individuals to monitor the performance of their test. When there is more than one operator, the method produces a unification of approach, to allow control over results, and allows discrepancies among performances to be identified. It also promotes the idea of "open" results that can be viewed by anyone, including outside scientists, interested in evaluating the status of a laboratory involved in providing results on which management decisions concerning disease control are made.

The method described here is not a deep statistical analysis of data. Rather, it attempts to visually assess results, so as to increase the awareness of operators about what they are doing on a daily, monthly, and yearly cycle of work. The most important feature of testing in a laboratory is that operators have a very good understanding of the principles of the test they are using, and that they fully understand the nature of their test results and the need to process data. There is no substitute for this understanding, but the charting method recommended is an aid to simplify the process of monitoring test performance. At a first glance, this approach may seem to be overcomplicated. However, it is to be assumed that people involved in testing have had some training and are running the assays on a fairly routine basis.

1.1. Principles of ELISA for Detection of Antibodies Against Rinderpest

Figure 1 shows the principles of the ELISA used. The basis of the test is the prevention of pretitrated monoclonal antibody (mAb) from binding to the rinderpest antigen on the wells of a microtiter plate by polyclonal antibodies in the samples (serum). The degree of prevention is measured with reference to controls with no sample added (Cm) in which maximum optical density (OD) values are observed, and to wells in which only the conjugate is added (Cc) where low color is observed. Percentage inhibition (PI%) values are calculated with reference to these values.

Control serum samples are provided in the kits, which give strong (C++) and moderate (C+) PI% values. These controls can be used for assessment of the test from plate to plate and day to day. The plate design for the kits is shown in **Fig. 2**. For each plate, 40 samples are examined in duplicate, at a single dilution, and the controls are placed as shown. Each PI% value is then calculated with reference to the controls of individual plates. Studies

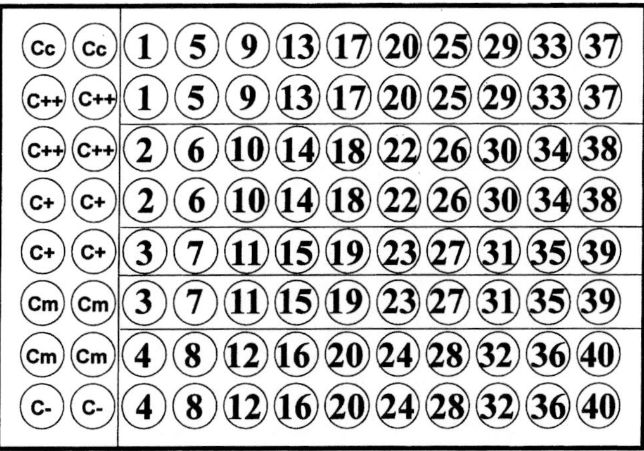

Fig. 2. Plate layout for rinderpest competition ELISA. Controls are C++ (strong antibody positive); C+ (weaker antibody positive); Cm (mAb control, no sample); and C– (conjugate control, no sample or mAb).

on large numbers of negative sera and experimentally infected animals have determined the PI% values that ascribe positivity to samples.

On receipt of the kits, operators should have everything to be able to perform the assay. The control sera enable operators to monitor the assay routinely, and the use of these data in control charts is the basis of this chapter. The necessary data for plotting on various charts is obtained through the calculation of the mean and standard deviation (SD), from the mean of control samples as raw OD data or PI% values.

2. Charts

Two kinds of charts are recommended: *(1)* Daily Detailed Data (DDD) charts, used to plot data from single plates; and *(2)* Summary Data Charts (SDC), used to plot data from all plates used on any day.

The use of such charts at various points of the rinderpest ELISA is illustrated in **Fig. 3**. The processing of data for plotting on the charts is important, and illustrative tables suitable for this purpose are presented in **Figs. 4–7**. Raw (nonprocessed) OD values, for each plate, are plotted for the Cm controls only on DDD charts and SDC charts. The PI% values are monitored for all controls on DDD and SDC charts. In terms of the practical use of these charts, a few rules can be given. These encourage the best use of the charts to allow easy monitoring and transparency of results to permit identification of problems on a continuous basis.

2.1. General Recommendations for Charting Methods

1. Charts should be displayed openly (on walls) and copies are also to be kept in a file.
2. A specific individual should be appointed to oversee the charts. This individual should ensure that all the people performing the assays fill in the tables and chart the results. This individual should ensure that only relevant data are added to the charts, for example, plates used for developmental work or research should not be included, but only those involved in running a routine assay be included.
3. The results on the charts should be discussed regularly with all those involved in laboratory testing, as well as any trends identified and appropriate action be taken.

2.2. Initial Examination of Kits

A great deal of care has been taken to ensure that the reagents and materials will work in laboratories worldwide with dif ferent local conditions, and that the kit will travel without deterioration

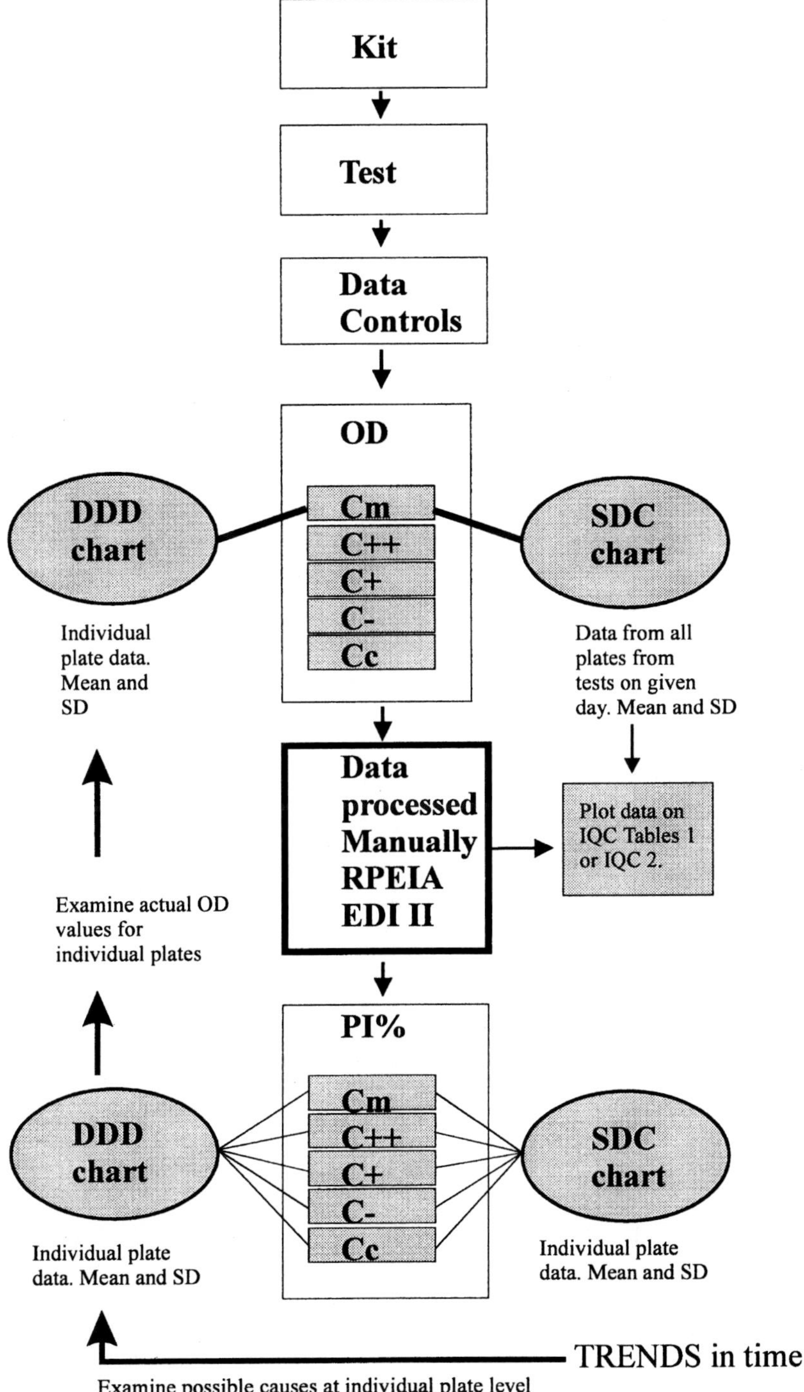

Fig. 3. Scheme for plotting data on charts.

of performance. On receipt of a kit, there are two initial questions: (1) How do we know that the kit reagents are working as expected? and, (2) How can we ensure that the kit keeps on working, i.e., the established diagnostic criteria are maintained?

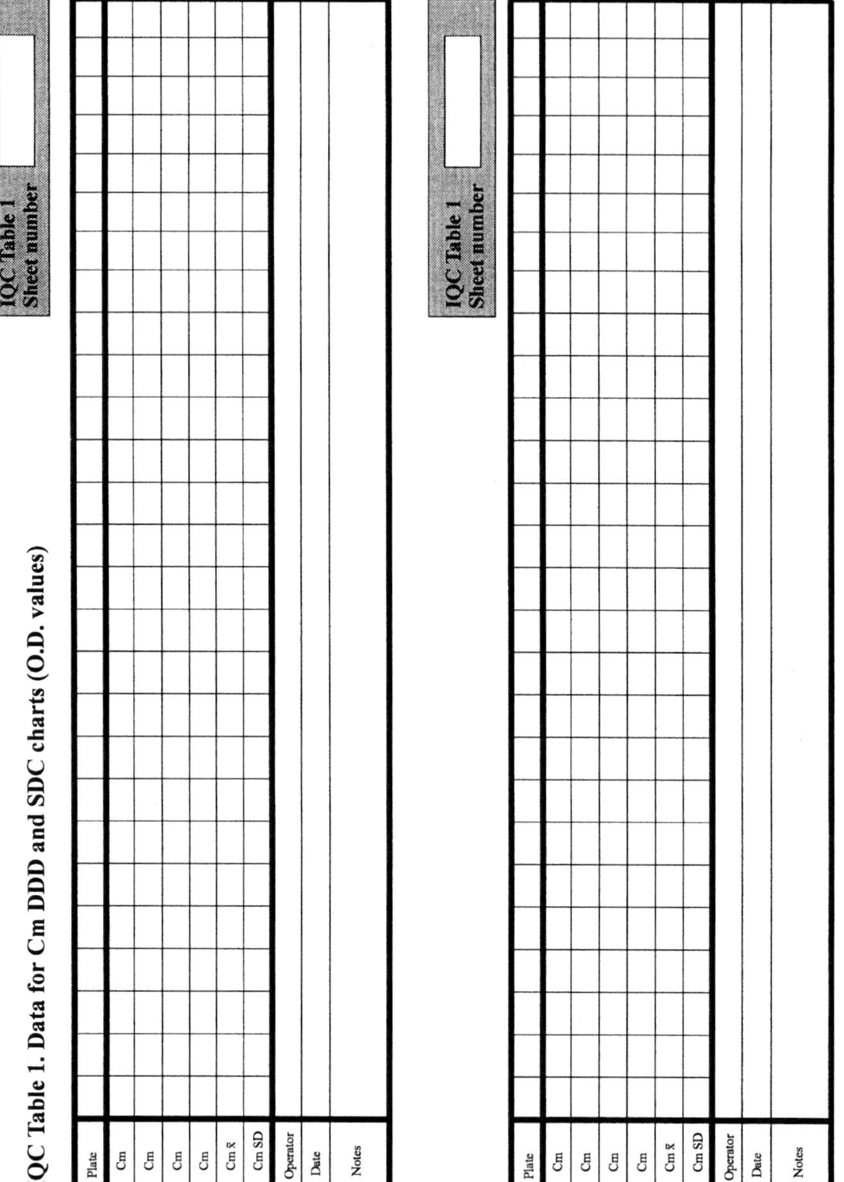

IQC Table 1. Data for Cm DDD and SDC charts (O.D. values)

IQC Table 1
Sheet number

Plate																												
Cm																												
Cm																												
Cm																												
Cm																												
Cm $\bar{x}$																												
Cm SD																												
Operator																												
Date																												
Notes																												

IQC Table 1
Sheet number

Plate																												
Cm																												
Cm																												
Cm																												
Cm																												
Cm $\bar{x}$																												
Cm SD																												
Operator																												
Date																												
Notes																												

Fig. 4. Tables of Cm controls as OD values for DDD and SDC analysis.

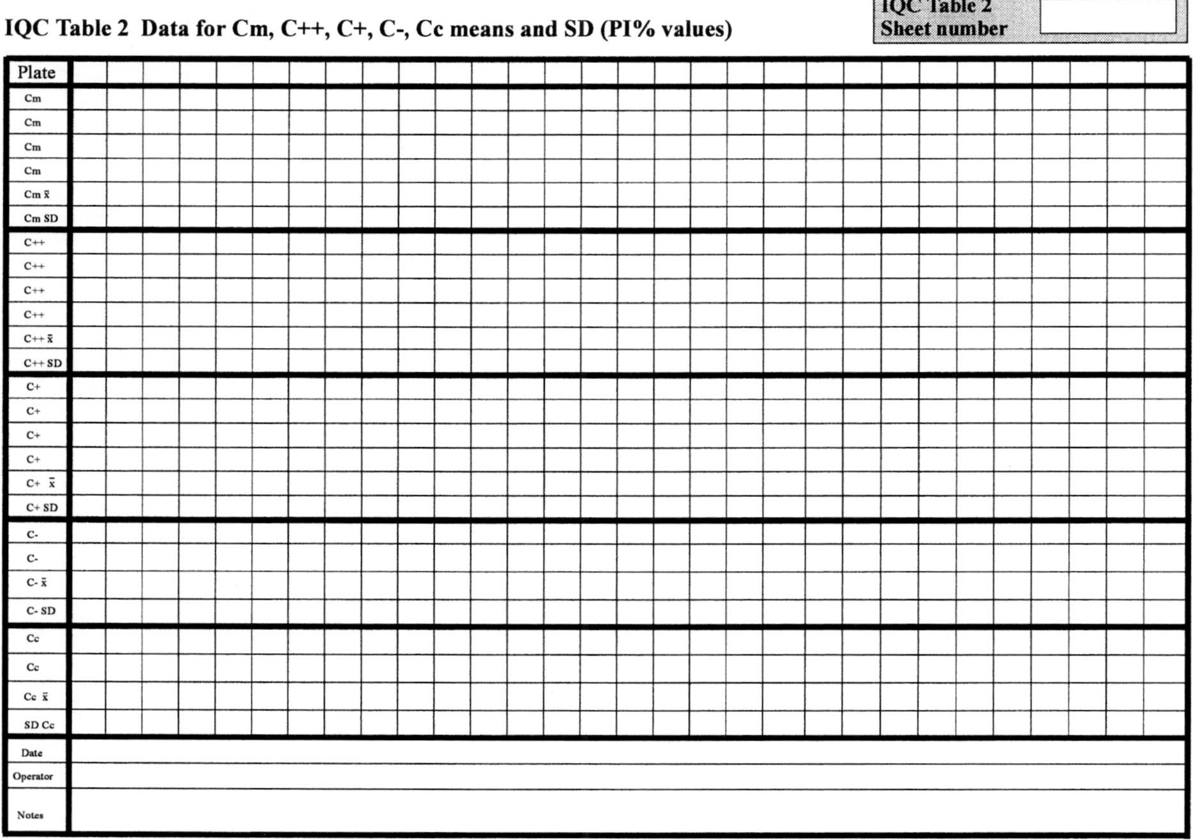

IQC Table 2 Data for Cm, C++, C+, C-, Cc means and SD (PI% values)

IQC Table 2
Sheet number

Plate
Cm
Cm
Cm
Cm
Cm $\bar{x}$
Cm SD
C++
C++
C++
C++
C++ $\bar{x}$
C++ SD
C+
C+
C+
C+
C+ $\bar{x}$
C+ SD
C-
C-
C- $\bar{x}$
C- SD
Cc
Cc
Cc $\bar{x}$
SD Cc
Date
Operator
Notes

Fig. 5. Table for data from Cm, C++, C+, C–, and Cc controls as PI%.

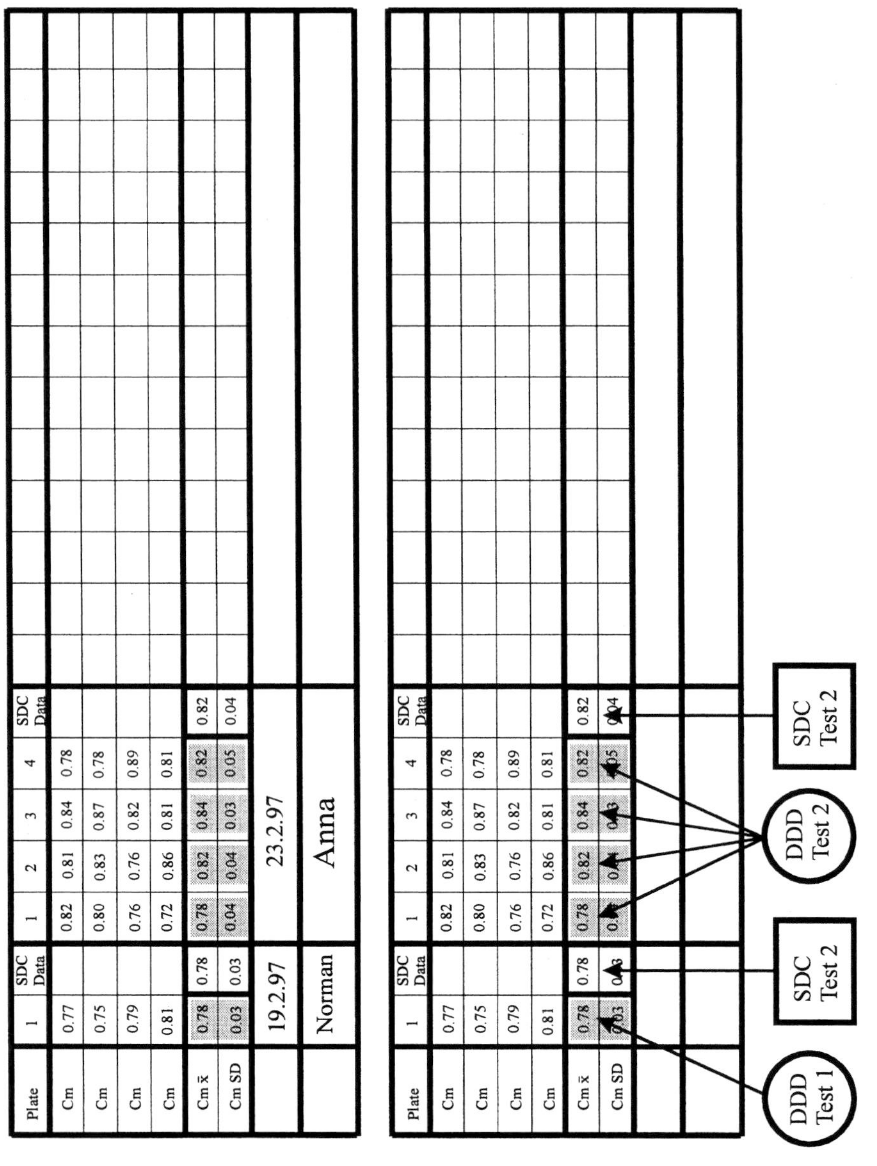

Plate	1	SDC Data	1	2	3	4	SDC Data
Cm	0.77		0.82	0.81	0.84	0.78	
Cm	0.75		0.80	0.83	0.87	0.78	
Cm	0.79		0.76	0.76	0.82	0.89	
Cm	0.81		0.72	0.86	0.81	0.81	
Cm x̄	0.78	0.78	0.78	0.82	0.84	0.82	0.82
Cm SD	0.03	0.03	0.04	0.04	0.03	0.05	0.04
	19.2.97		23.2.97				
	Norman		Anna				

Plate	1	SDC Data	1	2	3	4	SDC Data
Cm	0.77		0.82	0.81	0.84	0.78	
Cm	0.75		0.80	0.83	0.87	0.78	
Cm	0.79		0.76	0.76	0.82	0.89	
Cm	0.81		0.72	0.86	0.81	0.81	
Cm x̄	0.78	0.78	0.78	0.82	0.84	0.82	0.82
Cm SD	0.03	0.03	0.04	0.04	0.03	0.05	0.04

Fig. 6. Illustration of use of IQC Table 1 for obtaining DDD and SDC data.

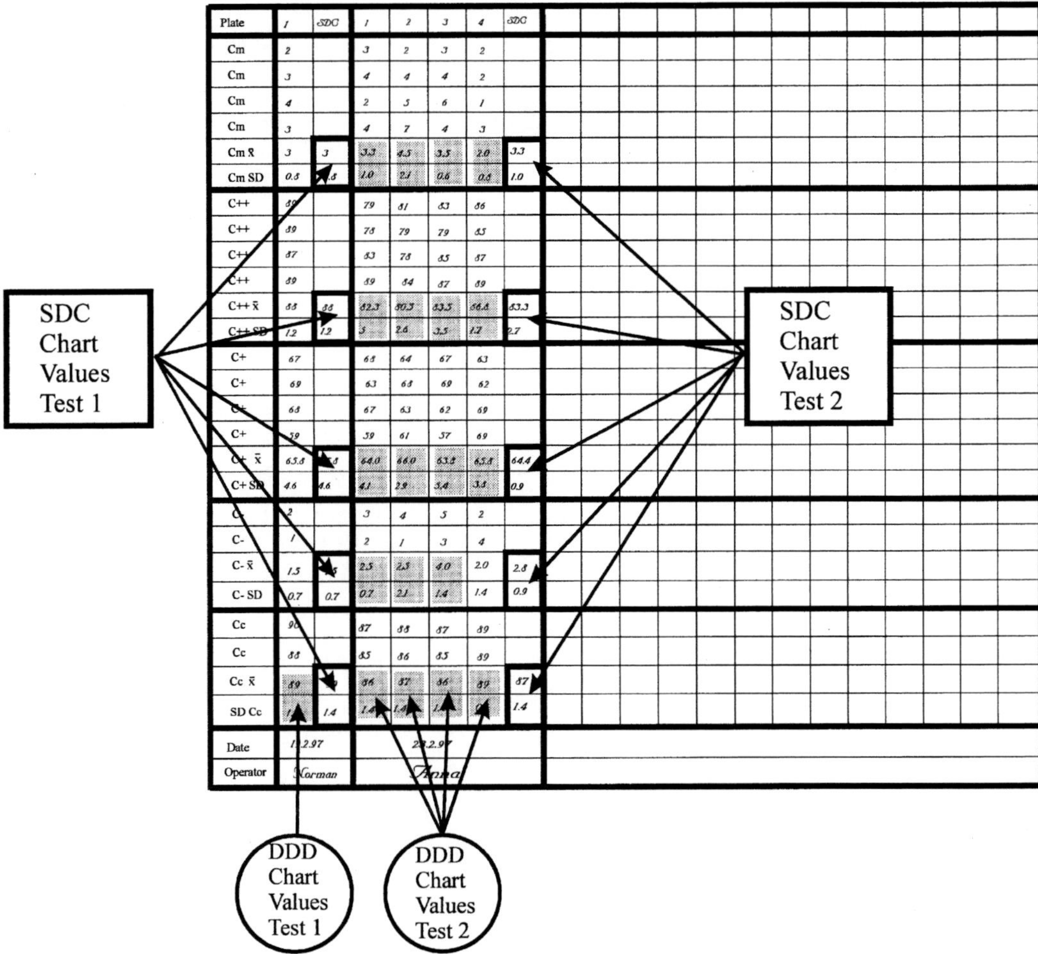

Fig. 7. Illustration of use of IQC Table 2 for processing data.

The first task then is to run an assay with the kit using available control reagents and to examine the results in the context of parameters given in the manual. This tells us whether the kit is performing as expected.

2.3. Running the Assay for the First Time

The following controls have been examined in the test. Test operators should familiarize themselves with the controls and their purpose. This information should be contained in the manual accompanying the kit.

Controls on ELISA plates are as follows:

1. Cm, mAb control.
2. C++, strong positive control.
3. C+, moderate positive control.
4. C–, negative serum control.
5. Cc, conjugate control (no serum/no monoclonal).

Note the following conditions of the test:

1. The results expected (and the limits allowed) have been worked out by the suppliers of the kits.
2. These controls have been assessed many times and the results examined statistically.
3. The results using the control reagents have fixed limits.
4. If the results obtained are the same or within allowable limits, then your test is good.
5. If the results are outside the limits, then something is wrong.

2.4. Data Processing Fundamentals

Let us deal with the fundamentals of what the data processing does. Initial checks should determine that the controls have been placed in particular positions on the plate as shown in **Fig. 2**. A typical set of OD data for the controls is shown in **Table 1**. The data is processed to calculate PI% values and are shown in **Table 2**.

Table 1
Data for control sera on one plate

Control	Data(OD)
Cc	0.010(0.009)
C++	0.077(0.063)
C++	0.072(0.071)
C+	0.278(0.296)
C+	0.313(0.280)
Cm	0.685(0.673)
Cm	0.636(0.641)
C–	0.668(0.667)

Table 2
Control samples data after processing

	OD_1	OD_2	OD_3	OD_4	$PI\%_1$	$PI\%_2$	$PI\%_3$	$PI\%_4$
C++	0.077	0.063	0.072	0.071	88	90	89	89.
C+	0.278	0.296	0.313	0.280	53	55	52	57
C–	0.668	0.667	—	—	–2	–2	—	—
Cc	0.011	0.09	—	—	98	99	—	—
Cm	0.685	0.673	0.636	0.641	–4	–2	–9	–8

The processing can be by hand (calculator) or through the use of dedicated software (as in the case of rinderpest ELISA). The formula for calculating the PI% value is as follows:

$$\text{PI\%} = 100 - [(\text{mean of replicate OD controls}/\text{median OD Cm}) \times 100]$$

2.4.1. Calculation of Mean and Standard Deviation

The mean for each control sample is obtained by adding up all the individual values and dividing by the number of values used (the number of values is usually ascribed the letter n). The sign for the average (mean) is x. Thus, for the previously cited example, the mean OD for the Cm is:

$$0.455 + 0.612 + 0.533 + 0.655 = 2.255/4 = 0.564.$$

The standard deviation (SD) in mathematical terms is the positive square root of the variance of the data. The variance is measured by subtracting the mean of the test wells, data ($\bar{x}1$, $\bar{x}2$, $\bar{x}3$, and so on) from the overall mean value (X) and squaring that value. Each of these squared values is then added. The resulting value is divided by the total number of datum points used minus one. We therefore have:

$$\text{Variance} = \frac{(X-\bar{x}1)^2+(X-\bar{x}2)^2+(X-\bar{x}3)^2+(X-\bar{x}4)^2}{n-1}$$

The SD is the square root of this value. As a demonstration, if we have OD data for Cm controls of 0.453, 0.612, 0.533, and 0.625, then we have for calculation of the mean and SD of OD values for Cm:

$0.565–0.453 = (0.109)^2 = 0.012$

$0.565–0.613 = (–0.048)^2 = 0.002$

$0.565–0.534 = (0.031)^2 = 0.001$

$0.565–0.656 = (–0.091)^2 = 0.008$

By adding up the values, we have 0.012 + 0.002 + 0.001 + 0.008 = 0.023. When we divide by n – 1 = 3, we have 0.023/3 = 0.0076. This is the variance. The SD is the square root of this, i.e., 0.0076 = 0.087. The Cm OD mean and SD are thus expressed as 0.564 ± 0.087.

This illustrates the principles of the calculation. In practice, this calculation is easily made using a statistical pocket calculator or using dedicated computer software associated with kits for a direct analysis of this data.

2.4.2. Recording Data in Tabular Form: before Plotting

The key to successful monitoring is attention to detail, the accurate manipulation of data, and the constant ability to check data. The next examples show how the data can be controlled by using tables, before plots are made. In this way, the operator can check the data as it is copied into the tables as well as be able to record the results of the calculations needed. The data can be stored in a file for instant reference in association with the charts.

We have to obtain the data for DDD and SDC charts. Two kinds of tables are shown to illustrate this:

1. IQC **Table 1** (shown in **Fig. 4**). This records the actual OD data for the Cm values as well as the mean and SD for each plate and the overall mean and SD for any given test.
2. IQC **Table 2** (shown in **Fig. 5**). This records the PI values for all the controls, the mean PI values and SD for each plate, and the overall mean and SD of all controls on any test.

Figure 6 illustrates filling in the data in the IQC **Table 1** and **Fig. 7** illustrates filling in the data in IQC **Table 2**. The relationship of the data according to DDD and SDC charts is shown in **Fig. 3**. This shows the necessary data needed to be plotted in terms of the controls. From **Fig. 5**, it can be seen that the data obtained in IQC **Tables 1** and **2** is in need for plotting at various times. Once in tabular form, the data can be easily plotted. Illustrations of plots are shown in **Figs. 8–20**. Tables can be filed for future reference..

The data in **Fig. 6** are described according to how it is to be plotted. Values and processed data from two tests with different operators are indicated. Column 1 shows the four Cm controls, the mean value calculated from these four controls in any single plate, and the SD of the data. The second column shows the data from a test involving a single plate. The mean value (0.78) and the SD (0.03) are put into relevant boxes after their calculation. These are plotted on the DDD charts (gray shaded boxes). The date and operator are added. The SDC value is calculated for the sum of all the mean values on all plates in a given test (in this case 1 plate so that SDC data are identical to the DDD data).

A second test is shown (four plates). Again the OD values are recorded and the mean and SDs calculated and placed in boxes along with the SD of data (shaded boxes). These are plotted on DDD charts.

The SDC data in this case is the value obtained after calculating the mean of all the individual plate PI means (DDD data means). Note that the SD of the SDC data is based only on analysis of the mean PI of individual plates; it is not the mean of the SD shown for each plate in the gray boxes.

Figure 7 shows data in the IQC **Table 2**. PI% results for two assay runs are shown. The two test days involved a single plate and four plates, respectively. The data required for SDC plots are shown in the thick lined boxes (overall mean and SD of results for all the plates run on that day). The data for the DDD charts (individual plate data) are also shown.

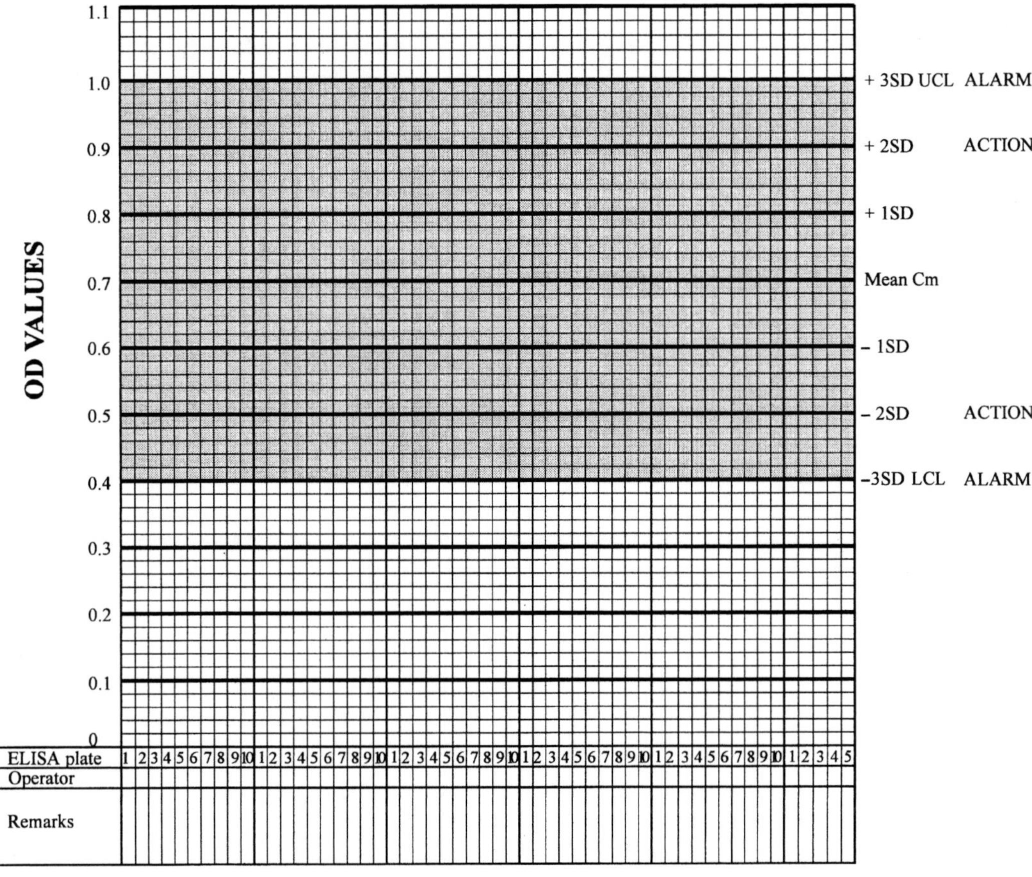

Fig. 8. Illustrative chart for DDD plots of Cm data.

3. Controlling the Assay Using Graphs: Plotting the Data

We make use of the fact that the same control sera are set up on each plate. We can examine the differences in results among the plates to keep a check on the test performance. Two kinds of data are available, as already indicated *(1)* actual OD readings, and *(2)* PI% values calculated by the software and used to assess samples.

Remember that a convenient method of viewing data is to plot values on a chart. This can be examined easily and can give a view of the data over a time period. Two kinds of charts are recommended for quality control.

1. A chart that keeps the actual data for various test parameters for each plate used. This is called a DDD.
2. A chart that summarizes data for any particular tests done on a given day. This is called an SDC.

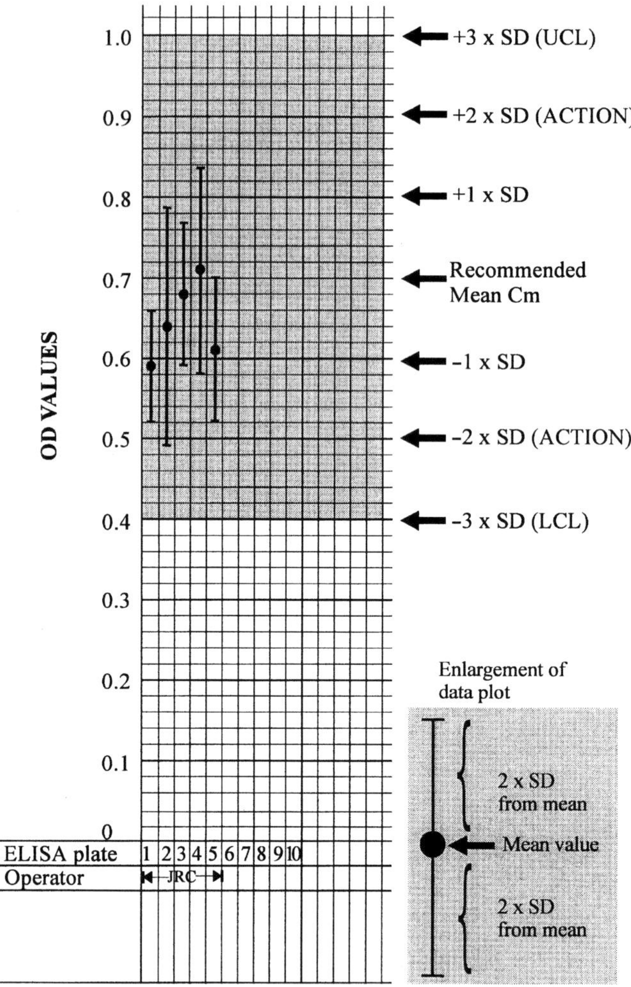

Fig. 9. Ilustrative close-up of plots of OD values on DDD chart for Cm.

3.1. Daily Detailed Data Charts

DDDs plot the OD data on the control Cm samples for each plate and the %PI values for other controls. Three charts are needed to cover all controls:

1. Cm: OD mean and SD.
2. C++ and C+: PI% mean and SD.
3. C– and Cc: PI% mean and SD.

3.1.1. Examples

Table 3 shows data from a test. Let us take the data of a plate read out as shown in **Table 3**:

cm data: 0.685, 0.673, 0.636, 0.641.

Calculate the Cm mean and SD of this data: mean = 0.659; SD = 0.024. Calculate the mean and SD for PI values given for C++, C+, C–, and Cc (*see* **Table 4**).

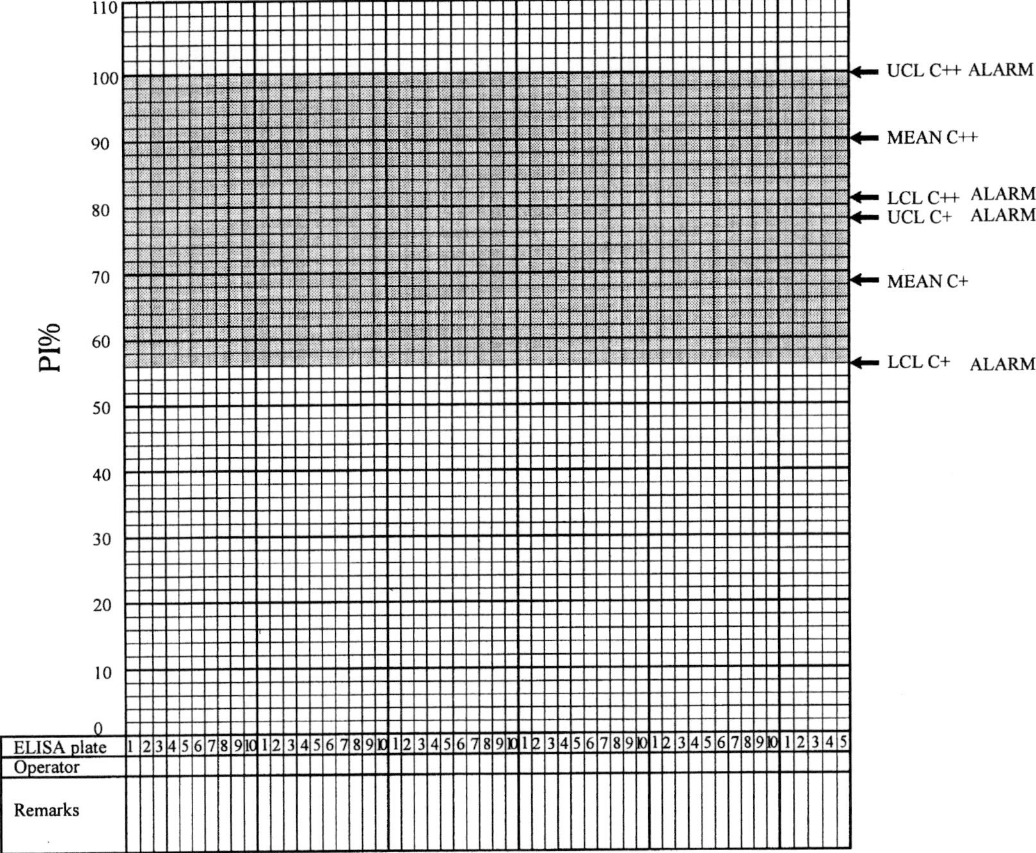

Fig. 10. Illusrative chart for DDD plots of PI% C++ and C+ data.

Multiply the SD by 2 and make a complete table as shown in IQC **Tables 1** and 2 (*see* **Table 5**). The calculation of SD gives information about the variation observed in the data and is important in assessing confidence about the calculated mean.

3.2. Plotting on DDD Charts

Note that we may have run more than one plate on any given day. The DDD charts examine the data from all the plates run so that reference to each plate can be made. Let us assume that we have run five plates on one day. The data in **Table 6** are an example of what might be expected from the five plates. The parentheses show the value of 2 × the SD for each point. Thus, for each plate the actual Cm values are noted and the PI values for each of the controls along with the SDs, are calculated. Now the data can be plotted.

3.3. DDD Chart Design

Figure 8 shows designs for plotting Cm OD. **Figure 9** shows an enlargement of an area with data plotted. **Figure 10** shows a design for a DDD control chart for PI% values. **Figure 11** illustrates an enlarged plot of data. Note that (1) the charts should

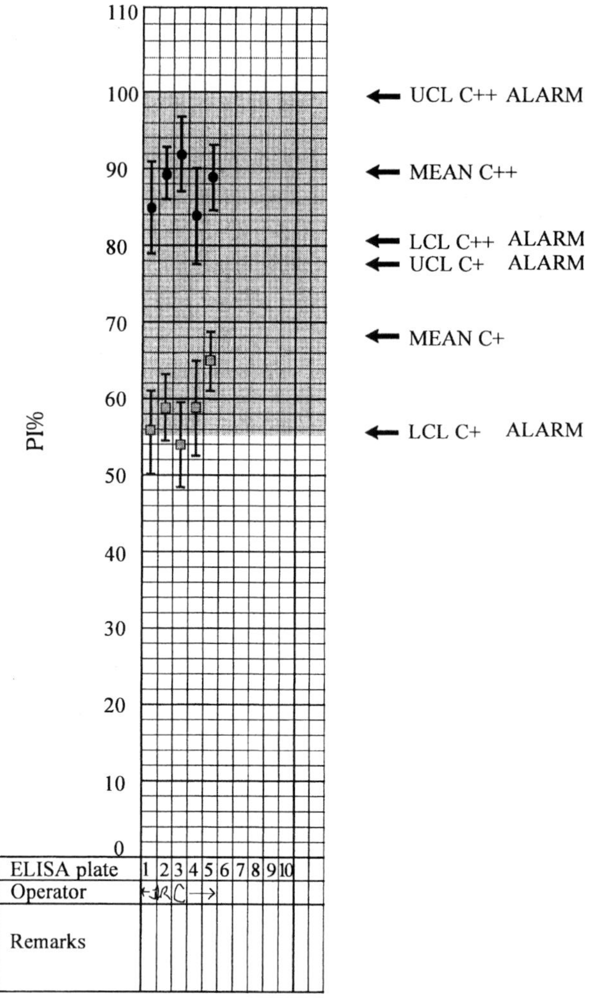

Fig. 11. Illustrative enlargement of chart for DDD plots of C++ and C+ PI% data.

be updated every time a test is made by each operator, and *(2)* the charts should be displayed preferably near where the tests are made/conducted.

In **Fig. 8**, the *y*-axis shows OD units. The *x*-axis contains columns, each one representing the data from a single plate. This chart is for plotting OD data from the Cm control. The expected mean of the Cm (given in the kit manual) and the allowed variation from the mean values are shown in the gray areas. This represents 1, 2, and 3 SD from the mean. The test values obtained on a plate should be within the ±2 × SD, preferably as close to the indicated mean as possible. The ACTION notice at ±3 × SD from the expected mean indicates that results are at too great a variance from the expected mean and that the test parameters should be examined. UCL and LCL are ALARM points representing the mean ±3 × SD values.

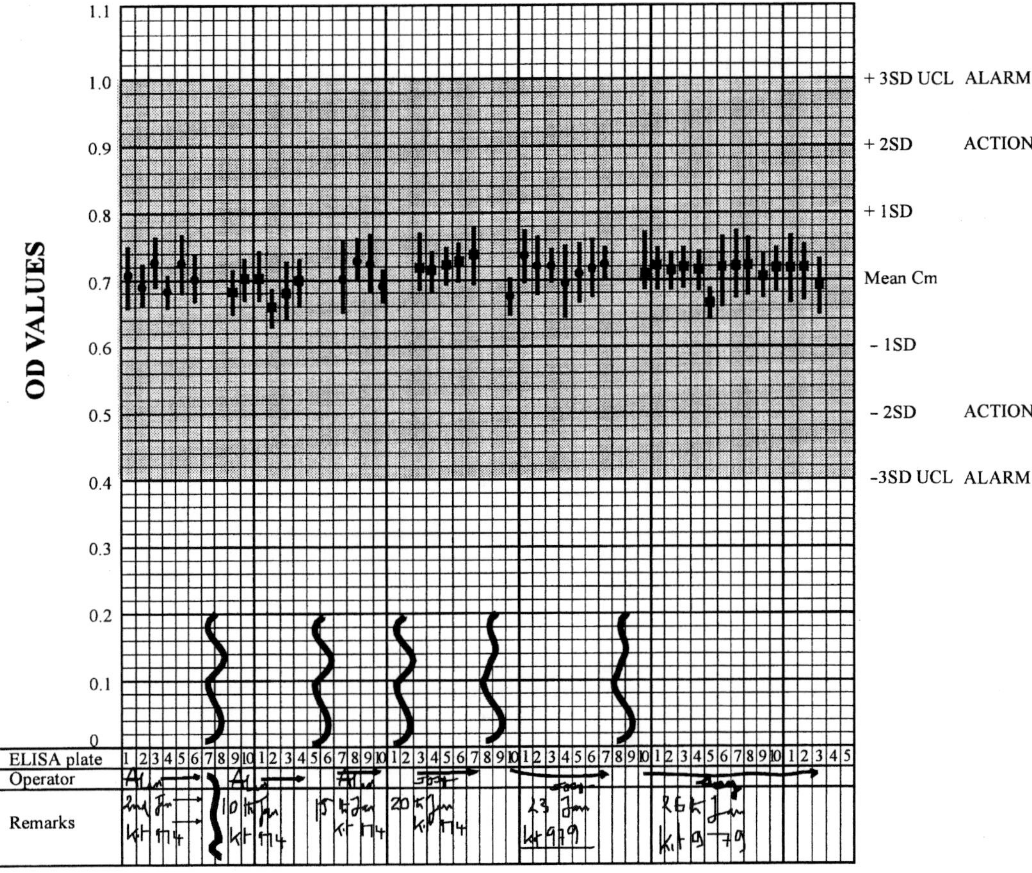

Fig. 12. Illustrative DDD chart for longer-term plots of several tests of Cm OD data.

Figure 9 shows an enlarged graph of the DDD chart with Cm data plotted. The data from the five plates examined above are plotted as mean and ±2 × SD from the mean Cm OD values. Note that the operator is indicated in the lower left-hand corner. This is important when tracing any problems (identifying specific problems to particular operators). Note also that this space should be used to indicate the date (to identify when the test was made). Similar considerations are shown in **Figs. 10** and **11**, in which the PI% values are shown. The limit values are also shown.

4. Summary Data Charts (SDC)

The DDD charts are plotted as an accurate reference of the test performance on each plate. The assessment of the whole test performed on a day-to-day, week-to-week, month-to-month, and year-to-year basis is examined by plotting data on SDC charts.

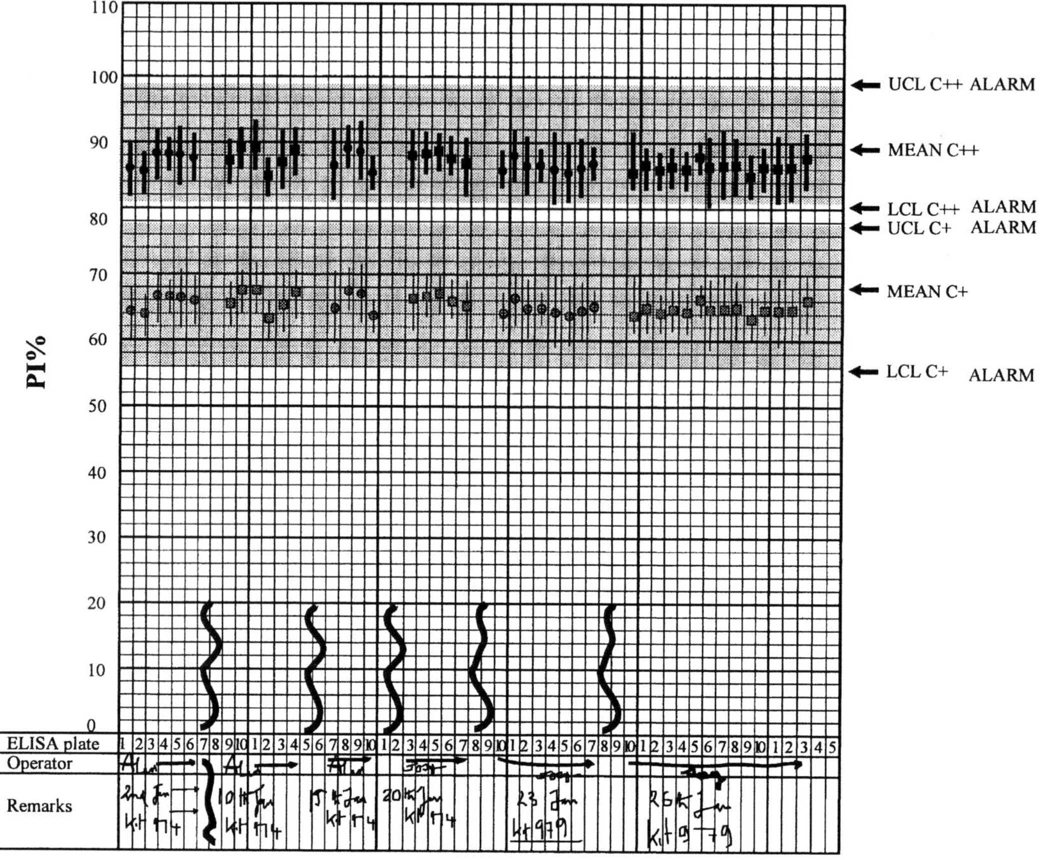

Fig. 13. Illustrative DDD chart for plots of C++ and C+ PI% data.

The SDC charts differ fundamentally from the DDD charts in that the data plotted represent the mean and variation from all the plates used in an assay is treated as a group. Thus, if only 1 plate is used on a particular day, then the data are used to plot the SDC chart points for that day. If 5 plates are used, then these will be used to obtain the SDC data for that day. If 35 plates are used, they will collectively give the SDC chart data for that day. If two series of tests are made on the same day, representing 5 and 6 plates, respectively, then the data from all 11 plates are processed to give the SDC data.

4.1. Data Processing for SDC Charts

Printouts from software packages or by-hand calculations give the PI% values for the various control sera used for each plate. Thus, we have PI% values for Cm, C++, C+, C–, and Cc. The SDC data are obtained by taking all the given mean values for any of the control sera and calculating the mean and SD of that data. The Cm OD data are also plotted on an SDC. The mean of

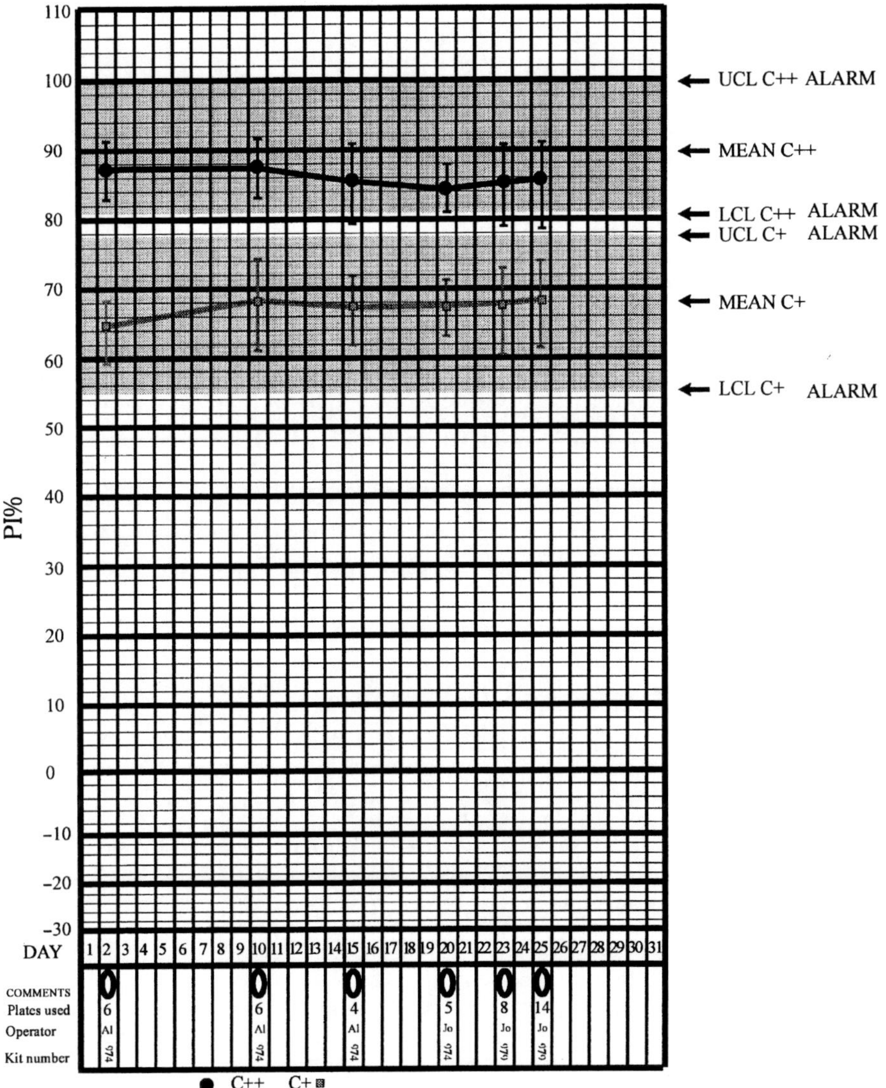

Fig. 14. Illustrative SDC chart for plots of C++ and C+ PI% data.

all the Cm values for a set of plates is calculated and the SD from this mean is plotted.

4.1.1. Example

We may have made a test on five plates. The mean PI% values on each plate are as given in **Table 7**. Calculate the mean and SD for each column (*see* **Table 8**).

4.2. Plotting Data

The values shown in **Table 8** are plotted on the SDC charts. As with the DDD, the plotting is split into different charts to cover the controls. The main idea here is to plot the summary data in real time.

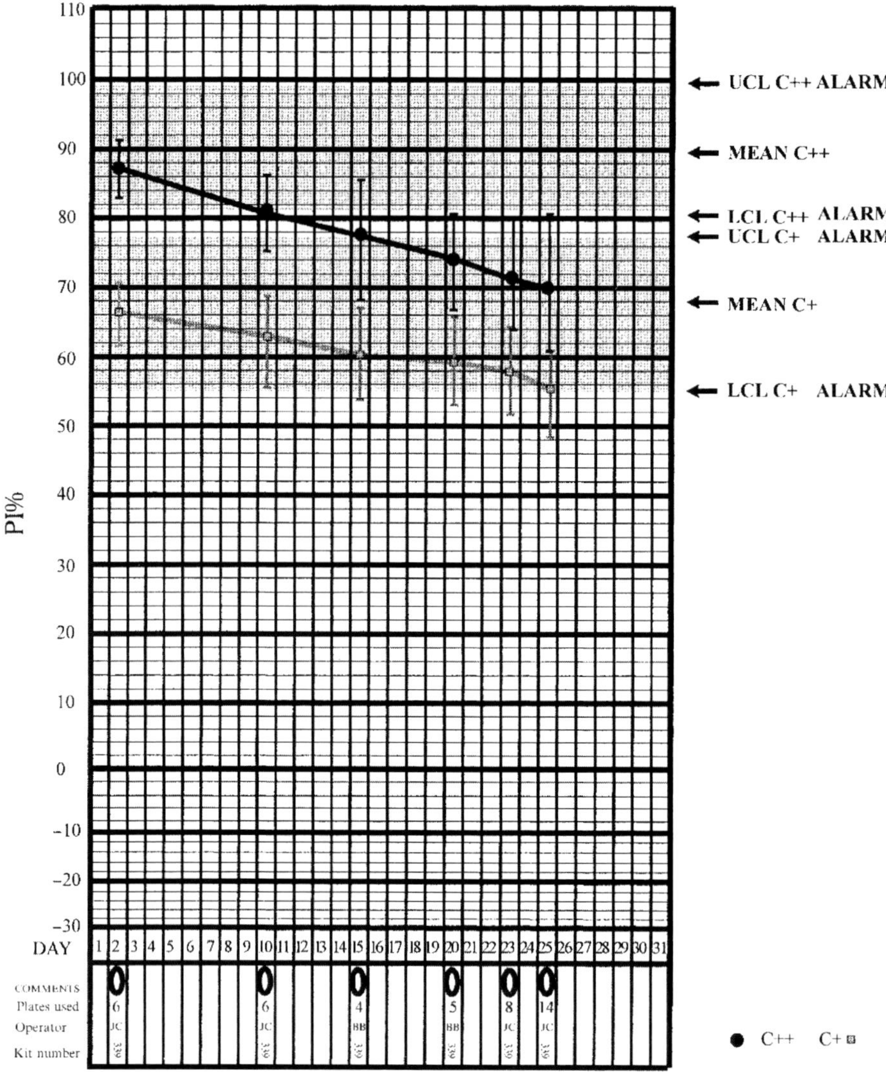

Fig. 15. Illustrative SDC chart of C++ and C+ PI% data showing downward trend.

The charts each have 31 days, so that the actual day in the month when the test is performed can be plotted:

1. Plot Cm data on one chart as summary OD values.
2. Plot C++ and C+ data on one chart as summary PI% values.
3. Plot Cc and C– data on one chart as summary PI% values.

The data are plotted on a calendar chart that measures the exact date when tests are performed. These data are first plotted on the example charts as shown. Each chart can plot data from day 1 of any particular month.

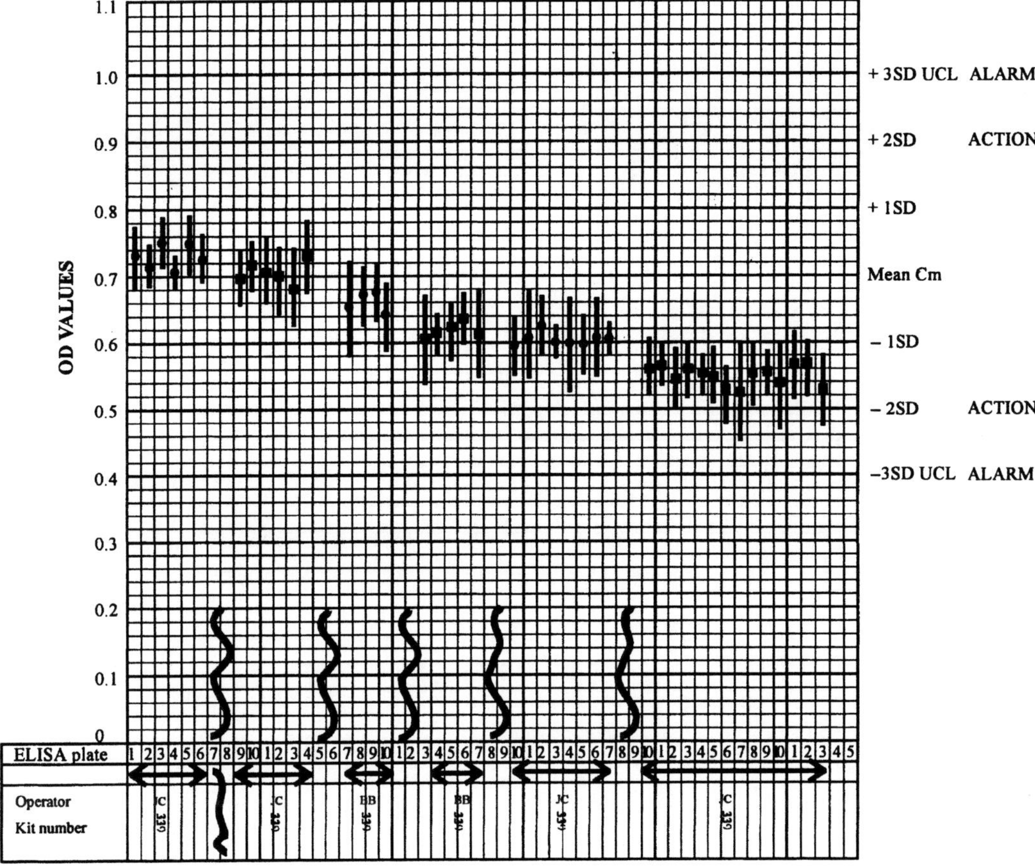

Fig. 16. Illustrative DDD chart for Cm OD values showing downward trend.

5. Interpretation of Charts

The purpose of charting the data is to help monitor the performance of the kit in its use to measure antibodies against rinderpest. The points of assessment are always with reference to the performance of the control sera and reagents supplied.

The data on these reagents have been obtained after multiple testing so that expected values and variation from these values have been recorded and calculated. The key assumption is that these are constants in the assay, i.e., that all the reagents and controls will remain the same, physically, throughout the time that they are used in the tests. Note that because of this assumption we have to be very careful not to handle the control samples carelessly, as they set the control limits of the assay.

The control serum samples represent sera containing an excess of anti-rinderpest antibodies (C++) and a relatively weak serum (C+) that should not give maximal inhibition but always

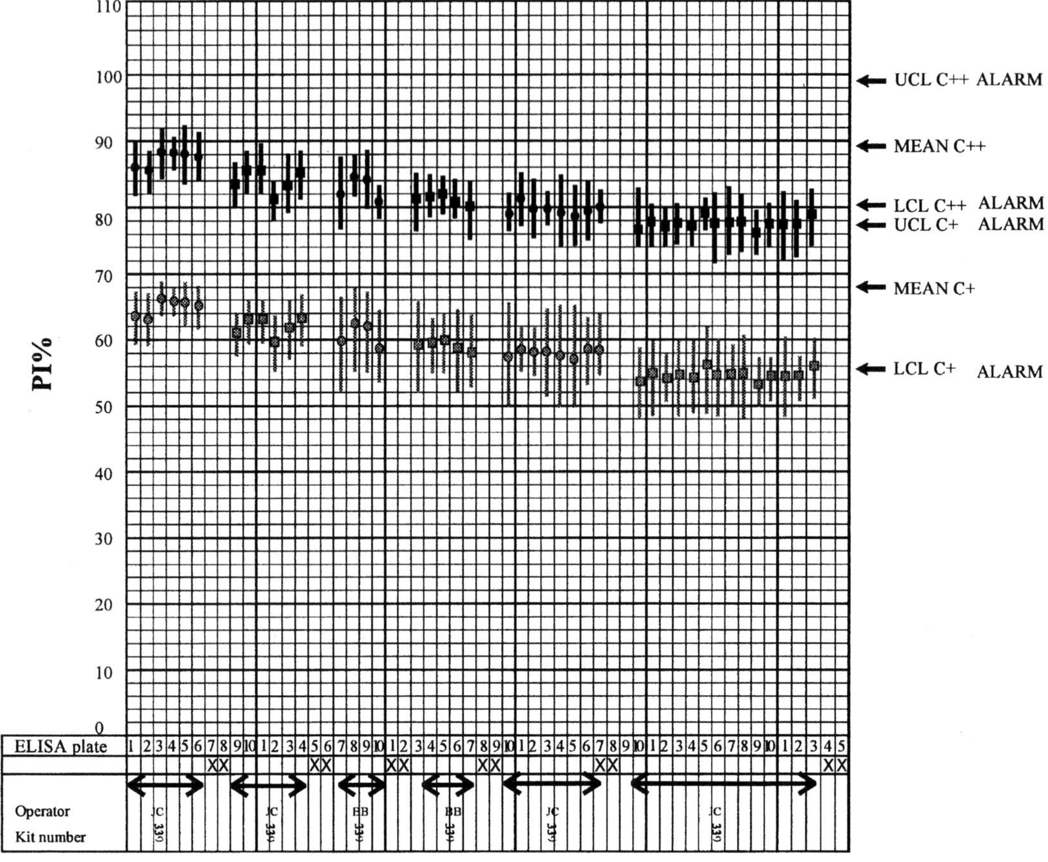

Fig. 17. Illustrative DDD chart for C++ and C+ PI% data showing downward trend.

be above the given cutoff value. We also have other "constants" that should be the same on each plate, i.e., the mAb (Cm), the C–, and the Cc.

5.1. Variation

There will be a variation in the results obtained in the tests. The variation will be from plate to plate, on the same day, from day to day, from operator to operator. The measurement of the variation is what the charts help the operator to investigate. We can (and have to) accept a degree of variation. The acceptance limits are those given in the manual. Thus, for the Cm:

1. A target mean OD reading is given.
2. Upper and lower limits for OD are given.
3. A target PI% value is given.
4. Upper and lower control limits for PI% are given.

For the C++, C+, C–, and Cc the mean and limits are expressed only in terms of the PI% figures.

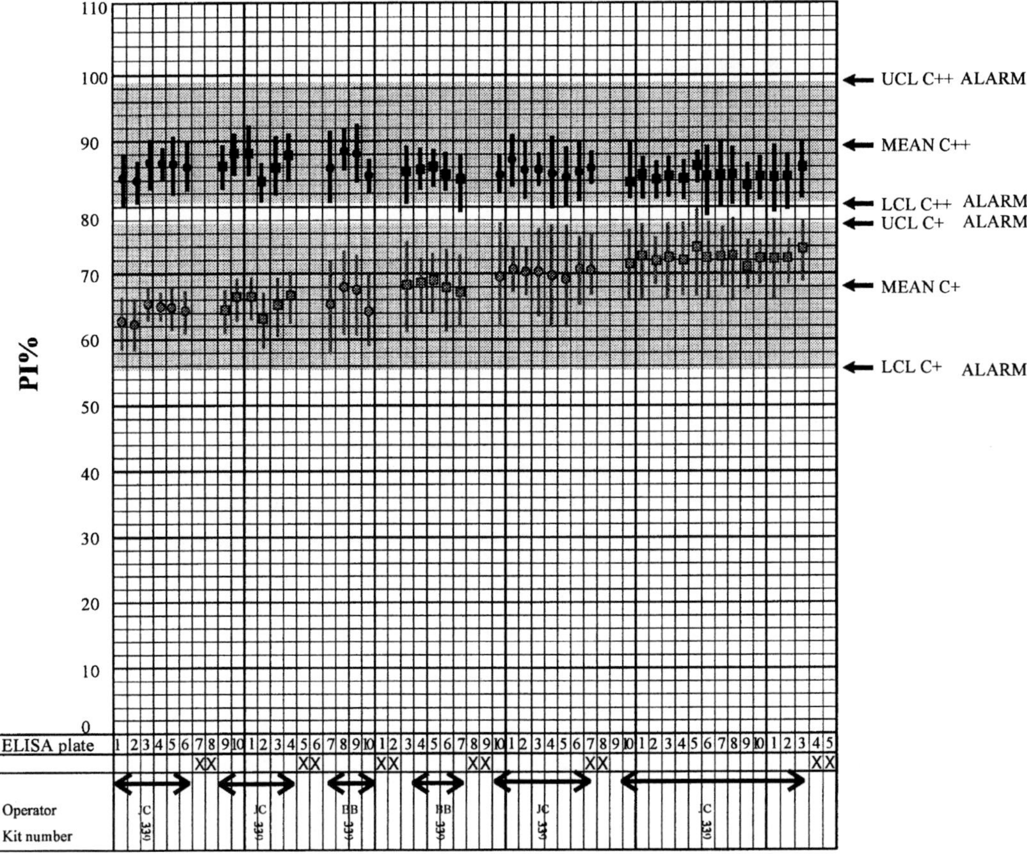

Fig. 18. Illustrative DDD chart for C++ and C+ PI% data showing upward trend for C+ and constant acceptable limits for C++.

Note that the first task when receiving a kit is to run the controls under the conditions described in the manual and to see what results are obtained. These should give mean values within the described limits in the manual.

Once this is established, the routine monitoring of the test on a daily, weekly, monthly, and yearly basis is vital to answer the question, Is the test the same each time? The charts merely plot the data that are generated each time a test is made. They are a visual representation of the data collected and concisely presented. The charts should be updated immediately. The charts should be in full view so that all individuals involved in the test can see them.

5.2. What Can We See from the Charts?

The main constant monitoring device is the SDC chart data. This gives a time-bound view of the test. Points can be drawn connecting data from one test day to another. This can give early warning of a trend in the test indicating that something is wrong.

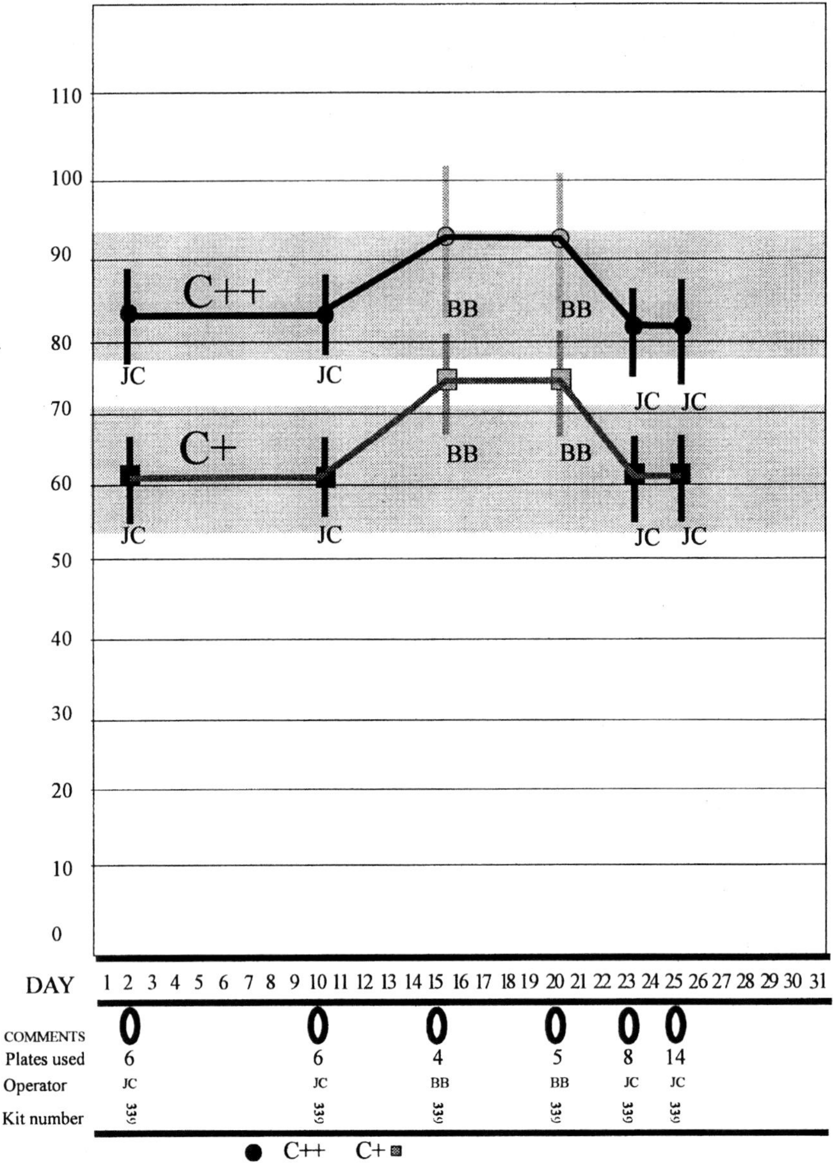

Fig. 19. Illustrative SDC chart for C++ and C+ PI% data showing effect of different operators.

This is illustrated under **Subheading 6**, where worked examples of different scenarios are examined.

The use of the DDD charts is important in that every single plate data is logged. A particular day's testing can be isolated for close examination from the SDC charts. The DDD charts can then be closely examined and reasons for excessive variation in the results examined. This is also examined under **Subheading 6**.

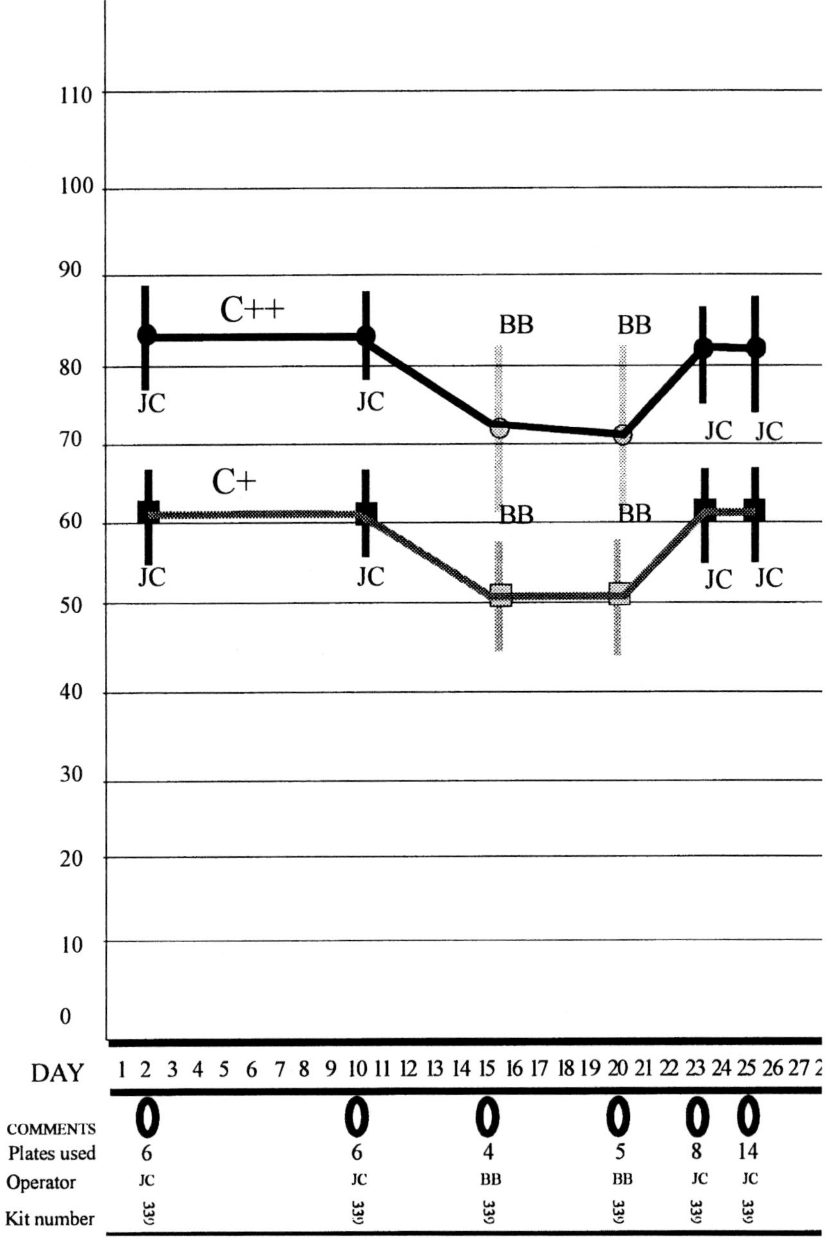

Fig. 20. Illustrative SDC chart for C++ and C+ PI% data showing effect of different operators.

6. Worked Examples on the Uses of DDD and SDC Charts

Several examples of what might happen in laboratories in time are given:

1. Good tests: no real problems.
2. Some worries: us test drifting?
3. Operator problems: ups and downs.

Table 3
Control samples data after processing

	OD_1	OD_2	OD_3	OD_4	$PI\%_1$	$PI\%_2$	$PI\%_3$	$PI\%_4$
C++	0.077	0.063	0.072	0:071	88	90	89	89
C+	0.278	0.296	0.313	0.280	58	55	52	57
C–	0.668	0.667	–	—	–2	–2	—	—
Cc	0.011	0.009	—	—	98	99	—	—
Cm	0.685	0.673	0.636	0.641	–4	–2	–9	–8

Table 4
Mean and SD for PI values of control data

	Mean	SD
C++	89.0	2.7
C+	55.5	2.7
C–	98.5	0.7
Cc	-1	0

Table 5
Completed calculation of mean and 2 × SD of control data

	Mean	*SD*	2 × *SD*
C++	89.0	2.7	5.4
C+	55.5	2.7	5.4
C-	98.5	0.7	1.4
Cc	-1	0	0

6.1. Good Tests: No Real Problems

Figure 12 shows a DDD chart with plots of the OD means and ±2 SD of the Cm for plates run by two different workers (Alan and Josy), on different days, with different kits (974 and 979).

Table 6
Example data from five plates with required parameters calclutated for inclusion in DDD charts

Plate	Cm (OD)	C++	C+	C–	Cc
1	0.59 (.07)	85 (6.0)	56 (5.0)	97 (1.8)	1 (0.2)
2	0.64 (.15)	89 (4.0)	59 (4.5)	94 (2.2)	2 (0.2)
3	0.68 (.09)	92 (5.2)	54 (5.5)	91 (3.2)	4 (0.1)
4	0.71 (.13)	84 (6.3)	59 (6.3)	89 (4.5)	5 (0.3)
5	0.61 (.09)	89 (4.5)	65 (3.9)	93 (6.8)	3 (0.4)

Table 7
Control data from five plates

	Cm	C++	C+	C–	Cc
Plate 1	–2	88	64	6	99
Plate 2	4	84	62	–3	91
Plate 3	3	87	59	–2	94
Plate 4	–1	89	63	4	93
Plate 5	–4	84	57	4	87

Table 8
Calculations of mean and SD from data in Table 7

	Mean	SD	2×SD
Cm	0	3.4	6.8
C++	86.4	2.3	4.6
C+	61.0	2.9	5.8
C–	1.3	4.4	8.8
Cc	92.8	4.4	8.8

6.1.1. Observations

1. The SD bars are of a similar length for all the plates and that the different operators have obtained similar mean values.
2. There are no large differences in SD or means for the kits.
3. The operators have identified themselves.
4. The operators have left a gap of two between different test days.
5. The operators have written on test dates.
6. The operators have denoted which kit was used. No further comments were worth noting.

The conclusion here is that the means of the OD values were near those specified in the manual and that there were no real differences between the operators' results. The same test's data was plotted as PI values on DDD charts. There were no large differences in SD or means for the kit controls. This would indicate that the samples analyzed on the individual plates would give good results within the expected limits.

Figure 13 shows an example of a DDD with data plots showing PI% means and ±2 SDs of the mean PI% of plates run by the two different operators, on different days, with different kits. The PI% values are plotted for each plate used. The operators are identified as well as the test kits. Gaps have been left between plates used in testing on different days. The key is to be able to identify individual plate data. Note that the variation is similar from plate to plate, irrespective of the kit used or the operator.

The workers have plotted SDC charts for the different days of testing (**Fig. 14**). Remember that they took the respective mean values required from all the plate data from tests performed on the same day. The results show that there is a clear difference between the C++ and C+ data. The means are in the expected range. There are no differences between the operators or the kits used (they had no effect on performance of tests). Data points have been connected to show any trend in data (going up or down).

6.2. Some Worries: Test Drifting

Figure 15 shows an SDC chart for a laboratory for the C++ and C+ controls. This is an example of an SDC chart with data plots showing PI% means and ±2 SDs of the mean PI% of C++ and C+ on six different days. The same kit is used throughout. Note that there seems to be a difference from the start of the month to the end. There was a gradual drift in the expected values from the first test in which the results were as expected to levels that are signaled as ALARM. The operators in this case should investigate the reasons that there is drift with reference to DDD chart data and examine operator differences and kit batch elements.

6.2.1. Examination of DDD Charts to Help Identify Problems

Reference to the DDD charts may highlight some reasons for the increased variation or drifting of an assay. Thus, the specific tests performed on the various days and plotted as overall SDC data can be examined in the light of individual plate data for any specific day's test.

Factors such as changes in conditions, operators, and kit batches also have to be examined, so that notes made on the charts highlighting these are important in this exercise. Note that the same kit has been used in the example, but by different operators.

The DDD chart in **Fig. 16** shows the actual OD data for the Cm for the plates shown in **Fig. 15**. The chart illustrates a situation in which there was an observed reduction in the mean of the PI values for the C++ and C+ in consecutive tests in SDC charts (**Fig. 15**). Thus, the reductions in OD observed in the raw data for Cm (**Fig. 15**) are matched with alterations in the control PI values. This indicates that the performance of the test is changing over a period of time; that is, the values are reducing with each test performed. Something has to be done to restore the recommended parameters with reference to the controls supplied. Again, the same kit was used for all tests so that differences cannot be ascribed to the change in reagents. The two operators had little effect on the reduction in expected PI values.

Figure 17 shows a DDD chart of C++ and C+ values of plates illustrating a situation in which there is a gradual reduction in values over a period of time (using the same kit). This shows actual individual plate data for C++ and C+ PI values. There is no great difference in the variation seen for any particular plate for either value (C++ or C+), but there is a gradual alteration in the mean from test to test. The observed reductions in actual OD for Cm are matched with reductions in expected PI values. The conclusion here would be that the test results obtained for the particular kit being used are not good. This is irrespective of operator factors; both obtain similar variation. There seems to be a gradual reduction in expected OD and PI values over a period of time. Both the C++ and C+ controls are now at ALARM levels even though the Cm OD values are just within allowable limits.

Reference to the DDD charts may also give a different picture in the context of having OD values observed for the Cm that are reducing.

The chart in **Fig. 18** illustrates a situation in which the reduction in actual Cm OD is matched by an increase in PI values, particularly for the C+. The variation in the tests is similar; that is, each test gives a mean with a similar variation. However, there is a continuous increase with time in the mean for the C+. This clearly indicates that as the test OD value goes down, the apparent sensitivity (ability to detect antibodies) goes up.

6.3. Operator Problems: Ups and Downs

Examination of the DDD and SDC charts can highlight operator problems. We can make the assumption that the kits generally remain stable. The most dominant factor in causing variation in test results is the operator. Whether this variation is acceptable or not can be decided after results are examined.

Figure 19 is an illustration of an SDC chart (shown diagrammatically, since we should now be quite familiar with the concepts from the previous more detailed illustrations). The data show PI values for C++ and C+ and indicate that there are different results according to the operator, because the same kit is being used. The reasons can be determined by an examination of all the control values plotted as DDD charts. Note also that operator BB has a higher variation in results as judged by the larger SD bars. In fact, operator BB has C++ and C+ values that are quite similar to each other, whereas there is a clear difference in the operator JC's figures. Operator BB has higher mean and variation values using the same kit than operator JC. Operator BB's values are unacceptable. Attention to the plate data on DDD charts will determine whether variation is general for any test or whether there is high variation in one or two plates tested. This is shown in **Fig. 20**.

Care should be taken in assessing SDC charts without reference to DDD charts. Remember, the SDC charts record all the results from a given test. They record only the sum of all the mean data and the variation inherent in that data. They do not consider the variation in each plate, so we could have a situation in which we have the correct mean (in limits) for SDC charts, but this had been arrived at through tests having very high and compensating very low control data means. The variation bars in the SDC charts will indicate whether this is inherent, so attention to the observed variation of the means is required, followed by specific examination of DDD charts.

Figure 21 shows DDD data for operator BB on tests performed on the 15th and 20th. Actual plate data of the mean and

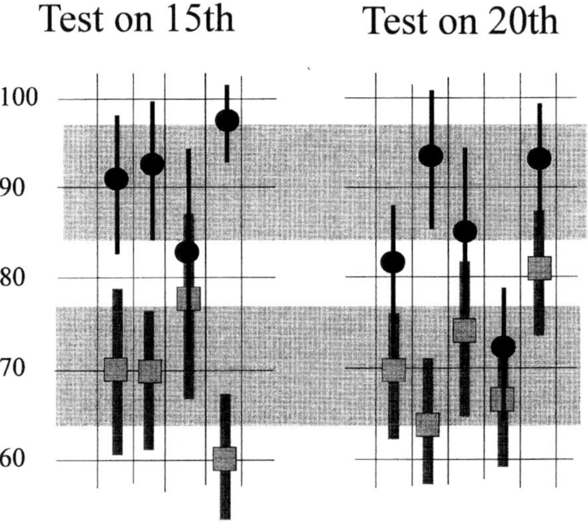

Fig. 21. Enlarged portion of DDD plots of PI% C++ and C+.

variation for each plate are shown. The gray areas denote limits for C++ and C+ controls. On the 15th, there were two plates out of limits for C+, one above and one below, although the actual mean of all the means for C+ (as plotted on the SDC chart) was about 70%. Thus, this operator had two plates that should be rejected. Similarly, on the same date two of the C++ controls were outside limits. On the 20th, we see a similar situation with two plates giving control C+ outside limits and three giving C++ outside limits. The overall conclusion should be that there is unacceptable variation in the tests of operator BB and that several of the plates used in the tests should have been rejected (not included in the testing). The plotting of all data in DDD charts immediately highlights this situation.

The chart in **Fig. 21** shows that the reverse trend for an operator can be seen, in which there is a reduction in expected PI values in comparison with other workers. The tests performed by one operator are not acceptable and asthe test was performed as expected by another operator, it must be a factor of the operator's that causes the problems with the assay.

7. Further Aid to Interpreting Charts

This section is intended to help the laboratory worker continuously interpret the charts as they are being plotted, i.e., as the "story" of the data unfolds. The rest of the kit's manual should be read first and the principles thoroughly understood. The intention here is to educate people in the ability to analyze charts to enable decisions to be made concerning day-to-day performance. The analysis infers that testing is being made over a significant time so that comparative results are obtained. This section uses "thumbnail" approaches at representing the different data that might be observed in practice. Analysis should lead to indications as to whether there is a need to take action and what actions are needed.

The advantages of charting data are that it can be viewed as a single entity and that trends and fluctuations can be rapidly observed through examination of SDC data and details at any point of time and can be expanded through examination of DDD data. This approach has already been explained. This section attempts to simplify likely scenarios in charts and indicate solutions where necessary, based on observations.

7.1. Examination of SDC Charts: Individual Points as Plotted

Individual plots summarize all data on a given day and test and relate the results in actual time so that trends or irregularities can be noted on a continuous basis.

1. The plots reflect the mean value of any control and its variation in all the plates examined in a given day's testing.
2. The bar plotted shows the variation.
3. The mean value and the error bars should fall within the given limits for the assay for the various control samples both for actual OD values and for the processed PI% data.

Thus, the SDC plots can alert operators to unacceptable means and errors, causing them to examine closely the individual plate data for that test to examine what factors produced the variation (which affects the mean value and size of error bars).

Figure 22 illustrates the various situations that could be encountered:

1. Plot A shows the mean to be within limits and the error bar to be short and also within limits. This is ideal with reference to the sample tested.
2. Plot B shows the mean to be within limits but one error tail of the bar to be out of limits. The error is probably higher than acceptable. Reference to individual data for that day may reveal the reason; for example, a single plate control could have been missed or given an out-of-limit result, which both reduces the overall SDC mean plot and increases error.
3. Plot C shows the mean to be out of limits and most of the error bar too. Reference to individual plate data will probably reveal that most of the plates gave mean values that were too low and that readings differ greatly. This is unacceptable.
4. Plot D shows the mean value to be too low and out of limits but that the error is small, indicating little variation in results for all the plates used. This is unacceptable. The data must

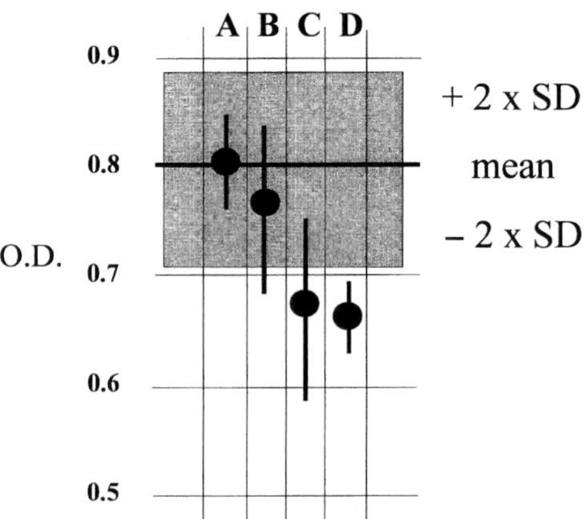

Fig. 22. Illustration of mean values and error bars in SDC OD plots. *Gray box* shows the upper and lower limits for values (plus and minus 2· SD) for the particular control sample examined.

also be examined with reference to other controls to determine whether the low value was reflected in other data. The reduction, say, of both mean values for SDC of strong and weak positive might indicate a systemic (general error), e.g., too short an incubations time with the substrate or a major general dilution error.

7.2. Examination of SDC Cm, C++, and C+ over Time

The SDC plots cover both the actual OD and the processed PI% values. It is important that both types of plot be examined together. Thus, the charts should be placed in close proximity. This should immediately alert operators to unusual fluctuations from the expected values in both charts as well as deviations in one chart but not in the other. When the Cm OD values are within limits, it is expected that the control serum values for OD and hence PI% will be within limits. When the Cm OD values do start to increase or decrease significantly (approach limits), it is possible that "alterations" in OD value are not mirrored by a significant change in the control PI% plots. In other words, when Cm OD values are showing trends, as shown in **Fig. 23**, the control C++ and C+ PI% charts should be consulted to measure the effect of the OD changes on the PI% values.

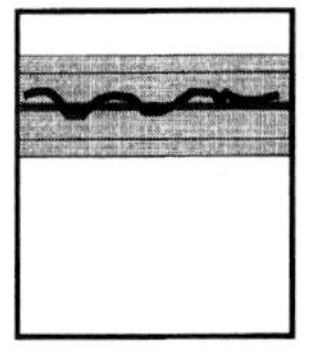

A. CONSTANT and IDEAL

Cm OD mean values all near ideal mean over time and regular (invariable).

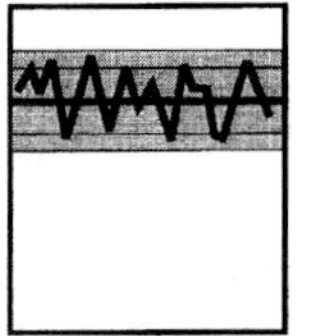

B. IRREGULAR WITHIN ACCEPTED MEAN LIMITS

Cm OD mean values all within limits over time but irregular (variable) not obviously associated with other

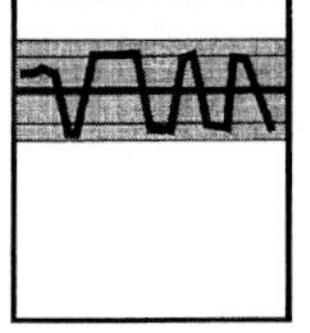

C. IRREGULAR (PATTERN) WITHIN LIMITS

Cm OD mean values all within limits over time WITH irregular (variable) data showing some pattern (possibly

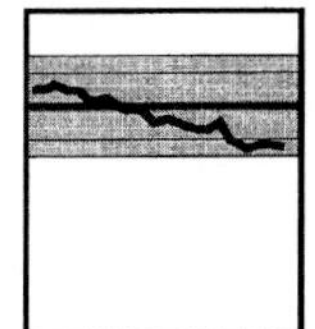

D. DRIFTING DOWN

Cm OD mean values all within limits over time but showing gradual reduction.

Fig. 23. (**a–d**) SDC plots in time showing different trends. The trends are observed in real time. Action points represent points where the expected means fall outside limits set and where the error bars begin to fall outside the limits at the upper or lower values.

As examples, the effect of a reducing OD value for 0% competition (maximum expected color from antigen binding to mAb [mAb control]) may (1) have no effect on the PI% results for the two control antisera, (2) affect both of these only when the OD falls below a certain level, or (3) only affect one control and not the other.

Figure 23 shows trends in time for SDC OD values for, say, the Cm, but would be pertinent to all plots of data for all controls. Basic large-scale trends are shown:

1. Situation A: This can be regarded as an ideal situation in which all means and error bars are within limits. The test values are constant, and it would not be expected that the test is altering in sensitivity.
2. Situation B: The curve is irregular with large swings in mean OD values throughout the time. This reflects a good deal of variation probably owing to differences associated with particular operators (differences in variability).
3. Situation C: The curve is irregular but contains areas of similarity of means. This can often be ascribed to changes in operators performing assays and/or notable changes in reagents. This type of curve should be analyzed in terms of identifying whether there are such factors that can be associated with the data.
4. Situation D: There is a fairly constant downward trend (or could be upward) irrespective of operators and probably signifies that the reagents are altering in time. This is particularly indicated when several operators perform assays. The retitration of certain reagents may be necessary to ascertain whether the accepted limits can be achieved. This identification also includes the necessity to obtain fresh reagents.

7.3. Control C++ and C+ PI% Data

C++ and C+ controls examine the competitive ability of the control sera with respect to the maximum reactivity of the mAb and antigen. They control the test and can be used to assess the test's performance in terms of analytical sensitivity. The actual OD data are related to the PI% data through processing with respect to the Cm control data.

Attention to examination of both OD SDC Cm and PI% SDC for the C++ and C+ is essential as already indicated. Figure 24 summarizes what might be observed with respect to SDC OD data and PI% data in the charts. The arrows reflect the overall trend observed as shown in **Fig. 23**:

1. The horizontal arrow indicates within mean acceptable values (as in situation A in **Fig. 23**).
2. The downward-angled arrow indicates a downward trend in values (situation B in **Fig. 23**).
3. The upward-angled arrow indicates an upward trend in results (not shown).

Irregular data are not shown. In **Fig. 24** the possibilities for SDC OD Cm data are represented by arrows (boxes 1–3), as well as all the possible, combinations of trends for the C+ + and C+ PI% data. **Figure 24** is meant to illustrate all combinations. The gray boxes represent the most likely combinations for SDC OD and PI% SDC data:

1. Box 1: The Cm OD values are within limits and constant. It is not expected that the C++ and C+ PI% values will be affected, and the expected trends in PI% are those indicated in box 1A. This situation is the one expected and mostly obtained. Box 1D shows a situation in which the C++ PI value is maintained but the C+ loses competing ability. This (increase in expected OD for C+) is a result of the control deteriorating and losing antibodies. The effect is not noted in the C++, probably because there is an excess of antibodies contained in the sample and the loss can be sustained without affecting the competing number of antibody molecules. Box 1E is also observed, but is more unusual, indicating that the C++ has lost antibody activity. This is most likely owing to the poor storage of that sample. The other combinations are unlikely.
2. Box 2: The Cm OD values are decreasing, possibly indicating that the antigen or mAb reactivity, or both, is being lost. The reduction in OD will be reflected by a relative increase in competing ability shown by the increase in PI% values. The results of PI% SDC will be most likely reflected as in box 2C, in which both controls increase in PI%. Although, since the C+ + contains an excess of antibodies, a situation as in box 2G is also possible.

SDC Cm OD Trends	SDC PI% Trends C++ and C+	A	B	C	D	E	F	G	H	I
1 →	C++	→	↘	↗	→	↘	↗	→	↗	↘
	C+	→	↘	↗	↘	→	→	↗	↘	↗
2 ↘	C++	→	↘	↗	→	↘	↗	→	↗	↘
	C+	→	↘	↗	↘	→	→	↗	↘	↗
3 ↗	C++	→	↘	↗	→	↘	↗	→	↗	↘
	C+	→	↘	↗	↘	→	→	↗	↘	↗

Fig. 24. Possible relationship of trends in OD SDC Cm and PI% SDC C++ and C+. Boxes 2–3 show trends observed in SDC OD data in time for Cm. Boxes A–I indicate possibilities in trends of PE% date for each of the controls C++ and C+ Examination of OD and PE% SDC trends together gives a clue as to the likely reasons for relationships. The gray boxes show most likely effects on C++ and C+ for respective Cm OD trends.

3. Box 3: The Cm controls increase in OD value in time. This would be unusual. However, here the increase in reaction could reduce both the C++ and C+ control sera's ability to compete as in box 3B. Again, the excess antibodies in the C++ might maintain the C++ PI% against that of the C+ as in box 2G.

An overall summary of the most likely scenario for the SDC OD and PI% relationship is shown in **Fig. 25**.

7.3.1. Irregular Plots

The same criteria for evaluating and comparing the Cm OD data and the C++ and C+ PI% data can be used to evaluate any time points plotted. This will establish any effects of the increase or decrease in Cm OD at any time on the expected PI% values.

When irregular results are obtained with high interest variation, one can note which of the results (at a given time) are affected most. Examination of the operator, methods, actual plate data, and day-to-day variables can be associated with good or bad results. Reference can be made to the individual plate data. Measures to solve the problems could then be used and results obtained after corrections compared.

7.4. Sources of Variation

As already stated, the kit is a complex association of reagents and equipment in the hands of different operators. The sources of variation thus come from these sources. Experience with this kit in many countries indicates that the chief source of errors (manifestation of variation) comes from the operators and not from the reagents. The continuous assessment of the kit is a good way to identify whether it is the reagents and/or equipment that are causing high variation as opposed to the operators. Some of the factors have already been examined, but still need to be emphasized.

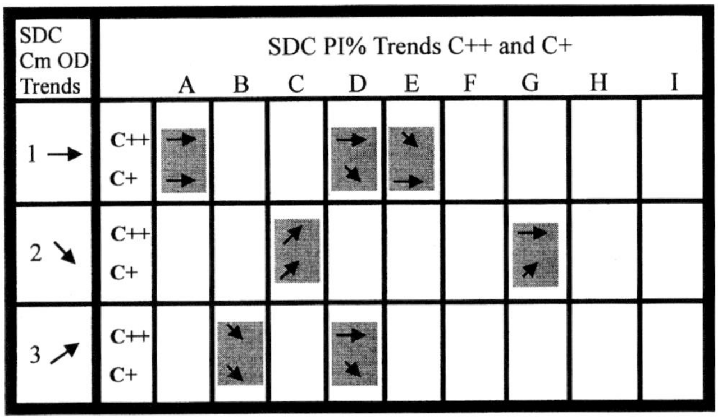

SDC Cm OD Trends	SDC PI% Trends C++ and C+	A	B	C	D	E	F	G	H	I
1 →	C++	→			→	↘				
	C+	→			↘	→				
2 ↘	C++			↗				→		
	C+			↗				↗		
3 ↗	C++		↘		→					
	C+		↘		↘					

Fig. 25. Summary of the most likely relationship of trends in OD SDC Cm and PI% SDC C++ and C+.

7.4.1. Elisa Readers

Cleaning

ELISA readers are seldom examined on a routine basis. The optical devices for reading the wells can become contaminated with chemicals and should be cleaned regularly. This is a simple process. They should not be cleaned with abrasive materials or those containing solvents affecting plastics.

Filters

Filters can deteriorate rapidly in humid conditions. They should be stored with the desiccant in a bag between uses. Machines with internal filter wheels have fewer problems. In cases in which there is a constant machine error indicating a failure to read, then another filter should be obtained. A spare filter should always be available (of appropriate wavelength). A careful check on the appropriate wavelength of the filter should be made initially. Some individuals use the wrong filter which, although allowing some OD to be measured (e.g., a 450-nm filter will give a readout for a 492 nm color, the readings will be very low as compared to those using the correct filter.

Od Readings

Individuals should know how the color they see relates to an OD readout. Some people have observed "good" color, which is in the expected range for the kit, but have then received very low OD readings from the machine.

7.4.2. Pipets

A chief source of error leading to variation is the use of pipets, which can be the chief cause of variation among operators. Even for an individual there is an "internal" bias toward pipetting in a certain way, either always having an amount slightly over or under. This assumption that pipets are calibrated properly (i.e., deliver the volume they are set for), is however, seldom the case. Greater care to standardize the pipeting technique will eliminate some variation in laboratories, particularly when several people are responsible for testing. This is particularly important in taking the samples from the field container to the wells in which a small volume is transferred. Care must be taken to allow an adequate time to pipet with an identical technique each time.

7.4.3. Reagents

The protocols given in the kit's manual should be strictly adhered to. Failure to maintain required minimal temperatures or to alter dilutions can severely harm the assay parameters. Such harm can be assessed with reference to the test performance before and after an identified abuse of reagent. However, such abuses are either not identified or not reported for other reasons. Note should be taken of likely susceptibilities of reagents to various physical conditions (*see* **Table 9**).

7.4.4. Water Quality

Water quality is consistently the chief source of problems in cases in which results (OD values) are generally much lower than expected. Attempts to obtain water from other sources should be made. The reasons for the alteration in color are not clear, and

Table 9
Possible problems with reagents

Reagent	Adverse parameters	Error	Effect
Ag for coating plates	High-temperature storage	Low Ag; low color	Change in sensitivity; test failure
H_2O_2	High-temperature storage; stopper left off; used at too high concentration	Reduced or no color	Test failure
mAb	High-temperature; denaturation; dilutions made up and used next day	Reduced color	Changes in sensitivity
Conjugate	High-temperature storage; changes; wrong dilution	Reduced color Increased or decreased color	Change in sensitivity
Blocking buffer	Wrong formulation	Color too high in controls	Test failure
Washing buffer	Wrong pH	Alteration in controls	High variation in controls

it is better to obtain water from other sources rather than waste time in curing an internal problem.

7.4.5. Poor Washing

Poor washing applies to washing tips and glassware and plasticware. It is better not to reuse anything that has had contact with an enzyme. When tips are reused, they must be acid washed and then very thoroughly rinsed in distilled water. The pH of the water should be checked because it can often be very acidic (poor plant-producing water). Poorly rinsed vessels in which original dilutions of reagents are made also adds to variation because activities can be reduced or totally destroyed in a highly alkaline or acidic pH range.

7.4.6. Mathematics

Errors in diluting reagents are a major problem. Calculations should always be checked and all bottles fetc., clearly labeled with the name of the reagent and dilution. The fundamental principles involved in good performance of ELISA should be learned through in-house training, external training, and reading of the literature. There is no substitute for training, which leads to improvements in practical skills and a thorough understanding of what one is doing.

7.5. More Problem Solving

Most problems are not really taken care of until it is too late. Operators must examine results constantly. The object of this section is to give in detail what should be done and when actions should be taken. The very reason for ICQ charts is to examine all results at all times. Actions are dictated by the results. **Figure 26** highlights measures to be taken when certain observations are made.

7.5.1. Stage 1: Running the Kit for the First Time

In stage 1, a single vial for the conjugate, Ag, and control C+ + and C+ as well as mAb is selected. The test should be conducted exactly as described in the kit manual. Results should be read and processed. The correct value for Cm OD, and allowable limits, are shown in the manual. The expected mean OD is 0.7, with the variation given at 1, 2, and 3 SDs from this mean expected value. The initial running of the reagents should give this mean, or a mean within the 2 × SD range recommended. Be concerned in cases in which the mean is outside the 2 × SD limits set, or when the mean is within the limits but when one end of the error bars plotted is inside the upper or lower mean or –3 × SD limits. Usually the OD readings are low when there is a problem.

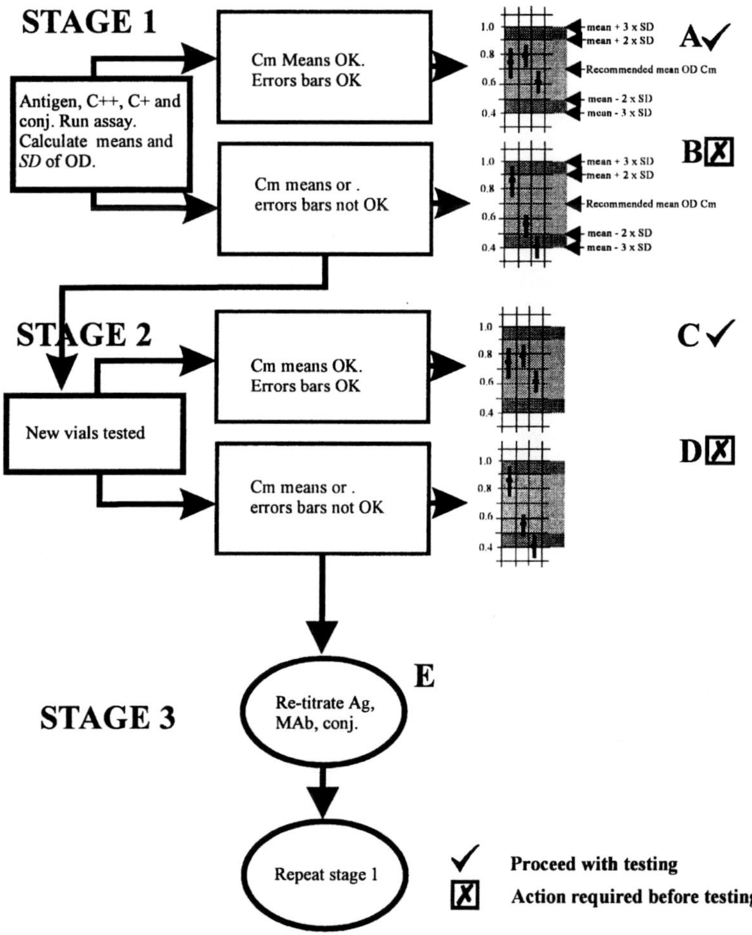

Fig. 26. Scheme for evaluating kits.

Situation A

In situation A, the results are good. The mean is between the 2 × SD limits. The extremes of the error bars are also within the 2 × SD limits. The reagents are performing well and testing can begin. The PI% values for C++ and C+ should be examined to check that they are within prescribed limits.

Situation B

In situation B, the means are either low or high. The usual situation is that they are too low. Even when the means are within the 2 × SD limits, note that we should be cautious when the error bars are in the 2–3 × SD range. Reasons for the low color may be that the reagent was not made up properly, either by incorrect dilution or losing material on opening the vial (freeze-dried material can be lost); that the reagents were damaged while being transported; or that the laboratory has poor water. A poor result means that stage 2 must be run.

7.5.2. Stage 2

In case there was a general poor dilution or problem of loss, it is good practice to select new vials of all reagents, and retest. The initial vials can be stored. Be extra cautious in diluting the new vial reagents accurately. Also be careful all material is solubilized and that none is lost when the vials are opened, or left on caps on dilution.

Situation C

If the results are good, then this points to the errors in stage 1 being dilution and making up reagents. Proceed with the testing.

Situation D

In cases in which there is no improvement, then some retitration and examination of the water in the laboratory is necessary in stage 3.

7.5.3. Stage 3

Simple First Checks

1. Are you using the correct filter? This should be 492 nm. If you have relatively strong color but the machine is reading only 0.1–0.4, then check the filter.
2. Make sure the substrate (H_2O_2) and chromophore *ortho*-phenylenediamine are made up properly. Check the viability by dipping the pipet tip into anti-mouse conjugate and putting the tip into freshly made up substrate/chromophore. This should turn dark brown very quickly.
3. Double-check all dilutions you are making from vials.
4. Check the pH of the substrate buffer after the addition of chromophore!

Obtaining Another Source(S) of Distilled Water and Repeating Stage 1

Water can have a limiting effect on color development. If replacement of water allows results as in "Simple First Checks" then proceed with a secured/pure source of water.

Retitrate the Antigen

Often there can be some lowering of antigen activity owing to denaturation (also on continued testing) and through aggregation. A simple examination of antigen can be made by keeping all other reactants constant.

1. Dilute antigen 1/25, 1/50, 1/100, and 1/200, as indicated in **Table 10**.
2. Coat the plates under standard conditions.
3. Wash.
4. Add mAb at the recommended dilution. Add C++ and C+ for reference. Cc is included in column 5.
5. Incubate.
6. Wash
7. Add conjugate.
8. Incubate.
9. Add substrate/chromophore.
10. Stop and read at 492 nm. Some possible results can be examined.

Result (A)

Table 10 presents possible results from titrations (a). If there is an increase of OD at 1/25 and/or 1/50, this indicates that there is a loss in activity of the antigen so that recommended dilution is not suitable.

Action

1. Use the antigen at a retitrated dilution that gives the mean OD for Cm within recommended limits. Check that the PI% values for C++ and C+ are within limits. In the example, a dilution of 1/50 is better.
2. Obtain a new batch of antigen.
3. Different results may be found as shown in result (b).

Table 10
Possible results from titrations (a)

	Diluted antigen[a]	1/25	1/50	1/100	1/200	0 No Ag
	Wells	1	2	3	4	5
A	mAb (Cm)	0.92	0.72	0.45	0.32	0.03
B	mAb(Cm)	0.91	0.69	0.43	0.34	0.04
C	C++	0.14	0.11	0.08	0.05	0.03
D	C++	0.15	0.12	0.06	0.04	0.04
E	C+	0.31	0.23	0.18	0.05	0.06
F	C+	0.32	0.24	0.15	0.06	0.07
G	0mAb	0.03	0.04	0.02	0.05	0.03

[a]mAb at recommended dilution

Result (B)

Table 9.11 presents possible results from titrations. Here, increasing the antigen concentration has no effect on increasing the OD.

Action: Retitrate the antigen, mAb, and the conjugate.

7.5.4. Retitration of Antigen, Conjugate and Mab

The antigen (Ag), mAb, and conjugate can be titrated on one plate (*see* **Fig. 27**). The antigen is diluted beginning at 10 times the recommended concentration into wells in columns 1 and 7. The antigen is then diluted in a twofold range over four wells (columns 1–4 and 7–10. Columns 5, 6, 11, and 12 receive only buffer. After incubation and washing, the mAb is added and then diluted beginning at 10 times the recommended dilution in rows

Table 11
Possible results from titrations (b)

	Diluted antigen[a]	1/25	1/50	1/100	1/200	0 No Ag
	Wells	1	2	3	4	5
A	mAb	0.40	0.41	0.43	0.32	0.03
B	mAb	0.43	0.40	0.41	0.34	0.04
C	C++	0.09	0.11	0.08	0.05	0.03
D	C++	0.08	0.12	0.06	0.04	0.04
E	C+	0.15	0.16	0.18	0.05	0.06
F	C+	0.16	0.17	0.15	0.06	0.07
G	O mAb	0.03	0.04	0.06	0.04	0.05

[a]mAb at recommended dilution

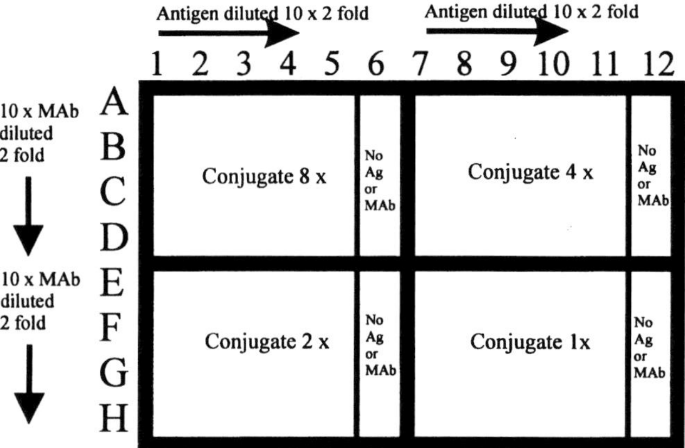

Fig. 27. Scheme for titration of all reagents.

A and E. The mAb is diluted in blocking buffer in a twofold range from A1–5, A7–11 to D1–5, D7–11; and E1–5, E7–11 to H1–5, H7–11, respectively. Columns 6 and 12 receive only blocking buffer. After incubation and washing, the conjugate is added in all wells of the four quarters of the plate indicated at four different dilutions representing 8, 4, 2, and 1 times the recommended dilutions. After incubation and washing, substrate/chromophore is added and the latter stopped at the recommended time. The color developed is then read at 492 nm. **Table 12** presents combinations of probable results. We have already assessed that under the standardized conditions, the antigen appears weak, so we are investigating mainly the probable situations in columns 5–8 in **Table 12**. However, the titration recommended will investigate all the scenarios. Sketch graphs of the plates as they might appear in the various scenarios are given below in **Figs. 28** (1–3) and **29** (4–6). The situations 7 and 8 are not illustrated since there is no color obtained and in this situation (which would be very unusual), new kit regents should be tested and the materials returned to source. From the pattern obtained it should be apparent where the problem is in the reagents.

7.6. Some Points to Help Testing

The following tips will help in testing:

1. *Check the antigen since it is the factor that most often causes problems.* Make sure that none is lost on opening a vial (also true for all other reagents), and that all is resuspended. Check that no reagent escapes or is stuck to lids.
2. *Check the pH of all buffers and if possible make up reagents.* The wrong pH for substrate/chromophore will affect color development.
3. *Practice good pipeting technique at all times.* There can be large errors when pipeting small volumes. This is particularly true when tests are first run by inexperienced operators. The variation in testing should go down on practice. This will be seen also with reference to data plotted on charts. The target maximum error between replicates is 10–15%. If there are many duplicates for controls and test sera with error > 10%, then

Table 12
Possible combinations of results[a]

1	2	3	4	5	6	7	8
Ag OK	Ag OK	Ag OK	Ag OK	Ag bed	Ag bed	Ag bed	Ag bed
M OK	M OK	M bed	M bed	M OK	M OK	M bed	M bed
C OK	C bed	C OK	C bed	C OK	C bed	C OK	C bed

[a]M mAb; Ag antigen C conjugate

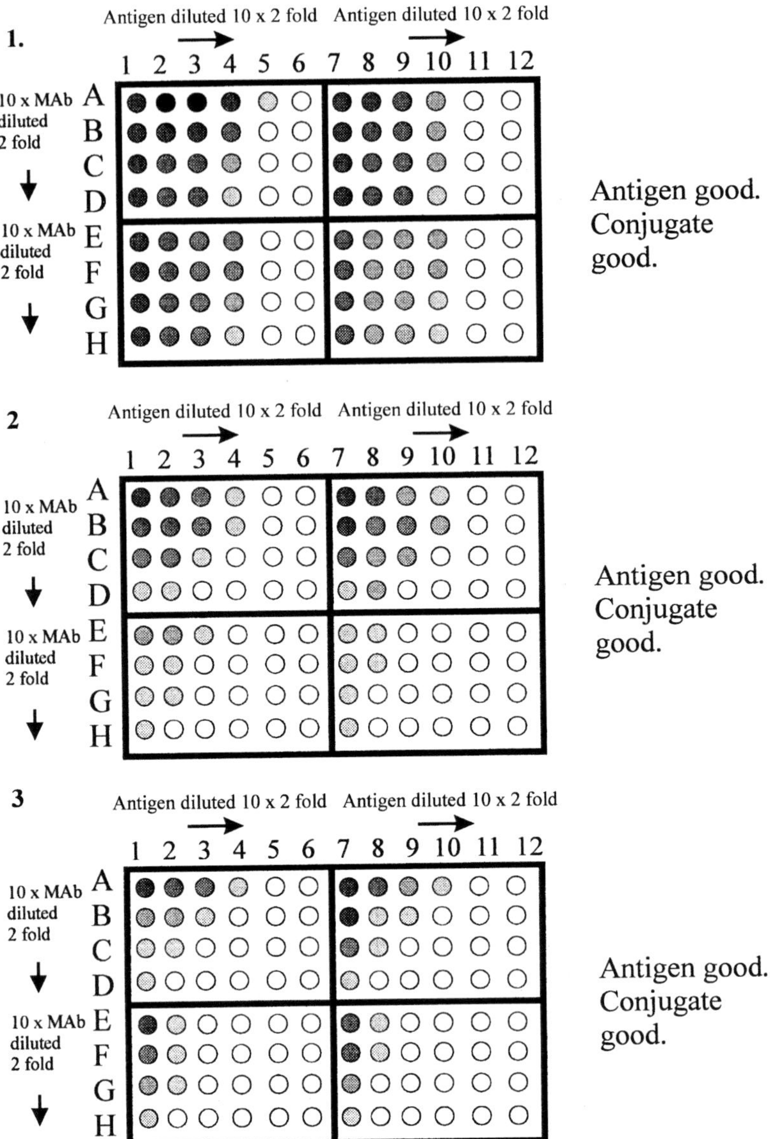

Fig. 28. Situations 1–3 on titration of reagents.

tighten up your technique for reagent transfer. Slow down the testing (transfer).

4. *Examine data obtained with respect to actual OD values generated (unprocessed).* Ignore the computer-generated processed data while examining OD values. Assess each plate by eye with respect to controls. Reject those in which Cm values are obviously too small. Reassess the processed plate data with respect to all results for all plates in a test. This can also be

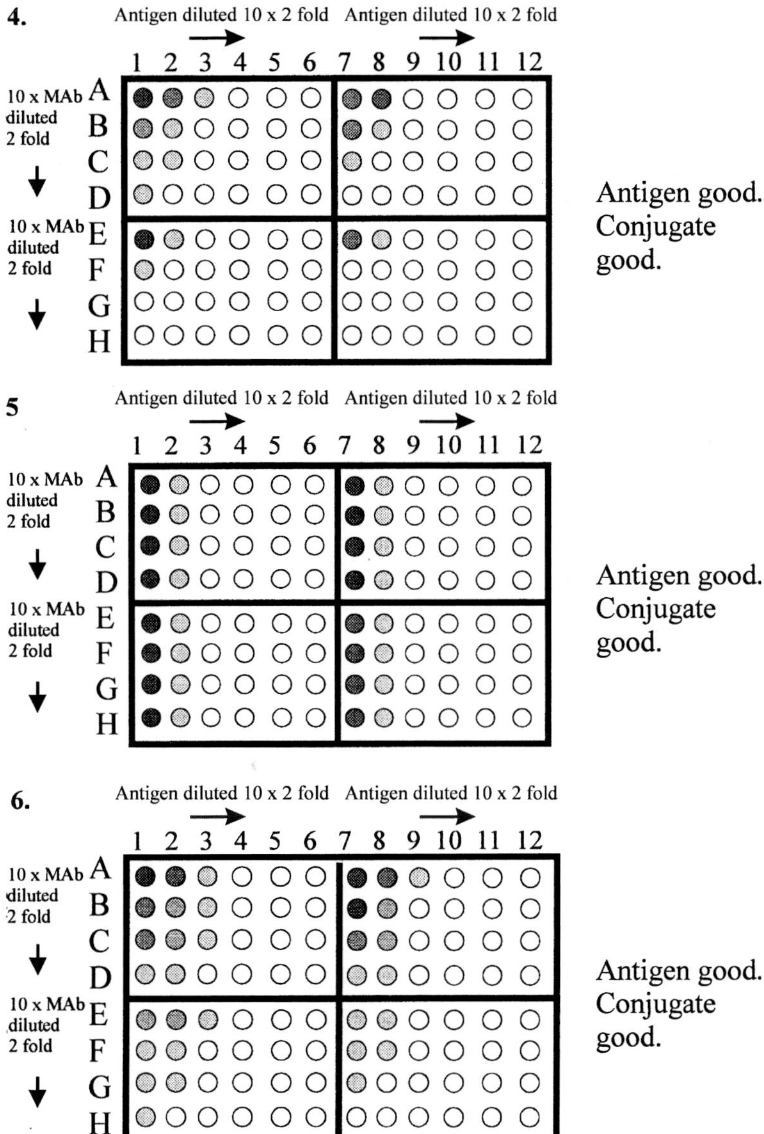

Fig. 29. Situations 4–6 on titration of reagents.

done when data are plotted on charts. Do you agree with the action recorded by software-processed data?

5. *What are the results fromthe sera tested?* Are you getting clear positive sera (high PI% competition of 80–100%), even when the Cm OD is low or out of limits? In this case, results may be acceptable, e.g., when in sero monitoring. However, attempt to increase Cm OD. Are you getting clear negatives (competition PI% values of –20 to 20%) even when the OD for Cm is low? Again, results may be acceptable. How many sera are in

the problem area (e.g., 40–55% PI) from the samples tested. All? A few? If there are many, then the whole system should be retitrated.

6. *Plot all processed data as they are processed on to the IQC charts.* The continuous examination and transparent recording of data is essential.
7. The methods described here should be used to routinely examine reagents throughout their lifetime of use as a kit for testing. When there is an identified drift to lower OD values for Cm, then the reasons can be investigated using the methods. The danger signals are when the mean OD of the Cm approaches the allowable mean 2 × SD limit. Remember to observe the lower limit of error bars (2 × SD error bar of Cm mean per plate). If this falls inside the or is within the mean Cm value –3 SD limits, then the system should be examined.

Chapter 10

Charting Methods for Internal Quality Control of Indirect ELISA

This chapter deals with control charts to monitor the performance of Indirect ELISAs. An Indirect ELISA kit for the detection of antibodies against Brucella is used to demonstrate the methods. Many of the features explained in Chapter 9 are relevant to this chapter; some repetition is intended, as this chapter may be read independently. **Figure 1** gives an overview of the indirect ELISA scheme used. The details of the procedure, which involves plotting the data graphically (charting methods), are explained. As a reminder, the objectives of charting data are as follows:

1. To keep a constant record of all data.
2. To monitor the assay from plate to plate in any one day's testing.
3. To monitor the tests made from day to day, week to week, year to year.
4. To allow rapid identification of unacceptable results.
5. To allow recognition of reagent problems.
6. To identify trends in results (increasingly poor performance).
7. To identify when a new set of kit reagents is necessary.
8. To allow identification of differences in operators of the assay.
9. To fulfill various criteria for good laboratory practice.
10. To fulfill necessary requirements for external recognition that tests are being performed at an acceptable level (increasingly important when results are used for international trading purposes).

John R. Crowther, *Methods in Molecular Biology, The ELISA Guidebook, Vol. 516*

DOI: 10.1007/978-1-60327-254-4_10

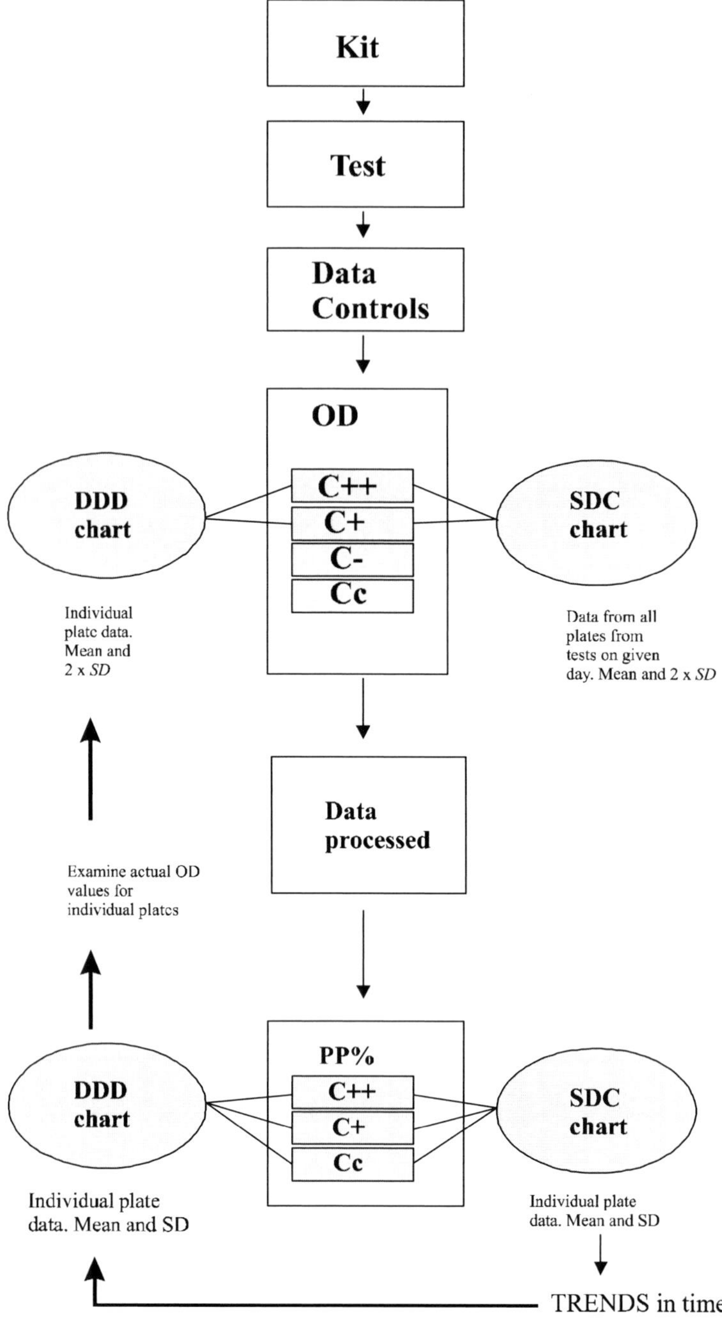

Fig. 1. Relationships of data management for Internal Quality Control of assays. The data obtained for various control samples can be expressed both as an average and as the variation from this average. The different controls can be used in different ways to monitor the performance of kits in time. The results are based on the manual calculation of means and 2 × SD values of data or through using the same principles on a spreadsheet analysis.

1. Good Practice of IQC

Internal quality control (IQC) methods allow test operators, as individuals, to monitor the performance of their test. When there is more than one operator, the method produces a unification of approach to allow control over results, and allows discrepancies among performance to be identified. It also promotes the idea of "open" results that can be viewed by anyone, including external scientists interested in evaluating the status of a laboratory involved in providing results on which management decisions concerning disease control are made.

1.1. Definition of a Perfect Kit

A kit should contain everything needed to allow testing, including software packages for storage, processing, demonstration, and reporting of data.

The reagents should be absolutely stable under a wide range of temperature conditions.

The manual describing the use of the kit should be "foolproof".

The kit should be validated "in the field" as well as in research laboratories.

All containers for reagents should be leakproof.

Internal quality control samples should be included.

External quality assessment should be included in the kit "package".

Data on relationship of kit results to those from other assays should be included.

Attention should be paid to ensuring that all equipment used in association with the kit is calibrated (spectrophotometers, pipettes).

Training courses in the use of kits should be organized.

Information exchange should be set up to allow rapid "on-line" help and evaluation of results where there are perceived problems.

The internationally agreed supply and control of standards used in kits should be maintained.

1.2. Good Practice of IQC

Test operators, as individuals, should monitor the performance of their test. Where there is more than one operator, the method produces a unification of approach to allow control over results, and allows discrepancies between performances to be identified. It also promotes the idea of "open" results, which can be viewed by anyone, including external scientists interested in evaluating the status of a laboratory involved in providing results on which management decisions concerning disease control are made.

The method described is not a deep statistical analysis of data; rather, it attempts to visually assess results so as to increase awareness of operators regarding what they are doing on a daily, monthly, and yearly cycle of work. The term "descriptive statistics" can be used. The most important feature of testing in a laboratory is that operators have a very good understanding of the principles of the test they are making, and that they fully understand the nature of their results and the need to process data.

There is no substitute for this understanding, but the charting method recommended is an aid to simplify the process of test performance. At first glance, the document may seem to be overcomplicated. However, it is to be assumed that people involved in testing have been trained to some level, and are running the assays on a fairly routine basis.

1.3. Charting - What This Document Describes

The charting method asks only for two extra pieces of manipulation of the data available from the multichannel spectrophotometer. The means and Standard Deviation (SD) from the means of control samples OD and the mean and SD of the PP (percentage positivity calculated with reference to a positive sample C++ mean) values are calculated, and certain values obtained above are plotted on two kinds of charts. These are:

1. Daily Detailed Data charts (DDD)
2. Summary Data Charts (SDC)

Tables A and **B** illustrate how data can be recorded before they are plotted. They are a device intended to induce operators to keep a careful record of data. They also serve to focus the minds of operators as to exactly what data are needed after each test. Thus, there is a systematic approach to data management that should impose a level of control on all laboratories involved with the same kit.

Charting imposes a system on all involved, and helps maintain the discipline needed to sustain the approach. The collection and storage of data in a fragmented way (for example, on bits of paper with calculations not recording time/date/operator for any given tests) should be avoided. The word transparency is meant to indicate that results and processed data are available to all for comment. Ultimately, a set of well-presented results is a credit to a laboratory, engenders good team spirit, and sustains interest in what can be a mundane task (continuous testing). Early indication of problems that can usually be easily solved (requisition a new kit, conjugate, change water, re-train operator) is a credit to the system used to assess performance, and ultimately saves a great deal of time and resources. In the past, assays using the kits have been poorly run in laboratories for a long time, and the results used in disease management. The late identification of bad assays destroys faith in the kit, reduces the trust of managers in the level of competence of laboratory staff and, worst of all, produces bad management decisions. There is everything to be gained by taking a little more time to examine, check, process, and display indirect ELISA results

1.4. Practical Approach to IQC Charting

Before going into detail, some elements of good practice are highlighted. A laboratory should:

1. Keep files with all IQC Tables A and B.
2. Plot all DDD and SDC and have these on show, preferably on a wall near to where the tests are performed.
3. Keep a copy of the charts on file.
4. Appoint an individual to "oversee" the charts. This individual should ensure that all people performing the relevant assays fill in the tables and chart the results. The individual should ensure that only relevant data are added to the charts, e.g., plates used for developmental work/research should not be included, only those involved in running routine assays.
5. The results on the charts should be discussed regularly with all involved in laboratory testing, and any trends identified.
6. The charts should always be discussed with managers involved in disease control, to increase their confidence in results.

1.5. Charting Process

The scheme in **Fig. 1** shows the data and where they should be plotted. The kit supplied has controls. The values of the controls are obtained as OD data from the spectrophotometer for each plate. The actual OD data are examined, as well as processed PP% data obtained for C+, Cc, and C-, with reference to the control C++ for each plate.

1.6. OD Data for DDD Charts

The required plots are obtained from the OD data of the C++ and C+ controls. On these charts, the mean OD of the four control values is calculated, along with the SD for each plate. Data from each plate are plotted on the DDD charts. Examples of how to calculate the mean and 2 × SD and plot values will be shown.

1.7. OD Data for SDC Charts

The data are obtained by taking the calculated overall mean values for all C++ and C+ respectively, for all plates used on a particular day, and then calculating the mean and 2 × SD of these means. Thus, if four plates are used, there are 4 mean OD values for C++, and the mean of these is calculated with the 2 × SD. If seven plates are used, then all seven mean C++ values are processed to obtain the overall mean and 2 × SD. These summary means and SD are plotted on charts with real-time x axis, so that the relationship of the results in time can be observed.

1.8. Plots of PP% Values

After plotting individual plate OD means and 2 × SD for C++ and C+ on DDD charts and their summary data on SDC, the data are further processed to obtain percent positivity results (PP%).

1. The PP% value is calculated with reference to the overall mean of C++ for each plate, as shown below.
2. The values of PP% for each of the wells (4 values) for C+, C-, and Cc are calculated for each plate.
3. The mean and the 2 × SD of the PP% values are then calculated for each control from individual plates for C+, C-, and Cc, and this is plotted on DDD charts.
4. Summary data from all plates with reference to PP% values for each control is then calculated.
5. The mean and 2 × SD of the entire individual mean PP% values from a specific test is plotted on SDCs, with an x axis in real time.

2. Indirect ELISA Kit for Antibody Measurement

The basis of the system used is shown in **Fig. 2**. A great deal of care has been taken by the supplier to ensure that the reagents and materials will work in laboratories around the world with different local conditions, and that the kit will travel without deterioration of performance.

On receipt of a kit, there are two initial questions:

1. How do we know that the kit reagents are working as expected?
2. How can we ensure that the kit keeps on working, i.e., the established diagnostic criteria are maintained?

Answering both of these questions is the focus of this chapter.

2.1. Validated Facts

Objective criteria are all that should be of interest to scientists performing tests. Although the following list may seem obvious, it is useful to review the facts surrounding kits.

The kits have been received. The following need to be verified:

1. Has the correct kit has been sent with latest manual?
2. Are all the reagents and materials present (with reference to a check list)?
3. Is the necessary infrastructure present in the laboratory?
4. Is an ELISA reader available?
5. Are power and water available?
6. Do the reagents work as expected?
7. Does the extent of training to allow performance of any ELISA need consideration?
8. Is data management understood (results processed manually or automated)?

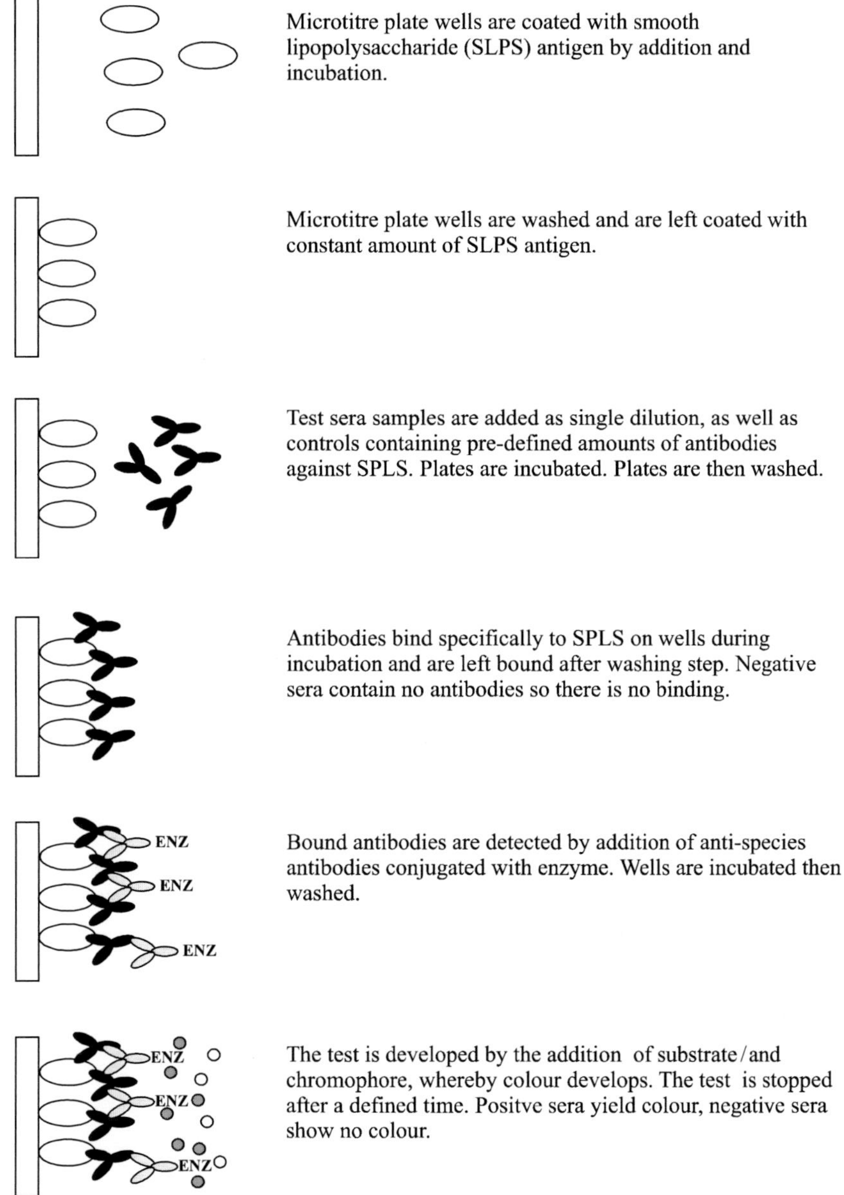

Fig. 2. Example of an Indirect ELISA – Brucellosis Indirect ELISA for antibody. The basis of the Indirect ELISA is that purified SPLS protein is attached passively to wells of microtiter plates. After washing away excess antigen, test and control sera are added and incubated. Antibodies specific for antigen bind. After washing plates, bound antibodies are detected by incubation with an enzyme conjugated anti-species serum. After washing, the test is developed by addition of substrate for the enzyme and a chromophore that changes color. Positive samples show color and negatives do not. The color developing is calculated with respect to the color developing in the strong control serum used.

9. Has a test been performed using controls?

The first task then is to "run" an assay with the kit, using available control reagents and to examine the results in the context of parameters given in the manual. This tells us whether the kit is performing as expected. This exercise also introduces the elements of charting.

2.2. Running an Assay for the First Time

We have used the following controls in the test. Test operators should familiarize themselves with the controls and their purpose. This information is contained in the manual.

1. C++ Strong positive control
2. C+ Moderate positive control
3. C- Negative serum control
4. Cc Conjugate control

The results expected (and the limits allowed) have been worked out and indicated in manual. These controls have been assessed many times, and the results examined statistically. The results using the control reagents have fixed limits. If the results obtained are the same or within allowable limits, then your test is good. If the results are outside the limits, then something is wrong!

The basis of the Indirect ELISA is that purified SPLS protein is attached passively to wells of microtiter plates. After washing away excess antigen, test and control sera are added and incubated. Antibodies specific for antigen bind. After washing the plates, bound antibodies are detected by incubation with an enzyme conjugated anti-species serum. After washing, the test is developed by addition of substrate for the enzyme and a chromophore that changes color. Positive samples show color and negatives do not. The color developing is calculated with respect to the color developing in the strong control serum used.

2.3. Data Processing

Assays should be performed exactly as described in the manual, using the control sample in the required positions for a test proper, taking care to note dilutions and storage conditions of reagents, as well as good laboratory practice and pipetting techniques. Conditions described should be rigidly adhered to, as any variation in methods produce variations in final results. Data are obtained from the plate reader.

Data may be managed (obtained, stored, and processed) using a software program. If no software is available, data are processed manually, with the help of a calculator.

2.4. Data Processing Fundamentals

Let us deal with the fundamentals of what the data processing involves.

Always check that:

1. The controls have been placed in particular positions on the plate.
2. The controls have been put in the correct position.

3. Altering the positions of controls and samples is not allowable if the EDI 2.3 software is processing data; as the data processed relies on the correct positioning of the controls, it is imperative to check that these are placed correctly, as shown in **Fig. 3**.

Table 1 shows the OD values that might be expected from a single plate in a test.

Table 2 shows the raw OD data and the PP values for controls (PP1 to PP4), and data after calculation of PP values.

Percent Positivity (PP) for controls are: Replicate OD value of each control/Mean value of C++ Control × 100

Percent Positivity (PP) values for tests are: Replicate OD value of Test Serum/Mean value of C++ Control × 100

Placement of controls and test samples on microtitre plates

Cc	Cc	1	5	9	13	17	20	25	29	33	37
Cc	Cc	1	5	9	13	17	20	25	29	33	37
C++	C++	2	6	10	14	18	22	26	30	34	38
C++	C++	2	6	10	14	18	22	26	30	34	38
C+	C+	3	7	11	15	19	23	27	31	35	39
C+	C+	3	7	11	15	19	23	27	31	35	39
C-	C-	4	8	12	16	20	24	28	32	36	40
C-	C-	4	8	12	16	20	24	28	32	36	40

Test serum samples 1-40 in duplicates

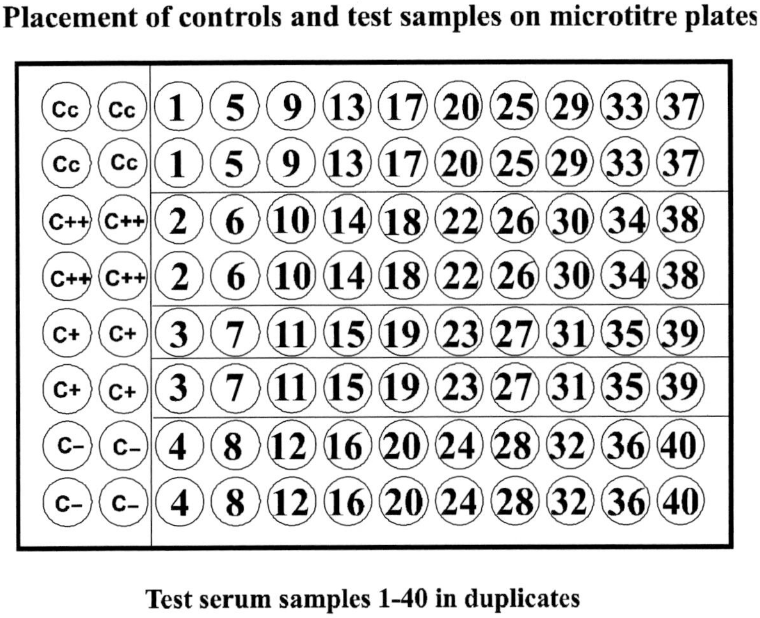

Fig. 3. Brucellosis Indirect ELISA for antibody detection, plate layout.

Table 1
Example of OD data for control sera on one plate

Controls	OD 1	OD 2	OD 3	OD 4
C++	1.020	0.986	0.980	0.956
C+	0.388	0.370	0.329	0.356
C-	0.005	0.025	0.002	0.007
Cc	0.134	0.015	0.012	0.009

Table 2
Processed data from Table 10.1

Controls	OD 1	OD 2	OD 3	OD 4	PP 1	PP 2	PP 3	PP 4
C++	1.020	0.986	0.980	0.956	104	100	100	97
C+	0.388	0.370	0.329	0.356	39	38	33	37
C-	0.005	0.025	0.002	0.007	1	3	0	1
Cc	0.134	0.015	0.012	0.009	14	2	1	1

For ICQ charting, consider all results for the controls and work out the PP% values with respect to the mean C++ value. These values should be calculated as shown below. Basically, we only need the unprocessed OD values for any plate to allow calculations.

As a reminder on how the mean and SD are calculated from first principles, we can use an example.

2.4.1. Example of Method of Calculation of Mean and Standard Deviation (SD) of Data

These values should be obtained using a calculator. However, it does no harm to examine the nature of the calculation briefly. The mean for each control sample is obtained by adding up all the individual values and dividing the figure by the number of values used (the number of values is usually ascribed the letter n). The sign for the average is $\overline{x}$.

As an example, we have data of 0.455, 0.612, 0.533, and 0.655 to process for a control.

The mean OD for the control is: 0.455 + 0.612 + 0.533 + 0.655 = 2.255 divided by 4 = 0.564

The Standard Deviation (SD) in mathematical terms is the positive square root of the variance of the data. The variance is measured by subtracting the mean of the test wells data ($\overline{x}_1, \overline{x}_2, \overline{x}_3$, etc.) from the overall mean value (X) and squaring that value. Each of these squared values is then added. The resulting value is divided by the total number of datum points used, minus one.

Therefore, in symbols we have:

$$\text{Variance}=((X-\overline{x}_1)^2+(X-\overline{x}_2)^2+(X-\overline{x}_3)^2+(X-\overline{x}_4)^2)/$$

In the above example we have:

$0.564 - 0.455 = (0.109)^2 = 0.012$

$0.564 - 0.612 = (-0.048)^2 = 0.002$

$0.564 - 0.533 = (0.031)^2 = 0.001$

$0.564 - 0.655 = (-0.091)^2 = 0.008$

Adding up the values, we have:

0.012 + 0.002 + 0.001 + 0.008 = 0.023
Divide by n–1 = 3: We have 0.023/3 = 0.0076

This is the variance.
The SD is the square root of this, i.e., $\sqrt{0.0076}$ = 0.087
The OD mean and SD are thus expressed as 0.564 ± 0.087

The calculation of the SD indicates far more than just analyzing the means. The value indicates how variable the data producing the mean is. Please refer to a textbook on statistics for a more detailed description of SD.

In examining the charts described later, the greater the SD for any mean value plotted, the greater is the variation, and the less confidence we can have in the data. The extent of the SD is examined with reference to the length of the bars drawn (representing 2 × the SD). Considerations of how much variation is "allowable" are not made here.

2.4.2. Processing OD Data for DDD and SDC Charts

From the OD data in **Table 1**, we have calculated the mean and SD of the controls, as shown in **Table 3**.

This would be calculated for each set of plate controls.

The C++ and C+ means and 2 × SD would be plotted on DDD charts.

A single point and 2 × SD bar for each plate used in a test are plotted. Thus, control C++ and C+ is recorded for every plate.

If only a single plate is used, then the SDC data is the same as the DDD data, and this would be recorded on the SDC chart. An example of OD data where more than one plate is used in a test is shown in **Table 4**. Here, the mean OD of each of the controls is calculated along with the 2 × SD.

Thus, for each plate, the C++ and C= mean and 2 × SD are plotted on DDD charts. The data for the SDC charts are calculated by taking each of the mean values for C++ and C+ for each

Table 3
Calculated mean and SD of Controls OD values from same data in Table 1

Control	Mean	SD	2 × SD
C++	0.986	0.026	0.052
C+	0.363	0.025	0.050
C-	0.009	0.010	0.020
Cc	0.043	0.061	0.122

Table 4
Illustrative results of mean OD and SD for C++ and C+ from 5 plates

	Plate 1 mean OD	Plate 1 SD mean	Plate 2 mean OD	Plate 2 SD mean	Plate 3 mean OD	Plate 3 SD mean	Plate 4 mean OD	Plate 4 SD mean	Plate 5 mean OD	Plate SD mean
C++	0.95	0.14	0.87	0.14	0.96	0.18	0.85	0.16	0.87	0.20
C+	0.38	0.012	0.45	0.014	0.32	0.010	0.34	0.006	0.39	0.012

Table 5
Calculation of overall test OD mean and SD for C++ and C+ for inclusion on OD SDC charts

Plate	C++ mean	C+ mean
1	0.95	0.38
2	0.87	0.45
3	0.96	0.32
4	0.85	0.34
5	0.87	0.39
Mean	0.90	0.38
2 × SD	0.10	0.10

plate and calculating their mean and 2 × SD. This is shown in **Table 5**.

2.5. Further Processing of Data to Calculate PP% Values for DDD and SDC Charts

2.5.1. DDD Charts

The establishment of the mean C++ value for a plate, as shown in **Table 3**, allows this value to be used to calculate PP% values for all controls for each plate. The calculation of PP% values is made for each well for the C+, C-, and Cc controls as well (as the test samples). The individual plate PP% values and 2 × SD are plotted on DDD charts; the overall mean and 2 × SD of this mean for all plates is plotted on SDC charts. Thus, in the example provided in **Table 3** , the calculation uses the mean value of the OD for C++ of 0.986 (0.99).

The formulae here are:

Percent Positivity (PP %) for controls: OD value of each control/Mean value of C++ × 100

Percent Positivity (PP %) values for tests: OD value of Test Serum/Mean OD value of C++ × 100

Table 6 shows the PP% values for the C+, C-, and Cc wells using the mean OD C++, as calculated by this method using data in **Table 3**.

Here the values of PP% can be processed and the mean and SD calculated for each control C++, C+, Cc, and C-. The means and SD*s* of the PP% values for the plate are shown in **Table 7**.

This data are plotted on DDD charts, and are obtained for each plate. For each plate, a DDD point is plotted with a corresponding 2 × SD bar.

For SDC charts, the PP% data from only C+, Cc, and C- are considered, as, by definition, the PP% for each plate is expressed as a percentage value of C++ (regarded always as 100%). The variation in PP% for C++ is viewed by examination of the OD and PP% DDD charts only.

2.6 Plotting PP% Data on SDC Charts

The C+, Cc, and C- results for PP% are recorded on SDC charts. Where a single plate is used in a test, the PP% values plotted are the same as those on DDD charts. Where there is more than one plate, the summary data for the controls are calculated. This is illustrated using data shown in **Table 8**, where results from 4 plates used in a test are shown.

Table 6
Calculations of PP% values using mean C++ OD value for a single plate (data in Table III)

Controls	OD 1	OD 2	OD 3	OD 4	PP1	PP2	PP3	PP4
C++	1.020	0.986	0.980	0.950	103	100	99.3	96.9
C+	0.388	0.370	0.329	0.356	39.3	37.5	33.3	36.1
C-	0.005	0.025	0.002	0.007	0.60	2.5	0.20	0.70
Cc	0.134	0.015	0.012	0.009	13.5	1.50	1.20	0.90

Table 7
Means and SD of PP% values

Control	Mean	SD	2 x SD
C++	99.8	2.5	5.0
C+	37.5	2.5	5.0
C-	1.0	1.0	2.0
Cc	4.3	6.1	12.2

Table 8
Results from 4 plates

	Plate 1	Plate 2	Plate 3	Plate 4	Mean PP% (SDC chart)	SD PP%	2 x SD PP% (SDC Chart)
C+	34	37	43	42	39.0	4.2	8.4
Cc	10	4	2	3	4.8	3.6	7.2
C-	1	1	3	4	2.3	1.5	3.0

Thus, the means of the PP% values for all plates are used to calculate data for SDC charts

Thus, the means of the PP% values for all plates are used to calculate data for SDC charts.

2.7. Initial Recording of Data

The key to successful monitoring is attention to detail, the accurate manipulation of data, plus a constant ability to check data. We have described the elements of what is needed to allow plotting of the charts. The next examples show how the data can be controlled by using tables, before plots are actually made. In this way, the operator can check the data as they are copied into the tables, as well as be able to record the results of the calculations needed. The data can be stored in a file for instant reference in association with the charts.

Remember, we have to obtain the data for DDD charts and SDC charts. Two kinds of table are shown to allow this. These are:

1. IQC Table A, which records the actual OD data for the control values; the mean and standard deviation for each plate, and the overall mean and SD for any given test (*see* **Figs. 4–6**).
2. IQC Table B, which records the PP% values for all the controls; the mean PP% values and SD for each plate, and the overall mean and SD of C+, C-, and Cc controls on any test (*see* **Figs. 7–9**).

2.8. Plotting Data on Charts

We make use of the fact that the same control sera are set up on each plate. We can examine differences in results between plates to keep a check on the test performance. As indicated earlier, two kinds of data are available:

1. Actual OD readings.
2. PP% values calculated by the software and used to assess samples.

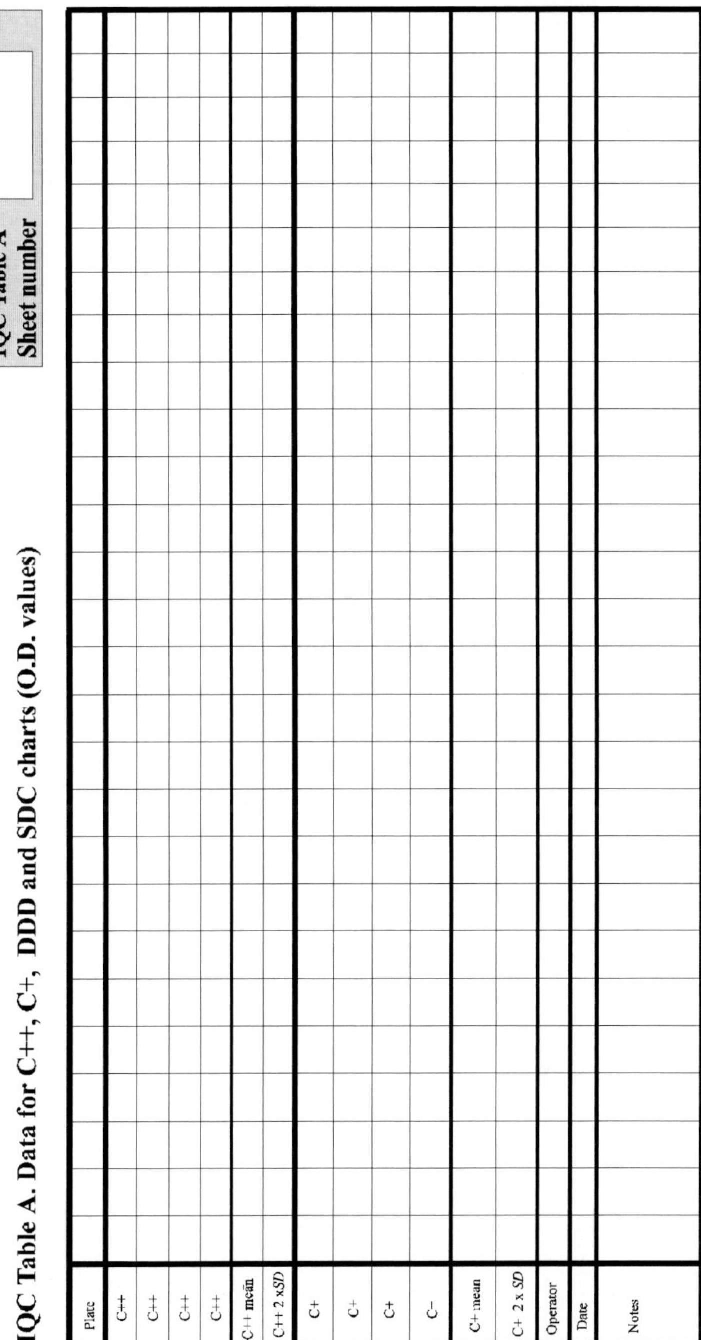

IQC Table A. Data for C++, C+, DDD and SDC charts (O.D. values)

IQC Table A
Sheet number

Plate
C++
C++
C++
C++
C++ mean
C++ 2 x*SD*
C+
C+
C+
C–
C+ mean
C+ 2 x *SD*
Operator
Date
Notes

Fig. 4. IQC Table A. No data.

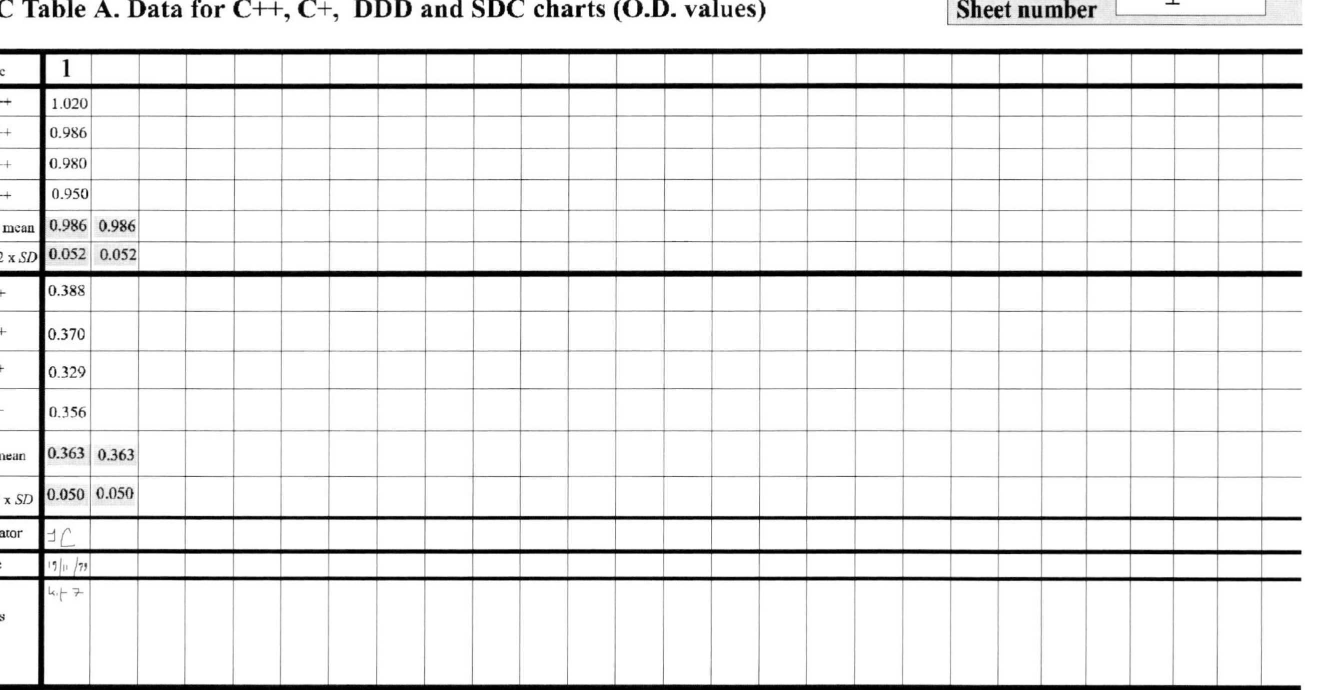

IQC Table A. Data for C++, C+, DDD and SDC charts (O.D. values)

IQC Table A Sheet number	1

Plate	1	
C++	1.020	
C++	0.986	
C++	0.980	
C++	0.950	
C++ mean	0.986	0.986
C++ 2 x *SD*	0.052	0.052
C+	0.388	
C+	0.370	
C+	0.329	
C−	0.356	
C+ mean	0.363	0.363
C+ 2 x *SD*	0.050	0.050
Operator	JC	
Date	19/11/79	
Notes	4+7	

Fig. 5. IQC Table with data from single test. Test using a single plate is processed for plotting on DDD charts. The DDD and SDC data (*gray boxes*) are the same as in the case of a single plate run.

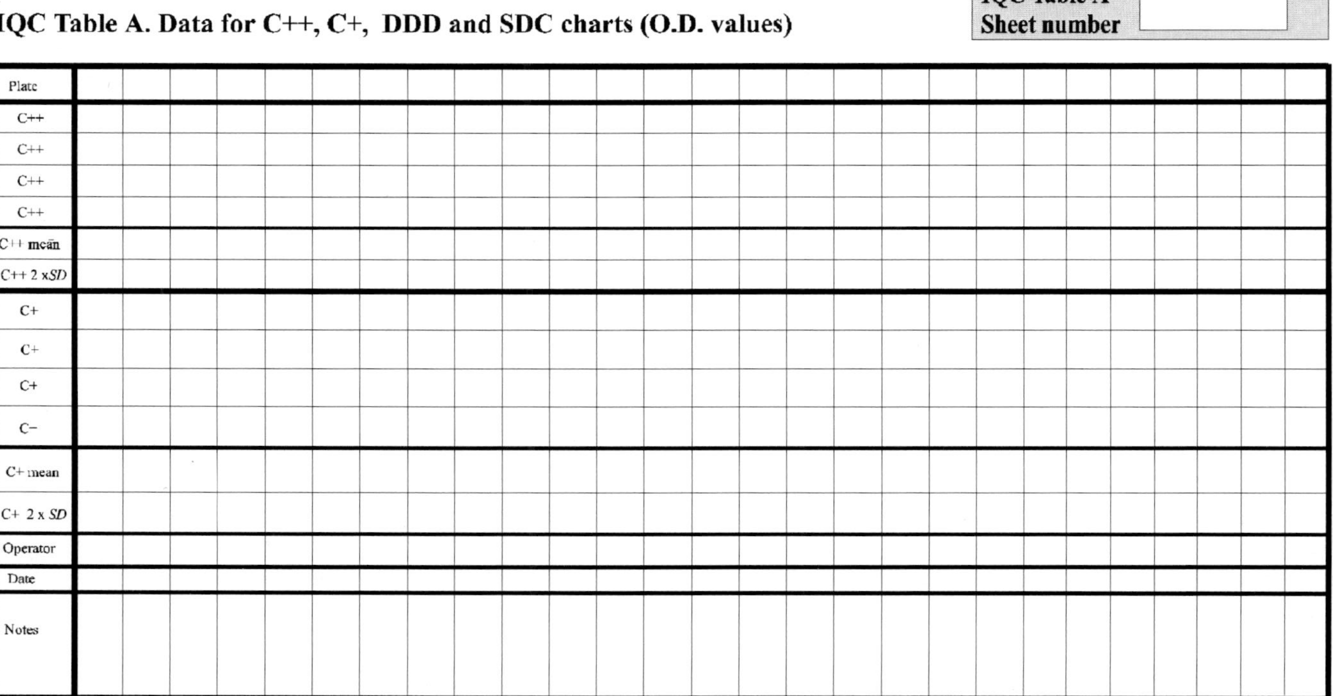

IQC Table A. Data for C++, C+, DDD and SDC charts (O.D. values)

IQC Table A
Sheet number

Plate																											
C++																											
C++																											
C++																											
C++																											
C++ mean																											
C++ 2 x *SD*																											
C+																											
C+																											
C+																											
C–																											
C+ mean																											
C+ 2 x *SD*																											
Operator																											
Date																											
Notes																											

Fig. 4. IQC Table A. No data.

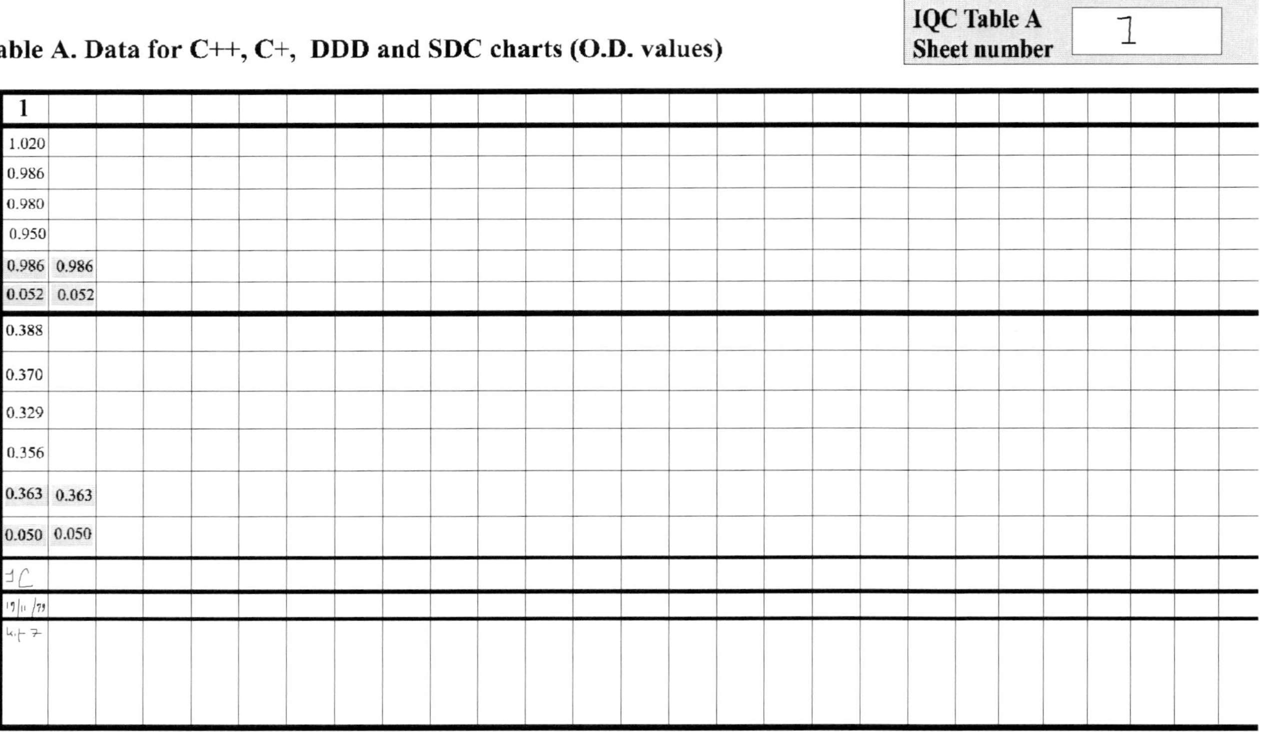

IQC Table A. Data for C++, C+, DDD and SDC charts (O.D. values)

IQC Table A Sheet number 1

Plate	1	
C++	1.020	
C++	0.986	
C++	0.980	
C++	0.950	
C++ mean	0.986	0.986
C++ 2 x *SD*	0.052	0.052
C+	0.388	
C+	0.370	
C+	0.329	
C–	0.356	
C+ mean	0.363	0.363
C+ 2 x *SD*	0.050	0.050
Operator	JC	
Date	17/11/79	
Notes	Kit 7	

Fig. 5. IQC Table with data from single test. Test using a single plate is processed for plotting on DDD charts. The DDD and SDC data (*gray boxes*) are the same as in the case of a single plate run.

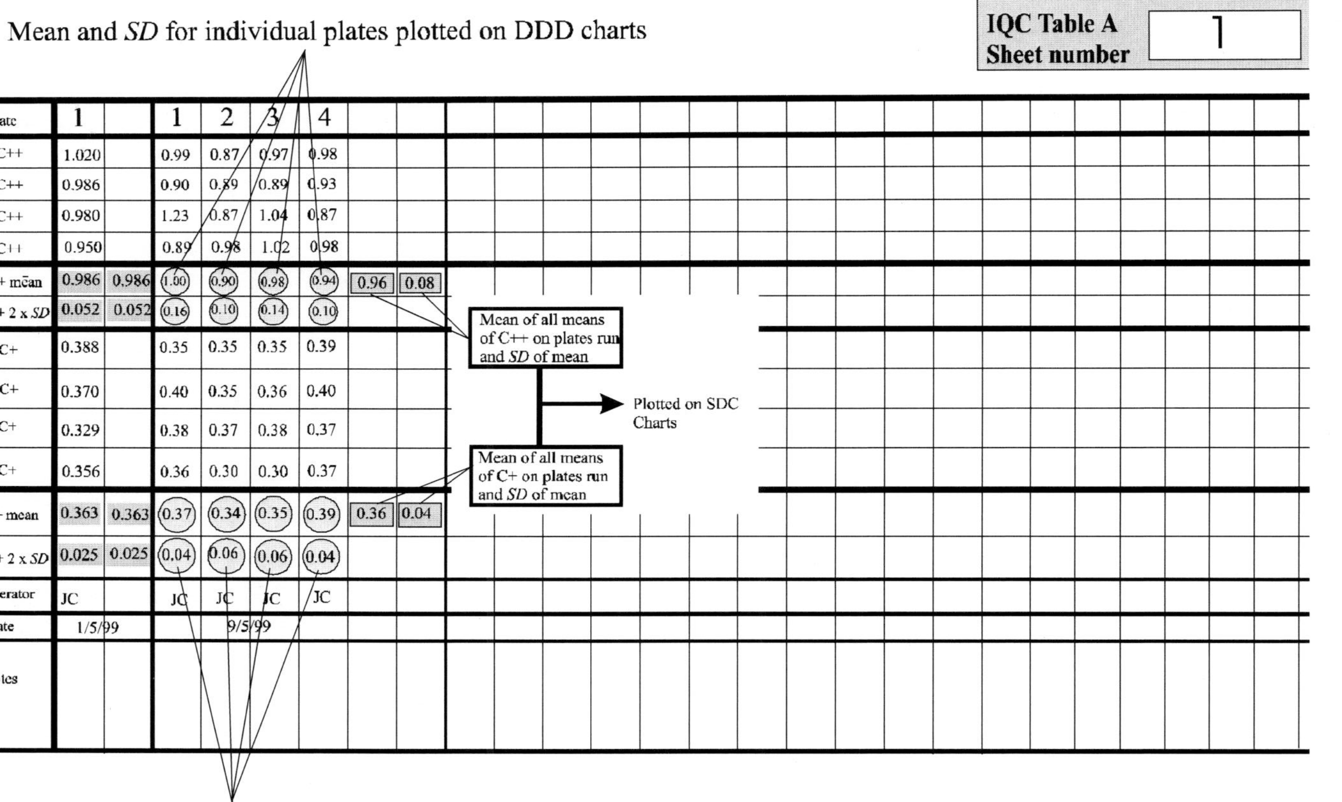

Plate	1		1	2	3	4		
C++	1.020		0.99	0.87	0.97	0.98		
C++	0.986		0.90	0.89	0.89	0.93		
C++	0.980		1.23	0.87	1.04	0.87		
C++	0.950		0.89	0.98	1.02	0.98		
C++ mean	0.986	0.986	1.00	0.90	0.98	0.94	0.96	0.08
C++ 2 x SD	0.052	0.052	0.16	0.10	0.14	0.10		
C+	0.388		0.35	0.35	0.35	0.39		
C+	0.370		0.40	0.35	0.36	0.40		
C+	0.329		0.38	0.37	0.38	0.37		
C+	0.356		0.36	0.30	0.30	0.37		
C+ mean	0.363	0.363	0.37	0.34	0.35	0.39	0.36	0.04
C+ 2 x SD	0.025	0.025	0.04	0.06	0.06	0.04		
Operator	JC		JC	JC	JC	JC		
Date	1/5/99			9/5/99				
Notes								

Fig. 6. Data (OD) from 2 tests. Two sets of data are on table. One set from a single plate test, and another set from a test involving 4 plates. Means and 2 × SD of means for each plate control C++ and C+ have been calculated, and these can be plotted on DDD charts (*grey circles*). The overall mean of the control means and the SD is also calculated (*grey boxes*). The mean values and 2 × SD are plotted in SDC charts. When only a single plate is used, the DDD and SDC data are the same.

ICQ Table B Sheet Number	

Plate		SDC																		
C++																				
C++																				
C++																				
C++																				
C++ mean																				
C++ 2 *SD*																				
C+																				
C+																				
C+																				
C+																				
C+ mean																				
C+ 2 *SD*																				
C–																				
C–																				
C–																				
C–																				
C– $\bar{x}$																				
C- 2 SD																				
Cc																				
Cc																				
Cc																				
Cc																				
Cc- $\bar{x}$																				
Cc- 2 SD																				
Date																				
Operator																				
Notes																				

Fig. 7. Table B provides for recording PP% data for C++, C+, Cc, and C-.

A convenient method of viewing data is to plot values on a chart. This can be examined easily, and can give a view of the data over a time period. As a reminder, we are plotting data on two kinds of charts that are recommended for Quality Control.

A chart that keeps the actual data for various test parameters for each plate used.

This is called a Detailed Daily Data Chart (DDD).

A chart that summarizes data for any particular tests done on a given day.

This is called a Summary Data Chart (SDC).

2.9. Daily Detailed Data Charts (DDD)

These are used to plot individual plate data for mean OD values and the SD from individual plates for C++, C+ controls.

One DDD chart is needed.

Note that we may have run more than one plate on any given day. We have already examined Table A for the recording of data for such plots. Now the data can be plotted.

ICQ Table B Sheet Number	1

Plate		SDC																		
C++	103																			
C++	100																			
C++	99.3																			
C++	96.9																			
C++ mēan	99.8																			
C++ 2 *SD*	5.0																			
C+	39.3																			
C+	37.5																			
C+	33.3																			
C+	36.1																			
C+ mēan	37.5	37.5																		
C+ 2 x *SD*	5.0	5.0																		
C–	0.6																			
C–	2.5																			
C–	0.2																			
C–	0.7																			
C–mean	1.0	1.0																		
C– 2 *SD*	2.0	2.0																		
Cc	13.5																			
Cc	1.5																			
Cc	1.2																			
Cc	0.9																			
Cc- mean	4.3	4.3																		
Cc- 2 *SD*	12.2	12.2																		
Date	19.11.99																			
Operator	John																			
Notes	Kit 12-146																			

Fig. 8. Table B with data for a singe plate recorded. The DDD chart data are the mean and 2 × SD of the control PP% for C++, C+, Cc, and C- values. Here, the DDD and SDC data are the same. No SDC data are recorded for the C++ PP% values.

2.9.1. DDD Chart Design - OD Plots

A design for the charts is shown in **Fig. 10**. A3 is the recommended size of the charts. Enlarged portions of the charts will be provided in the guide, to illustrate the plotting details (*see* **Figs. 11** and **12**).

The charts should be updated every time a test is carried out by an operator.

The charts should be displayed preferably near to where the tests are being carried out.

2.10. SDC Chart Design - OD Plots

Figure 13 shows a chart suitable for recording 3 months of data on SDC charts. On SDC charts, it is important to record the results related to the actual day they are performed. Thus, there is a temporal relationship established for the summary data

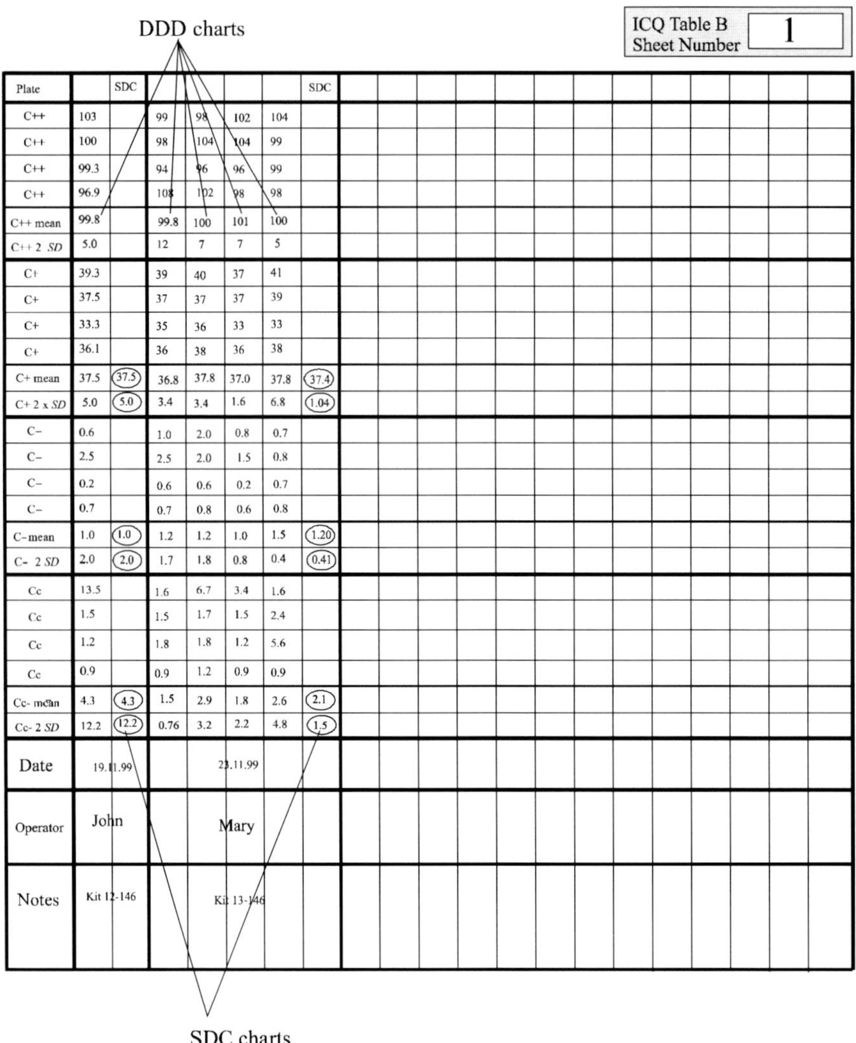

Plate		SDC					SDC
C++	103		99	98	102	104	
C++	100		98	104	104	99	
C++	99.3		94	96	96	99	
C++	96.9		108	102	98	98	
C++ mean	99.8		99.8	100	101	100	
C++ 2 *SD*	5.0		12	7	7	5	
C+	39.3		39	40	37	41	
C+	37.5		37	37	37	39	
C+	33.3		35	36	33	33	
C+	36.1		36	38	36	38	
C+ mean	37.5	37.5	36.8	37.8	37.0	37.8	37.4
C+ 2 x *SD*	5.0	5.0	3.4	3.4	1.6	6.8	1.04
C−	0.6		1.0	2.0	0.8	0.7	
C−	2.5		2.5	2.0	1.5	0.8	
C−	0.2		0.6	0.6	0.2	0.7	
C−	0.7		0.7	0.8	0.6	0.8	
C−mean	1.0	1.0	1.2	1.2	1.0	1.5	1.20
C− 2 *SD*	2.0	2.0	1.7	1.8	0.8	0.4	0.41
Cc	13.5		1.6	6.7	3.4	1.6	
Cc	1.5		1.5	1.7	1.5	2.4	
Cc	1.2		1.8	1.8	1.2	5.6	
Cc	0.9		0.9	1.2	0.9	0.9	
Cc- mean	4.3	4.3	1.5	2.9	1.8	2.6	2.1
Cc- 2 *SD*	12.2	12.2	0.76	3.2	2.2	4.8	1.5
Date	19.11.99			23.11.99			
Operator	John			Mary			
Notes	Kit 12-146			Kit 13-146			

Fig. 9. Table B with data for 2 tests recordedThe PP% DDD chart data are the mean and 2 × SD of the control PP% for C++, C+, Cc, and C- values (*grey boxes*). The SDC data are shown in *grey boxes.* No SDC data are recorded for the C++ PP% values, which are100% according to how the test is read. The variation of C++ is determined with reference to the DDD charts for individual plates for PP% data, and also by examination of the OD-DDD chart.

(**Figs. 14–16**). This is important to identify trends in time for the assay.

2.11. Resume on Charts

DDD charts are plotted as an accurate reference of the test performance on each plate. Individual plate data are plotted so that each plate can be identified and the data reviewed.

The assessment of the whole test (all plates) made on a day-to-day, week-to-week, month-to-month, and year-to-year basis is examined by plotting data on Summary Data Charts (SDC). These charts can graphically illustrate any large variations in data

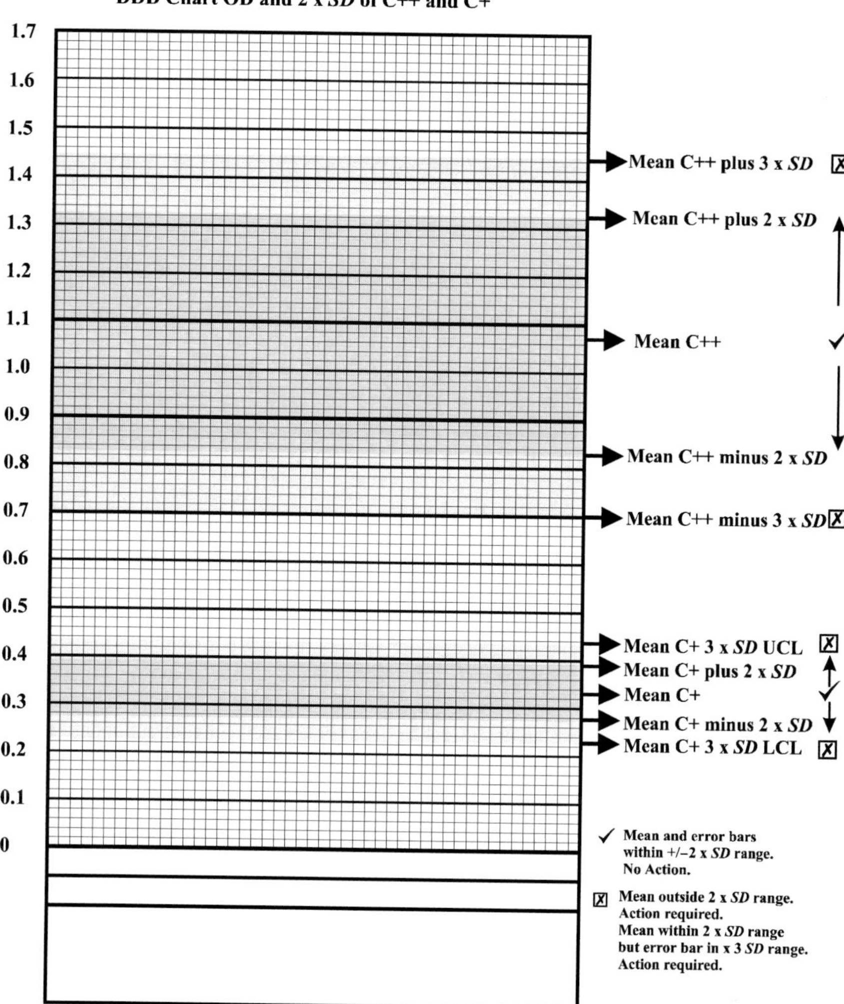

Fig. 10. Detailed Daily Data Chart for OD mean and 2 × SD plots of C++ and C+. The *y* axis shows OD units. The *x* axis contains columns, each representing the data from a single plate for C++ and C+. The expected mean and SD of the test controls (given in kit manual) and the allowed variation from the mean values are shown in the *grey areas*. This represents plus and minus 2 and 3 × SD from the mean. The mean test values obtained on a plate should be within the 2 SD (+/−), preferably as close to the indicated mean as possible. The tick at +/−2 × SD from an expected mean indicates that attention should be paid to results falling outside this range. If the mean falls within plus or minus 2 × SD but error bars fall inside 2–3 × SD, the test should be examined again.

(with reference to the error bars), so that individual plate data for that test can be reviewed.

SDC charts differ fundamentally from DDD charts in that the data plotted represent the mean and variation from all plates used in an assay treated as a group.

Thus, if only 1 plate is used on a particular day, then these data are used to plot the SDC Chart points for that day. If 5 plates are used, then these will be used to obtain the SDC data

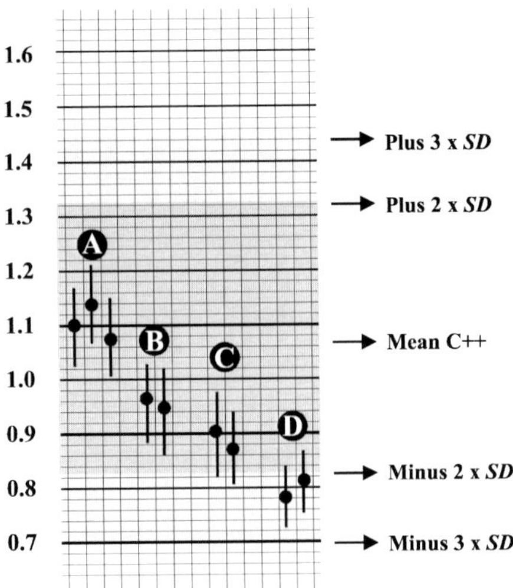

Fig. 11. Enlarged DDD chart showing some C++ plots. Individual plots for the C=++ OD values are shown. The error bars represent plus and minus 2 × SD from mean C++ OD for individual plates. In A, the points are close to the recommended mean, and the error bars are within the plus/minus 2 × SD limits. In B, the points are lower than the expected mean, but still within 2 × SD limits, and the error bars are also within the same limits. In C, the points are lower (approaching the 2 × SD limit), but still within limits; however, the lower limit of the error bars is between the lower 2 and 3 × SD limits. Caution should be used here. In D, the means are outside the 2 × SD limits and action should be taken. Note that the limits described for various plus and minus SD values may change according to the kit sent. The manual or notes sent should describe the limits. These can be set on particular charts. Each individual plate is plotted in this fashion. There should be a clear demarcation of the tests made. This is illustrated in Fig. 10.13, which shows three sets of test results.

for that day. If 35 plates are used, then they will collectively give the SDC Chart data for that day.

If two series of tests are made on the same day, representing 5 plates and 6 plates, respectively, then data from all eleven plates are processed to give the SDC data. All testing done is included.

It is important that OD data are in range, and that this is checked. It may be that results observed on PP% charts appear good, but that the OD values are actually out of range. This will be examined in the following section.

3. Interpretation of Charts

The purpose of charting the data is to help to constantly monitor the performance of the kit in its use to measure antibodies against Brucella. The points of assessment are always with reference to

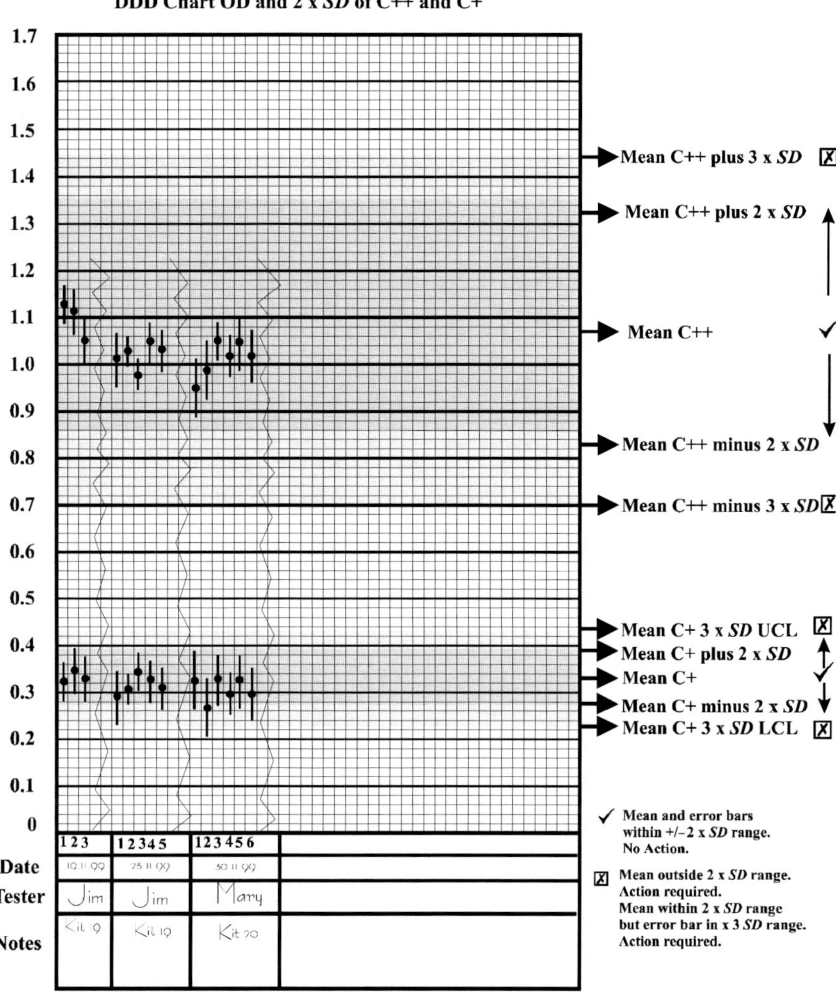

Fig. 12. DDD chart showing results from three tests. Note that there is a clear distinction made between tests (*zig-zag line*). The data, plate number, operator, and notes have been filled in.

the performance of the control sera and reagents supplied. The data should be on view to all, at all times, allowing the statistics of the test to be observed by eye (descriptive statistics).

The data on these reagents in the kit have been obtained after multiple testing, so that expected values and variation from these values have been recorded and calculated. The key assumption is that these are "constants" in the assay, i.e., that all the reagents and controls will remain the same physically throughout the time that they are used in the tests. Note that, because of this assumption, we have to be very careful not to handle the control samples badly, as they set the control limits of the assay.

The control serum samples represent sera containing a high level of anti-Brucella antibodies (C++), a relatively weak serum

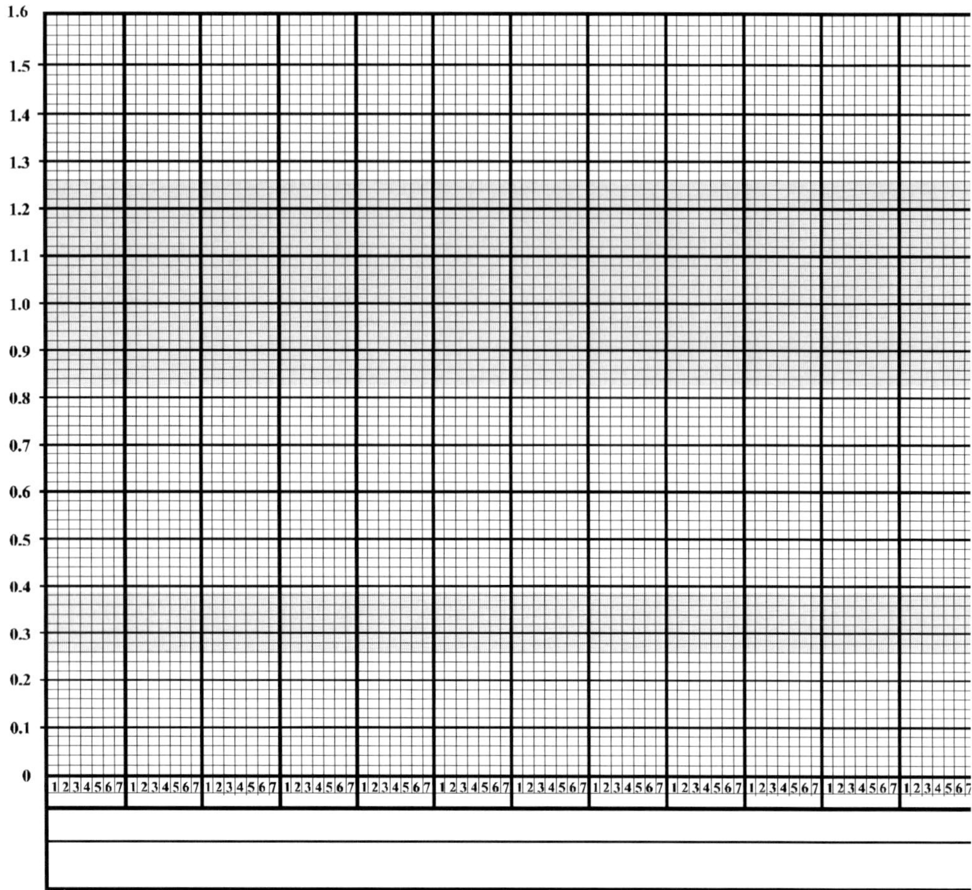

Fig. 13. Example of layout for SDC chart.

(C+) that should not give maximal reaction while representing ~30–40% of the value for the C++ inhibition, but which should always give results distinct from the C++ and C- controls.

3.1. Variation

There will be variation in the results obtained in the tests. The variation will be from plate to plate on the same day, from day to day, and from operator to operator. The measurement of this variation through calculation of the SD is what the charts help the operator to investigate. This variation is a result of the pipettes used, the operator's technique, the differences in reagent formulation, variable temperatures, the different kit batches used, water quality changes, and similar factors.

We have to accept a degree of variation. The indication of the acceptance limits are given in the manual. The point about the charts is that they reflect a degree of variation. When the test is

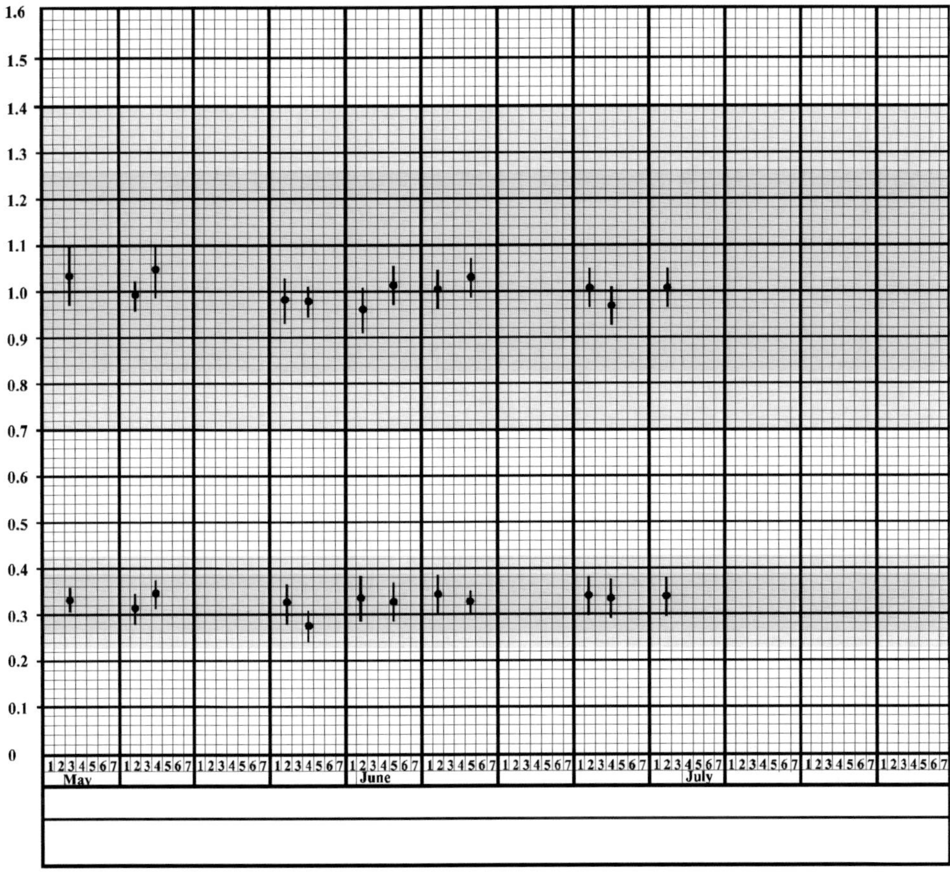

Fig. 14. SDC chart showing results plotted. C++ and C+ data plotted. *Dark grey area* = or −2 × SD and *light grey* = or −3 × SD from means.

within limits with respect to the control values observed, we are running an acceptable test. Constant monitoring allows a gradual change in data to be observed. When the limits are not observed, action is needed to rectify the situation, and clues on the nature of the problem are inherent in the data (e.g., a new operator can produce a bad result through bad technique, a new set of pipettes may not be accurate, or a new kit may have a reagent that has been badly affected in transit). The rapid assessment of data can aid the mass testing of samples to obtain meaningless results, and also allows comparison of results from different laboratories using the same kit. The processing of IQC data from different laboratories and the statistical comparison of results is part of any External Quality Assurance (EQA) practice.

For the controls:

1. A "target" or expected mean OD reading is given.
2. Expected upper and lower limits for OD are given (at the 2× and 3× plus and minus SD).

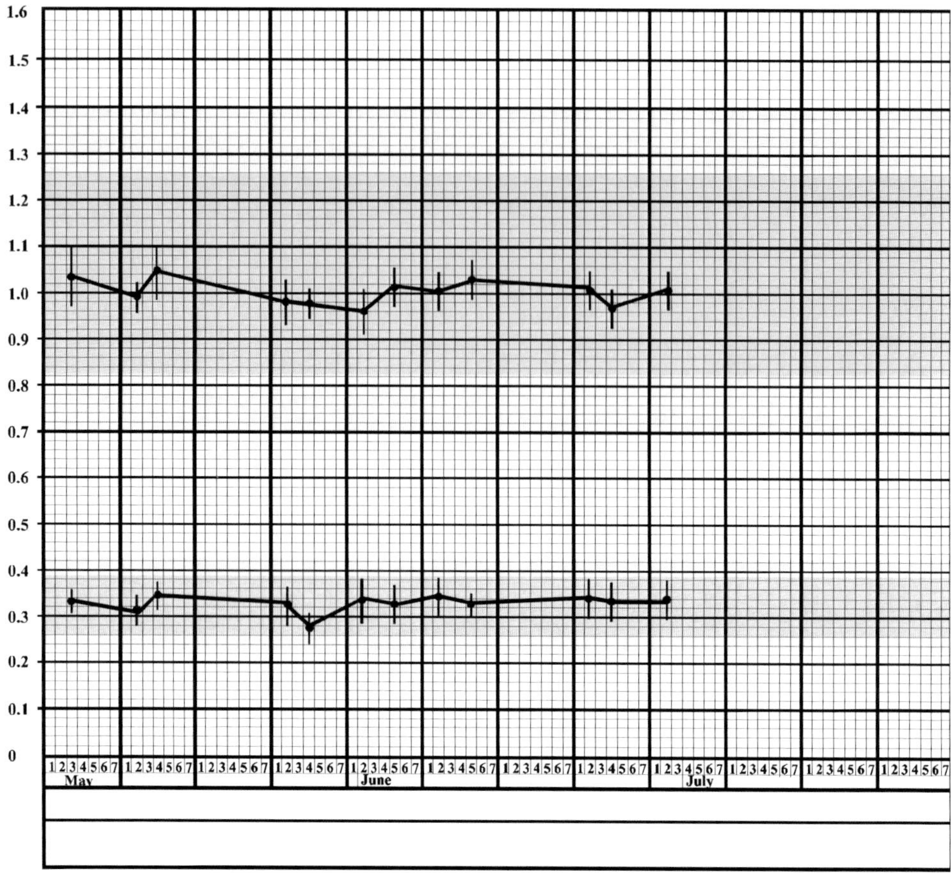

Fig. 15. SDC chart showing results plotted and connected by a line. C++ and C+ data plotted. *Dark grey area* = or −2 × SD and *light grey* = or −3 × SD from means.

3. An expected PP% for each control value is given.
4. Upper and lower control limits for each control value PP% are given (at the 2× and 3× plus and minus SD. To go back to the earlier part of this guide, the first task when receiving a kit is to run the controls under the conditions described in the manual and see what results are obtained. These should give mean values within the described limits in the manual. Once this is established, then the routine monitoring of the test on a daily, weekly, monthly, and yearly basis is vital to answer the question of whether the test is "the same" each time. The charts merely plot the data that are generated each time a test is conducted. They are a visual representation of the data collected and concisely presented. The charts should be updated immediately. The charts should be on full view for all involved in the test to see. Copies of the charts can be kept as well as those "on show".

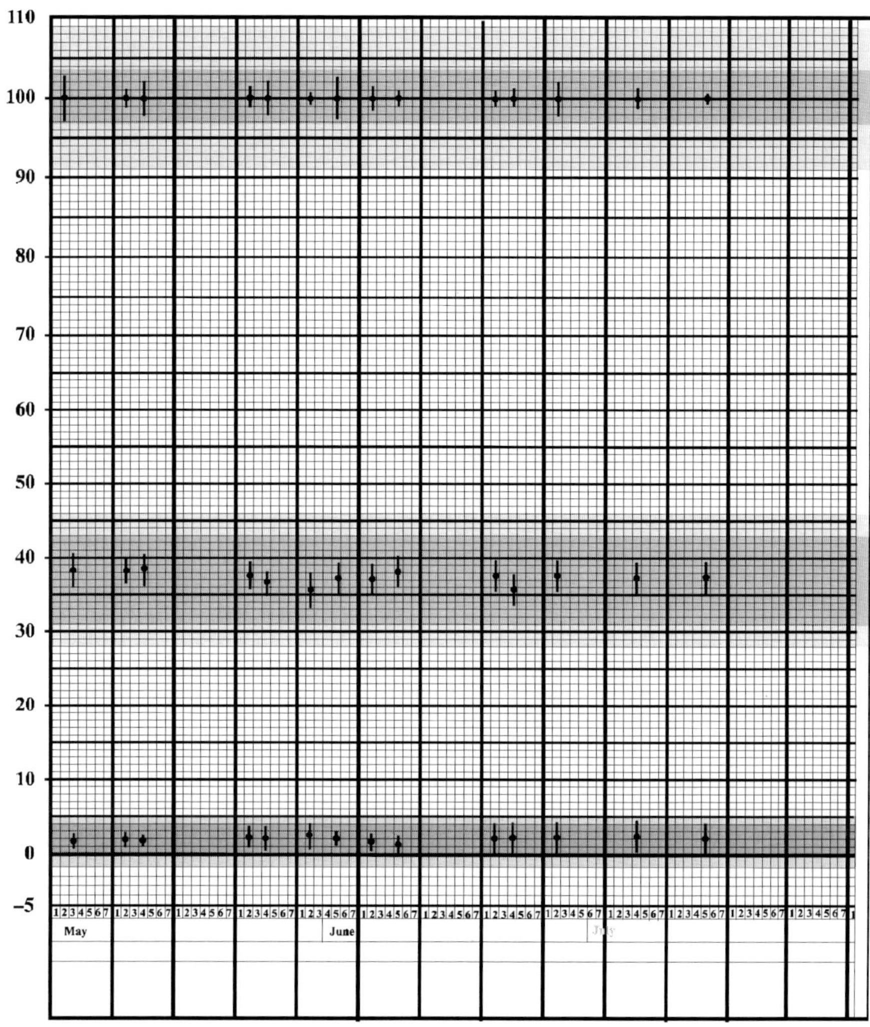

Fig. 16. SDC chart showing PI% results plotted. C++, C+, and C- data plotted. The C++ data are shown to illustrate that the variation can be easily observed, to indicate whether unacceptable mean C++ data are being included in tests. Reference to the DDD OD charts will identify "outlier" values, and it can be estimated whether such data should be included. The 2× and 3× SD is shown in *grey boxes*. These may vary according to "recommended" or calculated means and SD of particular kits.

3.2. What Can We See from the Charts?

The main monitoring device is the SDC chart, which gives a time-bound view of the test and highlights trends easily. Points can be connected to related data from one test day to another. This can give early warning of a "trend" in the test, indicating that something is wrong. This will be illustrated below where "worked" examples of different scenarios are examined.

The use of the DDD charts is important in that the data from every single plate are "logged", and a particular day's testing can be highlighted for close examination from the SDC charts.

Data are plotted as mean values with an error bar. Monitoring of tests is by observation that the means observed fall within limits, and that the means do not have too large an error. It is vital that the charts showing OD data are examined first and displayed, and not just PP% values on DDD and SDC charts. Where the OD values used to calculate PP% values are out of limits, it is possible that the "correct" PP% values can be obtained for certain controls.

Examination of error bars is also important where means are significantly different either as a group (as reflected in SDC charts) or as an individual mean in a group of plates on a single day's testing. Examination of the plate OD data for plates where error is high may indicate where the problem originates, e.g., the control serum for C++ or C+ may have been left out of a plate. Where a single result for a series of plates run on any day is seen to be "faulty" with reference to the other plates and accumulated data, then some adjustment to the data may be possible so that analysis of test samples from that plate can be made.

3.3. Examples of Use of DDD and SDC Charted Data

Examples of what might happen in laboratories in time will be given.

A. Good tests------------------------------No real problems.

B. Some worries-------------------------Is the test too variable, and why?

3.4. Good Tests (No Real Problems)

Testing begins with the initial running of the kit and kit controls. The prescribed values for the controls and the allowable limits are in the manual. If instructions have been followed accurately, then the kit function successfully. If the control OD values are within limits, then the kit is functioning as expected and test samples may be examined. Therefore, a good test begins with examination of the controls. Following this initial test, a good test is indicated where all the mean OD values of the controls are as expected (within 2 × SD limits prescribed) and the error bars do not overlap to the plus or minus 3 × SD areas.

3.4.1. Observations

Data from the initial running of a kit and two following tests are shown in **Fig. 17**. These are OD data plotted on a DDD chart. These data are all within limits with relation to the expected mean OD for C++ and C+ and the variation is similar, as judged by the length of the plus or minus 2 × SD bars. None of the bars are in the plus or minus 3 × SD areas marked on the charts.

Note that the SD bars are a similar length for all of the plates, and that the different operators have obtained similar means. Examination shows that:

1. There are no large differences in SD or means for the kits.
2. The operators have identified themselves.

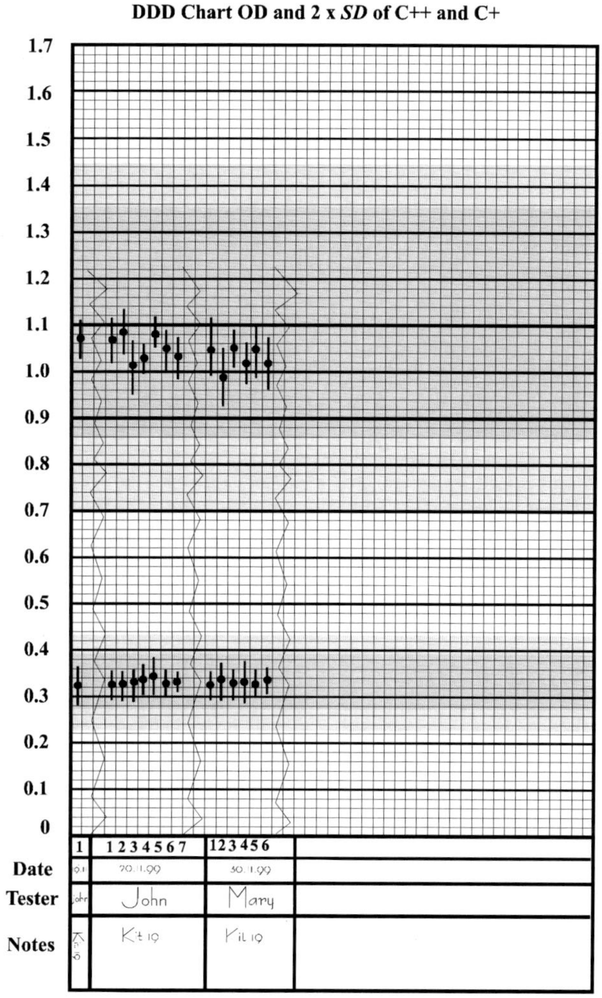

DDD Chart OD and 2 x *SD* of C++ and C+

1.7 1.6 1.5 1.4 1.3 1.2 1.1 1.0 0.9 0.8 0.7 0.6 0.5 0.4 0.3 0.2 0.1 0

	1	1 2 3 4 5 6 7	1 2 3 4 5 6	
Date		20.1.99	30.1.99	
Tester	John	John	Mary	
Notes		Kit 19	Kit 19	

Fig. 17. Example of a DDD with data plots showing PP% means and +/−2SD of mean.

3. They have left a gap of 2 between different test days.
4. They have written test dates in.
5. They have denoted which kit was used.

The OD values of plates run by the two different workers, on different days, with different kits, are shown. These represent no problems with respect to expected values and variations in tests. These data reflect the control values of each plate.

The SDC chart data for PP% for the same results, therefore, would not be expected to fall outside the range. This is shown in **Fig. 18**. The SDC plots are plotted in time.

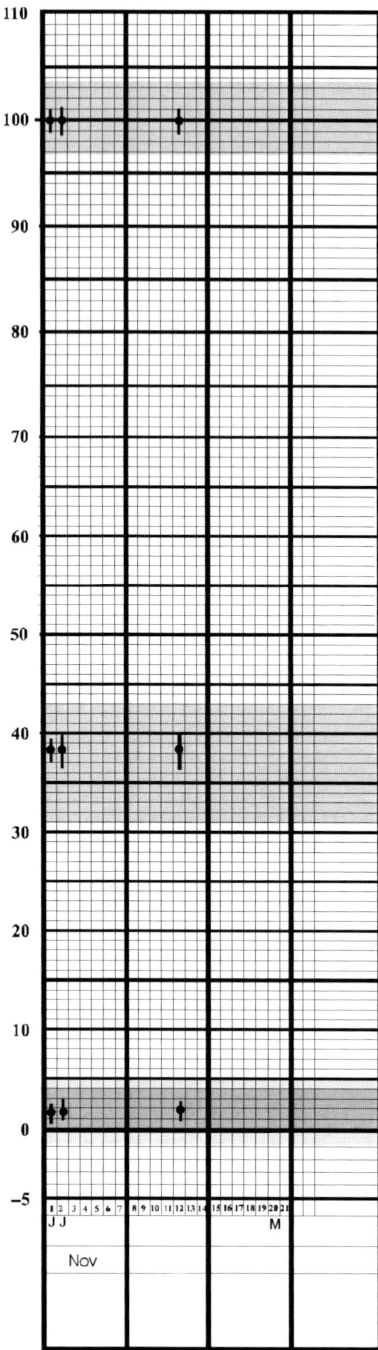

Fig. 18. Example of an SDC with data plots, showing PP% means and +/−2SD of mean. PP% of plates run by two different operators, on different days, with different kits. This test gives ideal values for means of controls and shows little variation, as judged by the length of the error bars. Note that the actual OD values on SDC charts should also be examined to see whether the test is within limits.

10.3.5 .Some Worries

10.3.5.1. Control Problems C++

The data in **Fig. 19** shows the C++ and C+ OD values for individual plates. Two operators performed the tests with the same kit reagents. Note that the OD values for the C++ are all too low, but that the error on each plate (as judged by the error bar length) is similar. The results for the Cc and C- were as expected (not shown). This would indicate that there is something wrong with the C++ control, and that both operators found a similar result. The C+ values are as expected. Translation of the OD values into PP% reveals that the C+ PP% are all out of range (as a result of the low C++ values). This is shown in **Fig. 20**.

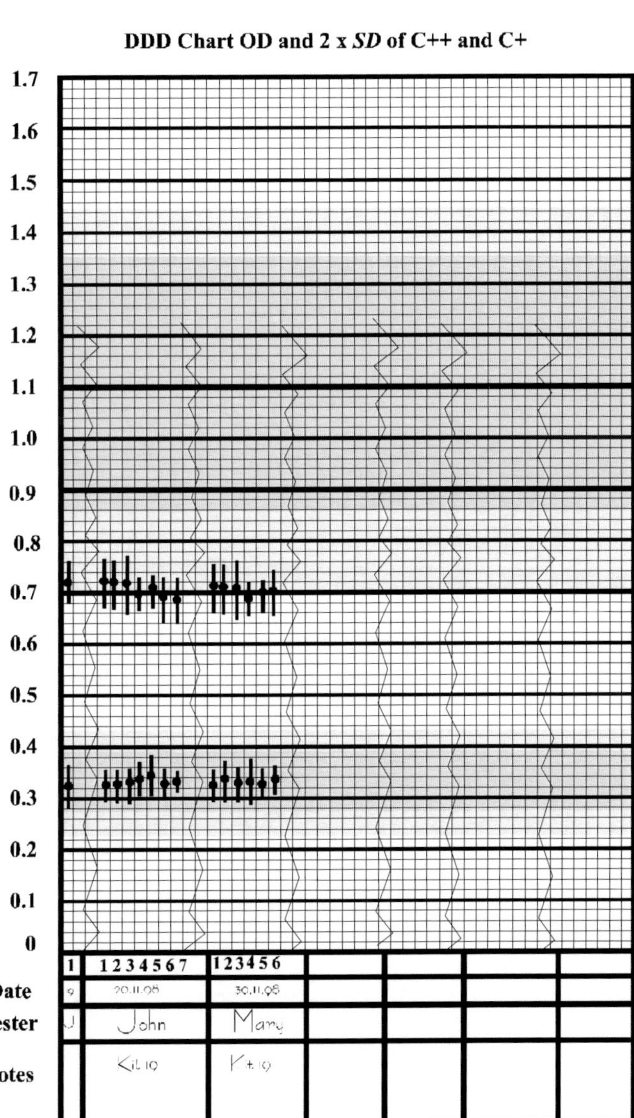

Fig. 19. DDD chart of OD data. Tests done on three days: the 9th, 20th, and 30th of a month. Two operators conducted the tests.

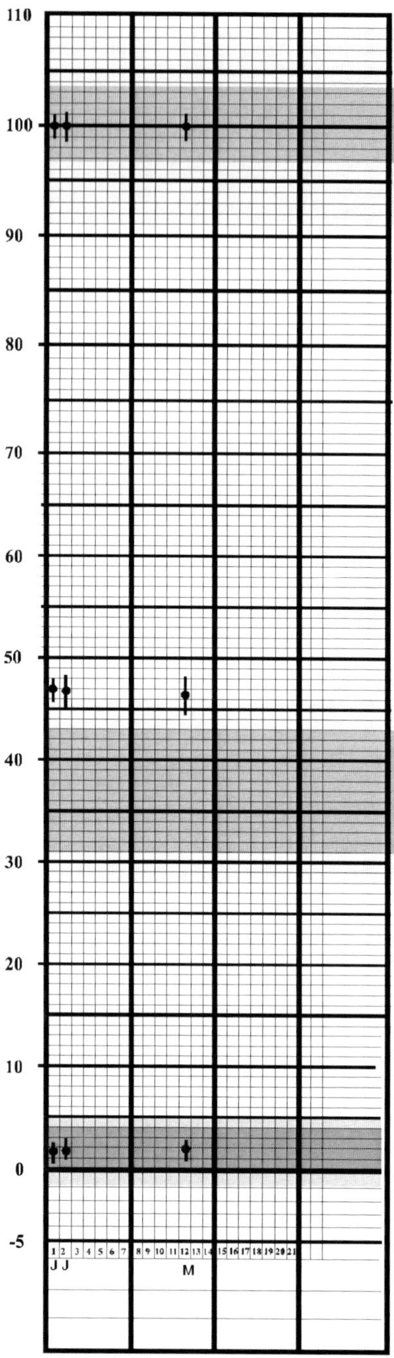

Fig. 20. SDC chart of PP% data in Fig. 10.18. Tests done on three days: the 9th, 20th, and 30th of a month. The Cc data are also included. Note that there is low variation in the overall tests, as judged by short error bars, even for the C++ data.

3.5.2. Control Problems C+

A similar picture is shown in **Fig. 21**; however, this time the C++ is as expected, whereas the C+ is lower than expected. Again, both operators used the same kit at different times, and the intrinsic variation with respect to the error bar length is acceptable. The C+ control in this case is not acceptable. The SDC of the PP% values is shown in **Fig. 22**.

3.5.3. High Errors on Single Plates in a Single Control

In a test, there may be one plate where the mean of a control OD value is obviously out of range, whereas the rest are as expected.

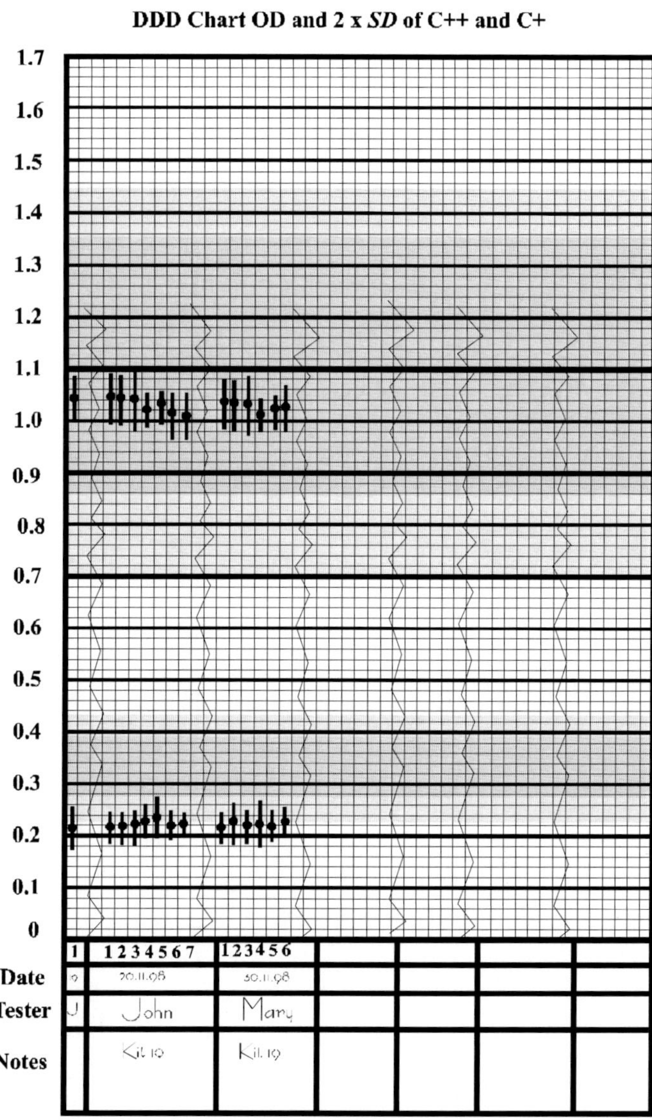

Fig. 21. DDD chart of OD data. Tests done on three days: the 9th, 20th, and 30th of a month. Two operators conducted the tests. The C+ values are too low and out of range as means. The error bars are acceptable. The C++ is as expected.

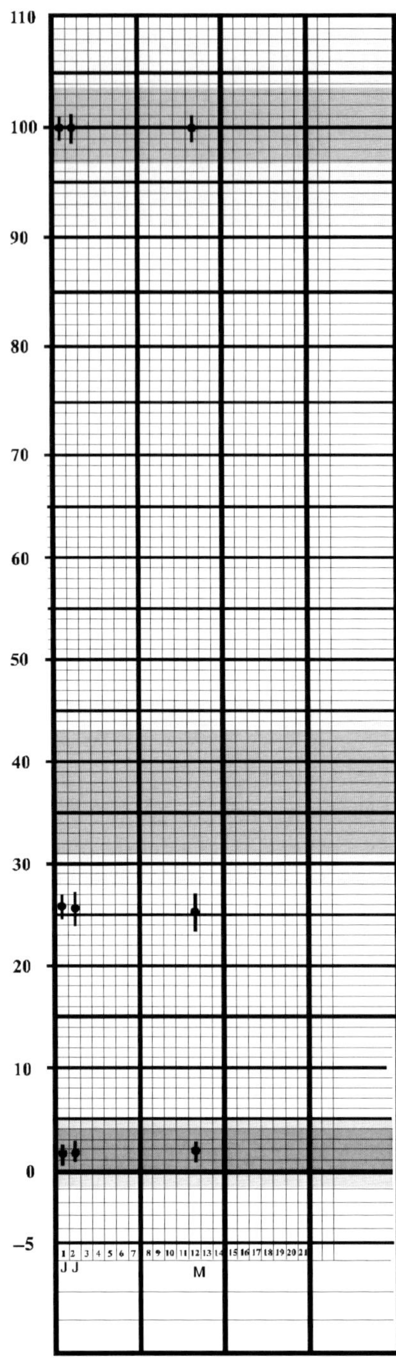

Fig. 22. SDC chart of PP% data in Fig. 10.21. Note that the C+ values are out of range.

There could also be a plate where the error is very high, but the mean is as expected. These are illustrated in **Fig. 23**.

The three situations A, B, and C, seen in **Fig. 23**, could also be present in the C+ controls on individual plates, with no problems with the C++.

A. The lack of variation indicates that similar conditions were present in each well of the respective control. In the context of all other plates in the test having expected values, this control

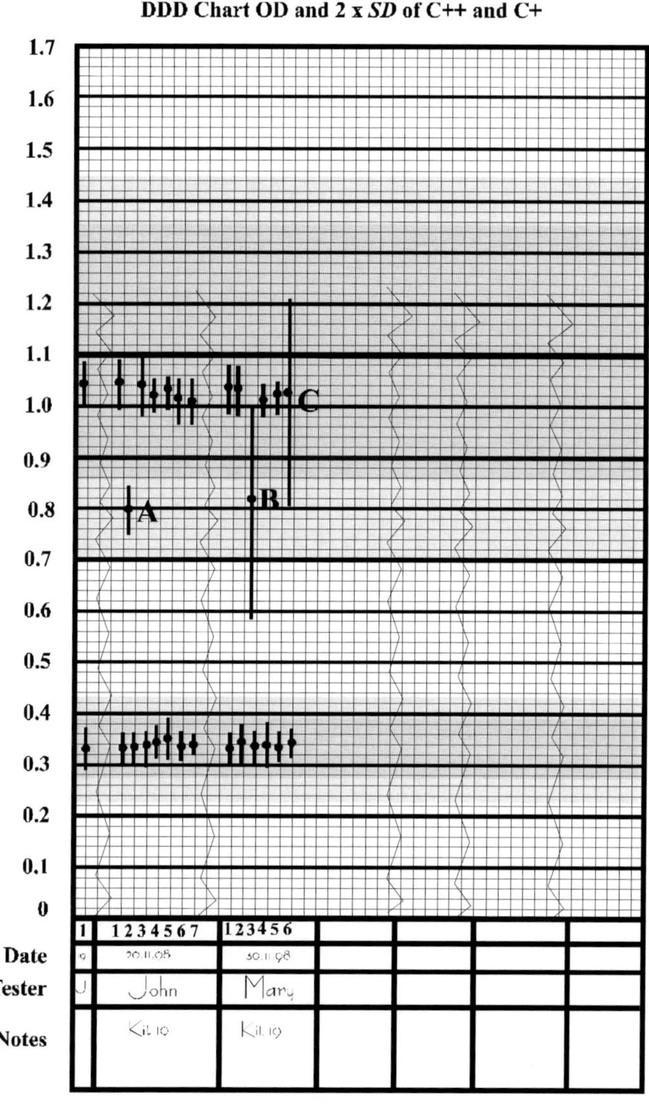

Fig. 23. DDD chart of OD data. The data (**A**) shows a mean which is unacceptable, but with an error similar to the rest of the test. (**B**) shows a large error (*long error bar*) and a mean that is unacceptable. (**C**) shows an unacceptable error, but an acceptable mean.

must be regarded as an operator error. To take an extreme situation, where the C++ was not added to a single plate, one would observe no color in that plate for that control. This would be obvious. If the wrong volume was added by error to the plate in question, the values obtained would be lower, but precise (in terms of error observed). In this situation, it may be possible to assume the C++ for that plate from the observed data from all plates run that day, and substitute this into the calculations of PP% for the aberrant plate.

B. A long error bar is seen, indicating high variation in the OD values in the controls. This should have been noted when tabulating the data. As we calculate the error based on all datum points and use the mean (not median), there is no "smoothing" of gross errors. The error in one well of a control, e.g., where no antiserum is added, can have a dramatic effect on the mean. If the data on the plates are revised, the "bad" OD can be ignored and the control OD revised in terms of the three wells showing the expected OD. This will reduce the error bar and restore the mean allowing calculations based on a more reliable estimate.

C. This shows a mean that might be expected, but with a high error. This is typical of a situation where there are at least two wells in a control showing discrepant values from the expected ones. Thus, the mean of a very high and very low result from two wells, along with two wells showing expected values, is approximately the expected mean. Again, this variation should be seen when tabulating data. The data for the plates showing high and low ODs should be reassessed. Note that the SDC plots of the OD for such plates, as in example B, might be affected by the low mean of the plates, whereas, the SDC plots for situation C would not be affected.

There could be an association where the effects described in situations A to C are observed in both the C++ and C+. This may be associated with an operator error with respect to the number of the plate processed in time. For instance, as an extreme example, it may have been the last plate in a test and the operator forgot to add the controls. Such an association is not common, and it is most likely that these kinds of variations are observed in controls on any one plate.

3.5.4. Variation of Means and Errors

A test could provide data where both the means and the errors vary. This would point to a problem with operator technique, e.g., inaccurate dispensing of reagents, or poor pipettes. **Figures 24** and **25** illustrate this kind of variation. Two operators, A and B, have made tests with the same kits. Operator A has results that are good, in that the means and the errors are all as expected. Operator B produces much more variation in the means and the

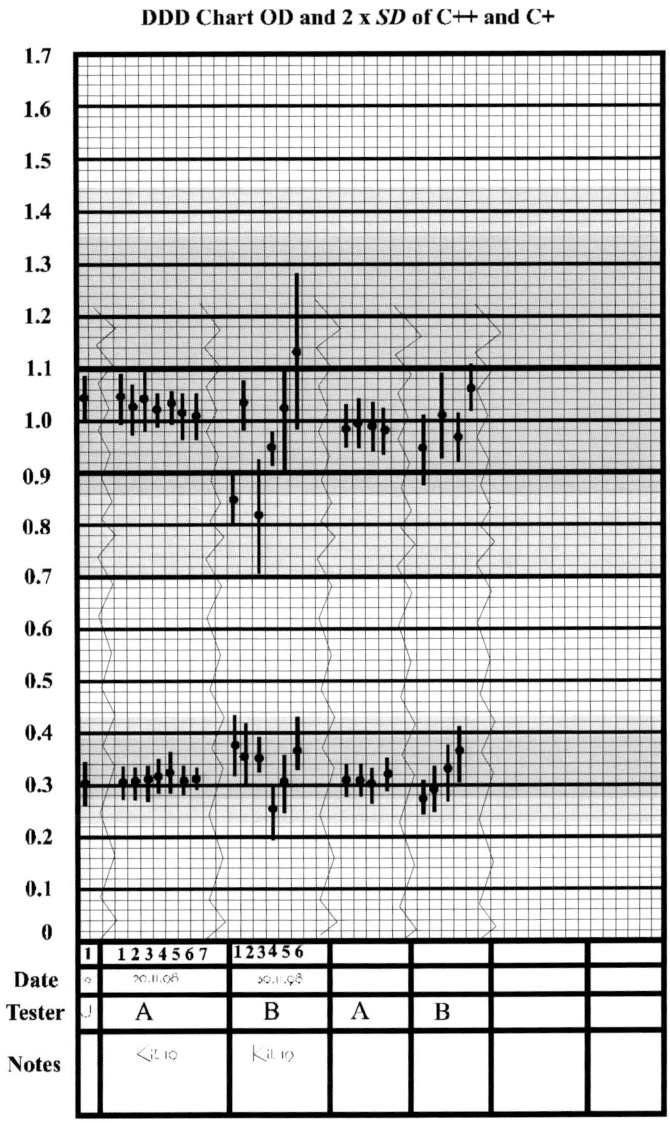

DDD Chart OD and 2 x *SD* of C++ and C+

Fig. 24. DDD chart of OD data. Operators A and B have used the same kit on different days. Operator A has good results throughout, with respect to means and errors. B shows higher variation in means, and has much higher error bars. This indicates operator error due to poor technique.

error bars. This indicates B's poor technique rather than reagent problems. There is an improved performance even in the second test performed by B.

Care has to be taken with regard to the use of only SDC charts of PP% and OD data in such cases. When tabulating data before plotting, such higher-than-expected variations in error bars and means from a single test can be easily observed. Note

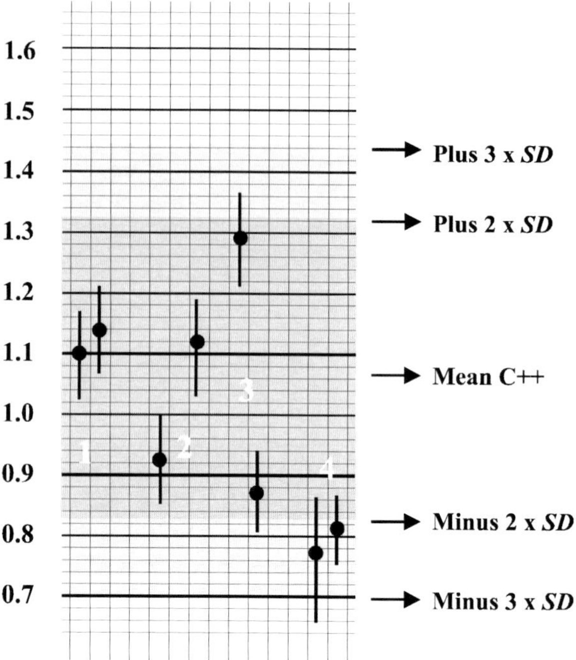

Fig. 25. Enlarged DDD chart of OD data. This illustrates allowable means and tolerance of allowable error bars. *1*, shows good test result with mean and error bars all within 2 × SD limits. *2*, shows more differences in means, but with the error bar still within 2 × SD limits. *3*, indicates possible problems, as the error bars are within the 2–3 × SD range. D is unacceptable data, as the means fall outside the 2 × SD range. *4*, shows unacceptable means.

that this type of variation is more generalized throughout a test, unlike the previously described single-plate anomalies.

3.6. Trends

Besides analysis of single datum points, there is a benefit from charts that show trends in overall data. This is relevant to all controls. The relationship of the trends within and between each control can establish the source of increasing errors in tests, so that action points can be identified and action then taken.

This section is intended to help a laboratory continuously interpret the charts as they are being plotted, i.e., as the story of the data unfolds. The section will use thumbnail approaches to represent the different data that might be observed in practice. Analysis should lead to indications as to whether there is a need to take action, and what actions are needed.

The advantage of charting data is that they can be viewed as a single entity, that trends and fluctuations can be rapidly observed through examination of SDC data, and that details at any point in time can be expanded through examination of DDD data. This approach has already been explained; this section will attempt to simplify likely scenarios in charts and indicate solutions where necessary, based on observations.

3.7. Examination of SDC Charts - Individual Points as Plotted

These charts summarize all data on a given day's testing, and relate the results in actual time, so that "trends" or irregularities can be noted on a continuous basis. The plots reflect the mean value of any control and its variation in all the plates examined in a given day's testing.

The bar plotted shows the variation. The mean value and the error bars should fall within the given limits for the assay for the various control samples, both for actual OD values and for the processed PP% data.

Thus, the SDC plots can alert operators to unacceptable means and errors, and cause them to closely examine the data on individual plates for that test, so as to examine what factors produced the variation (which affects the mean value and size of error bars). This entails examination of the data in DDD charts.

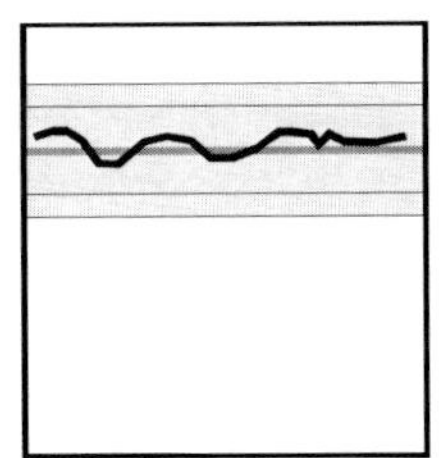

A. CONSTANT and IDEAL

C++ OD mean values all near ideal mean over time and regular (invariable).

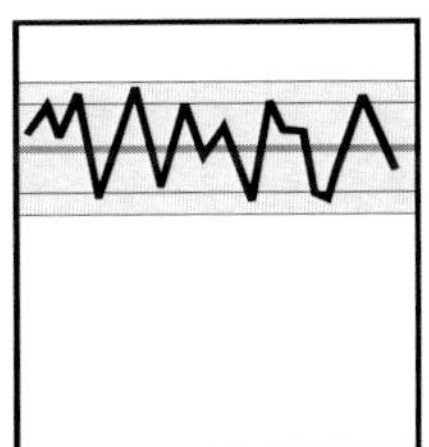

B. IRREGULAR WITHIN ACCEPTED MEAN LIMITS

C++ OD mean values all within limits over time but irregular (variable) not obviously associated with other changes in test e.g. different operators of specific kits used.)

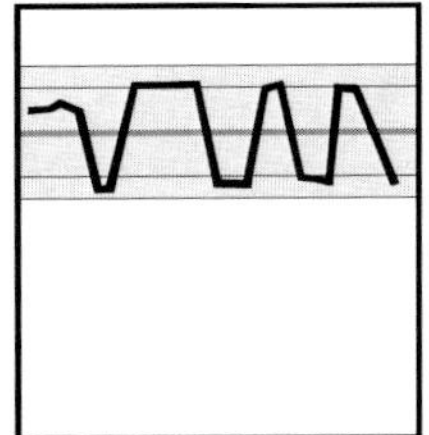

C. IRREGULAR (PATTERN) WITHIN LIMITS

C++ OD mean values all within limits over time WITH irregular (variable) data showing some pattern (possibly associated with other changes in test).

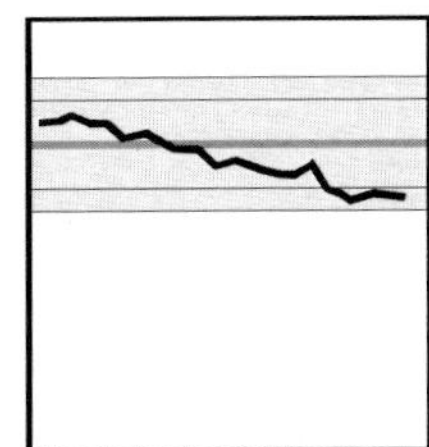

D. DRIFTING DOWN

C++ OD mean values all within limits over time but showing gradual reduction.

Fig. 26. SDC charts of C++ OD data, trends. This illustrates trends in data in time (**A**) Shows expected good results with no major variations. (**B**) Shows very irregular data, indicating irregular errors, probably due to operator variation and poor technique. (**C**) Indicates errors associated with operators, or change in kits or conditions. (**D**) Indicates that one of the controls is losing activity over time.

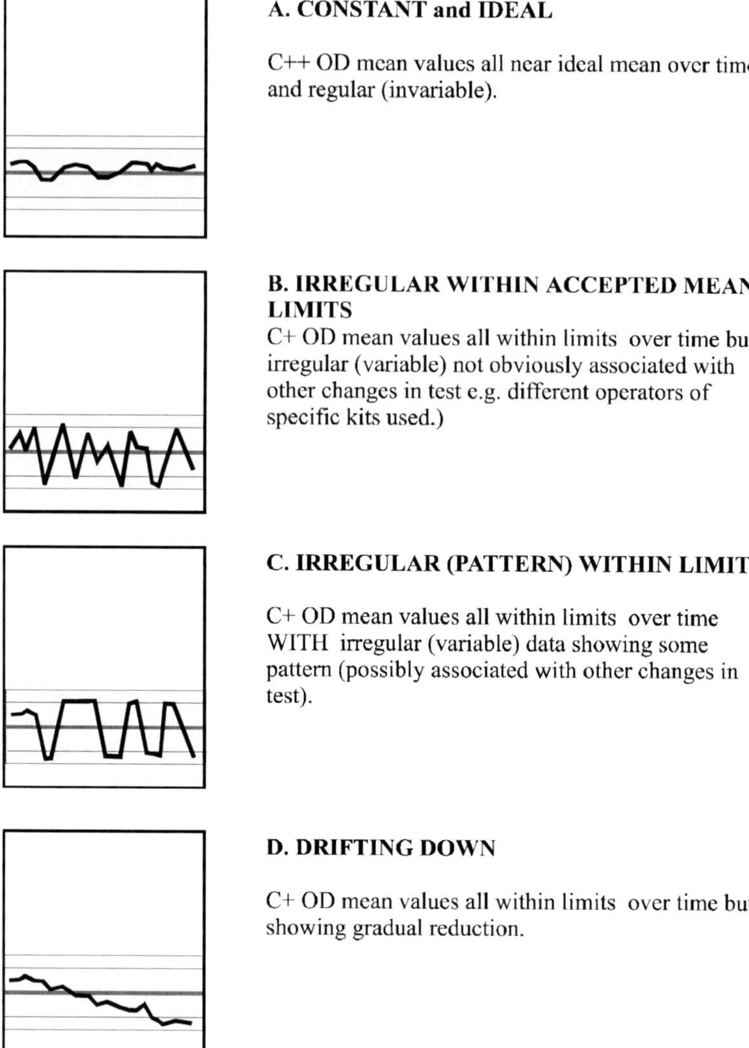

Fig. 27. SDC charts of C+ OD data trends. This illustrates trends in data in time. (**A**) Shows expected good results, with no major variations. (**B**) Shows very irregular data, indicating irregular errors, probably due to operator variation and poor technique. (**C**) Indicates errors associated with operators, or change in kits or conditions. (**D**) Indicates that one of the controls is losing activity over time.

The SDC plots cover both the actual OD and the processed PP% values. It is important that both types of plots are examined together, so the charts should be placed in close proximity. This should immediately alert operators to unusual fluctuations from the expected values in both charts, as well as deviations in one chart but not in the other. Where the OD values are within limits, it is expected that the control serum values for OD, and hence PP%, will be within limits.

Where the OD values change, they effect the PP% calculations. The trends in an assay may reflect that both the C++ and C+ decrease or (more unlikely) increase in OD value proportionally. Here, the correct PP% values are obtained, but the test may be out of limits eventually with respect to OD values. The changes or trends may only affect one control and not the other.

Figure 26 shows sketch diagrams of types of trends for C++ OD SDC charts. These represent C++ data. No error bars are shown. These illustrate major trends. Similar trends are illustrated for C+ in **Fig. 27**, and **Fig. 28** shows the most likely association of trends between C++ and C+ controls.

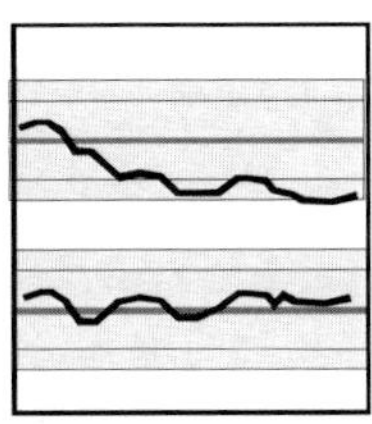
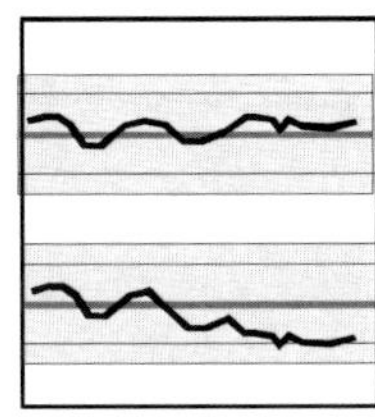

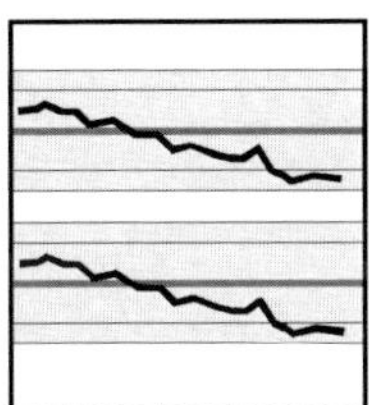

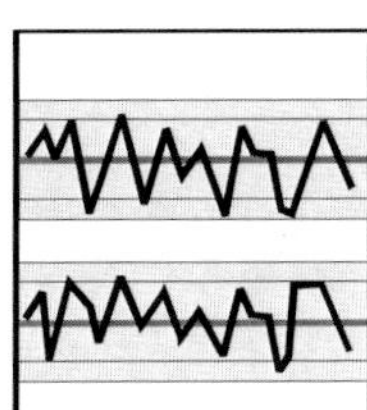

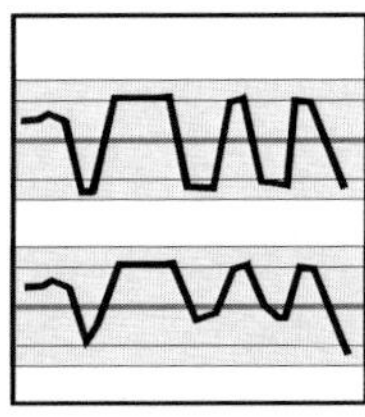

Fig. 28. SDC charts of C++ data trends. This compares trends with respect to most expected relationships. (**A**) Shows that either the C++ or C+ can remain constant and ideal whereas the other control can reduce in OD in time. (**B**) Shows a situation where both controls gradually reduce in OD. (**C**) Shows irregular results; usually, the inaccuracies inherent in such tests are reflected in both controls. (**D**) Shows that there is some consistency for accuracy in certain operators (or sets of conditions) compared to others.

4. Problem Solving

IQC results are obtained continuously, and should highlight problems as they arise. It is imperative that operators process and examine results constantly. Actions are dictated by the results. The object of this section is to detail what should be done and when actions should be taken. The following section highlights measures to be taken when certain observations are made. **Figure 29** illustrates stages in problem solving.

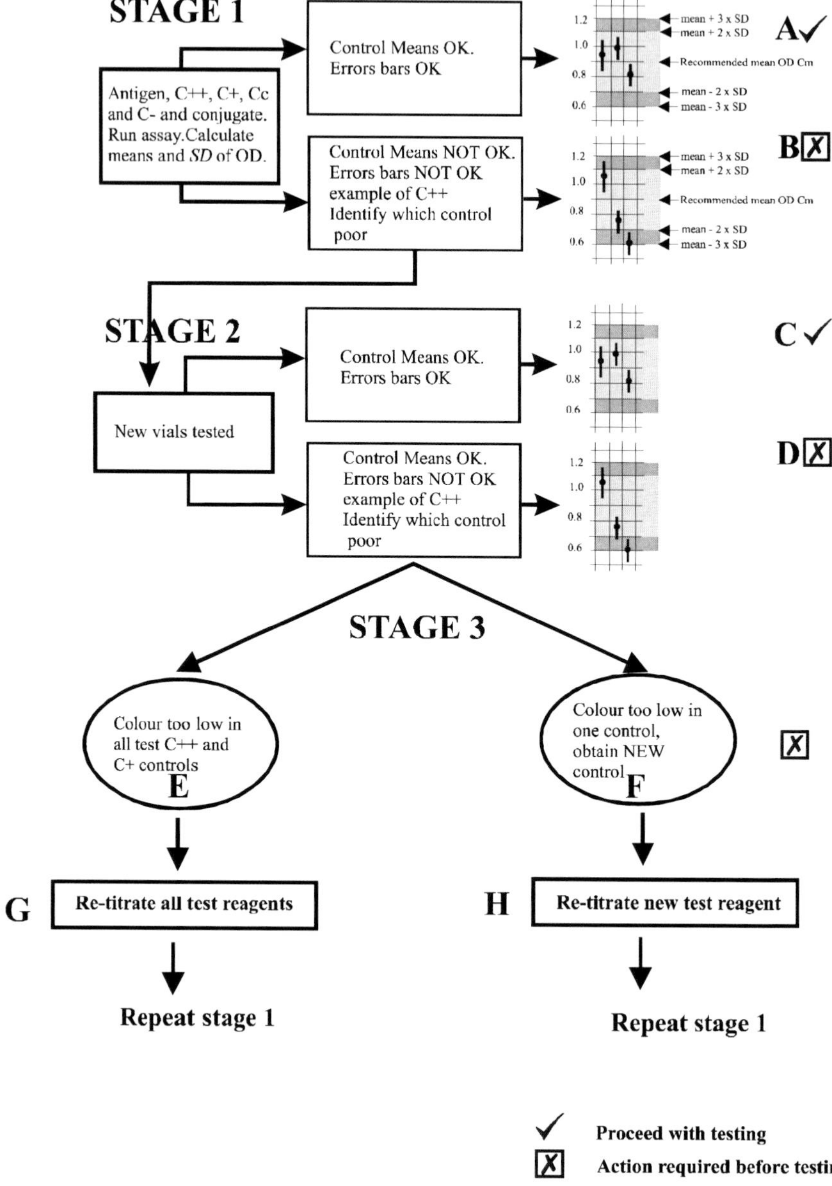

Fig. 29. Outline of steps in testing reagents for kit.

4.1. Stage 1

At this stage, the kit is opened and the reagents carefully made up as instructed. The test is performed exactly as described, and the control OD values and processed PP% values calculated. This can give rise to situations A and B.

In A, the test works exactly as "expected" with means and error bars in limits. There is no reason to postpone testing of test samples.

In B, one or more controls do not meet expectations, either with respect to the mean values or showing high errors.

4.2 .Stage 2

In the case of finding a problem with one or more controls, the test should be performed again with new vials of the reagents. Here again, the situation in C (equivalent to A), could be obtained on re-testing, and testing of samples can then be performed.

If, however, there are still problems (as shown in D), then Stage 3 should be examined.

4.3. Stage 3

This stage depends on the extent of the problems and on whether the problem can be associated with one particular control. In E, both C++ and C+ could be low (low color throughout). In this case, all the reagents (antigen, controls, and antibody conjugate) should be re-examined. This is expanded below in **Subheading 6. 2**. The colors in any control could also be high. Note that the situation in E could be observed in Stage 1 (as in B, for both controls). In this case, Stage 2 should still be performed, as there may well have been a common problem. In F, there is association of a color that is out of limits in only one control. Here, it is likely that, after obtaining the same result for two runs with separate vials of control, there is a fault in the control common to all vials. In this case, a new batch of that control should be obtained.

4.4. Use of Laboratory Sera

Where a laboratory has sera that have been proved positive in other tests, there is an opportunity to use this in the ELISA when problems with controls may occur. These may be used, for example, when the controls are both low, to ascertain whether the expected color can be obtained.

4.5. Re-Titration of Reagents

The ELISA system involves antigen, control antibodies, and a conjugate to detect bound antibodies. The kit instructions fix the dilutions of each of these. A simple method of testing each reagent in a range will help indicate whether there is a major problem with the activities of any of the reagents.

Figure 30 outlines a plate design to examine the three parameters of antigen, control serum, and conjugate using higher concentrations of reagents.

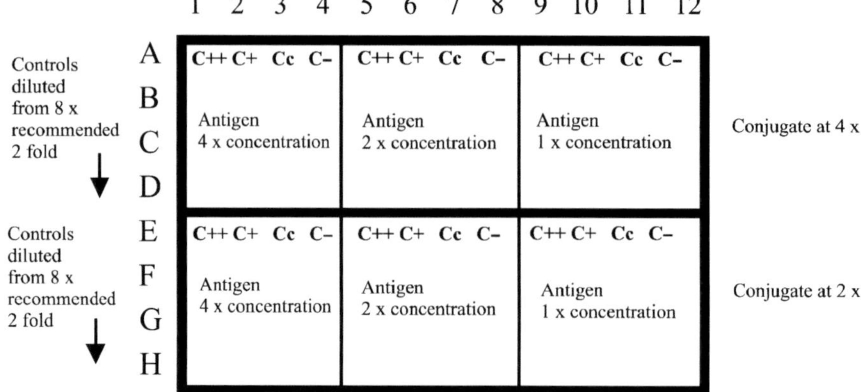

Fig. 30. Plate design for testing all reagents. The results of the test should indicate whether any of the reagents are not working. This does not account for the substrate, which will be examined later, should there be no color developing over the entire plate.

1. A plate is coated with antigen as shown. This is diluted at 4× and 2× of the recommended concentration, and at the recommended concentration.
2. The plate is incubated and washed.
3. The control sera are added as shown, starting with 8 times the recommended dilution, and diluted two-fold in blocking buffer.
4. The plate is incubated and washed.
5. The conjugate is added, as shown, in 2 blocks representing 4× and 2× of the recommended dilution.
6. After incubation, washing, and addition of substrate, the plate is stopped at the recommended time and read. Results are assessed.

Figures 31–33 highlight some of the results that could be obtained.

The procedures of testing reagents at elevated concentrations should highlight the problem areas. The single-plate procedure is not too expensive on reagents.

5. Sources of Variation

The kit is a complex association of reagents and equipment in the hands of different operators. The sources of variation thus come from these sources. Experience with this kit in many countries indicates that the chief source of errors (manifestation of

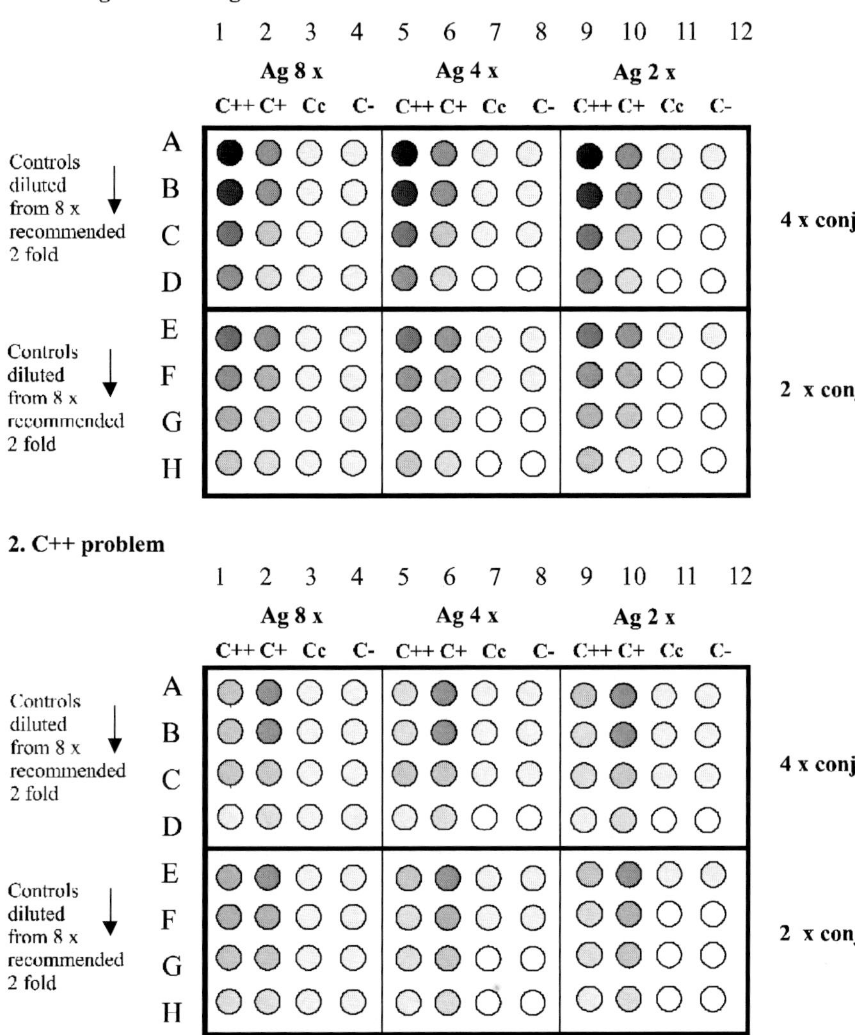

Fig. 31. Diagrammatic representation of plates. These show: *1*, a plate where there are no problems. *2*, a plate where there is a problem with the C++.

variation) comes from the operators, and not from the reagents. The continuous assessment of the kit is a good way to identify whether it is the reagents and/or equipment that is causing high variation, as distinct from operators.

5.1. ELISA Readers

Cleaning:

ELISA readers are seldom examined on a routine basis. The optical devices for reading the wells can become contaminated with chemicals, and should be cleaned regularly. This is a simple process. Readers should not be cleaned with abrasive materials or those containing solvents affecting plastics.

3. C+ Problem

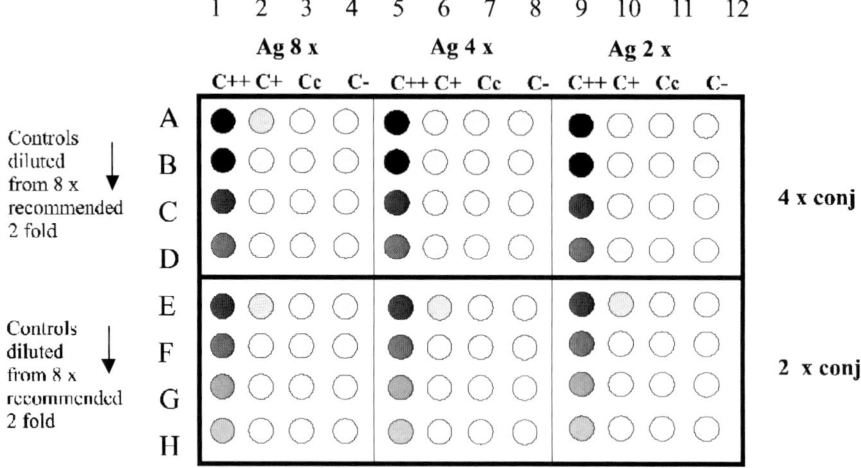

4. Conjugate problem

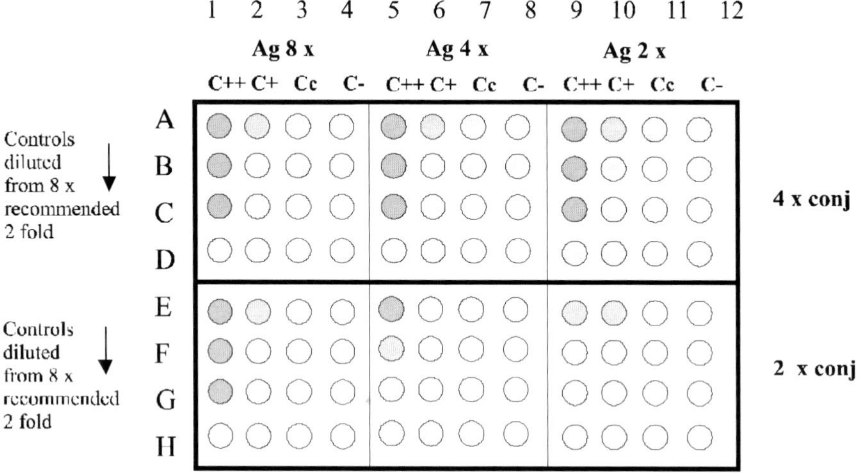

Fig. 32. Diagrammatic representation of plates. These show: *3*, a plate where there are problems with C+. *4*, a plate where there are problems with the conjugate.

Filters:

Filters can deteriorate rapidly in humid conditions. Between uses, they should be stored with a desiccant in a bag. Machines with internal filter wheels have fewer problems. Where there is a constant machine error, indicating a failure to read, another filter should be obtained. A spare filter (of appropriate wave length) should always be held.

Major errors come from not checking the simplest things. Two, in particular, are:

1. Checking that the appropriate wavelength of filter is being used. Some individuals use the wrong filter, due to which,

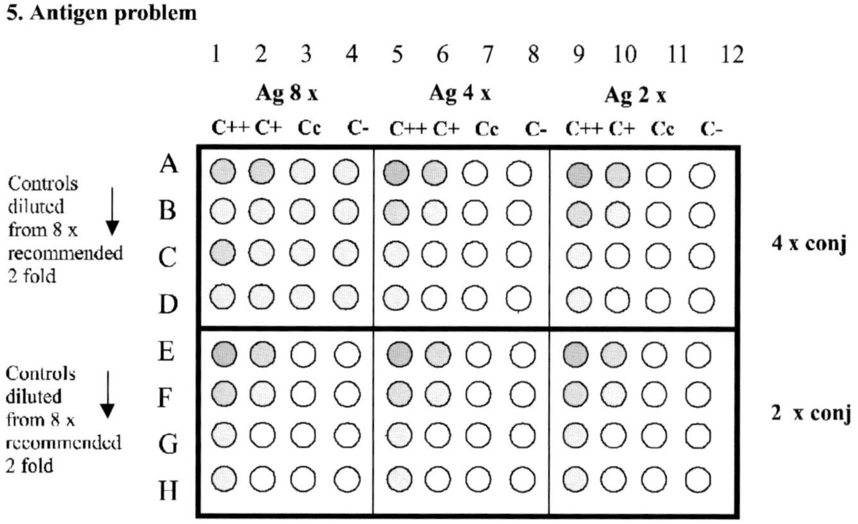

5. Antigen problem

1 2 3 4 5 6 7 8 9 10 11 12

Ag 8 x Ag 4 x Ag 2 x

C++ C+ Cc C- C++ C+ Cc C- C++ C+ Cc C-

A B C D E F G H

Controls diluted from 8 x recommended 2 fold

Controls diluted from 8 x recommended 2 fold

4 x conj

2 x conj

Fig. 33. Diagrammatic representation of plates. This shows: *5*, a plate where there are problems with the antigen.

although some OD can be measured, the readings will be very low when compared to those using the correct filter OD readings (e.g., a 450 nm filter will give a readout for a 492 nm color);

2. Individuals should know how the color they see relates to an OD readout. Some individuals observed good color, which is in the expected range for the kit, but have then received very low OD readings from the machine, due to the use of the wrong filter.

5.2. Pipettes

A chief source of error leading to variation is the use of pipettes. This can be the chief cause of variation among different operators. Even for an individual, there is an "internal" bias towards pipetting in a certain way, either always having a slight over or under volume. This assumes that pipettes are calibrated properly, i.e., they deliver the volume set for; however, this is seldom the case.

Greater care in standardizing pipetting technique will eliminate some variation in laboratories, particularly where several different people are responsible for testing. This is particularly important in taking samples from the field container to the wells where a small volume is transferred. Care must be taken to allow an adequate time to pipette with an identical technique each time.

5.3. Reagents

The protocols given in the manual should be strictly adhered to. Failure to maintain required minimal temperatures or to alter dilutions can severely harm the assay parameters. Such harm can be assessed with reference to the test performance before and after an identified reagent abuse. However, such abuses are either not identified, or not reported for other reasons. Note should be taken of likely susceptibilities of reagents to various physical conditions. These are shown in the **Table 9**.

5.4. Water Quality

Water quality is consistently the chief source of problems where results (OD values) are generally much lower than expected. Attempts should be made to get water from other sources. The reasons for the alterations in color are not clear, and it is better to obtain water from other sources rather than waste time in curing an internal problem.

5.5. Poor Washing

This applies to faulty washing of tips and glassware/plasticware. It is better not to reuse anything that has had contact with an enzyme. When tips are reused, they must be acid washed, and then very thoroughly rinsed in distilled water. The pH of the water should be checked, as this can often be very acidic (poor plant producing water).

Table 9
Sources of error

Reagent	Adverse parameters	Error	Effect
Antigen for coating plates	High temperature storage. Antigen is aggregated	Too little antigen. Expected color reduced	Sensitivity of assay changes (Low Cm values)
H_2O_2	High temperature storage. Stopper left off container. Too high a concentration used	Reduced or no color	Test fails. Cm values below lower range
Control sera	High temperature storage denatures antibodies. Dilutions made up and used next day	Reduced color	Sensitivity of assay changes
Enzyme conjugate	High temperature storage. Wrong dilution used	Too little color. Too strong a color. Too weak a color	Sensitivity changes
Blocking buffer	Wrong formulation	Too high a color in controls	Test fails
Washing buffer	Wrong pH	Alters expected colors in controls	Very variable results in controls

Poorly rinsed vessels in which original dilutions of reagents are made also adds to variation, as activities can be reduced or totally destroyed in a high alkaline or acidic pH range.

5.6. Mathematics

Errors in diluting reagents are a major problem. Calculations should always be checked, and all bottles and other equipment clearly labeled with the name of the reagent and the dilution.

The fundamental principles involved in good performance of ELISA should be learned through in-house training, external training, and reading of literature. There is no substitute for training, which leads to improvements in practical skills and a thorough understanding of what one is doing.

Chapter 11

Ruggedness and Robustness of Tests: Aspects of Kit Use and Validation

1. Background Information

When considering the use of any testsinformation about their performance under a defined set of conditions , that is, validation criteria, is necessary. My experience is with tests concerning animal diseases and as such there is involvement in helping to set up guidelines with the responsible International body, the World Organization for Animal Health or as it is also known, the Office International des Epizooties (OIE) in Paris.

The latest OIE guidelines for validation of tests, developed through cooperation with the scientific community, define stages of validation to be applied to a particular test's specific fitness for the purpose and form the basis of a peer-reviewed registration process and certification of tests with the OIE. While recognizing that validation is a continuous process, the OIE defines four stages *(1–4)* that gradually expand data to increase confidence that a test is valid for a wider range of countries and laboratories. The guidelines are extremely useful in determining the stage of justifiable validation claims, as well as starting development of tests. The OIE homepage can be consulted under links to Certification and Validation of Diagnostic Assays.

A major point to be realized is that tests, including ELISA, have to be considered as a part of a system designed for a specific purpose. The performance of a system can be affected by any component of the system, not just the chosen test method. Consequently, continuous assessment of the whole system is required.

John R. Crowther, *Methods in Molecular Biology, The ELISA Guidebook, Vol. 516*

DOI: 10.1007/978-1-60327-254-4_11

The major factors involved in assessment can be covered using the terms robustness and ruggedness. There is still debate concerning the definitions of the terms.

Most opinions seem to consider robustness as a measure of the resistance of a test to physical factors and ruggedness as to how a test performs under a wide variety of operational conditions. Ultimately, tests for use in diagnosis and surveillance have to be judged by their diagnostic performance which is measured in terms of diagnostic sensitivity (DSn) and diagnostic specificity (DSp). Here DSn refers to the proportion of known infected reference animals testing positive [TP/(TP+FN)], while DSp refers to the proportion of uninfected reference animals that test negative [TN/(TN+FP)]. (TP = true positive; FN = false negative; TN = true negative; FP = false positive).

The use of samples from representative populations is a major difficulty in validation. It is worth contrasting analytical sensitivity (ASn) and analytical specificity (ASp) measurements which are determined by better-defined reference materials (e.g., from experimentally derived samples). Here ASn refers to the ability of a test to measure the amount of analyte, such as antibody or antigen(s) in a reference material(s) and ASp the ability of a test to measure that analyte specifically in the presence of similar substances. Test DSn and DSp are factors of the performance only when an association of measurement is made to a population. The use of reference materials (standards) to keep track of a test to study the variation of ASn and ASp is more important in Internal Quality Control (IQC) to assess the functioning of the basic components of a test system to a required level of performance. Reliable kits must be resistant to physical forces and provide reagents and protocols that enable consistency to be maintained. These can be considered overall as stability factors.

1.1. Stability of kits/ Tests

The terms ruggedness and robustness deal with test stability from two angles:

- Physical factors affecting test performance (robustness)
- Factors affecting repeatability in a laboratory and reproducibility between laboratories (ruggedness)

1.2. Physical Factors Impairing the Biological Function of the Reagents

The major physical effects that influence test robustness are either during transportation to the end user (storage conditions, time of storage before receipt) or in the user's laboratory (storage and repeated use). These factors should be grouped under the term "robustness". So a robust test is one where the reagents are stable under a wide variety of physical factors during transportation and storage. A non-robust test would contain one or more elements that were easily affected by the same conditions. An example would be an enzyme conjugate whose activity was known to be drastically affected by relatively small increases in temperature above 4°C. Such a reagent might be shipped in ice but runs the risk of delays in transportation where the temperature cannot be maintained. This is even more marked where reagents have to be sent in dry ice. Although the sender may have supplied specific instructions for transportation, the test is in effect subject to deterioration. There may be several reagents subject to this and each element affected decreases the expected performance of the test (as it left the supplier) due to its "non ruggedness".

Assessing the stability of all reagents is not easy as all possible conditions cannot be predicted or tested. The sustained supply and successful use of a kit form a complex equation. The developmental stages are often part of the validation process *per se* and it is sometimes difficult to assess where exactly anyone is in the overall assessment of the stage of a kit. Some basic features of kit supply are shown in **Fig. 1.** Alternative pathways for supply are shown either as direct links between producer and user through transportation, or through links between producers and a distributor to the user. The kit has to be "fit for use" when it leaves either the producer with full quality control (QC) or the distributor (where QC testing may not be done). At this stage we regard the kit under "fitness for use" criteria, implying that the kit is formulated to achieve the defined performance when it leaves the producer's or distributor's premises. The possibility of a kit being affected by physical factors increases on each round of transportation.

Conditions during kit transportation are not under control and so are not as quantifiable as when kits are used in the laboratory. Conditions such as temperature, shaking, leakage, dehydration, UV, etc., that might affect the performance of a kit, are not easy to reproduce in suppliers' laboratories. Consequently, measuring this is not easy but features of the test reagents more inclined to be subject to temperature effects and time of storage under less than ideal conditions would tend to be less robust in practice. Although precautions to avoid such problems are advised, they are not always followed; or there is no admission, or knowledge, of adverse conditions. **Table 1** lists possible effects on biological reagents during transportation. Anything that affects a kit in this phase can be considered as dealing with the robustness of the kit.

In addition, once received by the user, the kit can be affected by laboratory variations in storage and handling and this should be considered under robustness. It might be useful to think about defining robustness in terms of "transport robust" and "laboratory robust". The same features affecting stability on storage and handling in a laboratory are present, but since conditions can be defined, any sudden failure of a test or slow deterioration in performance can be assessed with respect to known conditions through Internal Quality Control (IQC) (Internal laboratory proficiency). This will be discussed in detail later.

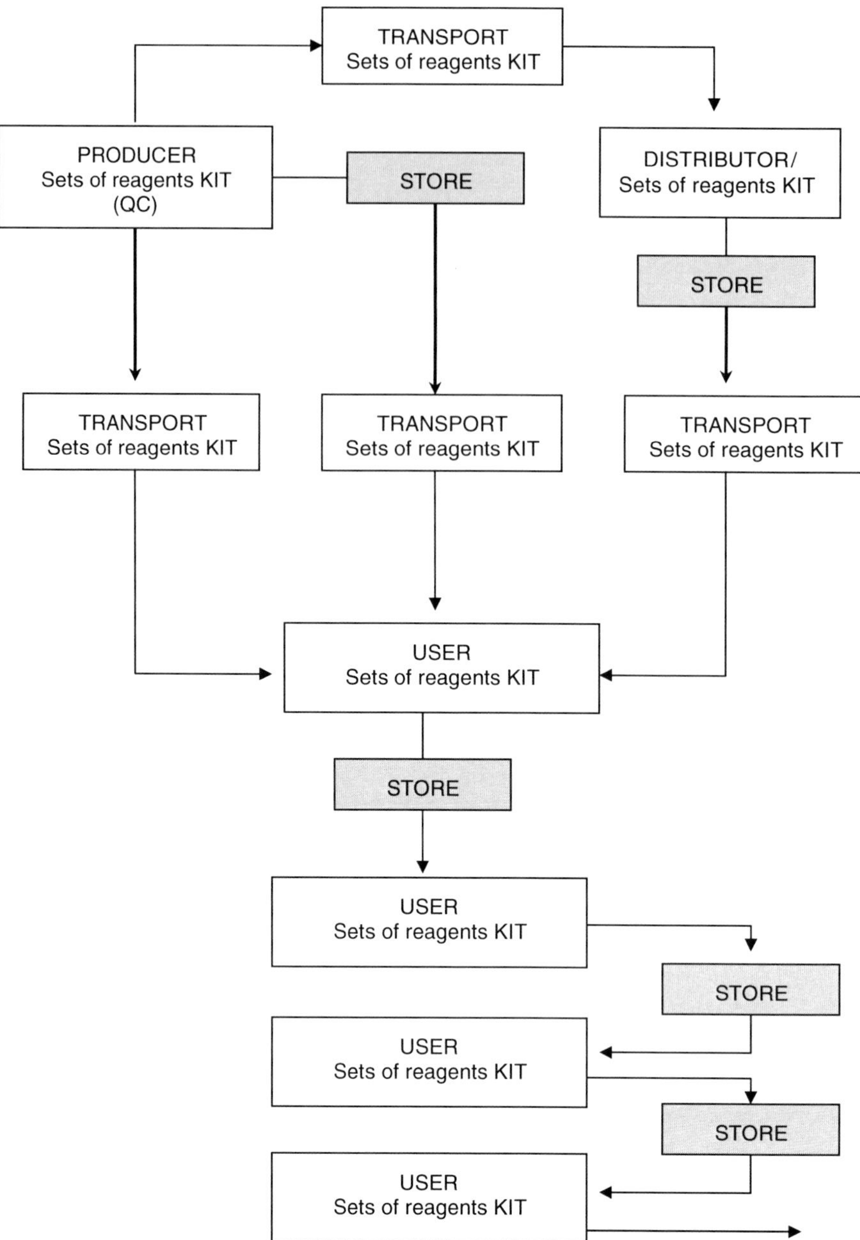

Fig. 1. Relationships of producer to end user in sending kits-robustness. The possibilities of affecting reagents are increased by the number of stages in transportation and storage.

1.3. Test Repeatability and Reproducibility in Terms of the Wide-spread Use of the Test in Conditions Which Are Variable and Less Than Ideal

Where a test functions as expected on receipt, features that resist change through the many possible variations in technique are features of ruggedness. The ultimate test is absolutely foolproof, can be done by totally untrained individuals, gives the same results for controls every day, every month, every year (highly precise) and can accommodate large variations in experimental handling and technique. In other words, ruggedness is a measure of resistance to user variables. It is not easy to monitor performance

Table 1
Factors affecting biological reagents in kits on transportation

Adverse Factors	Effects	Comments
Low temperature		
Freezing	Concentration Phase separation	Affects activity of reagents through errors in concentration
Freeze thawing	Denaturation proteins	Affects biological activity (both quantitative and qualitative)
	Coagulation	Clumping and aggregation can affect activities and increase dilution errors
	Inactivation enzymes	Reduces or eliminates biological activity
	Differential concentration of proteins	Affects concentration of reagents
High temperature	Denaturation proteins	Reduces or destroys biological activity. Can selectively alter quality of e reagents
	Inactivation complement and other factors	Affects results on variably heated samples
	Dehydration	Concentration of reagents. Could denature proteins
	Evaporation	Loss of fluid so test volumes too low
	Contaminant growth	Proteolysis, bacterial and fungal activity
	Hydration with humid conditions	Dilution
		Destruction of freeze dried reagents
Shaking	Frothing	Phase separation
	Vigorous shaking	Shearing effects on proteins (inactivation)
UV inactivation-sunlight	Inactivation	Biological activity altered or destroyed
Leakage	Loss of necessary volume	Reduces number of samples for test
	Contamination	Can lead to microbial degradation of reagents
Breakage	Loss of reagents	Reduces test numbers
	Contamination	Chemical or microbial breakdown/ inactivation
	Mixing	Cross contamination of activities
Re-hydration	Freeze dried reagents affected by moisture	Can destroy or alter biological activity directly or after microbial contamination

and cover the competence of staff to follow given instructions. Examination of the OIE validation criteria shows that at Stage 2 – repeatability and at Stage 3 – reproducibility are measured, i.e., ruggedness of the tests. It can be predicted that the more complex a test is and the more variables involved, the less rugged it is likely to be.

1.4. Samples Used for Diagnosis

The performance of any system is determined with reference to a defined set of reagents (e.g., kit). The function of tests is to do a job as summarized by OIE as "fitness for purpose". Kits provide reagents to users that should include the necessary controls to allow measurement of an analyte that can be translated into a conclusion, e.g., whether positive or negative. Attention should be paid in terms of ruggedness or robustness of any system as to the influence of taking a test sample and its storage and processing; this can have a profound effect on results. Where the conditions for sampling are very critical, this affects the ruggedness of a test. For instance, if a sample has to be taken and immediately placed in liquid nitrogen and held for exactly 11 h and 54 s then tested, plainly this is a ridiculous and totally untenable method. Such a test system is not rugged since the conditions cannot be met, or if attempted would fail. The taking of samples and their analysis by a test and the effect of different procedures should be taken care of in the validation data. For PCR, the sampling and processing (nucleic acid extraction) is extremely important to diagnostic sensitivity (DSn) determinations and slight alterations in technique or equipment used can greatly alter the diagnostic potential of a test.

2. Kits and Reagent Sets

Defining a kit is useful since reagents and protocols proclaiming to be kits can be very different and kit formulation can drastically affect their performance in terms of ruggedness and robustness and also in solving problems. Here there is a large distinction between the concepts of a kit for ELISA as against molecular methods; for example, PCR. The PCR will be discussed later since many laboratories now use this technique in conjunction with ELISA methods.

The definition of what comprises a kit rests on considerations on:

- Test validation
- The perceived objective of the kit

- The "market" or end-users who are to exploit the kit
- Factors involved in sustainability.

The equation for a kit is complex and involves technical performance, supply, profit motives, and continuity. Kits have to be accepted by international bodies to fulfil their ultimate role of standardization of a given approach to evaluate a given situation and allow harmonization with other tests measuring the same or similar factors.

The definition of an ultimate kit may be examined against kits that are already being used or to aid in designing better kits. Having said this, there is no perfect kit that deals with biological systems. The gathering of information from kits and the modification of reagents/conditions/protocols is necessary to account for the many variables which cannot be assessed at a single time point. Validation also involves the changes in the biological systems, such as alteration in the antigenicity of agents examined, which necessitates action.

2.1. A Perfect Kit

This has been examined in other Chapters but it is worth mentioning and expanding.

1. A kit should contain everything needed to allow testing, including software interfaces to facilitate storage, processing of samples, demonstration or training modules and analysis and reporting of data.
2. The reagents should be absolutely stable under a wide range of conditions of temperature.
3. The manual describing the use of the kit should be foolproof.
4. The kit should be validated "in the field" as well as in research laboratories.
5. All containers for reagents should be leak proof.
6. IQC samples should be included.
7. External quality assessment should be included in the kit "package".
8. Data on relationship of kit results to those from other assays should be included.
9. It is necessary to ensure that all equipment used in association with the kit is calibrated (spectrophotometers, pipettes).
10. Training courses should be organized in the use of kits.
11. Information exchange should be set up to allow rapid "on-line" help and evaluation of results where there are perceived problems.
12. The internationally agreed supply and control of standards used in kits should be maintained.

The establishment of these perfect conditions would greatly reduce problems in the ruggedness and robustness of tests. Some major criticisms of suppliers of kits are shown in **Table 2** where the points 1–12 refer to the perfect kit criteria given above. Not surprisingly, most of the features are expressed in the validation criteria required by OIE which deal with test performance.

2.2. Producer/End-User Responsibilities

Features of robustness and ruggedness are illustrated in **Figs. 1–4.** Various pathways for transportation of kits are shown in **Fig. 1.** A perfect scenario where a kit survives transportation and delivery as judged by the successful confirmation that the test works is shown in **Fig. 2.** On storage and reuse of the test there are no problems with reference to the controls provided. Here there are obviously no problems with transport robustness, laboratory robustness or ruggedness. The IQC monitoring of test performance is vital in assessing performance. A scenario where the kit is received but does not work is shown in **Fig. 3**, presumably because some of the elements are faulty. If the assumption is made that the quality control of the supplier was good and as the kit was labelled "fit for use", then it might be concluded that transportation may have affected performance (nonrobust). It is worthwhile for the user to repeat the test since it may have been an operator error leading to poor performance. The major cause of problems with a new kit (or even technology) is operator errors in dilution, manipulation, and nonadherence to protocols.

Table 2
Problem areas regarding available kits, e.g., ELISA

Perfect kit points	Available Kits performance
Completeness	Tips, water main problems for ELISA
Stable reagents	Some problems
Foolproof manual	Variable quality. Generally incomplete background
Field validated	Can be poor (related to need for OIE guidelines)
Leak proof	Good
IQC samples and methods	Some kits have necessary controls missing in their regime
EQA responsibilities	Poor
Relationship data to other tests	Not usual
Calibration equipment	Left to the user
Training courses	No
Rapid reporting problems	Not many systems in place
Standards	Poor

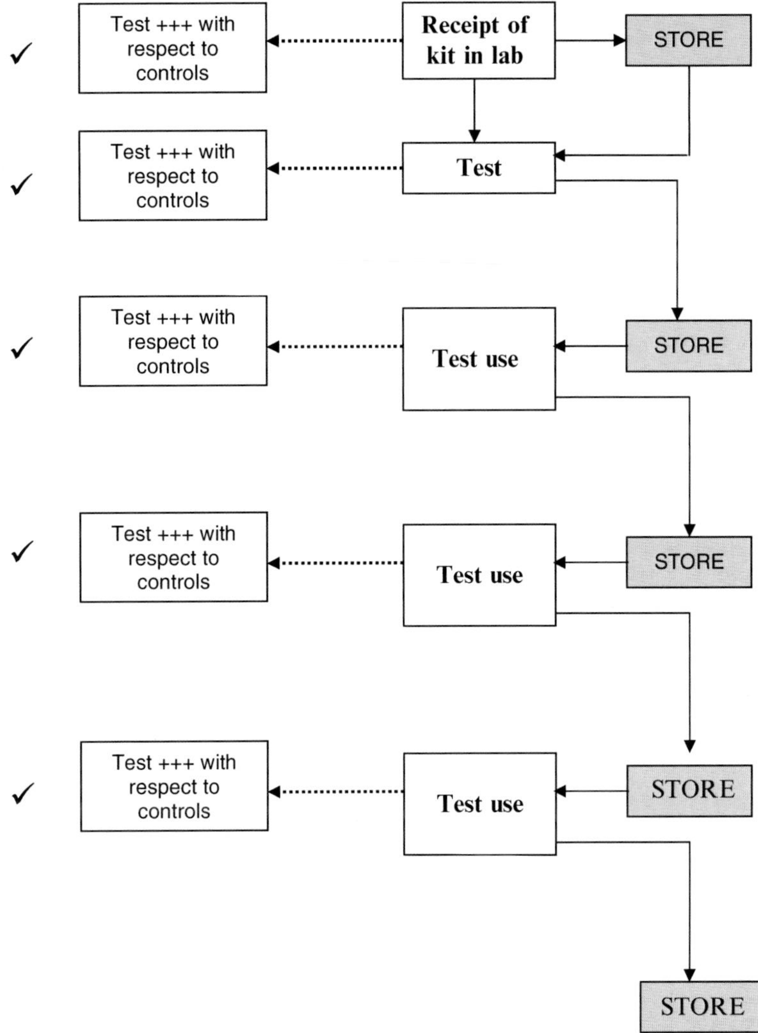

Fig. 2. Situation A. Receipt and use of a kit, no problems in robustness and ruggedness. The test is monitored with respect to controls and works every time. This is the role of IQC. ✓ *mark* indicates good test.

The kit performance is related to the controls given. On confirmation that something is wrong on receipt, there are choices for the user. He/she may contact the producer and report the finding to ask for help or a new kit. The responsibility to gather, respond, and update data on their test is that of the producer and this is inherent in the validation guidelines to achieve Stage 3 validation. The responsibility of the user is to provide data that is quality controlled and where great attention is paid to following the given protocols.

The user can also examine which of the test reagents is causing the problem(s) through trouble shooting. This requires a good level of understanding of the principles of the tests being used and the ability to think clearly and perform accurate experiments. This has been dealt with already in **Chapters 9** and **10** but an example of trouble shooting of an Indirect ELISA is repeated,

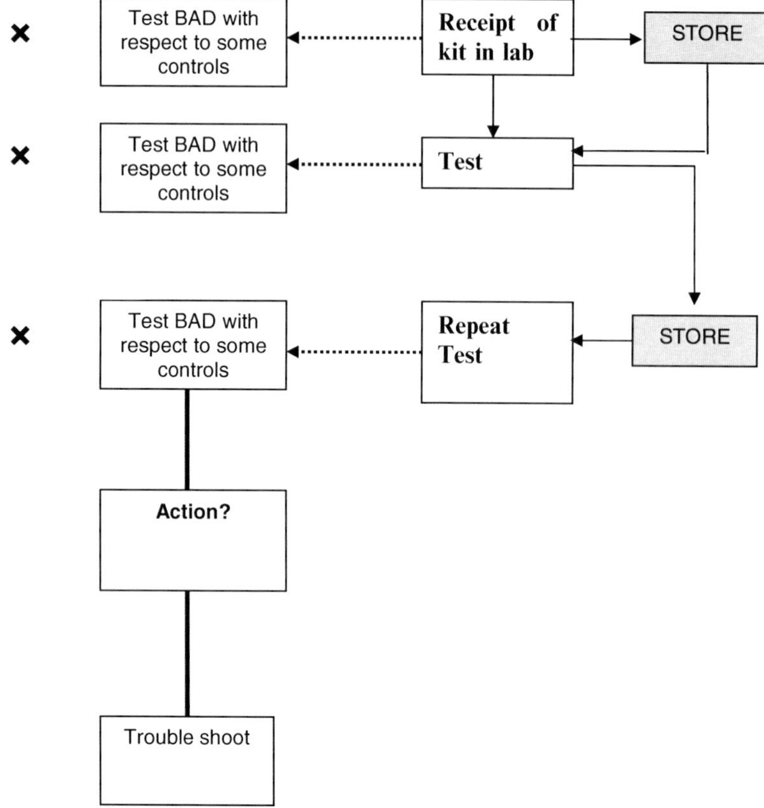

Fig. 3. Situation B. Receipt and use of a kit, ruggedness problem? A problem was identified on receipt of kit. Re-testing kit gave same result. Actions can be taken to investigate why the kit has failed with respect to controls, including examining the controls themselves, since not all may have failed. Trouble shooting may allow test reagents to be rescued but this depends on "skills" of end users, and ideal conditions as recommended by producer would not be met. × *mark* indicates bad test.

to illustrate that the process can be quick and not too expensive on reagents. The way forward then will depend on the results of the trouble shooting. If a single reagent is "faulty," e.g., has lost activity, then this might be replaced by the supplier or its concentration adjusted. If controls (one or more) are affected, it is difficult to replace these to achieve the producer-defined characteristics of ASn and ASp.

A result where a kit works initially, but fails at a later time- is shown in **Fig. 4.** The constant monitoring of a kit's performance with respect to controls is again emphasized, e.g., by the use of charting methods to continuously plot control data, so that trends in data can be seen. Failures may be progressive (through observation of a trend), or more sudden. Examination of reagents which affect a test performance is vital to ascertain what steps can be taken to bring the test back into use. As with the considerations above, single reagents can be obtained from the producer, e.g., controls. The use of in-house controls e.g., a

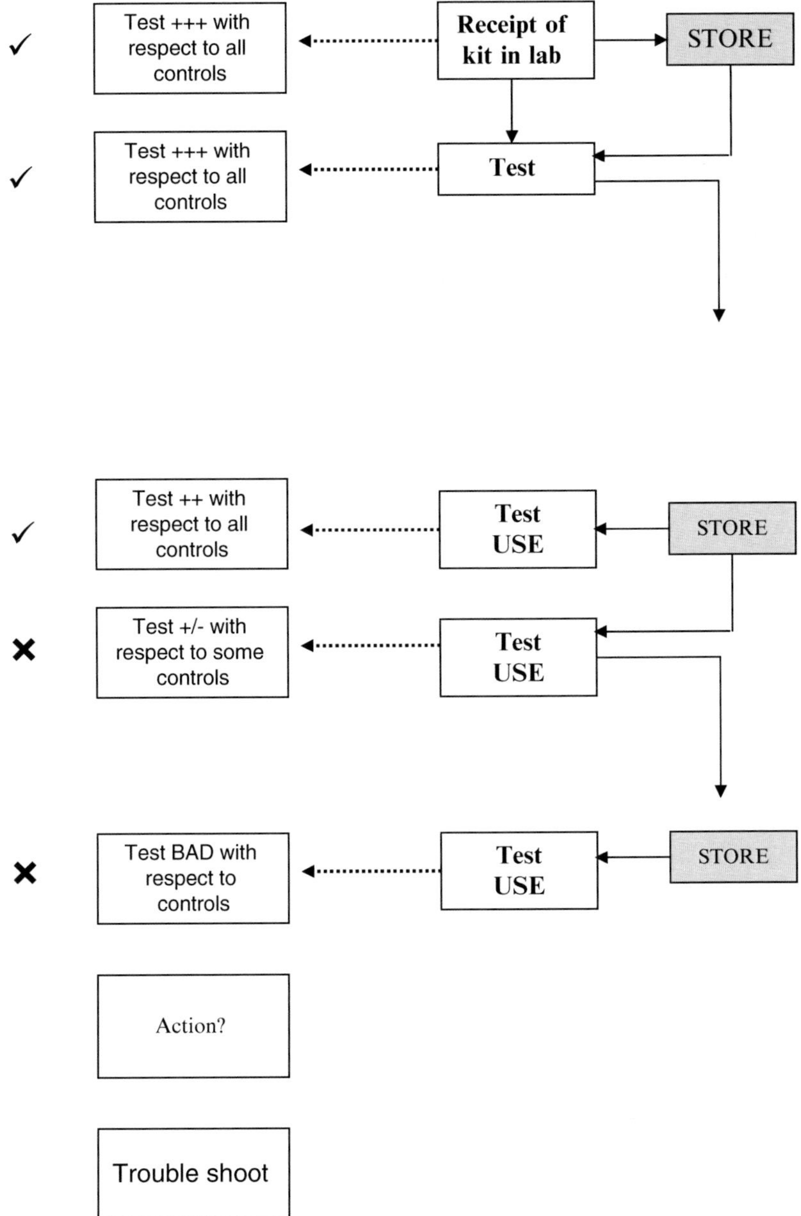

Fig. 4. Situation C. Receipt and use of a kit with gradual changes in performance. This is monitored through IQC with respect to given controls. The test performs well at the beginning but either gradually changes with respect to controls or is found to be failing at a specific time. Trouble shooting possibly identifies which reagent is failing and whether this can be compensated.

control positive serum, if included in tests as extra controls, can also be useful to measure given control activities. Thus the in-house control may retain its expected values whereas the given controls may have reduced values in time. Such aspects come under the heading of IQC. Robustness factors are more likely to be seen on delivery or soon after use. Ruggedness factors are linked strongly to good laboratory practice and the precision with which the kit functions under a wide range of variables.

2.3. Relevance of Ruggedness and Robustness to OIE Validation Pathway

The producer is responsible for robustness determination throughout transportation. Similar physical factors affecting robustness are present when the kit is received under the control and responsibility of the laboratory. Assessing robustness means assessing the stability of reagents over a range of conditions. Where a kit has been examined in many laboratories worldwide and attention has been given to stabilizing reagents for travel and storage in a laboratory, data will be available to measure the success of a test under those conditions. During development, the producer may have to adjust conditions to increase the stability of reagents and the eventual kit formulation can then be deemed robust. This is a major part of the validation process and can be costly in time and resources.

It is more difficult to obtain robustness data in the shorter term (predictive) though accelerating possibly adverse conditions. However, there is enough experience and practical demonstration of systems where robustness can be expected (but not initially tested). So, although no assumptions can be made until kits are sent out, the prediction that it is stable can be made.

In terms of the OIE guidelines, the question of how rugged and robust the kit is, is posed. Exactly what quantifiable data is needed here is not defined, leading to confusion and more subjective approaches. Data might best be shown from several sources and these are shown in **Table 3.**

2.4. Trouble Shooting ELISA

This has been looked at when considering charting methods in Chapters 9 and 10. Since a set of reagents in the form of a kit is sent to the user laboratory, the situations in **Figs. 1–3** could apply. In all cases, examination as to whether the reagents are behaving as expected by the producer is obtained with reference to given controls (at least initially) and through strict adherence to the given protocols. For simplicity's sake we can consider the evaluation of stages as shown in **Fig. 5.**

Stage 1

The kit is opened and the reagents carefully made up and/or used as instructed. The test is performed exactly as described and the control optical density (OD) values and processed values calculated. The situations A and B may occur.

A. The test works exactly as "expected" with means and error bars within limits. There is no reason to postpone testing of samples (situation in **Fig. 1**)
B. One or more of the controls do not meet expectations either with respect to the mean values or high variation (situation in **Fig. 2**); proceed with stage 2.

Stage 2

In the case of experiencing a problem with one or more of the controls, the test should be repeated with a set of new vials of the reagents. The situation in **C** equivalent to **A** could be obtained

Table 3
Quantifiable factors of robustness and ruggedness

Factor	Data
Experience with sending out kits	Time over which kits supplied (supplied by date-expire by date) Number kits sent and number batches sent Mode of transportation Adverse factors reporting e.g., delays at airports
Experience from single laboratory	Number labs where IQC good on receipt Number of labs where IQC not good on receipt Number of labs where IQC data alters from goods to bad
Cumulative data from one laboratory	Unprocessed data collected and analyzed IQC data analyzed Repeatability data
Cumulative data from many laboratories	Unprocessed data collected and collated External Quality Assurance data from supplier External Quality Assurance data from users Statistical analysis of data from number of laboratories Repeatability data compared (statistic) Reproducibility data shown (statistic)
Accelerated shelf life determination on one or more reagents	Data
Problems reported	Number and extent
Problems solved	Number and extent
Changes necessary in protocols to establish robustness and ruggedness	Show data on solving problems to achieve higher robustness and ruggedness
Sampling and samples	Data on variations in samples and extent they affect tests

on re-testing. If however, problems recur (as shown in **D**) then Stage 3 should be examined.

Stage 3

This depends on the extent of the problem(s) andwhether it can be associated with one particular control. For example, in E both the strong positive control serum given (C++) and moderate positive (C+) could have a low OD. In this case, all the reagents (antigen, controls, and antibody conjugate) should be re-examined. This is expanded in **Fig. 6** where a design to help troubleshoot all reagents in a single plate is given. The colors in any control could also be high. Note that the situation in E could be observed in Stage 1 (as in B for both controls). In this case Stage 2 should still be performed, as there may well have been a common problem. In F there is association of a color that is out of limits in only one control. Here, it is likely that, after obtaining the same result for two consecutive runs with separate vials of control, there is a fault in the control common to all vials. In this case, a new batch of that control, or a new kit, should be obtained.

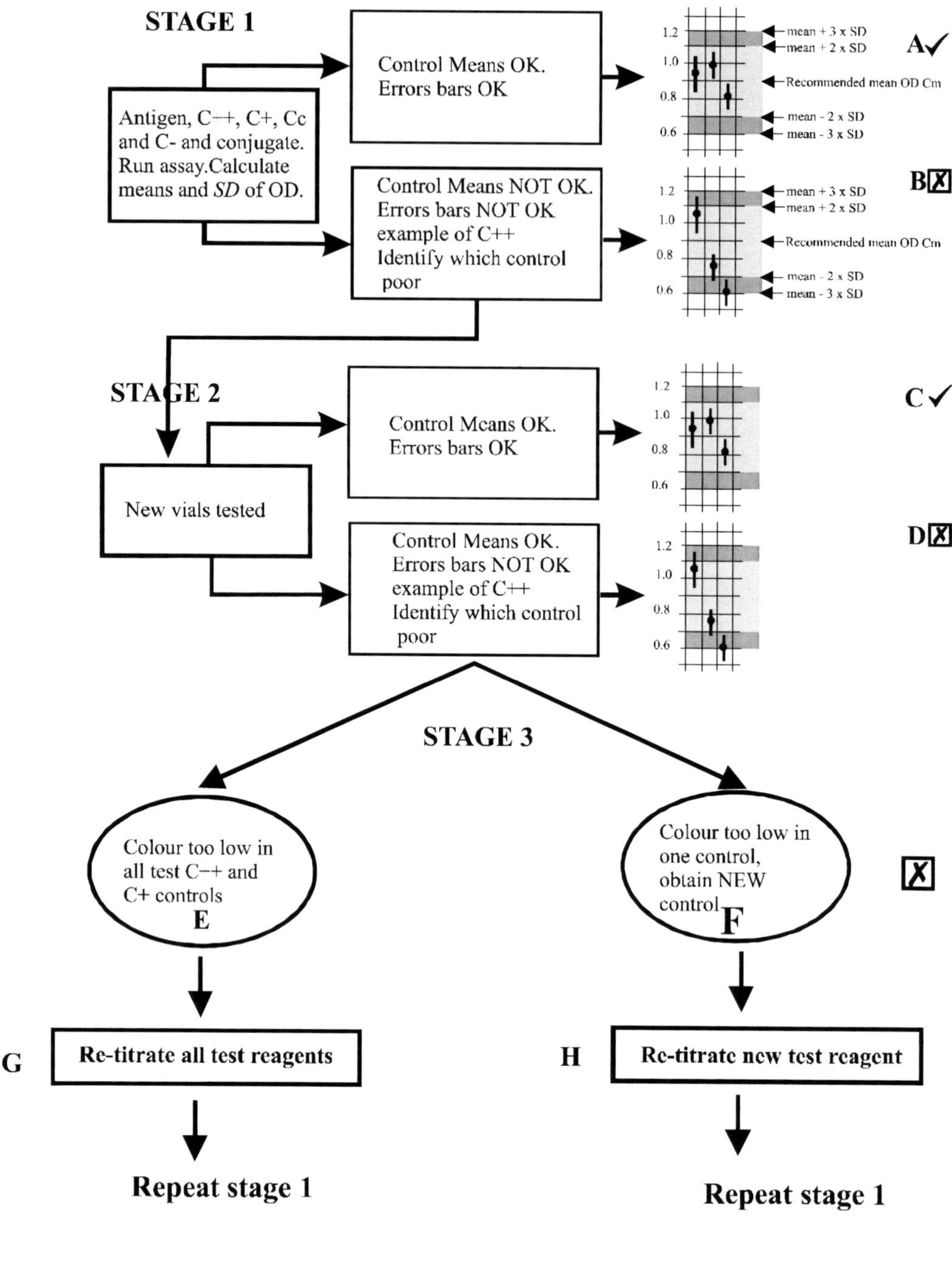

Fig. 5. Stages in examining an ELISA kit and consequences of different results. The results for the various controls are plotted. The limits recommended for the values are shown, as well as the mean and standard deviation from the mean of the results for controls. Such control charts are ideal for continuous monitoring (IQC).

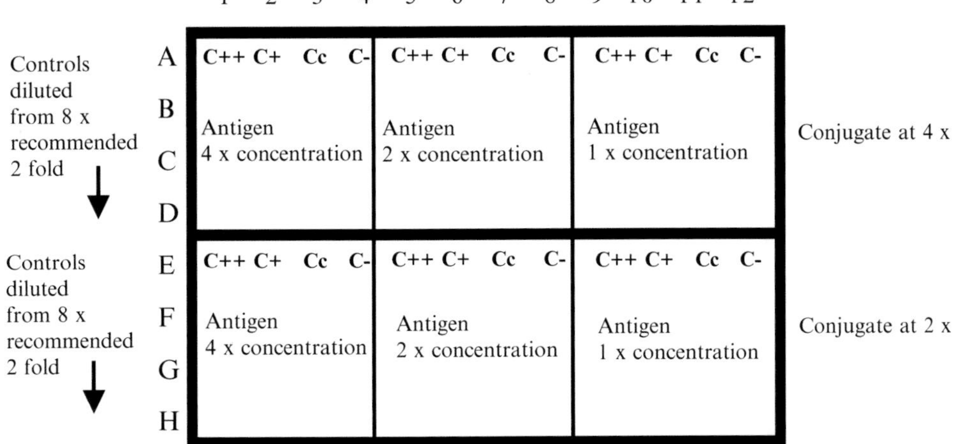

Fig. 6. Plate design assessing reagents for Indirect ELISA. Antigen is coated at 4× recommended concentration and twofold dilutions in respective areas of plate. After incubation and washing, control sera are added, diluted 8 times and twofold, in respective parts of plate. In this way, a mini-chess board titration of antigen and control sera is obtained. After incubation and washing, the conjugate is added 2× and 1× the recommended working dilution. After incubation and washing, the chromophore/substrate is added as recommended. On development the plate is stopped (if this is instructed). The patterns of reactivity should allow identification of single reagents where there is a possible concentration or qualitative problem. The assessment of the chromophore/substrate is not made here, but can be checked as a separate issue.

2.4.1. Evaluation of Reagents

A typical system for an indirect ELISA involves antigen, control antibodies and a conjugate to detect bound antibodies. The kit instructions usually fix the dilutions of each of these. A simple method of testing each reagent as a dilution range will help indicate whether there is a major problem with the activities of any of the reagents.

A microtitre plate design to examine the three parameters of antigen, control serum, and conjugate using higher concentrations of reagents is shown in **Fig. 6.**

1. A plate is coated with antigen as shown. This is diluted at 4×, 2× and one time the recommended concentration.
2. The plate is incubated and washed.
3. The control sera are added as shown, starting with 8 times the recommended dilutions and diluted twofold in blocking buffer.
4. The plate is incubated and washed.
5. The conjugate is added as shown in two blocks representing 4× and 2× the recommended dilution.
6. After incubation, washing and addition of substrate, the plate is stopped at the recommended time and read.
7. The results of the test should indicate whether any of the reagents are not working. This does not account for the substrate/chromophore failure where there would be usually no color developing over the entire plate, even on extended incubation. Possible results and conclusions to illustrate the usefulness of this system by endusers faced with a "failed" test are shown in **Figs. 7–11.**

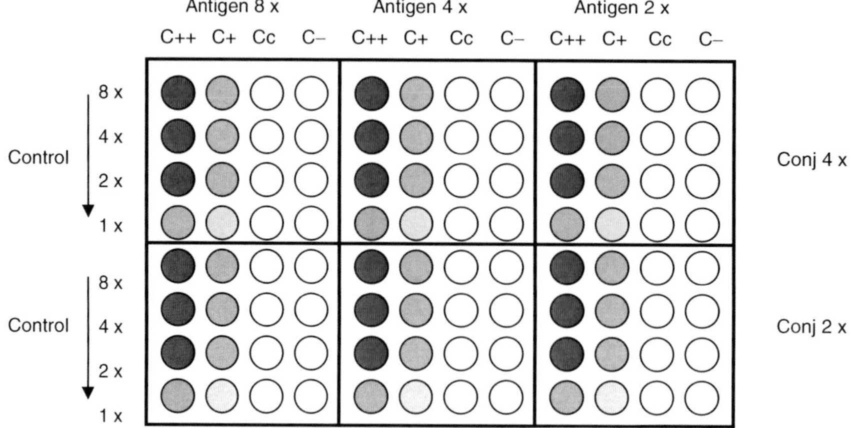

Fig. 7. No problems. Both controls show strong development of color reflecting increased concentrations of reagents.

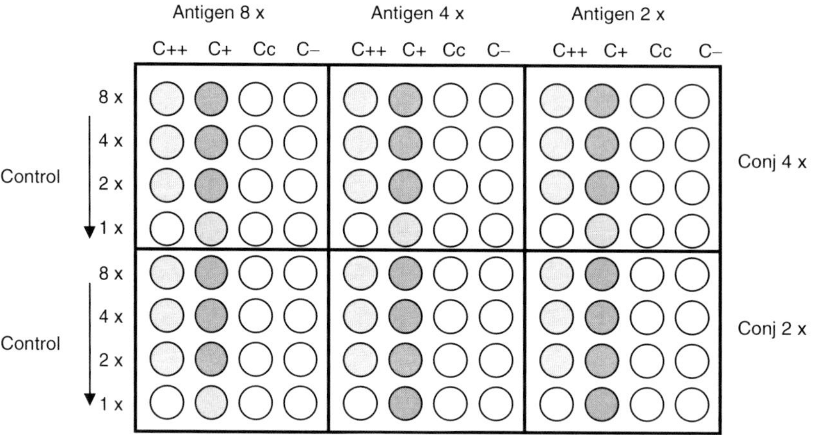

Fig. 8. C++ Problems. The OD for the C++ is too low. The C++ results are as expected.

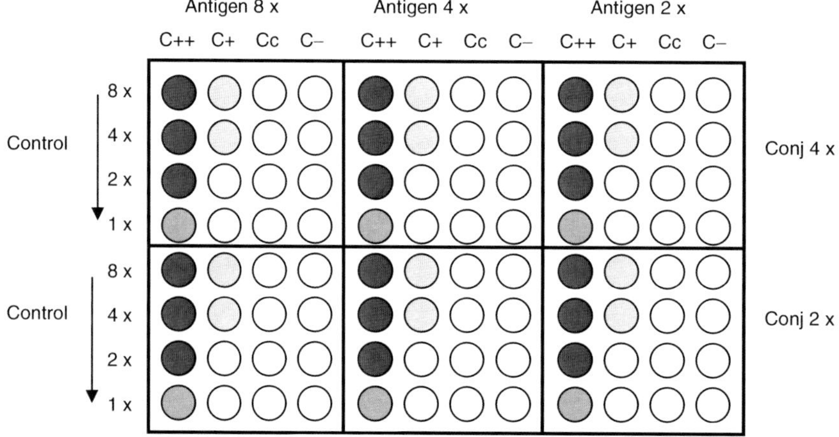

Fig. 9. C+ Problems.

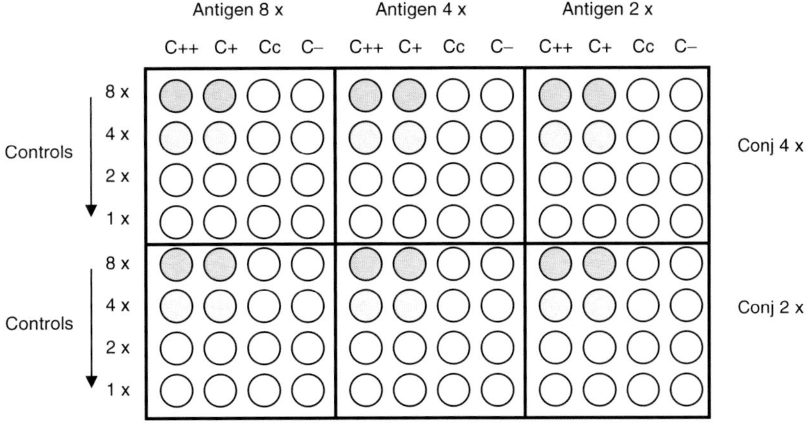

Fig. 10. Conjugate problems. There is little signal even for high concentrations of conjugate for both controls.

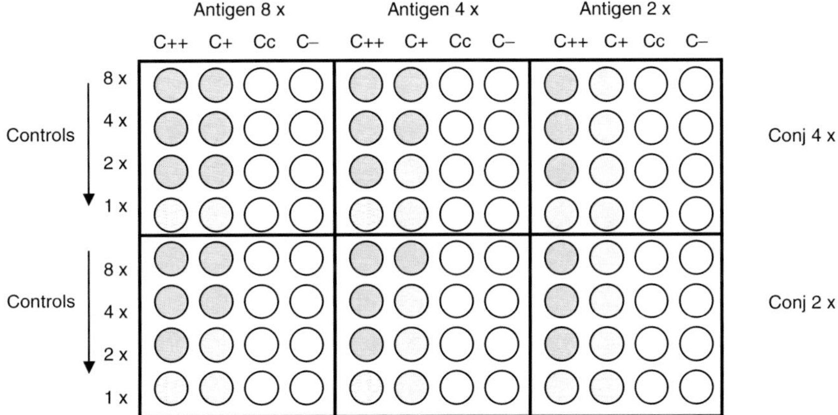

Fig. 11. Antigen problems. This can be confused with the conjugate problems but generally there would be more color and possibly a much reduced maximum plateau height for color even in excess controls positive sera and antigen.

2.5. Charting Methods

These have been dealt with extensively in Chapters 9 and 10 but will be re-emphasized here as part of a system to control testing. ICQ results are obtained continuously and should highlight problems as they arise. It is imperative that operators process and examine results constantly and actions taken as dictated by results.

Thus there is a systematic approach to data management that should impose a level of control on all laboratories involved with the same kit. IQC data are an integral component of the external quality assurance programme (EQAP) as the results from any laboratory can be examined and correlated with those obtained after an EQA exercise, whereby the same limited number of samples are assessed at given times by all laboratories involved in a network of sero-monitoring or sero-surveillance. Three examples of charting results are shown in **Figs. 12–14.**

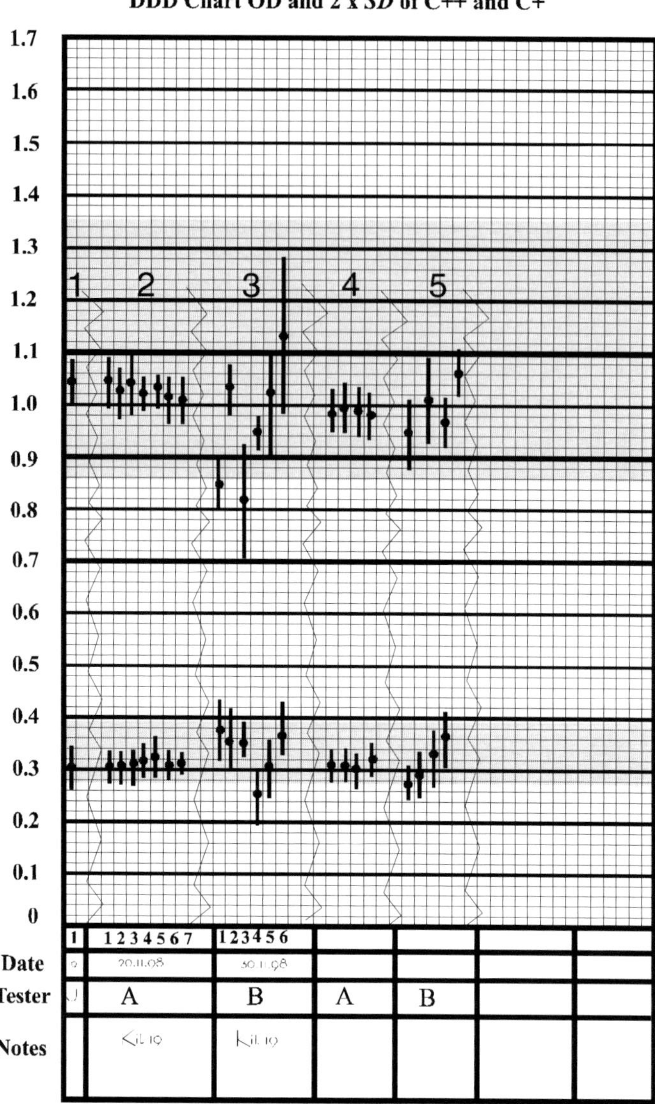

Fig. 12. DDD chart showing plots from five tests of an Indirect ELISA of control sera activity for strong control C++ and weaker control C+ sera. Each plate in a test has data plotted. The tester and date has been put on chart. Test 1 had 1 plate; test 2 had 7 plates; test 3 had 6 plates; test 4 had 4 plates and test 5, had 4 plates used. The mean value of the OD for the controls is shown for C++ and C+ for each plate. The allowable variation from the expected OD for the controls by the kit supplier is shown in *grey* for both C++ and C+. The mean values are plotted as *black points*. The *bars* show the plus and minus 2 × *SD* from the mean for each point (variation). Note in Test 3 there are problems with means out of allowable range for some plate controls as well as higher variation with respect to length of error bars.

3. Overview of Producer/User/National/Regional and International Responsibilities

Aspects involving the successful, sustainable supply of a kit and use of the kit to do a defined job are listed in **Table 4.** Although the players have been separated, the areas are interrelated and all

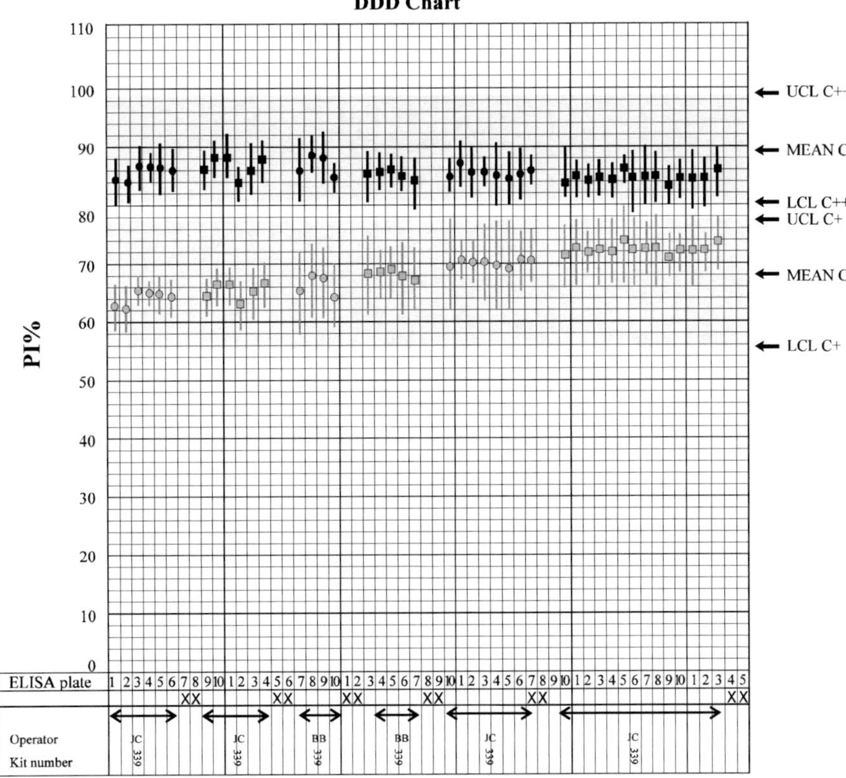

Fig. 13. DDD chart showing plots from six tests of an Competitive ELISA of control sera activity for strong control C++ and weaker control C+ sera. The data for each plate's controls (C++ and C+) is added (PI%). The C++ data for each plate is very similar for all tests and falls within the allowable limits of test (*grey areas*). However, the C+ data shows that there is a gradual drift in values higher (from around 60 to 74%) which alerts users to a problem either with that control, or with the relationship of C++ to C+ in terms of OD (which can be examined by consulting DDD charts of OD data).

factors have to be in place to optimize any use of kits to provide data to help in the control of diseases.

3.1. Training

The role of training is shown and this cannot be overemphasized. Kit supply without training is bound to fail. Training should concentrate on fundamental understanding of the principles of disease and of the relevance of data produced using kits to monitor the specific analytes produced by the disease process. (e.g., antibodies or antigens).Training in epidemiology is important to allow planning and assessment of the relevance of data, particularly where surveillance is involved. This is often poorly understood and the links between the epidemiologist and laboratory personnel (where different) should be strengthened to allow better planning and data management.

3.2. Reference Standards

Internationally accepted standards prove to be a difficult area for most diseases. A new assay may be measuring something for the first time so there is no reference preparation. Standards can be

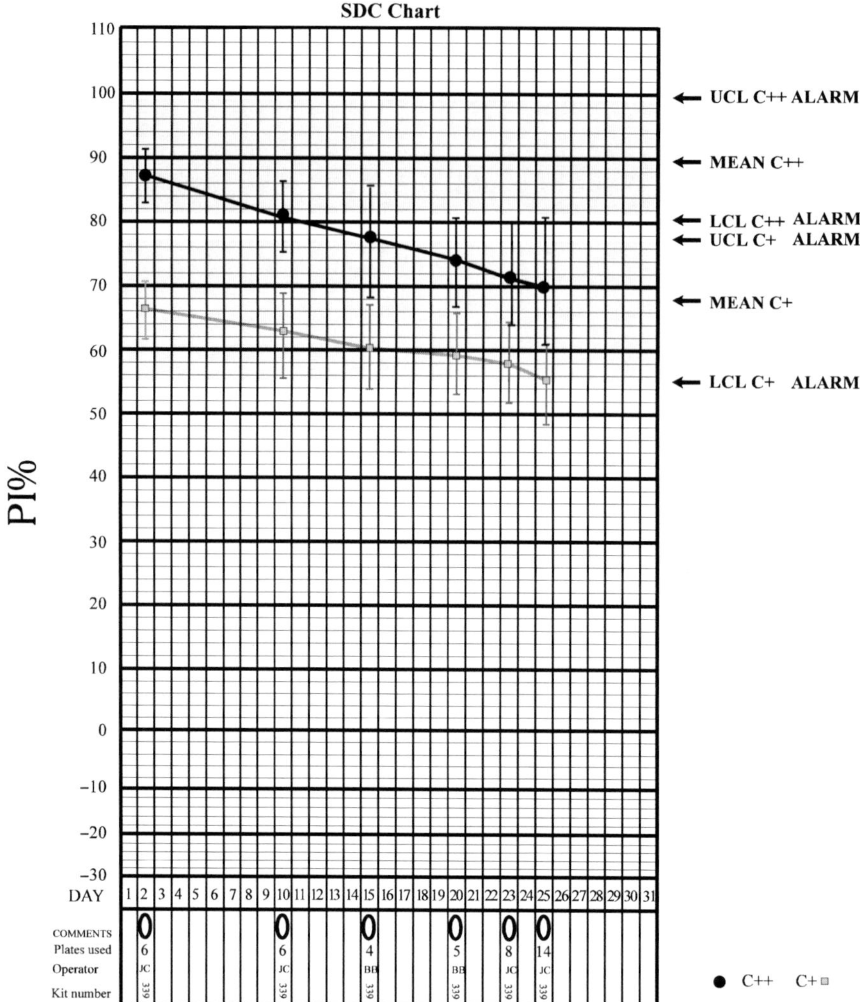

Fig. 14. SDC chart summarizes all plate data for two controls over time for a competitive ELISA. The results show percentage inhibition values for strong positive (C++) and weaker positive (C+) control sera). The times that the tests are done is shown in real time. The points represent the mean of the control values of the total plates run on each test (overall test variation). Each point refers to a test comprising one or more plates. The data from these individual plots can be looked at by consulting the relevant DDD charts to examine variation (length of error bars). In this case both controls showed a gradual decrease over time. *UCL* = upper control limit and *LCL* = lower control limit which are the limits of variation given by the producer. The LCL of the C++ is reached on the third set of tests, whereas the C+ reaches the LCL acceptable on the sixth test. The data indicate that there is loss of activity (competition) with both controls and that actions to remedy this are needed.

characterized for use at various levels and an overview is shown in **Table 5.** One key area in validating tests for diagnosis and surveillance data based on nonvalid criteria would support this stance. The OIE guidelines attempt to address this situation. The success of the implementation of the guidelines will be affected by resources. Where there have been large inputs into campaigns, there is a chance that properly validated kits will be available.

Table 4
Overview of responsibilities

Participant	Factor	Implications
Producer	Robust tests in kit form (complete) Fit for use on leaving supplier Rugged tests Defined fitness for purpose Produce good protocols Control (standards)? Data gathering and analysis-EQA? Response to problems (trouble shooting?) Help desk?	Validation pathway criteria followed
User	Collect and check kit Use kit/data process/report IQC (continuous and transparent) Trouble shoot/adjust/use Trouble shoot/report failure (links with producer maintained) Train and monitor staff	Effective use of kits in control programmes. Effective staff who understand principles and practice of tests
National	Train staff EQA (monitor laboratory) Adopt standards Plan with knowledge of tests (surveys) Accreditation pathway	Ensure capability of using tests most efficiently in well planned programmes.
Regional	Training Standardize (regional standards made and adopted) Harmonization exercises (proficiency testing, ring tests etc.) Collate and report results (epidemiology) EQA	Cooperation and coordination of efforts and maintenance of standards. Generate understanding and transparency
International	Harmonize tests Set standards (e.g., OIE) Monitor test developments Stimulate test development Fund test development Fund and perform training Management advice	Stimulation of good practice and effective testing. Consideration of needs of all countries in managing diagnosis and surveillance leading to better control and eradication of diseases

However, large inputs are not common, nor do planners even with large resources at their disposal, consider diagnostic and surveillance factors seriously. As an example, even the large-scale funded rinderpest campaign ignored these factors and kits for the measurement of antibodies for diagnosis; differential diagnosis and monitoring of the efficiency of vaccination were not planned and measures from a laboratory outside the planned project had to rescue this situation. Such kits have been largely instrumental in confirming the absence of rinderpest from the planet. Foot and

Table 5
Overview of standards for biological testing

Standards	Information
An International Standard (IS) Must be used to calibrate a new method for biological analyte Such standards are of limited quantity and usually associated with calibration of national or laboratory standards or reference materials An International Unit (IU) for activity is then assigned after extensive collaboration between several different laboratories. Such standards are usually regarded as the most reliable standards	Collected-tested-aliquoted under the responsibility of the accepted world body e.g., WHO International laboratory for Biological Standards These are then extensively tested for potency and stability Extremely rigorous standards are employed in preparation and storage of such preparations including Avoidance of contaminants with enzymes such as peptidases from source material. Prevention of adsorption by addition of carrier substances Avoidance of oxidation by containing the samples in an atmosphere of inert gas Limitation of moisture by desiccation, storage in the dark at –20°C
International Reference Preparation (IRP) Produced from IS	The IRP is regarded as a preparation which does not meet the demanding criteria of an IS but nonetheless is a useful in method to method standardization
Reference materials Not as extensively tested as IS Potency and purity data are provided by producer Valuable tools supplied by high level institutions involved in various disciplines	Such standards are very useful for substances that Unable to be characterized by chemical and physical means Heterogeneous materials Difficult to isolate samples Scarce or expensive samples Unstable or easily altered samples Expensive or difficult to prepare samples
In house working standards These are preparations produced by a laboratory performing assays or acquired without any reliable potency estimates	Frequently they are calibrated against an IS
Working standards Most important standard. Constitutes basis for accuracy of a routine assay. (e.g., in IQC)	Extensive validation and testing needed for introduction of a reference not normally necessary in the preparation of a working standard Laboratory must assume responsibility of maintaining standard's quality Larger volumes needed than reference standards

mouth disease (FMD) is a good example of the lack of direction in development. The use of nonstructural proteins of FMD virus in the measurement of antibodies to differentiate vaccinated from infected animals has gone on for about 12 years. There is still no agreed definitive test(s); no reference standards; large scale argument between different developers about the relative DSn and

DSp of various kits, and commercial operations selling kits for ill-defined or no fitness for purpose. Gradually this situation is being controlled through reference to the principles to the OIE guidelines; in fact it is hoped that suppliers will submit validation data to OIE so that there is a transparent dossier to be consulted by users to obtain the most appropriate kit for fitness for purposes that are needed for FMD.

Cost will be a major factor in any kit supply. Validation is expensive and accelerated approaches through large scale cooperation have to be paid for, so the cost of final kits will be high. This has the effect of turning countries towards cheaper kits with less of a validation profile, which could be damaging to national campaigns. The expenses of validated testing have to be realized and put into plans. Ultimately the economic advantage gained by international recognition of the absence of disease will determine whether this support is available.

A key international role is the control of testing with respect to the true identification of the stage of validation of a kit. The guidelines set the OIE standards and with these, it should be possible to judge the appropriateness of tests and make recommendations to use as well as further develop to attain a higher stage. Previously, the unleashing of tests that were not validated sufficiently, without the criteria for estimation of validation, had produced both apparent and more worryingly, inapparent insufficient data. It is expected that the OIE guidelines will increase the quality of testing and serve as a guide to users to expect more defined kits. The responsibility of the end user is to achieve levels of competence through training and experience in performing and understanding tests and the context of the results in control programmes is that most categories of what can be termed international (definitive) standards of activity are not available or not agreed to. This is partly because it is extremely difficult to produce standards of activity that can be quantified to reflect the effects of subtle qualitative differences in all biological situations and because the maintenance and distribution of such standards require great expertise and are very expensive. In the main, "in house" and "working standards" are used in biological testing. This leads to difficulties in assessing the relevance of data from a variety of test formats and complicates issues such as assessing DSn.

3.3. International Organizations

Some observations can be made from an international perspective to illustrate problems with the use of kits in the context of the OIE guidelines. Such examples illustrate factors influencing the use of kits, some of which are more politically motivated and which illustrate bad practice. The main criticism to date has been the lack of planning for fitness for purpose and validation. This is the main reason for the OIE guideline formulations. The transition from research-based reagents produced in institutions where facilities are good, to kits, has always been difficult and rather ad hoc. Validation has been mainly through trial and error, without adequate planned cooperative efforts.

Development of the sustainable supply of kits is difficult as there is a requirement for significant resources and the veterinary market is highly fragmented. Generally the level of quality management in diagnosis is poor in developed countries and even more so where developing countries do not support the veterinary field. There is also a danger that good levels of activity like sampling and testing that yield high amounts of data, are undoubtedly seen as productive and useful , whereas the mostly statistically nonviable data obtained is a waste of money in most control programmes.

4. Testing Involving Polymerase Chain Reaction (PCR)

So far the chapter has concentrated on the use of ELISA. The principles of validation of tests involving PCR (**Fig. 15**) as to fitness for purpose are the same as for serologically-based tests however, the components of the PCR require that a different emphasis be put on the various stages of testing, in particular when considering the role of kits. This poses problems in accommodating the technology for some of the statistical features required for validation of testing by serological methods as well as realizing the PCR result. The DSn is far more affected by sampling regimes and methods of nucleic extraction methods, than serologically based tests. The PCR also suffers from a technology hype where

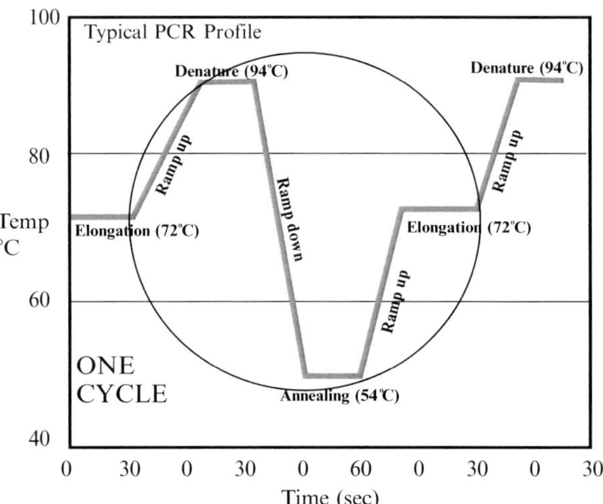

Fig. 15. Schematic illustration of a typical PCR temperature profile.

the undoubted exquisite ASn is more often than not extrapolated into an ultimate DSn without the necessary validation exercises to justify this. These two points indicate where the emphasis has to be placed in the validation pathway for PCR.

4.1. Interpretation of PCR Results

All PCR tests are performed together with suitable controls to assist in determining the reliability of the test results obtained. A positive PCR test result indicates that the nucleic acid genome of the pathogen was present in the sample analyzed. Furthermore, a positive PCR result does not necessarily indicate that the agent was present in a viable, proliferating, structurally whole or active form at the time of sample collection. A negative PCR test result indicates that the nucleic acid genome of the pathogen could not be detected under the test conditions used and suggests that the pathogen was either absent at the time of sample collection, or absent in the test material submitted, or present in sub-detectable quantities only. In a diagnostic application, a negative test result should therefore not be taken as a guarantee of the absence of the pathogen within the animal (or patient) sampled. A repeat submission of appropriate sample material may, therefore, be advisable. Note that when the recommended conditions of sample storage and submission, and sample preparation are not complied with, a negative effect (reduced sensitivity) on the outcome of the test may occur.

4.2. Validation of PCR

PCR measures the presence or absence of a disease agent through identification and quantification of specific nucleic acid. The PCR *per se* is probably accurate and precise through the use of standardized precise instrumentation and the availability of highly defined primers. Often PCR technology is examined and validation criteria assessed from more idealized samples generated in the laboratory under experimental conditions. However, care is needed to identify a test's purpose in this light, since diagnosis infers specific detection from samples taken under field conditions. The routine use of PCR to help diagnose diseases has to be considered as a package and the DSn and DSp have to be examined and challenged using field conditions. The DSn of the PCR is far more likely to be affected by sample volume, site of animal sampling, matrix and extraction methods, as compared to other assays. Generally factors of instrumentation, diagnostic primers and protocols offer less variability as compared to serologically based assays. Factors in the use of PCR for diagnosis are shown in **Fig. 16.** The factors (in grey boxes) must be considered more strongly in the validation of methods. This area can be associated with kits in the sense that specific methods using defined protocols, materials and equipment could be assembled. Thus a specific chemical to protect nucleic acid can be provided as well as nucleic acid extraction kits and control nucleic acid.

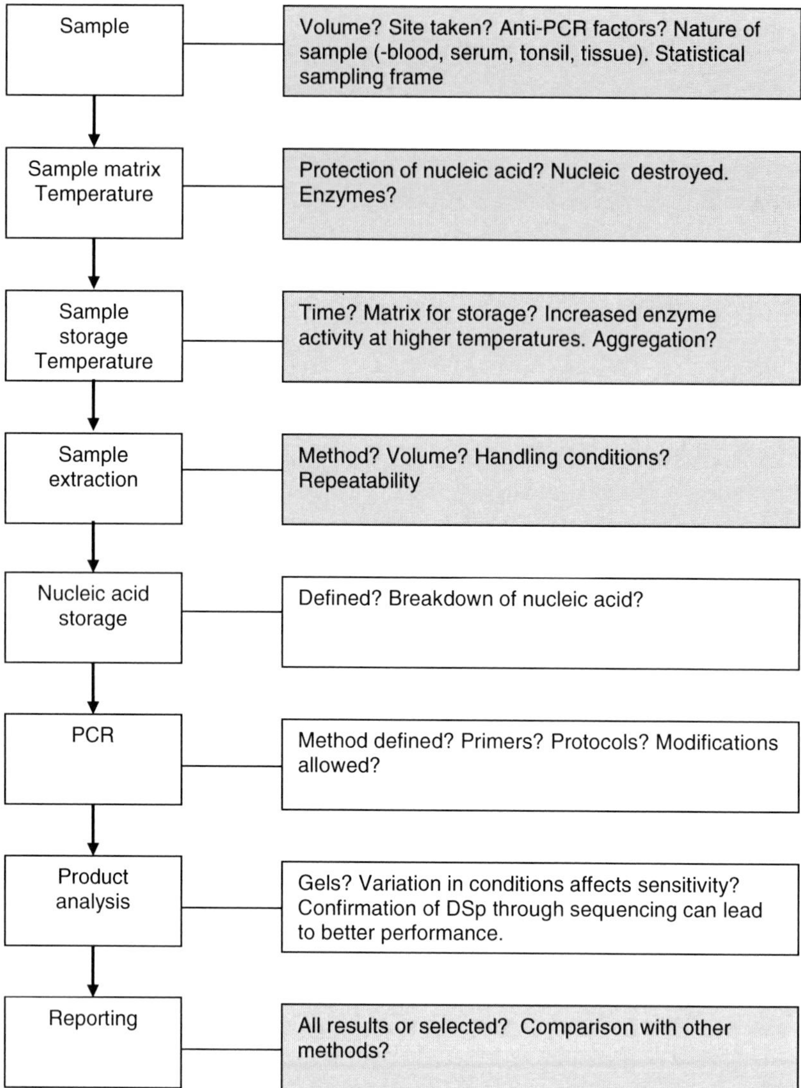

Fig. 16. Process of using PCR in diagnosis. The process of sampling and treatment/extraction are highlighted as having a major importance in assessing true the DSn of a PCR test.

In coordinated research programmes of the Joint FAO/IAEA division involving the use of PCR for diagnosing trypanosomosis, major factors influencing DSn proved to be the use of the appropriate sample collection, extraction methods and nucleic acid storage; i.e., sample handling before the PCR testing. The use of primers and primer sets was less of a variable since they can be defined exactly. However DSn is affected when protocols are tested in a wider range of countries due to slight variations in the sequence of field strains, e.g., when a test developed in Europe is used in Africa. The quality of amplicons (PCR products) can be assessed through sequencing and then better fit primers made to increase the DSn of some PCR protocols. Validation of primer sets under a variety of conditions is necessary so that DSn might be improved with reference to poor and non-specific products due to inexact primers (primers with mismatches) and sequencing during development can show the need to alter primers or conditions to allow better tests. A validation process can be summed up as follows and this might be incorporated into modifications of the OIE guidelines to better suit validation of PCR.

4.2.1. Stage 1 Validation

It involves a feasibility study to determine whether the assay can detect a range of agents (e.g., virus concentrations, virus serotypes/genotypes), without background activity. This stage includes all aspects of development and optimization of the test, including the identification of the test, the determination of the target template(s), the sequence determination of the primers and test conditions and criteria.

This involves the evaluation of the test against a panel of known positive and negative template samples to determine the ASn and ASp. It further involves the development and standardization of the assay in order to optimise all its components. Repeatability of results should then be established before continuing with the validation process (stage 2). In addition:

- ASn is needed to determine the smallest amount of analyte that can be detected using end-point dilution.
- ASp determines whether there is cross-reactivity with heterologous analytes not targeted for detection.
- IQC will involve the continuous monitoring of the assay for assessing repeatability and accuracy.

The following stages *(2–4)* are performed less frequently or otherwise less completely, although in the case of Stage 2, it is the most important component of the validation process.

4.2.2. Stage 2 Validation

This involves the determination of DSn and DSp as elucidated in the following section, where the infection status is determined by a relevant golden standard assay. In the case of serological assays, the OIE recommends that 300 reference samples from known infected animals and not less than 1,000 reference samples from known uninfected animals be included. It is even recommended that these values be increased to 1,000 and 5,000 respectively, to increase accuracy. In the case of PCR, these values have not been determined but will most likely consist of significantly lower numbers. We propose that the PCR test is validated using field samples and field conditions in parallel to determine the DSn and DSp.

The number of samples will depend on the type of disease; however, we propose that a minimum of 20 samples for rare pathogens and a minimum of 100 for more common pathogens would be an acceptable starting point to determine the confidence in a test with regard to diagnostic accuracy. The need to correlate the results with one or more other tests to add value to the PCR data is more pronounced at the early stages. As data increases, the cumulative effect will be to strengthen or weaken the argument that the PCR works "better" or "worse" than existing methods and help define the limits of the DSn and DSp. This often requires a rethinking of the epidemiology of some diseases, due in part to the easily demonstratable higher ASn of the PCR. Data from analysis of true field samples can be increased where the same method (standardized) is being applied in other laboratories. This is a very strong argument for encouraging early and sustained cooperation of laboratories in formally organized "networking" where the tests are harmonized to their ASn using agreed reference standards. The problem of a lack of viable number of field samples to allow validation is common to all tests where disease agents (antigens or nucleic acid) are being directly detected. Such situations require more attention to non-gold standard statistical methods where cumulative data under highly quality controlled conditions builds up sufficient data to allow confidence factors to be defined. Repeatability refers to the amount of agreement between replicates within or between runs. Reproducibility compares the same assay as performed between different laboratories. It is recommended that at least ten samples representing the full range of expected virus concentrations be tested in duplicate (known titres, low through high). The extent of agreement between a test value and the expected value for a sample of known virus concentration will reflect the accuracy of the assay.

4.2.3. Stage 3 Validation

This entails the continued monitoring of the validity of assay performance in the field by calculating the predictive value of positive or negative results based on estimates of prevalence in a target animal population. This can only be done satisfactorily if DSn and DSp data are available.

4.2.4. Stage 4 Validation

This involves the maintenance of validation criteria using internal quality controls. Frequent monitoring for repeatability and accuracy are needed. The OIE also recommends biannual ring-testing to determine reproducibility between laboratories, although annual testing is also described (see proficiency testing). A validated assay should consistently provide test results that identify animals as being positive or negative and accurately predicts the infection status with a predetermined degree of statistical certainty.

4.3. Proficiency Testing

Proficiency testing is the means used to determine the capability of a laboratory to perform the assay and effectively detect the agent (internal proficiency testing). Such testing will also contribute to ensuring that within or between laboratories performing routine diagnostic services, a specific assay is performed according to established international standards (external proficiency testing). It is also intended to achieve standardization of the assays in question. This will ensure that test results obtained are reproducible within and between laboratories and will therefore give a measure of confidence that the results obtained using such an assay are reliable and trustworthy.

- Internal proficiency testing

Internal proficiency testing is used to monitor the ability of members within a laboratory to produce repeatable and accurate results.

- External proficiency or ring testing

This is used for inter-laboratory comparisons and forms part of Stages 3 and 5 of the validation process as formulated by the OIE. This can be performed on a round-robin (continuous) basis. Although tedious and costly,, this process is necessary to achieve standardization of the PCR tests performed. The procedure here will be that a reference laboratory periodically sends each participating laboratory an external proficiency test, a panel of blind coded samples representing the full range of expected concentrations of the pathogen, as well as material derived from an uninfected source. Each participant then processes and tests the samples according to a particular assay method used in-house and (or at a following stage, using an agreed protocol). Statistical comparisons are then made among the laboratories.

The full range of relevant pathogens that might be encountered in a clinical specimen should be tested. Samples from uninfected sources which test positive in two or three of the laboratories can be discarded and may suggest mislabeled or contaminated samples. The goals of any clinical programme will also influence the criteria for proficiency.

5. Diagnosis – the Prevalence Paradox

Diagnosis and surveillance are aided by tests to measure the presence, parts, or evidence of a the disease agent through the detection of antibodies. The OIE guidelines demand a fitness for purpose for a test system. Data then must show how this fitness is proved though data obtained from studies of laboratory and field samples. Inherent in any validation studies are the errors due to variation of the biological, physical, and human elements. Any kit is subject to these errors and features of the effects of the errors have been discussed.

It is useful to put the errors in the context of epidemiological factors as ultimately this infers an understanding of disease in populations. This has relevance to validation as samples have to be examined from populations which are often not easy to define and thus produce degrees of uncertainty in data which are not easy to quantify with the required statistical confidence limits. Most difficulties in diagnosis come from the inadequacyof data on individuals to decide whetherthe test is positive (has disease/ had disease) or negative (does not have disease/has never had disease).

A major problem for all diagnosticians and people developing tests is the "prevalence paradox" where the performance of a kit is influenced by the number of animals at any time point that really have disease or in more epidemiological terms, the prevalence of a disease.

5.1. The Prevalence Paradox

The diagnostic performance of a test is related to prevalence through sampling and through estimated DSn and DSp of a test (data from validation studies). However, statistical analyses of factors in validation require the identification of populations with a known prevalence of true disease, so there is a major problem in the development of tests, a paradox where DSn and DSp rely on studies of a population of unknown prevalence.

5.1.1. Extremes of Prevalence

Two extremes can be used to illustrate the problem as shown in **Fig. 17.** This is an idealized situation which probably never exists. Population A has a high prevalence and therefore very few samples are needed to determine that the population is infected. Population B has an extremely low prevalence so that a very large number of samples are needed to establish any disease.

The risk of mis-diagnosis (false positive or false negative) is extremely high in B so that only tests with extreme specificity and sensitivity are acceptable. In A, the risk of a test missing a positive is very low and as most are positive, a few mis-diagnosed animals

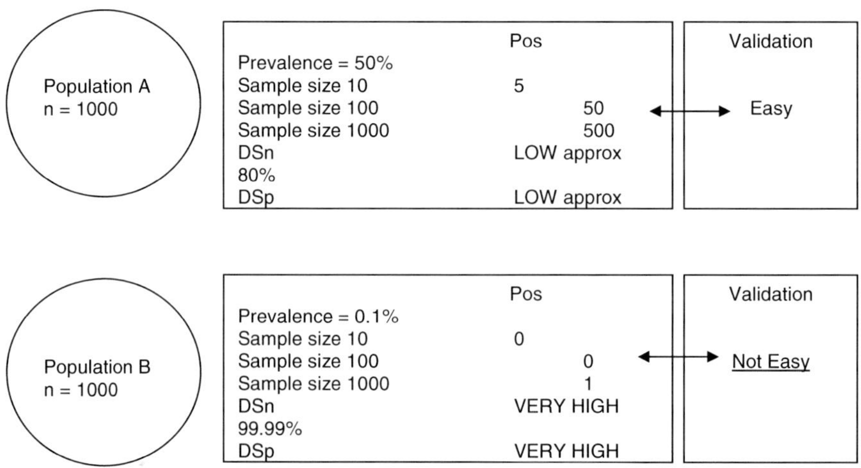

Fig. 17. Populations with very high and very low prevalences.

will not affect the population statistics much. In terms of individuals, in B, the risk of false positives is high unless the test is almost absolute in its specificity. In A, since most individuals are in fact positive the analysis that an animal is positive is correct in 5/10 cases so that an error rate for an individual at 80% DSp is low.

In practice, the definition of a population in the field is very difficult. Other signs of infection are sometimes useful to define an animal's status, but in time the population characteristic being measured by a test varies and infections are rarely synchronized, so that measurements of analytes are affected quantitatively and qualitatively (which can also affect quantitative measurement) due to specificity factors in the test. The populations are mixing, samples are mislabeled, people cheat and other interventions affecting tests are not recorded. It can be thus seen that trying to obtain a population with a characteristic whereby validation of fitness for purpose can be statistically defined is very difficult (particularly where disease produces low prevalence effects).

An attempt to solve the paradox is often made through laboratory experiments whereby animals are infected under controlled conditions and test formats examined with well-defined samples. Here, as a reminder, the Analytical Sensitivity (ASn) and Analytical Specificity (Asp) of tests can be established, and samples used to compare a developing test result with an established test and with other control standards. The calculated sensitivity should reflect DSn, and different formats can be used to analyze relative analytical sensitivities.

Extremes of disease prevalence show that the need for DSn of tests is very different. Validation with a very low prevalence is badly affected by tests with a low DSn and populations are extremely difficult to find to act as pools for samples in validation exercises.

The DSn of a test is often determined by analysis of negative populations where a particular disease has never been recorded. This offers a solution to estimating DSp but still suffers from the fact that the populations do not exactly reflect the particular geographical area or breed and other field factors associated with disease. In most cases the epidemiological situation for a disease is highly variable. This depends on many factors such as disease transmissibility, geographical location, animal husbandry and density and animal movement control and knowledge. This variability can be examined and statistical confidence in data increased by repeat testing and increased studies on populations, but this is expensive and needs a great deal of organization. The relation of DSn, DSp and prevalence is shown in **Fig. 17.** This is a rather simplified illustration of their relevance to test validation criteria. The variability of a population is shown by the width of the grey bars which relate prevalence to DSn and DSp requirements. The necessary values of DSn and DSp are also variable. Most situations with regard to disease prevalence fall into the areas defined in 1 and 2, particularly the latter. Here accuracy can tolerate a relatively wide DSn and DSp. As the prevalence reduces, the DSn and DSp become far more critical for "true" diagnosis. Such reductions in prevalence are obviously encouraged to show a reduction, and final elimination, of a disease. Classically, in the elimination of brucellosis the stages in elimination take prevalence rates from 5 to 0.5% relatively easily. The real difficulties come in taking this final 0.5% to zero and proving it with a test(s) without undue intervention and the culling of many false positive animals.

5.2. Present Situation with Kits

The validation status of most kits being used is strongly in question. It is probably true to say that most report DSn ranges of 90–99% and DSp of 95–99%. This means that for most herd diagnostic purposes (*see* **Fig. 18**) the majority of kits get away with some fitness for purpose criteria, although these are seldom defined. However, kits are often used for studying populations where prevalences are unknown or widely wrong or a great deal lower than expected. In this case the kits are not valid and results should be held in great suspicion. Such suspicion starts with suppliers' figures for DSn and DSp. Care must be taken to examine data to assess whether the figures tally with the studies. This is one overriding aim of the OIE guidelines. So the use of criteria for DSn and DSp for inappropriate populations and worse still, individuals of any population, is a common failing of diagnosticians.

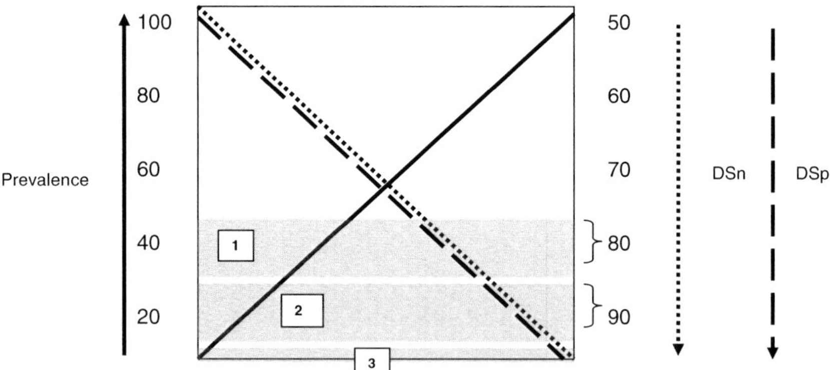

Fig. 18. Relationship of prevalence to DSn and DSp. The relationship of required DSn to prevalence is shown in the graph. The range of 0–50% for DSn is more arbitrary and meant to illustrate the principle involved since any test should be better than a toss of a coin (50% correct). The zones of uncertainty for prevalence (unknown prevalence) affecting measurement of DSn are shaded in *grey*. The range of uncertainty for each zone is reflected by the width of the *greyed bands*. This is the area of paradox where one determination relies in the other and neither can be measured to a defined confidence. As the prevalence is reduced (real or apparent) then the need for a high DSn is more and more marked. There are few problems where the prevalence is higher than 10% (areas 1 and 2) and problems increase as the prevalence approaches and falls below 1%. The lower the prevalence the greater the DSp affects determinations of DSn. Note that at 100 prevalence there is a need for a minimal (on scale provided) DSn, but that a 100% DSp would be needed to rule out false positive reactions.

5.3. Accumulation of Data

The true status of DSn and DSp of any test therefore often relies on a more cumulative statistical approach in development where a test is used to analyze populations based on whatever sampling frame is used. This in turn leads us to point out the importance of well-conducted data management, collection and analysis, where kits are used in a wider context to increase validation data. Data can then be from rather poorly planned sources. On analysis of data, tests can be modified to meet requirements for increased or decreased DSn and DSp. The continuous nature of validation is then stressed along with data capture, analysis, and modification of conditions and re-assessment of fitness forpurpose. The problem with this is that tests have to be released at some point so that reaching a total understanding about the performance of a test for all situations is impossible. Emphasis on the user can be made at this point, as he /she has the necessary reagents to evaluate against the local samples. The laboratory has the possibility of altering values of the test (e.g., cutoff estimates) to revise DSn and DSp characteristics within the context of planned sampling frames for a particular disease.

The validation process should be promoted by users reporting such studies to international organizations as well as the producer, so that other users can benefit and producers can respond by developing new systems satisfying better the needs of laboratories. There is no formal arrangement, or portal, for this type of development. Some companies do encourage reporting and will act on data, others do not care. The level of understanding of tests, and their use and flexibility, is also very poor and without this there is little chance that tests can be maximized in their use, nor will the controlled flow of validation data be possible. The development of a web-based portal to retrieve data from laboratories using kits would be beneficial. This would act as a source of data to allow increased validation and would encourage laboratory personnel to participate. Problems could be solved on-line in a more public forum and developments suggested or protocols agreed, which extend uses or statistically better qualify data.

6. Conclusions

The terms ruggedness and robustness have been defined and their importance in the validation of tests emphasized. Robustness was determined as the resistance of a kit or set of defined reagents to reduced performance due to any physical factors on transport or in the laboratory. Ruggedness involves resistance to variations in laboratory technique and effects of sampling. The responsibilities of the producer and end user in supply and use of kits were examined and helpful advice made to improve methods for testing and continuous monitoring of kits, such as charting methods to record IQC data; troubleshooting of problems with kits and reporting problems. The end user should be trained enough to be able to determine which parts of a kit are non functioning and take steps to eliminate the problem or at least report findings for action by the supplier. End users should also have the skills to adapt tests to local conditions and produce quality controlled data to justify findings. In turn the supplier should take steps to gather data continuously and act on any problems. This is seen as part of validation.

The difficulties in validation were examined from the perspective of the prevalence paradox where populations used for validation are variable so that "true" DSn is not easy to measure with any confidence. The importance of obtaining data from well-run tests and collation of data to increase the validation criteria was stressed. A key area to increase quality is agreement, production, and characterization of reference samples. This is not an easy task due to the particular problems of variation seen in biological systems, the heterogeneous nature of analytes, the variation in the needs for hard-to-define populations and the cost of maintaining and distributing materials. International organizations have, so far, played a major role in facilitating the development of kits to be used in the control of disease; supplying training to allow the materials to be used efficiently and seeking to keep quality issues uppermost in obtaining data. This process suffers from discontinuity of funding and poor coordination of planning in the medium and long term. Diagnostic and surveillance activities are often forgotten in the planning process at national and certainly regional levels. If followed, the OIE guidelines, possibly with modifications concerning PCR testing, would solve many of the problems associated with the supply of kits used in diagnosis and surveillance. An overview of the aspects of validation is shown in the literature review *(1–16)*.

References

1. Wright P.F., Nilsson E., Van Rooij E.M.A., Lelenta M. & Jeggo M.H. (1993). Standardization and validation of enzyme-linked immunosorbent assay techniques for the detection of antibody in infectious disease diagnosis. *Rev. Sci. Tech. Off. Int. Epiz.* 12, 435–450.
2. Zweig M.H. & Campbell G. (1993). Receiver-operating characteristic (ROC) plots: a fundamental evaluation tool in clinical medicine. *Clin. Chem.* 39, 561–577.
3. Jacobson R.H. (1998). Validation of serological assays for diagnosis of infectious diseases. *Rev. Sci. Tech. Off. Int. Epiz.* 17, 469–486.
4. Wright P.F. (1998). International standards for test methods and reference sera for diagnostic tests for antibody detection. *Rev. Sci. Tech. Off. Int. Epiz.* 17, 527–533.
5. Office International des Epizooties (2000). Standard for management and technical requirements for laboratories conducting tests for infectious animal diseases. *In:* OIE Quality Standard and Guidelines for Veterinary Laboratories: Infectious Diseases (2002). Office International des Epizooties (OIE), 12 rue de Prony, 75017 Paris, France, 1–31.

6. Greiner M., Gardner IA. (2000). Epidemiologic issues in the validation of veterinary diagnostic tests. *Prev. Vet. Med.* 45 (1–2), 3–22. Review.
7. Greiner M., Gardner IA. (2000). Application of diagnostic tests in veterinary epidemiologic studies. *Prev. Vet. Med.* 45 (1–2), 43–59. Review.
8. Enoe C., Georgiadis M.P. & Johnson W.O. (2000). Estimating the sensitivity and specificity of diagnostic tests and disease prevalence when the true disease state is unknown. *Prev. Vet. Med.* 45, 61–81.
9. Greiner M., Pfeiffer D. & Smith R.D. (2000). Principles and practical application of the receiver operating characteristic (ROC) analysis for diagnostic tests. *Vet. Prev. Med.* 45, 23–41.
10. Crowther J.R. (2000). Validation of Diagnostic Tests for Infectious Diseases in: The ELISA Guidebook: Methods in Molecular Biology. *Humana Press, Totowa, NJ*, Chapter 8, pp. 301–345.
11. Crowther J.R. (2000). Charting Methods for Internal Quality Control in: The ELISA Guidebook: Methods in Molecular Biology. *Humana Press, Totowa, NJ*, Chapter 9, pp. 347–394.
12. Office International Des Epizooties (2002). OIE Guide 3: Laboratory Proficiency Testing. in: OIE Quality Standard and Guidelines for Veterinary Laboratories: Infectious Diseases. OIE, Paris, France, 53–63.
13. Sampling Methods. Manual of Diagnostic Tests and Vaccines for Terrestrial Animals. (2004). Terrestrial Manual 5th Edition, Parts 1 and 2, Chapter I.1.1.
14. Quality Management in Veterinary Testing Laboratories Manual of Diagnostic Tests and Vaccines for Terrestrial Animals. (2004). Terrestrial Manual 5th Edition, Parts 1 and 2, Chapter I. 1.2.
15. Principles of validation of diagnostic assays for infectious diseases. Manual of Diagnostic Tests and Vaccines for Terrestrial Animals. (2004). Terrestrial Manual 5th Edition, Parts 1 and 2, Chapter I.1.3.
16. Validation and Quality Control of Polymerase Chain Reaction Methods used for the Diagnosis of Infectious Diseases. Manual of Diagnostic Tests and Vaccines for Terrestrial Animals. (2004). Terrestrial Manual 5th Edition, Parts 1 and 2, Chapter I.1.4.

Chapter 12

More Advanced Statistical Methods for Quality Assurance, Test Validation, and Interpretation

1. Background

This chapter examines statistical factors involved in assessing tests for their usefulness in diagnosis. Some of the terms have already been introduced and discussed, but here fresh directions and analyses are examined to aid understanding, and to help with the more difficult areas of interpreting results and the mathematical background. The data are based on an excellent document *(1)*, which should be consulted by those interested in the more detailed mathematical background to the principles and in extensive referencing. Some of the abbreviations used differ from other chapters where terms are transposed into mathematical equations.

Diagnostic tests for diseases determine specific properties of a specimen that lead to a decision as to whether a sample is positive or negative. The extent to which the test result is correct depends on the true status of the sampled animal/human, and is expressed as the diagnostic accuracy. There is a paradox here, as some other assessment of the disease state has to be inferred to allow validation of a serological test such as the ELISA. This problem is at the root of the diagnostician's job, and statistical parameters involving sampling and comparative testing are constants. Defining an ELISA in terms of diagnostic accuracy is part of an overall process of validation, which produces continuous data in time and where the target population of an assay changes. As described in previous chapters, diagnostic sensitivity (DSn) and diagnostic

John R. Crowther, *Methods in Molecular Biology, The ELISA Guidebook, Vol. 516*

DOI: 10.1007/978-1-60327-254-4_12

specificity (DSp) are both factors in assessing overall diagnostic accuracy.

No test is 100% correct, and the job of the diagnostician is to monitor the performance of a test in time and to understand the inherent errors and the factors influencing the test, such as sampling. Some sources of error are shown in **Table 1** and these have to be measured from day to day, operator to operator, and from sample to test result. Logically, the more the work done in analyzing samples from as wide a possible set of situations, the more can be understood regarding test performance under more variable conditions. This validation process is continuous, as already indicated, and establishing performance criteria is at the core of assigning statistical parameters to test results. One main difficulty is defining, in terms of sample number and distribution, the minimum requirements for establishing a test's performance, leading to complications arising from the simple question: "Is the sample positive or negative?"

Table 1
Sources or errors for testing

Error	Example
Pre-test errors	Misidentification of animals
	Mixing up samples
	Contaminating samples
	Cross contamination of samples
	Poor storage conditions
Analytical errors	Pipetting, measurement (dilutions etc.)
Random and systematic errors	Instrumentation calibration and faults
	Reagent deterioration and unmeasured effects on storage
Post-analytical errors	Sample identification.
	Poor interpretation of data.
Sources of errors in laboratory data, statistical	Random error: an observed deviation from the true result in an unpredictable direction
	Bias-deviation from the true value in a specific direction
Sources of errors in laboratory data, operational	Factors that interfere with the measuring process
	Biological factors that affect the measurement of the analyte concentration in vivo

2. Test Evaluation

Test evaluation is any study that measures the performance of a diagnostic test, and the term validation is sometimes used as a synonym. Validity describes the degree of agreement between a quantity measured by a method and the presumed true quantity of interest. Based on this information, it should be possible to decide whether or not the inferences from test results under the given circumstances of application are valid. The term evaluation should be used for the process of generating quantitative measures of validity (performance measures) and the term validation should be used for the final decision as to whether the performance criteria justify the application of the test in a given situation. The most commonly used parameters for test evaluation are precision and accuracy (*see* **Fig. 1**). These have already been looked at in other chapters, but it does no harm to revisit them. The two terms represent independent features of a diagnostic test. A test can be precise (producing the same results, with only little variation) but non-accurate (producing only false results). On the other hand, even correct test results may be non-precise (i.e., more than 10% variation between sub-samples).

2.1. Rules

Evaluation and validation results apply first of all to the given application, which can be characterized according to three main settings: test procedure, test population, and test purpose (internal

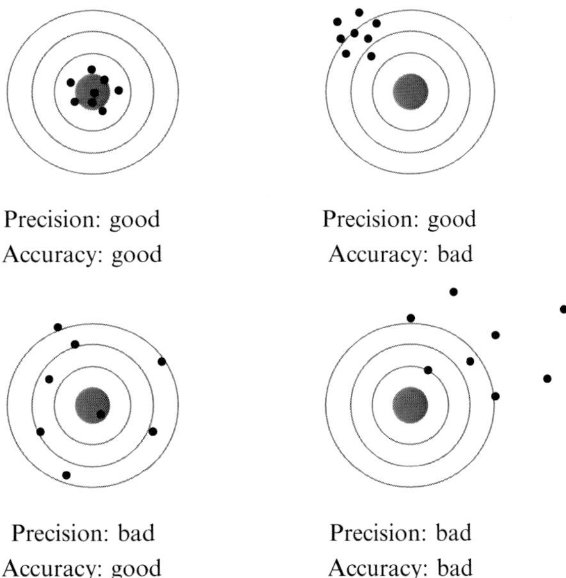

Fig. 1. A reminder about the difference between precision and accuracy using 8 trials on a shooting target.

validity). Extrapolation to other applications (changes in one or more of the factors) is less reliable, and depends on how representative the conditions of the study are when applied to other settings (external validity). (*See* Chapter 11 for other considerations of the responsibilities.)

3. Basic Concepts of Quality Assurance (QA)

The golden aim of the QA system is to incorporate classical tools such as calibration, assay validation, intra-run and inter-run controls, and internal and external quality control into integrated components of a total quality management (TQM) scheme that additionally has pre-analytic and reporting methods, as well as preparatory and common laboratory procedures. The goal of TQM is the international harmonization of laboratory performance and improved cost effectiveness. The ISO 9000 series standards issued by the International Organization for Standardization serve as a guideline for implementation of TQM, and provide a basis for laboratory certification.

Quality is relative, and requires external goals and standards for definition and assessment. Quality has been defined as fitness for the intended use. Quality critically depends on the precision/accuracy of the method, but always refers to clinical and decision-making requirements that need to be translated into laboratory QA.

The total error budget refers to the maximal allowable laboratory error from the clinical or decision-making point of view, and includes biological (within-subject) variation, systematic errors, and random errors. The goal of QA, through application of Quality Control (QC) measures, is to establish a system for routine laboratory procedures that copes with the quality requirements and alerts the technician when the system fails to meet the requirements.

3.1. Classical Tools of QA

- Calibration of working standards (in-house internal reagents; denoted as tertiary standards) against National Standard Reagents (National Reference Preparations or secondary standards, which are calibrated against international standards, i.e., primary standards), or inclusion of standards supplied with commercial test kits
- Inclusion of samples for QC (denoted as controls, from now on) in each run of an assay. Controls are usually calibrated against standards
- Rules for the validation of single samples (usually based on their coefficient of variation) and series (usually based on the deviation from the expected value of internal controls)

- Control charts (e.g., Levey-Jennings)
- Control limits

3.2. Levey-Jennings Control Charts and Their Application

This type of control chart is commonly used and involves:

1. Plotting control limits of mean values ±2 and ±3*s* (*s* here = SD) with the expected value (mean, *m*) for a control sample or samples, using horizontal lines (*see* **Fig. 2**).
2. Plotting internal controls for each run.
3. Accepting assay runs only if the control value of the run is within *m* ± 2*s*. The run is then "in-control" or "valid."
4. Rejecting runs where the control value of the run is outside *m* ± 2*s*. The run is then "out of control" and results cannot be reported for unknown test samples in this run. The problem must be fixed and the run repeated. This is known as the 1_{2s} rule because one control value is outside the 2*s* limit. This procedure is not very efficient in detecting shifts. Several control values in direct sequence exceeding the same control limit are useful in detecting systematic error (shift). Such a systematic bias may increase with time (drift). Appropriate rules to detect shifts and drifts include two controls in sequence (i.s.) exceeding the 2*s* limit (2_{s2}), four controls i.s. exceeding the 1*s* limit (4_{1s}), or ten controls i.s. exceeding the mean (10_x).
5. All decisions, remedial actions, and results of troubleshooting must be documented! Remember well: "You have not done what you have not written down".

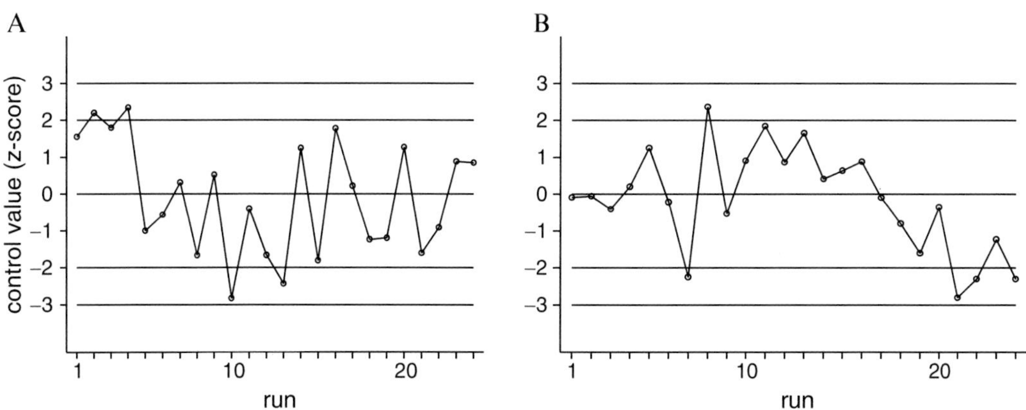

Fig. 2. Levey-Jennings control charts of hypothetical control value data over 24 analytical runs. (**a**) The 1_{2s} rule is violated four times (warning rule). 2_{2s}, 6_x, 8_x, 10_x are not violated (no systematic error), 1_{3s}, R_{4s} are not violated (no random error). (**b**) The 1_{2s} rule is violated five times (warning rule). 2_{2s} is violated (run 21, 22), 6_x is violated (run 10–15; drift), 8_x is violated (run 17–24; drift), 10_x is not violated, 1_{3s} is not violated, R_{4s} is violated (run 7, 8).

3.2.1. How are Control Limits Established?

Control limits are established through:

1. Choice of appropriate controls (internal controls are acceptable where no recognized controls exist).
2. Inclusion and measurement in the test of an internal control preparation (preferentially calibrated according to international reference preparations) in analytical runs over 10–20 working days, under routine conditions, with the collection of at least 20 measurements.
3. Establishing mean (m) and standard deviation (s) of the repetitive measurements. The control limits are given as 95% confidence interval of the measurement ($m \pm 2s$).
4. Updating calculations for each new measurement of the internal control preparation.

4. Generation of Laboratory Data

Test results can be binary, semi-quantitative, and quantitative, as indicated in **Table 2.** Note that it is generally possible to express test results using less informative scales. For example, quantitative data can be classified as negative/intermediate/positive or negative/positive. This is associated with loss of information.

4.1. ELISA Data

Scoring of results by visual inspection can give qualitative or semiquantitative results that may be suitable for field applications in peripheral locations. Here, there should be suitable controls to assess the ability of operators to read tests; however, the ELISA usually gives continuous OD data from a photometer, and this is considered next. Data are from:

- Titration methods that give semiquantitative data where the highest reciprocal serum dilution in which the analyte is still detectable is reported as endpoint titer.
- Titration methods that give quantitative data where derivation of a numerical measure from a model is fitted to a standard curve.
- Single dilution methods can give quantitative data (referred to as absorbance method), and numerical corrections using internal standards are possible. This is the method of choice where high samples are processed, e.g., for serosurveys and serosurveillance.
- Kinetic readings that yield quantitative data through measurement of the enzyme-substrate reaction over a defined time

Table 2
Some features of data obtained by diagnostic and serodiagnostic methods

Type of test	Type of scale	Possible outcomes (examples)	Methods (examples)[a]
Qualitative (binary)	Categorial (binary)	Test negative, –, 0 Test positive, +, 1	Direct detection (microscopy, culture, PCR)
Semi-quantitative	Categorial (ordinal)	Negative – 0 Intermediate +/– 1 Weak positive + 2 Positive, ++ 3 Strong positive, +++ 4 Reciprocal titers (e.g., 64, 128, 256, 512, 1024, 2048,...)	ELISA (titration), IFAT, CFT Somatic cell count in mastitis diagnosis Tuberculosis skin test
Quantitative	Continuous (interval or ratio)	[min, max] Where min and max is the minimum and maximum value, respectively Each value between min and max may occur	ELISA (single-dilution)

[a]PCR = polymerase-chain reaction,
ELISA = enzyme-linked immunosorbent assay,
IFT = immunofluorescence test,
CFT = complement fixation test
[b]Not for comparison of tests

interval, with results expressed as a measure of the slope of OD values in a defined time.

Some ELISA-specific flaws:

- Edge effects introduce technological bias occurring at the outer wells of an ELISA plate, probably due to temperature gradient, and this may invalidate both single-dilution and titration assays.
- Data censoring where physical lower and upper bounds exist for the photometer reading, so that observations that exceed the machine limits are still used to report a test value. These values should be censored, as they are not allowable. Titration assays give censored values if the true endpoint dilution is not observed. This is practically relevant, because often only a limited number of dilutions are tested. The problem is to fit any theoretical distribution to the data that include an unknown fraction of censored observations.

4.2. Corrections, Standardization, and Units (example related to ELISA)

The interpretation of test results using unprocessed OD ELISA data (usually referred to as raw data) is not recommended for reporting and interlaboratory comparison. For use of single dilutions of samples, it is common practice to express results of samples with respect to reference values (normalization, indexing, or ratio methods).

References may be:

- Non-antigen controls (netto-ELISA), where the OD value of a non-antigen control is subtracted from the sample OD. This may be useful for virus serology where the virus antigen is presented in a matrix of host tissue material, but there is a risk of over-correction; it is more expensive on materials, and difficult to standardize.
- Plate blank values, which correct bias for the run, and can be a control for charts; there is a risk of over-correction.
- Cut-off values, which have an inherent meaning, but there is no bias correction when cut-off values are not run-specific, and a lot of material is needed for controls if cut-off is run-specific.
- Internal negative standard (signal-to-noise-ratio), which can mean that division by a small number (negative) introduces unnecessarily variability.
- Internal positive standard (sometimes referred to as percent positivity – PP); here, internal standards should be adjusted to national or international reference preparations). This gives some bias control for the run; the test results have an inherent meaning, and arbitrary ELISA units can be established. There is a risk of over-correction, and control charts are still necessary.
- Negative and positive standards. For example:

$$\text{Index}_{\text{sample}} = \left(\text{OD}_{\text{sample}} - \text{OD}_{\text{neg}}\right) / \left(\text{OD}_{\text{pos}} - \text{OD}_{\text{neg}}\right)$$

or back-transformation:

$$\text{OD}_{\text{cor r}} = \text{Index}_{\text{sample}}\left(\text{mean OD}_{\text{pos}} - \text{mean OD}_{\text{neg}}\right) + \text{mean OD}_{\text{neg}}$$

This gives bias correction for the run, but risks over-correction, and control charts are still necessary.

- Mean and standard deviation of negative controls (referred to as standardized deviation ratio)

$$\text{SDR} = \left(\text{OD}_{\text{sample}} - \text{mean OD}_{\text{neg}}\right) / \text{standard deviation OD}_{\text{neg}}$$

This result has an inherent meaning, but there is no bias correction when cut-off values are not run specific, and a lot of material is needed for controls if cut-off is run-specific. Reference samples included for the purpose of standardization (normalization) are denoted as standards. Reference samples included for QC purposes are denoted as controls. Samples calibrated against standards may also serve as controls.

5. Diagnostic Evaluation of a Test

A characteristic of diagnostic tests is that the inferences from the test results are of interest, rather than the observed test values. For example, the specific antibody concentration of a serum sample may be examined with the intention of finding out whether or not an animal is infected. Other inferences from serodiagnostic tests include measuring the level of protective immunity or the transition between disease stages (follow-up investigation). The test result should correlate with the disease status of the tested animal; however, test result and disease status are not necessarily in complete agreement. All testing samples may give false-positive or false-negative results. Consideration to the true concentration of the analyte (e.g., specific antibody) only, is not the goal of testing, but instead there has to be a comparison of the test result with the true status of the patient. This approach is referred to as diagnostic evaluation. The standard for presenting the results of such a study is the 2 × 2 table (**Table 3**).

5.1. Prerequisites

The disease status of each individual that is tested for evaluation purposes must be known. The reference method used to establish this "true" disease status of each individual is referred to as the gold standard. Practically speaking, the gold standard is the most reliable diagnostic method available, but may be a combination of the results of more than one reference test. Of course, the

Table 3
Contingency (2 × 2) table for cross-tabulation of test results and the true state of disease

	Diseased (D+)	Non-diseased (D–)
Test positive (T+)	True positive (TP)	False positive (FP)
Test negative (T–)	False negative (FN)	True negative (TN)

results of the test being evaluated must not be a part of the definition of the reference status.

5.1.1. The Five-Stages Model for Test Validation

This has already been discussed in Chapter 8, but is worth reiterating. Test validation is a continuous process that can be divided into five components:

1. Feasibility studies that involve preliminary studies to assess the technical feasibility of an assay. This requires the selection of control samples and selection of an analytical method.
2. Assay development and standardization, which involves classical optimization procedures such as checkerboard titration and refinements of the protocol. The benchmark for optimal test conditions is the analytical sensitivity (Asn) and analytical specificity (Asp), precision, and differentiation of known control samples.
3. Estimation of test performance characteristics. Here, consideration of the prevalence of the disease is needed for test validation, and has an important impact on the predictive values of test results.
4. Monitoring of assay performance needs to address the prevalence of disease in the target population.
5. Maintenance and enhancement of test validity involves QA, and internal as well as external QC procedures. It also includes revalidation after changing the test environment (target population, technical factors, reagent replacement, and the like).

5.2. Test Performance Parameters

Precision and accuracy are independent features of any diagnostic test. A test can be precise (producing the same results with only little variation) but non-accurate (producing only false results). On the other hand, even correct test results may be non-precise (i.e., more than 10% variation between sub-samples). Precision is the ability of a test to give constant results.

Measures of precision are:

- Repeatability: degree of variation between results within one laboratory (within the assay, from day-to-day, run-to-run). Expressed by the standard deviation or other useful measures of variation.
- Reproducibility: degree of variation of results between laboratories. Expressed by the standard deviation or other useful measures of variation.

5.3. Diagnostic vs. Analytical Evaluation

The terms sensitivity and specificity describe the analytical accuracy of a test. They are associated with the ability of a test to detect small quantities of the analyte, but not cross-reactive substances. The challenge is to select putative cross-reactive substances; respectively, samples from sources free from the infection of interest but with other relevant clinical conditions.

5.3.1. Accuracy

Accuracy is the ability of a test to give correct results (agreement with the reference method).

Measures of accuracy:

- Sensitivity (Se) is the probability of a test to give a positive result when the disease is present (diagnostic sensitivity). It can be estimated as relative frequency of positive test results in infected individuals.

$$\text{Sensitivity} = \text{TP}/(\text{TP} + \text{FN})$$

- Specificity (Sp) is the probability of a test to give a negative result when the disease is not present (diagnostic specificity). It can be estimated as the relative frequency of negative test results in non-infected individuals.

$$\text{Specificity} = \text{TN}/(\text{TN} + \text{FP})$$

5.3.2. Some Terms Used in Measuring Accuracy

Efficiency (Ef)

Efficiency is the probability of a test to correctly classify non-infected and infected individuals of a study population with a given prevalence. The efficiency depends upon the prevalence!

$$\text{Efficiency} = (\text{TN} + \text{TP})/(\text{TN} + \text{FN} + \text{TP} + \text{FP})$$

Youden's index (J) is the probability of a test to correctly classify non-infected and infected individuals. The Youden index does not depend upon the prevalence!

$$J = \text{Se} + \text{Sp} - 1$$

Likelihood ratio of a positive test result (LR+) is the ratio of the probability of disease to the probability of non-disease, given a positive test result.

$$\text{LR}+ = \text{Se}/(1 - \text{Sp})$$

Likelihood ratio of a negative test result (LR–) is the ratio of the probability of disease to the probability of non-disease, given a negative test result.

$$\text{LR}- = (1 - \text{Se})/\text{Sp}$$

5.3.3. Sensitivity and Specificity Depend on the Cut-Off Value

In a quantitative test, a cut-off value must be selected. Note that sensitivity and specificity are inversely related when the cut-off value is consequently changed; there is no absolute single true sensitivity and specificity. By changing the cut-off value, one can obtain any desired sensitivity or specificity.

5.4. Planning of Validation Studies

The planning phase of a validation study is concerned with the selection of a study design and the determination of sample size or sizes. The quality of the validation study will depend largely upon these settings.

5.4.1. Study Design (Sampling)

The reference population of animals used for an evaluation study should be representative of the target population. Many biological factors (e.g., age, sex, nutritional and immune status, and other infections) influence test results. Therefore, the results of an evaluation study may not be valid when the test is applied to another population. Although experimentally infected animals may not be representative of any natural animal population *per se*, they have been suggested for validation purposes. This is reasonable when there is no clear knowledge concerning populations, and experimental samples can be generated with the epidemiological niches in mind, as far as possible.

5.4.2. Pre-Stratified Sampling

In pre-stratified sampling designs, the subpopulations of infected and non-infected individuals are sampled separately, and sample sizes for the two groups are fixed arbitrarily. Therefore, the sample prevalence is also arbitrary; e.g., 50% prevalence if 100 negative and 100 positive controls are sampled. It is reasonable to assume that this prevalence differs from the actual prevalence in the target population. Thus, prevalence-dependent measures of accuracy can only be extrapolated to real situations if they are formally corrected for the appropriate prevalence in the target population. Pre-stratified sampling designs are often realized by defining clinical groups, e.g., healthy blood donors or clinically advanced cases of the disease in question. Ideally, groups should represent the real target populations. Evaluation studies sometimes consider additional subpopulations with related disease states. Moreover, the positive and the negative reference groups may be stratified according to some biological data. Sensitivity and specificity for such designs should be separately established for the different groups. If the test parameters differ among the subgroups of infected individuals (e.g., disease states, age), between the subgroups of non-infected individuals (e.g., other diseases/infections, exposure, age), the resulting overall sensitivity and specificity depends upon the distribution of these strata in the target population. If information on the respective structure of the target population is lacking, it is not possible to obtain unbiased estimates of the overall sensitivity and specificity. Nevertheless, such detailed information would be useful for a technical optimization of the test.

5.4.3 Post-Stratified Sampling

The situation is quite different if the gold standard is applied to a non-stratified sample of the target population. For such post-stratified sampling designs, the prevalence, according to the gold standard in the evaluation sample, is taken as the unbiased estimator of the real prevalence in the target population. Moreover, the sample can be assumed to be representative with regard to those factors that may modulate the sensitivity and specificity of the test. Thus, measures of test accuracy would not need any correction for prevalence or biological factors. The estimates of sensitivity and specificity derived from post-stratified sampling designs are *per se* more reliable than their counterparts from pre-stratified studies. In the case of post-stratified designs, the prevalence is a random variable, and therefore the variances of sensitivity and specificity will be greater than in pre-stratified designs.

5.4.4. Partial Verification

If the reference test is very expensive or invasive, one may use the new test as a screening device and confirm all positive test results, but only a part of the negative results, with the reference method (partial verification). This yields a 2 × 3 table in which the third column displays the number of non-verified subjects (**Table 4**).

Using the notation indicated in **Table 4**, we define the proportion of individuals that receive verification given a positive test result as $c_1 = (a + b)/n_1$ and the corresponding proportion given a negative test result as $c_2 = (c + d)/n_2$. If the sampling proportions are unequal ($c_1 \neq c_2$), the naive estimates of sensitivity ($Se_{nv} = a/(a + c)$) and specificity ($Sp_{nv} = d/(b + d)$) are biased (verification bias), because the numerator and denominator refer to different sampling proportions. We presume that the selection of (c+d) animals for the reference test does not depend on their true infection state (conditional independence assumption). In this case, bias-corrected estimates of sensitivity (Se_{corr}) and specificity (Sp_{corr}) are given as:

Table 4
Cross-tabulation of the results of a validation study with partial verification

		Gold standard test			
		D+	D−	unverified	
New test	T+	a (46)	b (1)	e (0)	n_1
	T−	c (17)	d (30)	f (106)	n_2

Notation is T+, T−, D+, D− for test positive, negative, gold standard positive, negative, respectively. (numbers in parentheses are used for illustration of calculations in the text)

$$\text{Se}_{\text{corr}} = (\text{a} / c_1) / (\text{a} / c_1 + \text{c} / c_2)$$

and

$$\text{Sp}_{\text{corr}} = (\text{d} / c_2) / (\text{d} / c_2 + \text{b} / c_1) \text{ respectively.}$$

In our example, 47 T+ animals ($c_1 = 1$) but only 47 of 153 T– animals ($c_2 = 0.307$) receive the gold standard test. The naive estimates were $\text{Se}_{\text{nv}} = 0.73$, $\text{Sp}_{\text{nv}} = 0.97$, and bias-corrected estimates were $\text{Se}_{\text{corr}} = 0.45$, $\text{Sp}_{\text{corr}} = 0.99$.

5.4.5. Sample Size

The sample size (n) needed for an evaluation study depends upon the desired precision of the concerned parameter (P). The standard approach assumes simple random sampling and states:

$$n = P(1 - P) / (d / 1.96)^2$$

where P denotes an *a priori* estimate of the concerned parameter (e.g., Se, Sp, Ef) and d denotes the acceptable deviation according to the 95% binomial confidence interval of the parameter CI95%.

$$(P) = P \pm d.$$

Consider an ELISA with unknown sensitivity (assume the worst-case scenario of P=0.5). To estimate sensitivity with a precision of ±5% (d=0.05), we need:

$n = 0.5(0.5)/(0.05/1.96)^2 \approx 385$ animals with confirmed disease.

This is only a rough guideline. In practice, it is desirable to include even more samples in the reference populations for three reasons:

- The *case mix* (i.e., the stage and severity of disease and biological influencing factors) in the sample can often be improved by increasing the sample size.
- A larger sample size compensates for intra-herd correlation when the sample includes animals from different herds.
- The formula above is only an approximation. Exact confidence intervals established based on the calculated sample size will not have the desired coverage.

5.4.6. Consensus on Validation

- The cut-off value and the accuracy measures should be established using the same set of negative and positive reference samples. Theoretically, this leads to a resubstitution bias (accuracy estimates that are too optimistic). From an epidemiological viewpoint, it is desirable to optimize the cutoff by considering the resulting accuracy parameters of the target population.

- Subpopulations (e.g., vaccinated, non-vaccinated livestock) need to be considered.
- Sensitivity estimates based on experimentally infected or vaccinated animals are preferable.

From the epidemiological viewpoint, Se estimates are regarded as potentially biased when established under experimental conditions. The measures so established are internally valid, but may not be used on a population basis for further inferences (predictive values and prevalence estimates; see forthcoming sections).

- In cases where diagnostic Se cannot be compared under the conditions outlined above, relative Se may be compared using samples from infected herds/flocks. Selection of infected herds/flocks may be based on epidemiological, clinical, and serological evidence, but samples from all animals in the herd/flock should be used in the comparison

The true infection status of every animal in the study should be known.

- Comparative test validation in different laboratories should be based on a proper standardization of assay conditions
- The test validation should include the assessment of potential cross-reactions

Panels of sera with various diagnostic statuses are extremely useful, but should not replace the representative sample from the target population.

5.5. Bias in Test Validation

Validation studies also need to be valid. Internal validity is achieved if the study represents an unbiased estimate of test performance measured under the given conditions (test protocol, reference samples, and laboratory).

Bias to be considered for internal validity include:

- Diagnostic review bias: The result of the reference test is influenced by the result of the test. Remedy: Blind testing, where sample identity and control identity is unknown until the end of testing.
- Test review bias: Interpretation of the results is influenced by the knowledge of the disease status. Remedy: Blind results of the reference test.
- Incorporation bias: The test result is actually used as one of the (reference) diagnostic criteria. Remedy: Avoidance.
- Information bias: Reference test procedure is not appropriate; e.g., the new test is supposed to be more accurate than the reference test. Remedy: The bias may be corrected if Se and Sp

of the reference method and the prevalence in the evaluation sample are known.

- Work-up bias: The efforts to verify the disease are more serious in test-positive than in test-negative subjects. Remedy: Blind testing.
- Verification bias: The selection of reference samples is influenced by the test result. Remedy: All individuals receive verification or analytic correction.
- Resubstitution bias: Considered a mild bias and usually negligible. Remedy: Optimization of the cut-off value and estimate of the accuracy measures using independent samples.
- External validity: The extent to which the result of a study can be extrapolated to other target populations may be compromised through a selection bias. The reference population is not representative of the target population. Remedy: Make the sample representative. The distribution of known biological factors should not deviate substantially between the evaluation and target population. Analytical correction is possible if the impact of biological factors on Se and Sp can be modeled.

6. Cut-Off Values

The cut off value:

- Is a test value that classifies the results as test-positive and test-negative
- Partitions the results of non-infected individuals into true-negative (TN) and false-positive (FP) results, unless the test is perfectly specific (in which case we would only observe TN results)
- Partitions the results of infected individuals into false-negatives (FN) and true-positive (TP) results, unless the test is perfectly sensitive (in which case we would only observe TP results)

As a result of biological and interfering factors, the measurement results of animals with and without the specific infection overlap. For example, assume that the ELISA PP values were normally distributed for negative and positive controls and have the mean values m_{neg} and m_{pos}, respectively (**Fig. 3**). In order to draw diagnostic conclusions, it is necessary to define a threshold value (cut-off or critical value), at which results can be differentiated into test-positive and test-negative.

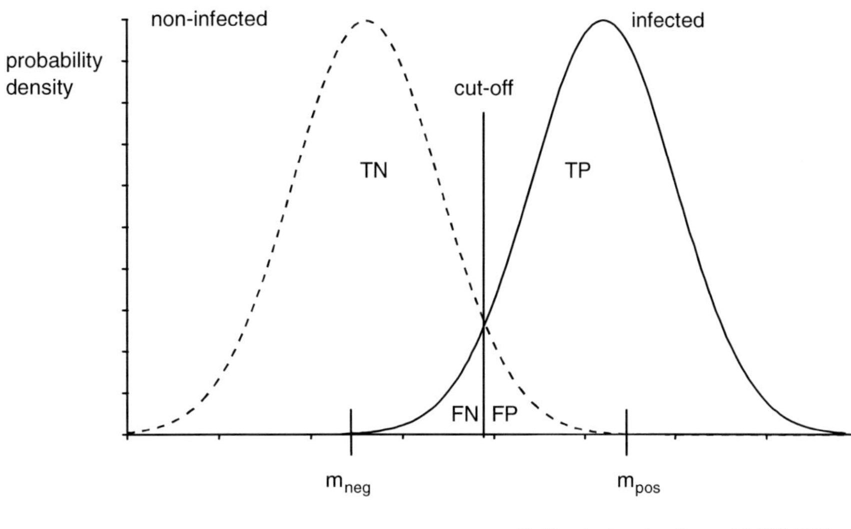

Fig. 3. Hypothetical distribution density of ELISA results of subpopulations of non-infected (*left*) and infected (right) individuals

Due to the overlapping of values, it is not possible to find any cut-off value that perfectly discriminates between infected and non-infected. As can be seen from the intersection of the curves with the cut-off, we have now subdivided our negative control population into true-negative (TN) and false-positive (FP) results. At the same time, the cut-off differentiates the positive control group into the false-negative (FN) and true-positive (TP) fractions. These so-called decision fractions are of fundamental importance for establishing sensitivity and specificity, and the cut-off is a prerequisite for diagnostic decisions.

6.1. Selection Procedures

The cut-off value is a selected threshold value used to differentiate between test values of two subpopulations with known diagnostic accuracy. Both test parameters, sensitivity and specificity, should be considered for the selection of the cut-off value.

6.1.1. The X-Bar-plus-2s and Other Arbitrary Methods

It is common practice to define the cutoff as the mean plus 2 or 3 SD of the negative control group. The rationale is that, under the assumption of a normal distribution, the mass of these negative samples (97.5%, given the fact that ~915% of normally distributed observations could be expected within a range of $\bar{x} \pm 2s$) would test negative.

If the negative control group is sampled representatively, 97.5% of non-infected individuals of the target population could also be expected to give negative test results. This approach obviously has its drawbacks. For one, normal distribution is not always realized; for another, the distribution of positive controls is completely neglected.

The most critical flaw is that it only takes into account specificity and completely disregards sensitivity. Conceptually, the x-bar-plus-2s procedure results in a reference value of the upper confidence limit of a diagnostic variable as determined by using specimens from a reference population (non-infected or non-diseased "normal"). Obviously, the reference value does not allow a complete control of test parameters, and therefore can be referred to as an arbitrary approach. Another arbitrary approach is to select a fixed test value as cut-off. Arbitrary methods in selecting cut-off values are valid if the resulting diagnostic performance is evaluated in a consecutive step. In this context, however, "arbitrary" may have a positive connotation, as it describes the possibility to select as a cut-off any value that realizes the preferred performance criterion.

Other approaches using the highest value observed or twice the mean value of the negative reference group as the cutoff value are less statistically orientated. Such approaches are valid, but the disadvantage is that they do not allow control of sensitivity and specificity. Sometimes the cut-off is not statistically well motivated, expressed in terms of the mean value plus z·s of the negative controls, with z greater than 3. In these cases, the formula is the result of the arbitrarily selected cutoff value, rather than the other way round. Keeping in mind that any value within the measurement range may be selected as the cutoff value, we know that the resulting test accuracy is the benchmark, and not the mathematical elegance of the selection procedure. More sophisticated approaches to cutoff selection are briefly discussed next.

6.1.2. Select a Low Cut-Off Value and You Get a Good Sensitivity

In certain situations, it is desirable to minimize the probability of false negative results by setting a low cut-off. Consequently, the test becomes more sensitive. Some examples are:

- Where it is extremely important not to miss any case of infection/disease and false-negative results are not acceptable; e.g., in a surveillance program
- Where false-positive results are acceptable to a certain extent because a second, more specific test is used to confirm the test result (sequential testing: screening, confirmatory test)
- Where the consequences associated with false-positive test results are not very severe. A false-negative result, however, would have a more negative impact in terms of costs and animal welfare
- Where the disease can be treated, as opposed to fatal untreated cases

6.1.3. Select a High Cut-Off Value and You Get a Good Specificity

Setting higher cutoffs increasing the test's specificity means that positive reactions are more reliable than the negative. Investigations aimed at confirmation of a clinical suspicion or the diagnosis of a fatal disease are examples of such a situation.

Examples of setting high cutoffs are:

- Where false-positive results are not acceptable, and it is extremely important not to misclassify any non-infected individuals as infected/diseased; e.g., in surveys with an emphasis on conservative estimates of seroprevalence
- Where false-negative results are acceptable to a certain extent because a second test is applied in parallel. The interpretation rule (positive if both or only one of the tests gives a positive result) will increase the overall sensitivity
- Where the consequences associated with false-negative tests results are not very severe. A false-negative result, however, would have a more negative impact in terms of costs and animal welfare
- Where the disease is severe, but its confirmation has only little impact in terms of therapeutic, preventive, and other measures

6.1.4. Selection of Cut-Off Values Using Negative and Positive Reference Sera

Three steps are essential in the classical procedure for cut-off selection:

1. Pre-selection of the parameter of interest (sensitivity or specificity).
2. Selection of a cut-off value that realizes this parameter.
3. Establishing the resulting parameter for the given cut-off value. However, it is more practical to optimize both test parameters at the same time.

The approach is straightforward if sensitivity (Se) and specificity (Sp), the prevalence in the target population (P), and the costs associated with misclassifications are known. In this case, the cut-off is chosen so that the misclassification costs term (MCT) becomes minimal. Note that costs in this context can be seen in terms of money, or medical, social, or other disadvantages associated with false test results.

$$\text{MCT} = (1 - P)(1 - \text{Sp}) + r\,P(1 - \text{Se}),$$

where r denotes the ratio of costs attributable to false negative and false positive results, respectively.

The MCT represents a summary index of accuracy, weighted for the prevalence and for misclassification costs, and is related to the test efficiency. Plotting MCT versus the selected cut-off value results in a graph from which an optimal cut-off can easily be read (**Fig. 4**). Software is available for such graphical analysis under arbitrary defined conditions regarding prevalence and misclassification costs.

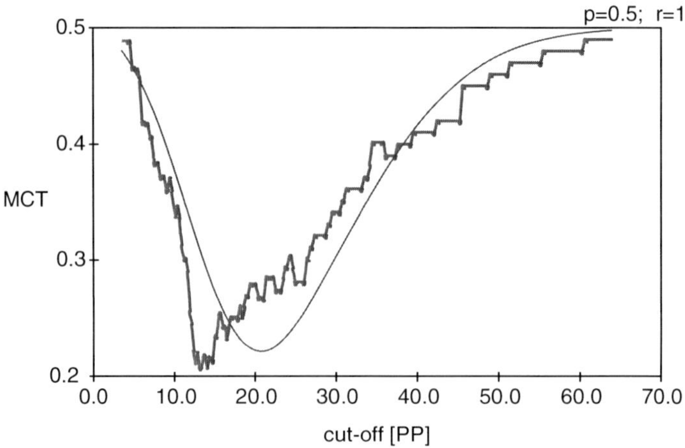

Fig. 4. Cut-off optimization using the misclassification cost term (MCT) for a *Borrelia* antibody ELISA for dogs

Cut-off values ranging from 12 to 15 PP minimize the overall misclassification cost. The two curves represent MCT values based on nonparametric (empirical graph) or parametric (function graph) estimates of sensitivity and specificity, respectively *(2)*. Optimized cut-off values can also be obtained from a receiver operating characteristic (ROC) function.

6.1.5. Intermediate Test Results

There is need for caution if a diagnostic decision is based on a test result falling very close to the cut-off value. It is common practice to refer to such results as borderline or intermediate, grey or fuzzy zones. Confirmation of the diagnosis by re-testing after a certain time interval often clarifies the matter. Standardized analytical approaches (six-cell matrix) to the utilization of non-negative, non-positive test results for test evaluation are available. Statistically, the intermediate range may be defined as the range of cut-off values that would result in a sensitivity or specificity less than a predefined level of accuracy. The intermediate range may cover a considerable proportion of the measurement range (**Fig. 5**). The proportion of the remaining range of clearly negative or positive results is referred to as a valid range proportion, and can be used as a measure of the diagnostic test performance.

The intersection point of the two graphs (sensitivity – Se and specificity – Sp) represents a cut-off at which equivalent test parameters (Se = Sp) could be achieved (based on observed proportions). Using two cut-off values (solid vertical lines) as limits of an intermediate range (IR), 90% Se and Sp could be achieved if results to the right of IR are considered negative and results to the left of IR are considered positive. Parametric estimates can be inferred from the diamonds on the horizontal line (*from* **2**).

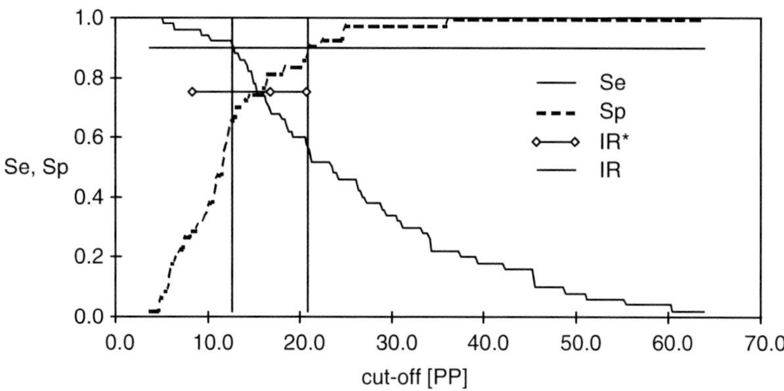

Fig. 5. Cut-off selection by "Two-Graph Receiver Operating Characteristic" (TG-ROC) for a *Borrelia* antibody ELISA for dogs.

6.1.6. Variable and Stratified Cut-Off Values

A further dimension to be considered is time, as time-dependent changes occur in the target population. The standard deviation ratio (SDR) is a method that accounts for time drifts by updating the cut-off value from run to run.

Test sera below a critical threshold of SDR are defined as negative, and their values are included in the negative reference group. Thus, the threshold value will be recalculated for every run of the test. The procedure is probably restricted to applications with only little variation in the negative group (small *SD*) and quite stable prevalences below 30%. In order to warrant a consistent diagnostic performance, SDR-based tests should be re-evaluated from time to time.

6.1.7 Intrinsic Cut-Off Values

A notorious problem of diagnostic testing in both medical and veterinary disciplines is test validation in the absence of available reference methods (gold standards). The interpretation of results from non-validated tests in a clinical or epidemiological setting remains vague and may not justify the application of expensive tests. The methods that deal with the problem of unavailability of gold standards are usually based on latent class models, and require multiple tests per subject.

In the epidemiological context, prevalence estimations based on a single test are the problem. The lack of reliable estimates of sensitivity and specificity invalidates the Bayesian approach of correcting the apparent prevalence. A new approach of prevalence estimation based on a single quantitative test by mixture-distribution analysis has been recognized in the OIE Manual of Standards for Diagnostic Tests and Vaccines *(3)*. The method involves a so-called "intrinsic cut-off" value *(4)*, which is the cut-off that differentiates the two components of bimodally-distributed test data.

7. Meta-Analysis of Diagnostic Tests (MADT)

Meta-analysis is a tool for risk assessment studies when data is derived from either multicenter studies (planned meta-analysis) or published studies. Data from individual studies are either pooled or treated as units of statistical analysis, with the objective of obtaining overall estimates for the concerned risk factors. The evidence for the diagnostic accuracy of a test is usually based on multiple primary validation studies, rather than on a single study. As multiple studies cover a wide range of conditions such as reference populations, study design, and laboratory proficiency, they possibly give more reliable test performance parameters. Planned multicenter validation studies and the systematic review of published studies are important realizations of multiple-study-based test validation, and differ in the extent to which the involved primary studies can be controlled for marginal conditions. Various methods are described for a quantitative summary of multiple validation studies, which is referred to here as meta-analysis of diagnostic tests (MADT).

7.1. The Objectives of MADT

MADT has several potential applications:

- Evaluation of the accuracy of a diagnostic test based on multiple primary validation studies (for planned multicenter studies and quantitative literature reviews)
- Investigation of the association between study characteristics and the results of the primary studies (validity)
- Investigation of the association between characteristics of the study population (or populations) and the results of the primary studies
- MADT may become increasingly important in the context of quality assurance concepts for evaluation studies.

7.2. Heterogeneity

The variability of sensitivity (Se) and specificity (Sp) between primary studies is due to:

- Host-pathogen-analyte systems
- Technical details (test principle and modification, with its inherent analytical precision and accuracy)
- Laboratory proficiency
- Study population (or populations) and sampling procedure
- Study design (e.g., blind testing)
- Weighting of Se and Sp (implicit through informed cut-off selection, or explicit through arbitrary cut-offs)

7.3. Meta-Analytic Summary 18easures of Test Accuracy

The methods to summarize accuracy measures across individual primary studies include the summary receiver operating characteristic (sROC) analysis, weighted mean values of sensitivity and specificity, relative risk, and standardized mean difference (SMD). The methods for MADT usually presuppose that each primary study contributes exactly one combination of Se and Sp to the summary estimate. Below, the two most important summary measures of accuracy are briefly described (*see* **Figs. 6** and **7**).

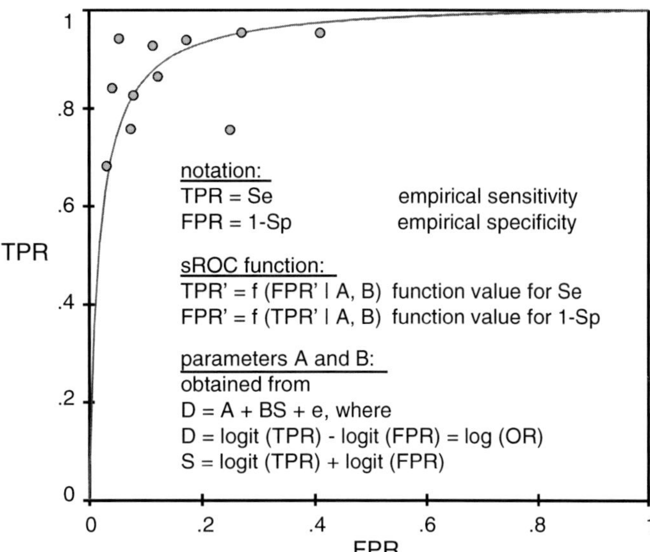

Fig. 6. Notations, formulae, and graphical representation of the sROC method for MADT, according to *(5)*.

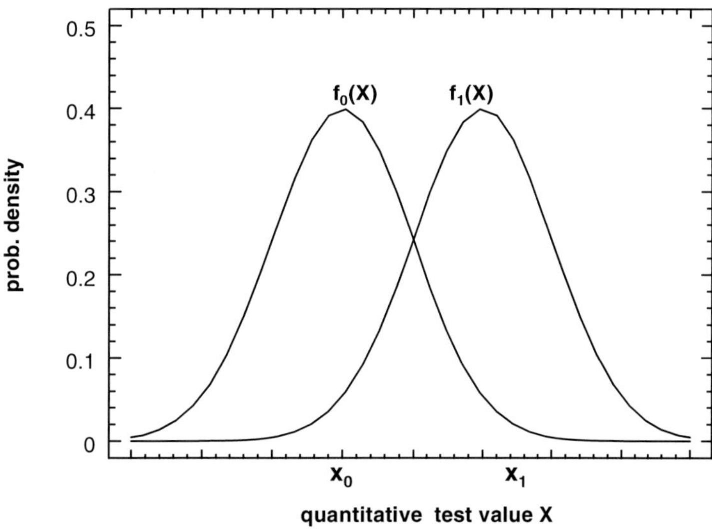

SMD = $(x_1-x_0)/s$, where s is the common standard deviation

SMD = 0.5513 (logit Se + logit Sp)
= 0.5513 log OR

The summary measure is the weighted sum of SMD accross all primary studies.

Fig. 7. Notations, formulae, and graphical representation of the SMD method for MADT, according to *(6)*.

Mixed effects logistic regression models have been described to account for multiple estimates of Se and Sp per publication, where the effects of covariates (as fixed effects) could be investigated despite lack of independence of the primary study units across the publications (Greiner et al., 1998).

8. Bayes Theorem

When an individual serum sample arrives in the laboratory for serodiagnosis, a test should only be motivated by clinical suspicion, to prevent what has been called a diagnostic cascade effect. The estimate of the likelihood of infection (or disease) is independent of the test result, and therefore referred to as prior or pre-test probability. Prevalence, risk factors, clinical history, clinical findings and symptoms, and other information (including subjective insights and beliefs, as well as previous test results) may be relevant factors involved in the pre-test probability.

After performing a test, the pre-test probability may be updated by the information of the test, and the new estimate of the probability of infection (or disease) is the posterior or post-test probability.

The algebraic basis of this approach is known as the Bayes' theorem. The objective for its application in diagnostic tests is to increase the overall information by combining clinical and test-derived evidence. The link between the patient-specific pre-test and post-test probabilities is the likelihood ratio (LR). The likelihood ratios are summary measures of sensitivity and specificity, and are often understood as test-specific values invariant to changes in the source population (which is an oversimplification).

According to the Bayesian approach, a probability (e.g., that a test-positive animal is truly infected) is conditioned on another probability (e.g., the pre-test probability). This is the fundamental principle for understanding and deriving the parameters often used in the interpretation of test results, such as the predictive values and the approximately unbiased estimator of prevalence (see below).

9. Predictive Values

It is essential to know that the predictive values are functions of the prevalence of the disease. This can be seen from the expression of the predictive values in terms of the pre-test probability, prevalence, sensitivity, and specificity (**Table 5**). As the pre-test probability of disease in individuals has a higher information level

Table 5
Expected probabilities of the four possible outcomes: true positive (TP), true negative (TN), false positive (FP) and false negative (FN) of a diagnostic test

	Diseased	Non-diseased
Test positive	Se P	(1–Sp) (1–P)
Test negative	(1–Se) P	Sp (1–P)

than the population prevalence, it can be easily seen that PVs are especially meaningful for clinical serodiagnosis.

9.1. Factors of the Pre-Test Probability

- Disease prevalence.
- Clinical symptoms.
- Likelihood of disease when anamnestic information is considered.

The integration of the pre-test probability and the test result (positive or negative) can be derived from Bayes' theorem, which can be simplified as follows.

The predictive value of a positive test result, the positive predictive value (PPV), is the probability that a positive test result is from an infected individual. This value can be estimated as the proportion of infected individuals in all individuals with a positive test result, and depends on the pre-test probability P of disease (prevalence, etc.)

$$\text{PPV} = \text{TP}/(\text{TP}+\text{FP})$$

$$\text{PPV} = (P)\text{Se}/[(P)\text{Se}+(1-P)(1-\text{Sp})]$$

The predictive value of a negative test result, the negative predictive value (NPV) is the probability that a negative test result is from a non-infected individual. This value can be estimated as the proportion of non-infected individuals in all individuals with negative test results, and depends on the pre-test probability P of disease (prevalence, etc.)

$$\text{NPV} = \text{TN}/(\text{TN}+\text{FN})$$

$$\text{NPV} = \frac{(1-P)\text{Sp}}{\left[(1-P)\text{Sp}+(P)(1-\text{Se})\right]}$$

Interpretation of the predictive values:

- PVs are prevalence-dependent measures that characterize a test result, rather than the test itself
- PVs can be used to indicate the likelihood of disease in an individual with a given test result.

- PVs can be used to estimate the proportion of FP and FN results when the test is applied to the test population
- PVs are important to understand that test results may have different meanings for different subgroups of a population
- PVs cannot be obtained by the standard 2 × 2 table when the prevalence of true positive samples is not in agreement with the actual prevalence in the target population

9.2. The Rogan-Gladen Estimator

If infection prevalence is estimated using the results of a diagnostic test, i.e., the apparent prevalence (AP) is known, we can get an approximate unbiased estimate of the true infection prevalence (P) in the form of the Rogan-Gladen estimator (P_{RG}):

$$P_{\mathrm{RG}} = (\mathrm{AP}+\mathrm{Sp}-1)/(\mathrm{Se}+\mathrm{Sp}-1)$$

This estimate provides a Bayesian estimate of infection prevalence conditional on the test sensitivity (Se) and specificity (Sp). It has been recognized that P_{RG} is left-censored for values smaller than 0 (0.0) and right-censored for values greater than 1 (1.0). Moreover, it is not defined for Se + Sp = 1.0.

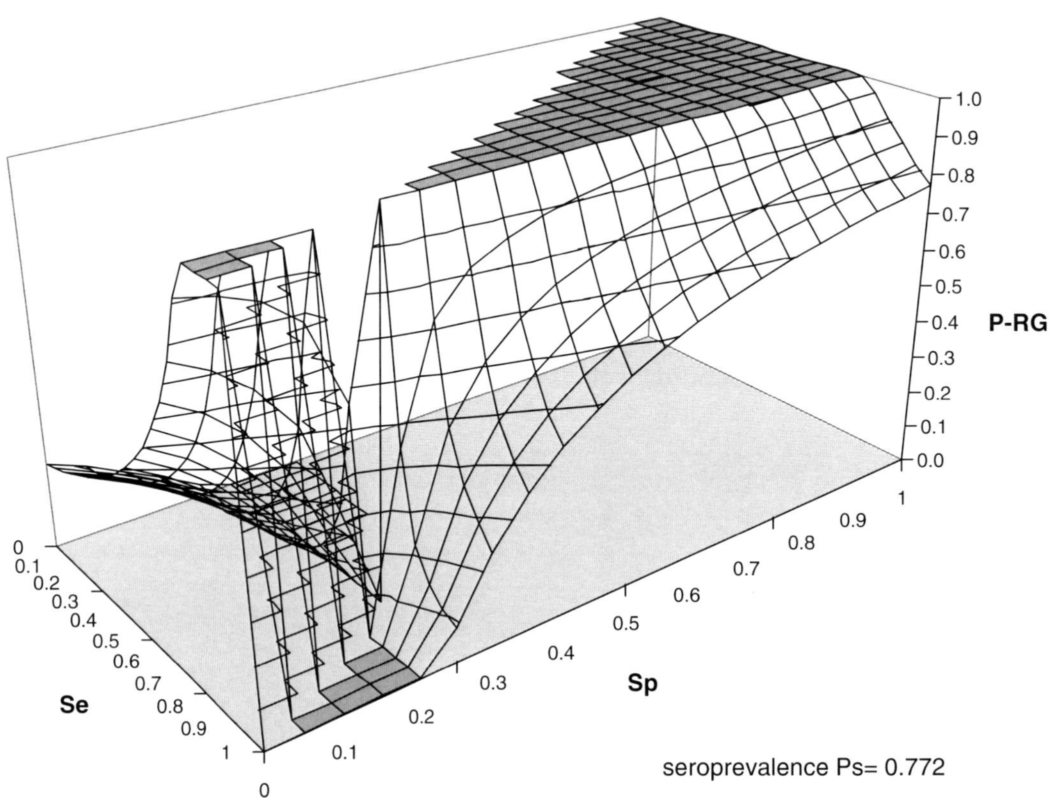

Fig. 8. The Rogan-Gladen estimator (P_{RG}) as a function of Se and Sp and with the observed value for the apparent prevalence (Ps = 77.2%).

If we plot the P_{RG} values against a range of test Se and Sp, we get a visual impression of the properties of P_{RG} (**Fig. 8**).

A drawback is the relative lack of statistical precision. The variance of P_{-RG} is larger than that of direct prevalence estimates, because it includes uncertainty about the diagnostic parameters Se and Sp.

10. Data Analysis and Hypothesis Testing

Worked examples are ideal for demonstrating principles. Sets of data with headings were used, as shown in **Table 6**, then plotted in various ways to examine the relationships of data. The actual data are not given, and the results are only shown to illustrate graphical and analytical methods. The key here is to translate the data with similar properties (e.g., "pos" or "neg", or titer or OD values) into similar exercises.

Table 6
Results using different tests and systems on 100 cattle sera

Variable name	Meaning	Categories/values	Corrections and data processing (check all data for plausibility and consistency)[a]
AnID	Animal identification no.		
Sex		"male", "female"	could be coded 0, 1
Breed		"local", "cross", exotic"	could be coded 0, 1, 2
T1	reference test	"pos", "neg"	should be coded 0, 1
T2	IFT	titers	find the base 2 log
T3.1, T3.2	ELISA (A)	OD values of two replicates[b]	find the mean value
T4	ELISA (B)	OD values	
T5	ELISA (C)	Titers	find the base 2 log
T6	ELISA (C)	OD values at dilution 1/200	
T7	Agglutination test (A)	"–", "+/–", "+", "++", "+++"	recode using 0, 1, 2, 3, 4
T8	ELISA (D)	OD values	
T9	ELISA (E)	OD values	
T10	Agglutination test (B)	0, 1, 2, 3	

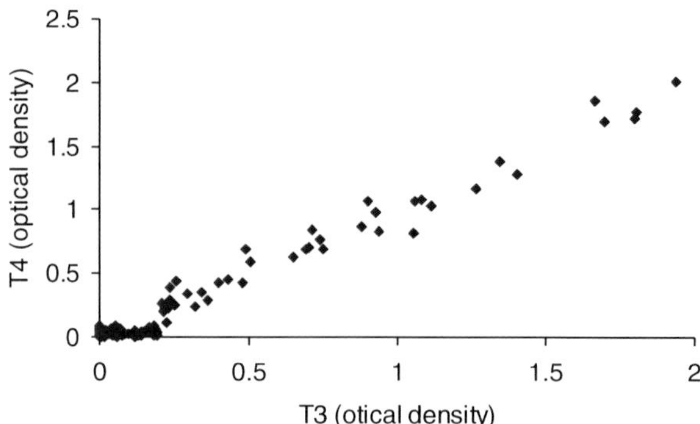

Fig. 9. Scatter plot of T4 versus T3 optical density (OD) values (n = 100 matched pairs, no missing values).

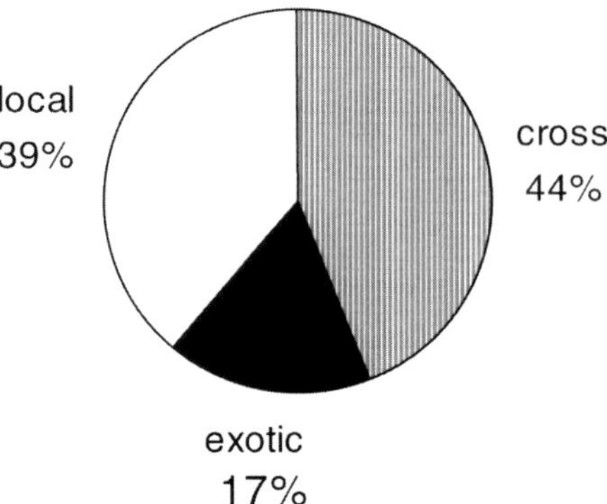

Fig. 10. Pie chart of the distribution of breeds in the sample (n = 100, no missing values).

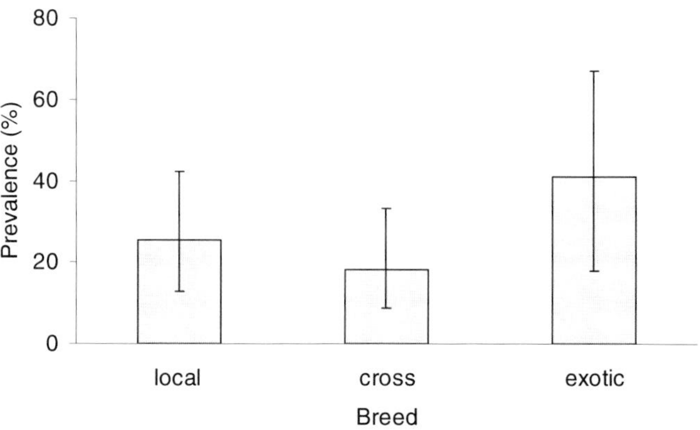

Fig. 11. Bar chart of the prevalence estimates according to T1 (with 95% binomial confidence limits) for local (n = 39), cross (n = 44), and exotic cattle (n = 17).

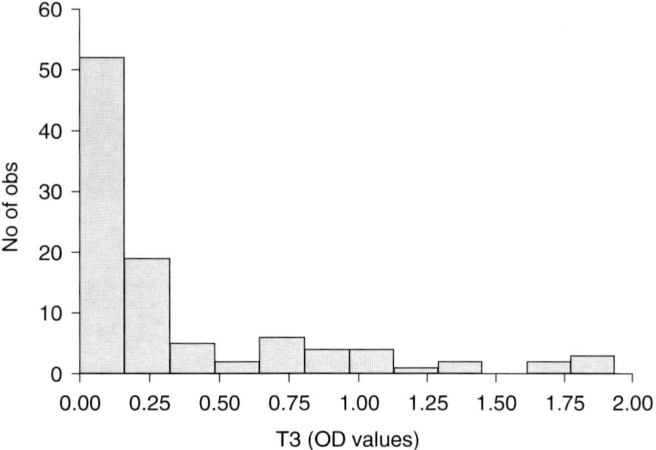

Fig. 12. Histogram of T3 optical density (OD) values ($n = 100$, no missing values).

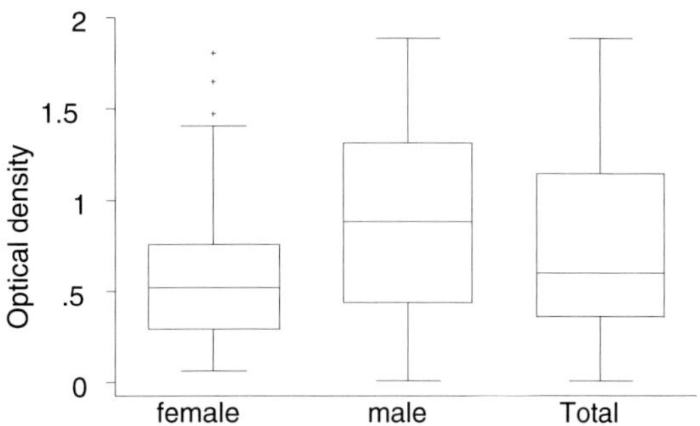

Fig. 13. Box plots of T8 data for female ($n = 51$) and male ($n = 49$) cattle. The box extends from the 25th (x_{25}) to the 75th (x_{75}) percentile (interquartile range, IR). The median value is indicated as a horizontal line. The whiskers extend to the upper and lower adjacent values, which are defined as the largest value less than or equal to $x_{75} + 1.5$ IR, and the smallest value greater than or equal to $x_{25} - 1.5$ IR, respectively. More extreme values than the adjacent values are plotted individually.

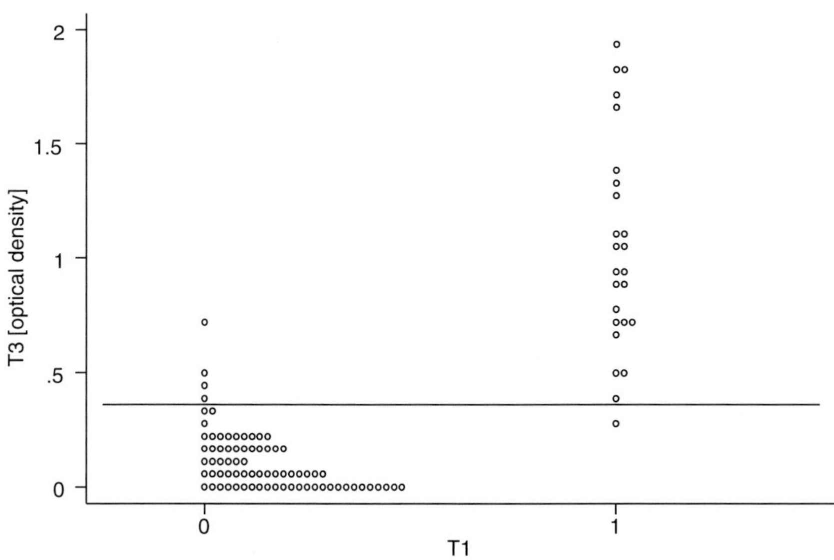

Fig. 14. Dot plot of T3 data grouped by T1 ($n = 100$, no missing values). Note that T3 is considered as the reference test. A useful cut-off value for T3 is indicated (OD = 0.36).

10.1. Graphical Methods

For graphical methods, *see* **Figs. 9–14**.

10.2 Precision Profile

Precision profiles are used for test optimization and characterization procedures (**Fig. 15**). In principle, it is a plot of a measure of variation of replicate readings (e.g., standard deviation) against the mean values, and it is especially useful for a number of replicates greater than 5.

10.3. Numerical Methods

- Establish useful statistics for the data
- Optimize cut-off values (where appropriate) for tests T2–T10, using T1 as the reference test (gold standard)
- Calculate the sensitivity, specificity, likelihood ratios, and predictive values (the latter for 1%, 50%, and 90% prevalence)
- Calculate the sensitivity and specificity with exact confidence limits for each test (T2–T10)
- Calculate the prevalence for each test (T2–T10)

10.3.1. Geometric Mean Value

A useful measure of the central tendency for titers is the *geometric mean* (GM).

Version 1 (looks simple, but may be hard to compute)

$$GM = \log_2 x = \{1,2,3,4,5,6,7,\ldots,10\}$$

Example using data:

$$GM = \sqrt[18]{64 \cdot 128 \cdot 128 \cdot 128 \cdot 128 \cdot 1024 \cdot 256 \cdot 512 \cdot 512 \cdot 256 \cdot 512 \cdot 512 \cdot 256 \cdot 1024 \cdot 64 \cdot 128 \cdot 512 \cdot 1024}$$

Version 2

$$GM = \text{antilog}_{10}\left(\frac{1}{n}\sum_{i=1}^{n}\log_{10} x_i\right)$$

Example using IFT original titers:

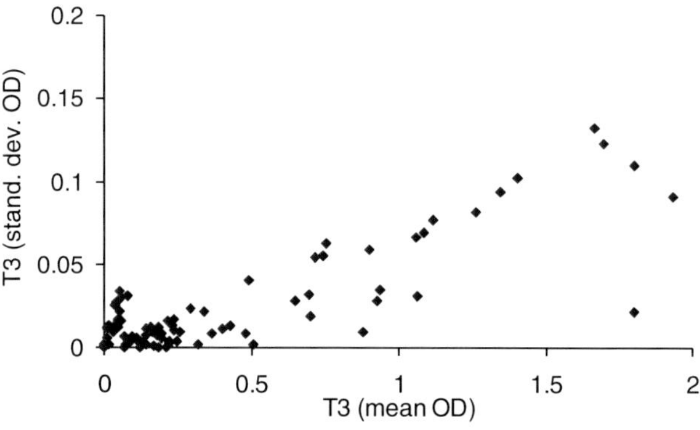

Fig. 15. Example of a precision profile for T3.1, T3.2 (twofold) replicates.

$$\begin{aligned}GM = \text{antilog}_{10}[(&1.806 + 1.806 + 2.107 + 2.107 + 2.107 \\ &+ 2.107 + 2.107 + 2.408 + 2.408 + 2.408 \\ &+ 2.709 + 2.709 + \text{antilog}_{10}[2.4414] = 10^{2.4414} \\ &= 276.4\end{aligned}$$

10.3.2. Some More Notes on Titers (Ref. 8)

1. In titration assays, the serum samples are usually diluted following a base 2 geometric series.

   The reciprocal titers can be given as, for example:

$$x = \{2, 4, 8, 16, 32, 64, 128, \text{to } 1024\}$$

   Consequently, one may argue for a transformation using the base 2 that would result in

$$\log_2 x = \{1, 2, 3, 4, 5, 6, 7, \ldots, 10\}$$

The GMT can then be expressed as GMT = antilog$_2$

$$\left(\frac{1}{n}\sum_{i=1}^{n}\log_2 x_i\right)$$

   Example using test 6 original titers:

$$GM = \text{antilog}_{10}\begin{bmatrix}(6+7+7+7+7+10+8+9+9+8+9+9+8 \\ +10+6+7+9+10/18\end{bmatrix}$$

$$= \text{antilog}_2\,[8.11] = 2^{8.11} = 276.3$$

2. Animals showing no reaction, even with undiluted sera, do not have any titer, according to $\log_2$ coding. A reciprocal titer of 1 would be coded "0" ($2^0 = 1$) and represents the smallest possible value. Consequently, $\log_2$ coded data describe only animals with observable, positive reactions.
3. Furthermore, the comparison of $\log_2$ coded data for animal groups involve two statistics: the proportion of animals with positive reactions ($\log_2$ titer 0) and the GMs.
4. The limitations (2.-4.) do not hold true for titers expressed using arbitrary ordinal scales.
5. The coded titers may occasionally be assumed as normally distributed if a reasonable range of titers has been observed (i.e., sera have been titrated to their real endpoint titers).
6. The testing of only a few titer steps results in data censoring. In this case, the distribution of titers is ordinal.

10.4. Hypothesis Generation

Questions arise, such as: "is there a difference of OD values between male and female animals, or is this difference only due to chance?" This question translated into statistical language reads:

The null hypothesis (no difference) is tested against the alternative hypothesis (there is a difference), using an appropriate statistical test.

10.4.1. Hypothesis Testing - Comparison of Prevalences Between Groups

The translation of human language questions into statistical hypotheses and the selection of an "appropriate test" is the domain of the statistician.

Example: analysis of T1 data for an effect of sex and breed (**Tables 7–14**).

- Establish the prevalence (based on T1) for the gender and breed groups
- Is there a significant impact of sex and breed on the prevalence?

Table 7
Data on sex and breed related to results

Sex	T1	0	1	Total
Female		3 7	14	51
Male		38	11	49
Total		75	25	100

The prevalence is 27.4% (15.9–21.7% exact binomial confidence interval, CI) and 22.4% (11.8–36.6% CI) for female and male cattle, respectively. The difference is not significant (chi-square; df = 1; $p = 0.56$)

Table 8
Data on sex and breed related to results

Breed	T1	0	1	Total
Local		29	10	39
Cross		36	8	44
Exotic		10	7	17
Total		75	25	100

The prevalence is 25.6% (13.0–42.1% CI), 18.2% (8.7–33.2% CI) and 41% (18–67% CI) for local, cross, and exotic cattle, respectively. The difference is not significant (chi-square; df = 2; $p = 0.17$). More appropriate methods (e.g., logistic regression) exist that account for possible interactions between the variables

Table 9
Data on sex and breed related to results *(1)*

Equality of populations (Kruskal-Wallis Test)

Breed	Observed	Rank sum
Local	39	1919.00
Cross	44	2135.50
Exotic	17	995.50

The null hypothesis that all three groups are from the same population of titers (no difference between the breeds) cannot be rejected (chi-square = 1.59, df = 2, $p = 0.45$). There is no significant difference between the groups

Table 10
Data on sex and breed related to results *(2)*

T2

Breed	0	1	2	3	4	5	6	7	Total
Local	5	16	11	4	1	0	1	1	39
Cross	3	13	5	9	1	2	6	5	44
Exotic	2	3	2	0	0	1	4	5	17
Total	10	32	18	13	2	3	11	11	100

The null hypothesis of an equal distribution of titers between the three groups (homogeneity) can be rejected (chi-square = 26.4, df = 14, $p = 0.023$). The titers of the three breeds are not from the same distribution. Note that the procedure (1) has less statistical power than (2)

Table 11
Data on sex and breed related to results *(3)*

Breed	**0**	**1**	**Total**
0	37	2	39
1	31	13	44
2	7	10	17
Total	75	25	100

Pearson chi2(2) = 19.0711 Pr = 0.000. T2r (T2 recoded; 0 = negative, 1 = positive, using the cut-off 4.5)

Table 12
One-way analysis of variance *(1)*

	One-way analysis of variance		
Sex	**Mean**	**Std. dev**	**Freq.**
Female	0.61962353	0.42453208	51
Male	0.90076531	0.51277515	49
Total	0.757383	0.48832472	100

Table 13
Analysis of variance *(1)*

	Analysis of variance				
Source	**SS**	**df**	**MS**	**F**	**Prob > F**
Between groups	1.97522705	1	1.97522705	8.95	0.0035
Within groups	21.6324154	8	0.220738933		
Total	23.6076425	9	0.238461035		

Table 14
Comparison of populations *(2)*

Sex	**Obs**	**Ranksum**
Female	51	2,175.00
Male	49	2,875.00

10.4.2. Comparison of Titers Between Groups

Different options exist, including:

1. The comparison of the mean values of log-transformed titers using nonparametric statistics
2. The comparison of observed frequencies of titers using the chi-square test. Example: analysis of T2 data for an effect of the breed (**Table 9**)

Is the result of (2) important? To answer this question, we would compare the prevalences between the groups (**Table 11**).

The null hypothesis of equal T2 prevalences of the three breeds can be rejected (chi-square = 19.1, df = 2 p < .05).

The point estimates (and 95% binomial confidence limits) of the local, cross, and exotics were 2/39 = 0.051 (0.06 0.173), 13/44 = 0.295 (0.167 – 0.452), and 10/17 = 0.588 (0.329 – 0.815), respectively. The confidence intervals are partially non-overlapping (local versus exotics). Thus, the results of the chi-square test (under the null hypothesis of no difference) confirm the evidence from non-overlapping confidence intervals (under the alternative hypothesis of differences). These results are consistent with (2).

We conclude that there is a difference between the outcomes of T2 between the breeds. It appears that the nonparametric Kruskal-Wallis test (1) did not have sufficient power to detect the difference.

10.4.3. Comparison of Mean Values (cContinuous Data) Between Groups

Various options exist, including: (1) parametric and (2) nonparametric tests.

1. Example: analysis of T8 data for an effect of the sex (**Tables 12** and **13**). The null hypothesis of equal mean T8 (ELISA D) values between male and female cattle can be rejected (ANOVA, $p < .05$). There is a significant difference between the groups.
2. Equality of populations (Kruskal-Wallis test) (**Table 14**). The null hypothesis of equal mean T8 (ELISA D) values between male and female cattle can be rejected (ANOVA, $p < .05$). There is a significant difference between the groups.

10.5. Basic Principles and Features of ROC Plots

The underlying assumption of ROC analysis is that a diagnostic variable (e.g., degree of suspicion, measurement value) is to be used as a discriminator of two defined groups of responses (e.g., test values from diseased/non-diseased or infected/non-infected individuals).

ROC analysis assesses the diagnostic performance of the system in terms of sensitivity (Se) and 1 minus specificity (1 – Sp) for each observed value of the discriminator variable assumed as the decision threshold (cut-off value to differentiate between the two groups of responses). For tests that yield continuous results, such as ELISA, the cut-off value is shifted systematically over the range of observed values, and Se and 1 – Sp are established for each of these, say, k different operating points. The resulting k pairs {(1 – Sp), Se} are then displayed as the ROC plot. The connection of the points leads to a staircase trace that originates from the upper right corner and ends at the lower left corner of the unit square. The interesting feature of this plot is that it characterizes the given test by the trace in the unit square, irrespective of the original unit and range of the measurement. ROC plots can therefore be used as a universal tool for test comparison, even when the tests are quite different in their cut-off values and in their units and ranges of measurement. ROC traces for diagnostic tests with perfect discrimination between negative and positive reference samples (no overlapping of values of the two groups) pass through the co-ordinates {0;1}, which is equivalent to Se = Sp = 100%. Consequently, the area under such ROC plots (area under curve, AUC) would be 1.0. As indicated earlier, the probabilities (1 – Sp) and Se are estimated by the respective proportions of the false positive and true positive fractions. The most important statistical feature of the ROC plot is the area under the curve (AUC).

10.5.1. Plotting ROC Curves in Practice

ROC plots can be generated using simple spreadsheet programs such as EXCEL, using the steps described below:

1. Generate a grid of possible cut-off values. For discrete test data, each observed value is one grid point. For continuous data, the range is divided into, say, 100 intervals. The interval limits are the grid
2. For each grid point assumed as the cutoff value, establish sensitivity (Se) and 1 minus specificity (1 – Sp)
3. Plot Se against (1 – Sp) for all grid points

The ROC plots presented below were constructed using the MedCalc program (MedCalc Software, Belgium). ROC analysis is also featured by commercial statistical program packages (SAS, Stata, Simstat, Testimate, AccuROC, GraphROC, and S-PLUS), sometimes in the form of user-defined macros. Shareware and public domain software exists, too (CLABROCW, LABROC1, LABMRMC, PEPI, AUROC, ROCNPAR, ROCWIN, TG-ROC, ROC-&-ROL). The program CMDT, which offers ROC analysis along with other statistical tools in the diagnostic test context, is available from the web site listed in the References.

Example: Estimation of the AUC for T3 using T1 as a reference test:

$$A = (1.04 - 0.11)/0.47 = 1.97$$

$$B = 0.13/0.47 = 0.276$$

$$R = 2{,}864;\ \mathrm{U} = 2{,}575 + 75(75+1)/2 - R = 1{,}861$$

$$\mathrm{AUC}_1 = 1{,}861/1{,}875 = 0.9925$$

$$\mathrm{AUC}_2 = \phi\left[1.97 / \left(1 + 0.13^2\right)^{0.5}\right] = \phi[1.953] = 0.9745$$

Thus, the nonparametric and parametric estimates of the area under the ROC curve for T3 data are 0.9925 and 0.9745, respectively.

10.5.2. The Area under the ROC Curve (AUC)

The theoretical exponential function that underlies the empirical ROC plot can be estimated under the assumption of normally distributed values for the two groups of responses *(binomial distribution assumption)*. The ROC function is then characterized by the parameter *A*, which is the standardized mean difference of the responses of the two groups, and the parameter *B*, which is the ratio of the standard deviations. *A* and *B* are also referred to as the separation parameter and the symmetry parameter, respectively (Metz, 1978). For example, consider a set of test data for a negative and a positive reference group with the mean values $\bar{x}_0$ and $\bar{x}_1$, where $\bar{x}_0 < \bar{x}_1$, and with the standard deviations $\bar{x}_1$ and s_1, respectively.

$$\mathrm{A} = \bar{x}_1 - \bar{x}_0 / s_1$$

$$\mathrm{B} = \mathrm{s}_0 - \mathrm{s}_1$$

The area under the ROC curve (AUC) can be estimated with and without assumptions concerning the distribution of test results. The nonparametric approach is based on the fact that the AUC is related to the test statistic U of the Mann-Whitney rank sum test (Hanley and McNeil, 1982).

$$\mathrm{AUC}_1 = U/n_1 n_0 \qquad (12.1)$$

with $U = n_1 n_0 + n_0(n_0 + 1)/2 - R$

and R = rank sum of the negative sample.

Alternately, the parametric approach considers the parameters *A* and *B*, as indicated above, and the term Φ (z)/], which is the cumulative frequency distribution function of the standard normal distribution (Obuchowski, 1994)

$$AUC_2 = \Phi[A/(1+B^2)^{0.5}] \qquad (12.2)$$

From **Eq. 12.2**, we can see that AUC = 0.5 if A = 0. Equal mean values of the negative and positive reference population indicate a non-informative diagnostic test. In this situation, A = 0 and AUC = 0.5 applies. Theoretically, AUC < 0.5 if A is negative. In practice, such situations are not encountered or, respectively, the decision rule is converted to obtain positive values for *A*. The binomial assumption may not be justified for a given set of test data. Therefore, alternative methods were developed, based on maximum likelihood estimates of the ROC function and the AUC (Dorfmann and Alf, 1969). It has been pointed out by Zweig (1993) that study design effects, and specifically the representativeness of the reference populations, should also be considered for ROC analysis. The interested reader is referred to Greiner et al. (2000) for further details regarding ROC analysis.

If a ROC plot is constructed using a single cut-off value, the trapezoidal AUC is (Se + Sp)/2.

10.5.3. Optimization of Cut-Off Values Using ROC Curves

Geometrically, the point of the ROC plot with the greatest distance in a northwesterly direction from the diagonal line (Se = 1 – Sp) represents the optimal pair of sensitivity and specificity that can be achieved with the test. Smith (1991) points out that the optimal cut-off value is a function of the true prevalence (p), the costs of false positive (CFP), and costs of false negative (CFN) test results. His recommendation is to select a cut-off value at which the slope of the ROC curve equals [(1 – p) CFP]/[p CFN].

10.6. Plotting ROC Curves in Practice

ROC plots can be generated using simple spreadsheet programs such as EXCEL, by following steps 1–3:

1. Generate a grid of possible cut-off values. For discrete test data, each observed value is one grid point. For continuous data, the range is divided into, say, 100 intervals. The interval limits form the grid
2. For each grid point assumed as a cut-off value, establish sensitivity (Se) and 1 minus specificity (1 – Sp)
3. Plot Se against (1 – Sp) for all grid points

ROC plots presented below were constructed using the MedCalc program (MedCalc Software, Belgium). ROC analysis is also featured by commercial statistical program packages (SAS, Stata, Simstat, Testimate, AccuROC, GraphROC, S-PLUS) – sometimes in the form of user-defined macros. Shareware and public domain software exists, too (CLABROCW, LABROC1, LABMRMC, PEPI, AUROC, ROCNPAR, ROCWIN, TG-ROC, ROC-&-ROL). The program CMDT, which offers ROC analysis along with other statistical tools in the diagnostic test context, is available from the web site listed in the References.

Example: Estimation of the AUC for T3 using T1 as a reference test.

$$A = (1.04 - 0.11)/0.47 = 1.97$$

$$B = 0.13/0.47 = 0.276$$

$$R = 2{,}864;\ \mathrm{U} = 25\ 75 + 75(75{+}1)/2 - R = 1{,}861$$

$$\mathrm{AUC}_1 = 1{,}861/1{,}875 = 0.9925$$

$$\mathrm{AUC}_2 = \phi\left[1.97 / \left(1 + 0.13^2\right)^{0.5}\right] = \phi[1.953] = 0.9745$$

Thus, the nonparametric and parametric estimates of the area under the ROC curve for T3 data are 0.9925 and 0.9745, respectively (**Fig. 16**). For T7 and T10 data, *see* **Fig. 17**.

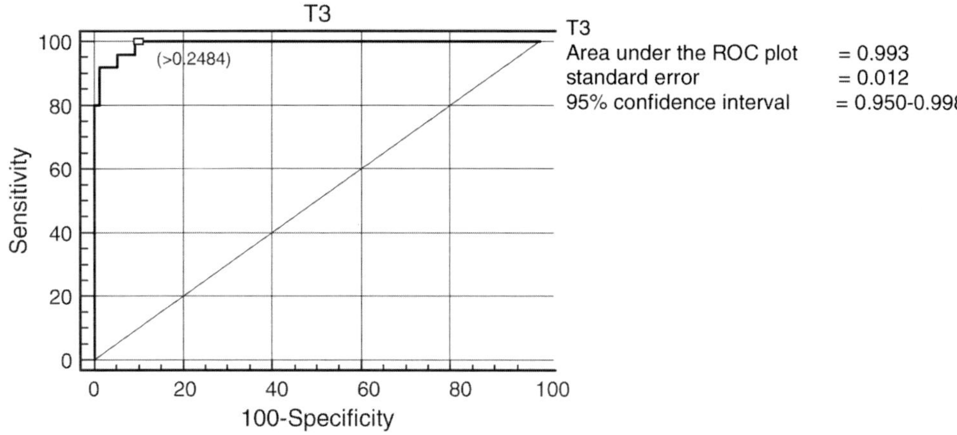

Fig. 16. ROC plot for T3 data (T1 assumed as the reference test, $n = 100$).

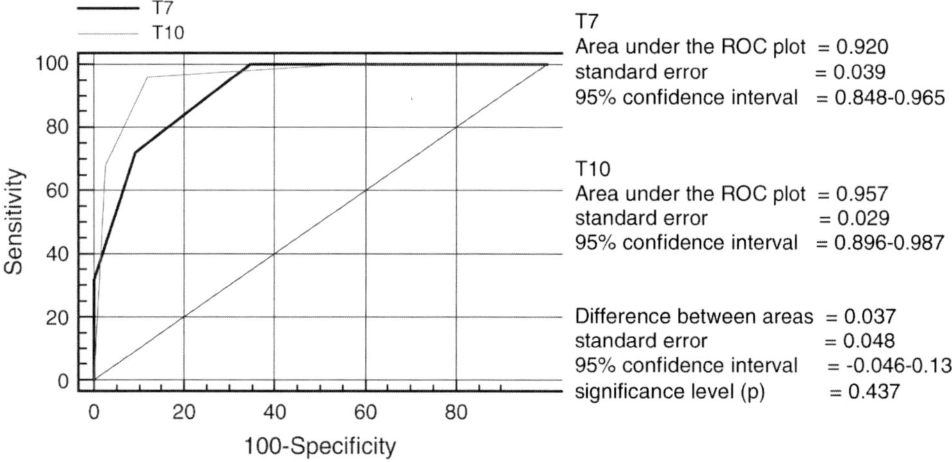

Fig. 17. ROC plots for T7 and T10 data (T1 assumed as the reference test, $n = 100$).The difference between the areas under the two ROC curves is not significant ($p = .437$).

11. Test Comparison

In diagnosis, the types of questions are exemplified by analysis of the following data.

Results of 6 diagnostic tests (A–E) for 5 animals are given below:

$$A = \{0.42, 0.87, 1.21, 0.00, 2.26\}$$

$$B = \{1, 1, 1, 0, 1\}$$

$$C = \{+, +, -, \ -, +, +, \}$$

$$D = \{64, 128, 1024, 32, 2048\}$$

$$E = \{\mathrm{N, N, P, N, P}\}$$ \right\}

$$F = \{15.3, 25.0, 47.9, 5.8, 88.2\}$$

How do we compare such results?

11.1. Complications

The comparison of two or more diagnostic tests is not a trivial matter. The choice of a statistical method depends on the nature of the test result. At least nine situations can be distinguished (**Fig. 18).** A flow chart of nine possible situations of a comparison of diagnostic tests (boxes) is shown. The horizontal dotted lines indicate the possibility of using a test on a lower scale (to the right) for comparison if the scale type is changed accordingly.

We may compare different tests even in the absence of the gold standard. Test comparison usually addresses one of the following questions:

1. Is there an agreement between the results of methods A and B?
2. Is there a correlation between the results of method A and method B? Or, more practically, is it possible to predict the result of one method by the results of the other? If yes, which factors may be used for the prediction?

The drawback of test comparison is that with respect to *(1)*, the null hypothesis of no agreement is often not satisfactory; with respect to *(2)*, no standards exist that allow us to judge the minimum correlation required before attempting to replace one method by another one. The separate analysis of correlation for diseased and non-diseased animals is useful to assess the conditional dependence between two tests (Gardner et al., 2000).

Examples of two diagnostic tests are provided below.

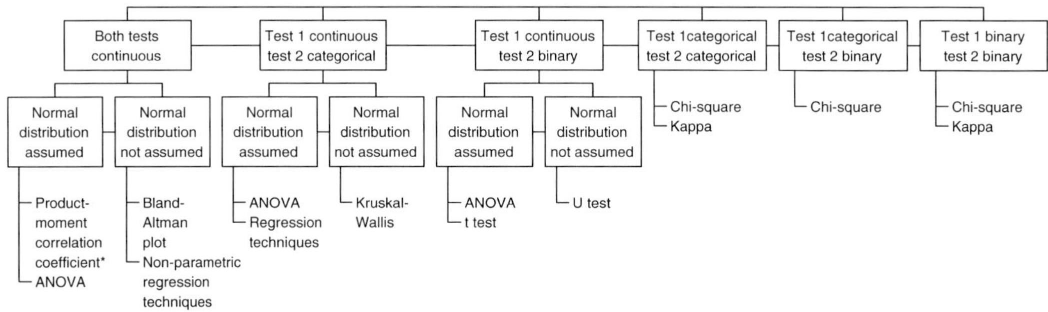

Fig. 18. Flow chart of nine possible situations of comparison of diagnostic tests *(boxes)*. The *horizontal dotted lines* indicate the possibility of using a test on a lower scale (to the *right*) for comparison if the scale type is changed accordingly.

11.1.1 Two Continuous Tests

A comparison of T6 and T8 by ANOVA requires:

(a) Pooling results of both tests (new variable "T68" with $n = 200$)

(b) Defining a variable that indicates the matched pairs (new variable "replicate"; range is from 1–100). An ANOVA of "T68" for the grouping variable "replicate" yields **Table 15**.

Thus, there is no statistical agreement between the T6 and T8 data (ANOVA, $p = .783$). The null hypothesis of equal variances could not be rejected (Bartlett's chi-square = 107; df = 99; $p = .27$).

The plot of the differences between individual samples measured by two methods against their mean value investigates the variance across the level of the analyte.

Confidence limits for the deviation (mean plus/minus 1.96-fold the standard deviation of the differences) can be constructed (**Fig. 19**). This graphical method is recommended, as there is no violation of any statistical assumption. *(8)*.

Table15
Analysis of variance between groups

Analysis of variance

Source	SS	f	MS	F	Prob > F
Between groups	25.3338927	9	0.255897906	0.85	0.7833
Within groups	29.9592711	00	0.299592711		
Total	55.2931638	99	0.277855094		

Bartlett's test for equal variances: chi2(99) = 107.0468 Prob>chi2 = 0.27

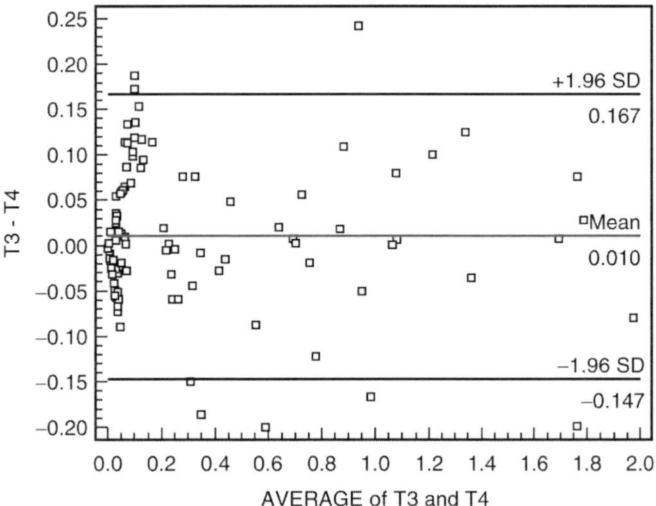

Fig. 19. Bland-Altman plot for comparison of T3 and T4 results ($n = 100$).

11.1.2. Two Categorical (or Binary) Tests

The kappa test is applicable to squared matrices comparing an equal number of categories for each test, often used for the comparison of two binary tests. However, situations with more categories are possible. The kappa index indicates the level of agreement beyond chance between two tests. A kappa index of null indicates that the observed agreement can be explained just by chance. Refer to Thrusfield *(9)* for more details.

12. Diagnosis at the Herd Level

Serological tests are applied to a sample of the animals from an infected herd. Questions arise as to the factors involved in the probability that the herd is correctly diagnosed as infected.

12.1. Background

Logistical and budgetary constraints limit the scope of surveys, and some kind of cluster sampling is usually done where animals are drawn at random from the primary sampling units (such as herds, flocks, litters). Typical objectives of the sampling and testing include:

1. Estimation of the proportion of infected herds (herds are the units of concern).
2. Estimation of the within-herd level of prevalence (e.g., for herd certification).
3. Estimation of the prevalence of infection on animal-level across herds (involves cluster sampling).

No standard sampling design accommodates these different objectives.

Subheading 12.1.1. concentrates on the first objective, where, in addition to the misclassification problem of the diagnostic test (sensitivity Se < 1; specificity Sp < 1), there is an additional uncertainty due to sampling error. Some threshold value (c) is require65, that denotes the maximum number of test-positive cases that are accepted for the diagnosis of non-infection at the herd-level. The value for c may be null. In this situation, a single test-positive animal would result in a classification of the herd as infected. $c = 0$ is not very useful, unless the serological test is very specific. We are interested in the herd-level sensitivity and specificity, and assume that we don't have any better information about the true number of infected animals in the herd than the population prevalence (p). If the number of infected animals per herd was exactly known, the derivations below should be based on the hypergeometric rather than on the binomial distribution.

12.1.1. Herd-level Sensitivity and Specificity

Initially, we forget the herds and recall the probability of a positive test result, which we denoted as apparent prevalence (AP) and is given as:

$$\Pr(\mathrm{T}+) = p\,\mathrm{Se} + (1-p)(1-\mathrm{Sp})\text{which we denote as AP.}$$

If none of the animals in the sample is infected (p = 0), the probability of a (false-) positive result is AP = 1– Sp.

If all animals in the sample are infected (p = 1), the probability of a (true-) positive result is AP = Se.

Assuming independence of observations, we conclude that the probability of finding exactly c positive test results out of a sample of size n is just (the binomial density):

$$\Pr(x = c \mid \mathrm{n}, \mathrm{AP}) = \binom{n}{x} \mathrm{AP}^{c} (1-\mathrm{AP})^{n-c}.$$

The probability of finding up to c positive cases (i.e., x = 0, 1,…, c) is given by the cumulative binomial distribution function:

$$\Pr(x \le c \mid n, \mathrm{AP}) = \sum_{x=0}^{x=c} \binom{n}{c} \mathrm{AP}^{x} (1-\mathrm{AP})^{n-x}.$$

We assume that some animals of the herd are truly infected (p > 0). The herd-level sensitivity (HSe) is the probability of finding more than c animals that test positive, and is given as:

$$\mathrm{HSe} = 1 - \Pr(x \le c \mid n, \mathrm{AP})$$

The same applies to negative test results; the probability of a negative test result is given as:

$$\Pr(\mathrm{T}-) = p(1-\mathrm{Se}) + (1-p)\text{which we denote as } (1-\mathrm{AP}).$$

If none of the animals in the sample is infected (p = 0), the probability of a (true-) negative result is (1 – AP) = Sp.

If all animals in the sample are infected (p = 1) the probability of a (false-) negative result is (1 – AP) = 1 – Se. Assuming independence of observations, we conclude that the probability of finding exactly d negative test results out of a sample of size n is just (the binomial density):

$$\Pr(x = d \mid n, 1-\mathrm{AP}) = \binom{n}{d} (1-\mathrm{AP})^{d} \mathrm{AP}^{n-d}.$$

The probability of finding up to d negative cases (i.e., $x = 0, 1, \ldots, d$) is given by the cumulative binomial distribution function:

$$\Pr\left(x \le d \mid n, 1 - \mathrm{AP}\right) = \sum_{x=0}^{x=d} \binom{n}{x} (1 - \mathrm{AP})^x \, \mathrm{AP}^{n-x}.$$

We assume that no animal of the herd is truly infected ($p = 0$; $(1 - \mathrm{AP}) = \mathrm{Sp}$). The herd-level specificity (HSp) is the probability of finding less than or equal to c animals test positive (or, we could also say, d or more animals test negative; $d = n - c$) and is given as:

$$\mathrm{HSp} = 1 - \Pr\left(x \le d - 1 \mid n,\ 1 - \mathrm{AP}\right)$$

13. Quantitative Risk Analysis (QRA)

This is very important, as it tries to assess the impact of diagnostic results. The type of questions raised can be best illustrated with an example.

Ten horses are to be shipped from Europe to the US. A complement fixation test for *Babesia* antibodies gave negative results for all the horses. What kind of information is needed to estimate the risk of importing at least one animal with equine babesiosis, despite the negative test results? The relevant information may be uncertain (not precisely known). How can we deal with the uncertainty? Imagine you were responsible for risk assessment from the importation point of view. Which of the diagnostic parameters (sensitivity or specificity) would be more of a concern for you?

13.1. Background

Decision making is frequently concerned with an assessment of the risk of unfavorable situations. "Unfavorable" means that the situations may cause costs, harm, and social or economic disadvantages. Official organizations such as the World Trade Organization (WTO) and Office International des Epizooties (OIE) encourage national authorities to use standardized methods and measures for a quantitative risk assessment (QRA). A systematic approach to a quantitative risk assessment includes hazard identification, hazard characterization, exposure assessment, and risk characterization *(10)*. In **Subheading 13.1.1**, one typical scenario of QRA, where serodiagnostic tests are involved, is examined.

An important feature of QRA methods is that calculation of "point estimates" is not completely satisfactory. The likelihood of having at least one infected horse in the group of ten animals despite negative test results depends on various factors, such as disease prevalence in the country of origin, sensitivity, and specificity of tests. These factors may not be known precisely and, in practice, some expert opinions are needed about the minimum, most likely, and maximum value of the involved factors. Thus, the outcome of interest is a distribution of possible values rather than a single value.

13.1.1. Scenario

A country free of equine babesiosis wants to import horses from an endemically infected (with low prevalence) country. Importation would depend on the results of a prescribed test (complement fixation) for babesiosis. One or more seropositive animals would render the whole group ineligible for importation (rejection).

1. The first objective is to estimate the risk of importing one or more Babesia-infected horses in a shipment of ten animals, should all animals be seronegative.
2. We are also interested to know the probability that all animals are uninfected, although we have one animal (or two or three animals) with positive test results in the shipment.

13.1.2. Selection of a Model for QRA

It is reasonable to assume that the sensitivity (Se) and specificity (Sp) of the diagnostic test and the prevalence of babesiosis in the country of origin (p) are involved in our model. We further assume that the horses were not selected for export based on their babesiosis status, and that no better information on the number of infected animals in the shipment is available than that given by p.

Thus, we assume equal prevalence in the country of origin and in the shipment. Furthermore, we assume that the shipment will be rejected if at least one test-positive animal is found. The number of positive test results allowed for maintaining the declaration of the lot as free from infection is c = 0.

13.1.3. Risk of Disease Introduction

Here we are concerned with false-negative test results.

The probability of infection (D+) in one horse with a negative test result (T–) can be written as:

$$\Pr(\mathrm{D+}|\mathrm{T-})$$

Note that this probability is related to the negative predictive value (NPV = Pr (D– | T–)):

$$\Pr(\mathrm{D+} \mid \mathrm{T-}) = 1 - \Pr(\mathrm{D-} \mid \mathrm{T-}) = 1 - \mathrm{NPV},$$
$$\text{where NPV} = (1-p)\mathrm{Sp} \,/\, \left((1-p)\mathrm{Sp} + p(1-\mathrm{Se})\right)$$

The probability of having $x = 0, 1, 2, \ldots, 10$ horses with false-negative test results in the shipment of size $n = 10$ is given by the binomial distribution:

$$\Pr\left(x \mid \mathrm{n}, 1-\mathrm{NPV}\right)=\binom{n}{x}\left(1-\mathrm{NPV}\right)^{x}\mathrm{NPV}^{n-x}. \tag{3}$$

The only "favorable" outcome is to have no false-negative results in the sample ($x = 0$). In this case **Eq. 3** can be simplified:

$$\Pr(0|10, 1\text{–NPV}) = \mathrm{NPV}^{10}$$

This is the probability of having no false-negative results in a sample of $n = 10$. Therefore, the probability of having at least one false-negative horse (probability of introduction of the disease) is just:

$$\Pr(\text{introduction}) = 1-\mathrm{NPV}^{n} \tag{4}$$

13.1.4 Risk of Unnecessary Rejection

Here we are concerned with false-positive test results. The probability of no infection (D–) in one horse with a positive test result (T+) can be written as:

$$\Pr(\mathrm{D}-|\mathrm{T}+).$$

Note that this probability is related to the positive predictive value (PPV = Pr (D+ | T+)):

$$\Pr(\mathrm{D}-|\mathrm{T}+) = 1 - \Pr(\mathrm{D}+|\mathrm{T}+) = 1\text{–PPV},$$

$$\text{Where PPV} = p\,\mathrm{Se}/(p\,\mathrm{Se}+(1-p)(1-\mathrm{Sp})).$$

We again use binomial distribution to find the expected probability of observing x false-positive cases out of m positive test results (note that x now has a different meaning than above):

$$\Pr\left(x \mid m, 1-\mathrm{PPV}\right)=\binom{m}{x}\left(1-\mathrm{PPV}\right)^{x}\mathrm{PPV}^{m-x}.$$

Economic losses occur if all m test-positive animals are false-positive. The probability of having x = m horses with false-positive test results out of m horses with positive test results is given as:

$$\Pr\left(\text{false rejection}\right)=\Pr\left(x=m \mid m, 1-\mathrm{PPV}\right)=\left(1-\mathrm{PPV}\right)^{m}. \tag{5}$$

Eq. 5 is only defined if there is at least 1 positive test result (m 1). That should be clear. Where we do not have any positive test result, there is no risk of having false-positive test results.

Table 16
Risk assessment of disease introduction through importation of live animals. Hypothetical range of possible values for variables involved in the models

Input variable	Minimum value	Most likely value	Maximum value
Se	0.60	0.85	0.99
Sp	0.90	0.95	0.999
p	0.0001	0.02	0.20

13.1.5. Input of Information

For all models, the rule "rubbish in-rubbish out" applies. Misspecification of the model may occur if the real scenario is not appropriately translated into a schematic pathway. Another problem is uncertainty of values to be used for the computation. We may get estimates of the involved parameters from different sources (own study, published information, consultation with experts, meta-analysis) but precise information may not be available, so usually a range of possible values are used in the model (or models), rather than point estimates. **Table 16** shows possible values for the variables involved in our models.

The values are inserted into the models (**Eqs. 4** and **5**) in the form of random numbers drawn from triangular distributions, with parameters (minimum, most likely and maximum value), as indicated in **Table 16**.

In practice, a computer program can be used for automatic re-calculations. This approach is referred to as a Monte-Carlo simulation, and the generation of one set of random numbers is called iteration. A correlation between variables can be considered. A high number of iterations, say 10,000, would generate 10,000 random numbers from the specified sampling distributions and produce 10,000 values for the outcome variable. The distribution of the latter can be used to interpret the risk for all plausible combinations of input variables.

13.1.6. Output of the Model-Risk of Disease Introduction

The point estimate of the probability of having at least one horse with a false-negative test result in the group of 10 horses (based on the most-likely values of **Table 9**) is $1 - [0.9968]^{10} = 0.032$. This means that the risk of introducing a carrier animal of equine babesiosis is 3.2%. The range of possible values for this risk uncertainty of the involved parameters is indicated in Table 16. A simulation study is conducted with 10,000 iterations, and the outcome-variable- risk of disease introduction is shown in the form of a frequency distribution histogram (**Fig. 20**), where the large majority of possible outcome values are below 0.5, leading to the conclusion that the risk of disease introduction is essentially

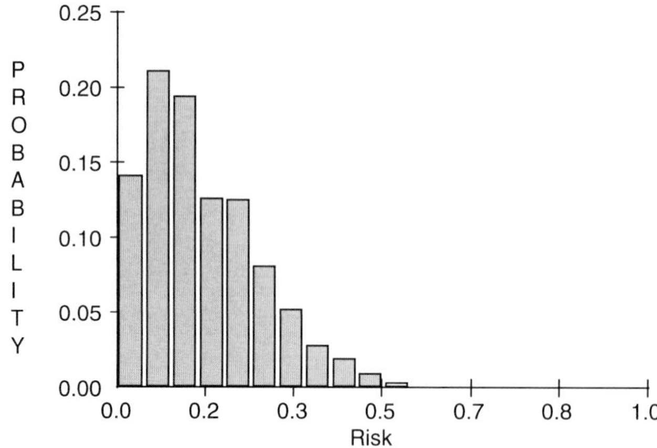

Fig. 20. Distribution of the risk of introducing equine babesiosis by importation of at least one out of ten horses with a false-negative test result.

below 50%. This finding thus also shows the considerable risk of disease introduction. Measures to reduce this risk can be put forward (some of which may not be realistic), such as importing fewer horses, using a more sensitive test, and minimizing the probability of infection through careful selection of horses from areas with low prevalence. These conditions could be identified if the correlation between risk and the influencing parameters is investigated, and this is called sensitivity analysis.

13.1.7. Output of the Model - Risk of Unnecessary Rejection

The point estimates of the probability of having exactly one, two, three, or four false-positive test results in the group of 10 horses, based on the most-likely values of **Table 16**, are:

$$[0.7424]^1 = 0.7424, [0.7424]^2 = 0.5512, [0.7424]^3 = 0.4092 \text{ or } [0.7424]^4 = 0.3038, \text{respectively.}$$

This means that the risk of unnecessarily rejecting the shipment of 10 horses depends on the actual observed number of positive test results. There is a high risk of 74% if only one positive test is observed.

Conversely, when four positive test results are obtained, there is only 30% risk of unnecessary rejection.

The range of possible values for these risks is the key. A frequency distribution histogram for the possibility of a situation where there are two positive test results is shown in **Fig. 21**. This indicates that the risk of unnecessary rejection is more than 50% in the case of rejection based on a single positive test result ($c = 0$ rule).

This would mean that half of the export permits would have to be unnecessarily withheld (no true infection). However, this

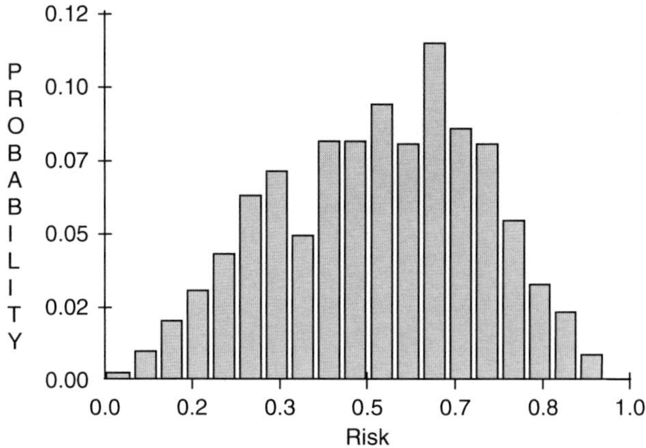

Fig. 21. Distribution of the risk of an unnecessary rejection (no true infection) of a group of ten horses, based on two positive test results. Data from a stochastic risk mode for hypothetical data. See text and **Table 18** for the definition of the model and the input variables.

Table 17
Herd-level sensitivity and specificity for a diagnostic test with sensitivity = 96% and specificity = 94.67% and the prevalence 5% applied to a sample of *n* = 20 animals with the decision rules of classifying the farm as negative if not more than *c* = 0, 1, 2 positive test results occur

Herd-level sensitivity and specificity	c = 0	c = 1	c = 2
HSe	87.5%	60.0%	31.5%
HSp	33.4%	71.1%	91.2%

rule favors the importing country, because the probability of infection in non-rejected groups of animals is low. The probability of unnecessary rejection (no true infection in the group) decreases with the number of positive test results. These scenarios show that rules with $c > 0$ reduce the probability of unnecessary rejection.

The risk analyst is interested in the distribution of the outcome value rather than in the point estimates, because this ensures that appropriate decisions are still valid when there is uncertainty regarding the input parameters.

Examples:

We found that for test T3 (at cut-off 0.36) Se = 96% and Sp = 94.67%. We assume that the test is to be used for the detection of infected farms, with a sample size (n) of 20 animals. We further assume that the true prevalence (p) is 5%. What is the herd-level sensitivity and specificity if we choose c = 0, 1, and 2 animals as thresholds to define the herd as non-infected? (*see* **Table 17**)

$$\Pr(T+) = AP = p\,Se + (1-p)(1-Sp) = (.05)(.96) + (.95)(.0533) = 0.0986$$

$$\Pr(T-) = 1 - AP = p(1-Se) + (1-p)Sp = (.05)(.04) + (.95)(.9467) = 0.9014.$$

References

1. Gardner, I. A, Greiner, M. *Advanced Methods for Test Validation and Interpretation in Veterinary Medicine.* 2nd ed. Berlin, Universität Berlin and the University of California Davis, 2000. 102 p.
2. Greiner, M., Sohr, D., Gobel, P. A modified ROC analysis for the selection of cut-off values and the definition of intermediate results of serodiagnostic tests. *J. Immunol. Methods*, 185(1):123–132, 1995.
3. Jacobson, R. Principles of validation of diagnostic assays for infectious diseases. In: *Manual of Standards for Diagnostic Tests and Vaccines*, edited by Office International des Epizooties (OIE), Paris, 1997, p. 8–15.
4. Greiner, M., Böhning, D. Notes about determining the cut-off value in enzyme linked immunosorbent assay (ELISA) -reply. *Prev. Vet. Med.*, 20:307–310, 1994.
5. Moses, L.E., Shapiro, D., Littenberg, B. Combining independent studies of a diagnostic test into a summary ROC curve -data-analytic approaches and some additional considerations. *Stat. Med.*, 12:1293–1316, 1993.
6. Hasselblad, V., Hedges, L.V. Meta-analysis of screening and diagnostic tests. *Psychol. Bull.*, 117:167–178, 1995.
7. Greiner, M., Kumar, S., Kyeswa, C. Evaluation and comparison of antibody ELISAs for serodiagnosis of bovine trypanosomosis. *Vet. Parasitol.*, 73:197–205, 1997.
8. Bland, J.M., Altman, D.G. Statistical method for assessing agreement between two methods of clinical measurement. *Lancet*, 1:307–310, 1986.
9. Thrusfield, M.V. *Veterinary Epidemiology*, London, Blackwell Science, 1995.
10. Ahl, A.S., Acree, J.A., Gipson, P.S., McDowell, R.M., Miller, L., McElvaine, M.D. Standardisation of nomenclature for animal health risk analysis. *Rev. Sci. Tech. OIE*, 12:1045–1053, 1993.

Chapter 13

Internal Quality Control and External Quality Management of Data in Practice

In this chapter, the use of control charts to both continuously evaluate testing in individual laboratories as well as provide data for external monitoring is examined in detail. The data is based on the publication by D. E. Rebeski· et al., "Charting methods to monitor the operational performance of ELISA method for the detection of antibodies against trypanosomes" in *Veterinary Parasitology*, 2001, 96, 11–50, and is a detailed example of the investigation of the performance of four indirect ELISAs for the detection of antibodies against trypanosomes using *Trypanosoma congolense* and *T. vivax* antigen-precoated plates in 15 veterinary diagnostic laboratories in Africa and Europe. The study shows the practical use of charting methods with respect to assessing the operational performance of each ELISA.

Data from standardized internal quality control (IQC) samples were used to assess ELISA performance indicators with reference to expected upper and lower control limits, as determined from studies by the kit producer (tentative values). Based on unprocessed (optical density) and normalized absorbance values (calculated as a percentage positivity of a control), dispersion of values from the expected data range were estimated though plotting the location and deviation of the values.

In addition, assay precision was estimated by plotting the distribution of coefficients of variation <10% of the IQCs. Binding ratios of various controls were calculated to estimate the assay proficiency with respect to the accuracy of assessing whether the IQC samples tested positive or negative in the test proper. The graphical analysis of dispersion of absorbance values in combination with assay precision and proficiency criteria were considered satisfactory to allow

John R. Crowther, *Methods in Molecular Biology, The ELISA Guidebook, Vol. 516*

DOI: 10.1007/978-1-60327-254-4_13

the evaluation of the operational performances of the ELISAs, and provide useful decision-making criteria for plate acceptance and rejection. The establishment of standardized and transparent IQC data charting methods for the indirect ELISAs provided an increased measure of confidence to national laboratories with respect to their reports on disease occurrence. Moreover, the relative assay performances among all laboratories were examined, using summary data charts, with reference to the performance criteria described. The IQC data were also examined using modified Youden plot analysis, demonstrating that indirect ELISA methods can be successfully applied at diagnostic laboratories in the tropics for monitoring trypanosomosis control programs.

1. Introduction

Work on serological methods has demonstrated that the ELISA is the most suitable method for complementary use with traditional parasitological techniques, to refine routine control and diagnosis of *Trypanosoma congolense*, *T. vivax*, and *T. brucei* in livestock *(1)*. Indirect ELISAs have been evaluated for antibody detection in serum samples using crude trypanosomal antigen preparations, or purified antigen fractions originating from rodents or *in vitro* cultures *(2–5)*. For the detection of circulating trypanosomal antigens in serum samples, direct sandwich assays were developed, exploiting monoclonal antibodies *(6)*. However, these efforts have not led to the distribution of a robust, sustainable, and internationally recognized ELISA. For international trade, prescribed tests for detection of tsetse-borne trypanosomosis by the Office International des Epizooties *(7)* are based on methods for agent identification using direct examination and concentration of parasites, rather than antigen detection ELISA methods, although it has been demonstrated that parasitological techniques provide low sensitivity with a high specificity. For antibody detection, the indirect fluorescent antibody test (IFA), rather than the ELISA method, is recommended for use as an alternative test.

Four indirect ELISAs had been developed, and their robustness and diagnostic performance evaluated *(8–11)*. In addition, a standardized, transparent control system monitoring the operational performance of the ELISA within specified limits has been developed, and examined for implementation as a routine application in diagnostic laboratories in the tropics.

The objective of the study was to obtain data on the quality control of four ELISAs for detecting antibodies against trypanosomosis through the use of charting methods. Such methods ensure the constant control and monitoring of the operational performance of ELISAs with respect to the tentative control data ranges determined during the assay development stages at the FAO/IAEA Agriculture and Biotechnology Laboratory. The data were obtained from standardized IQC samples *(12)*, and processed using Shewhart-like charts *(13)*. The methods provided immediate visual monitoring, and helped in controlling the operational performance from plate to plate and day to day. The overall operational performance of the assays was compared among 15 laboratories in Africa and Europe. The results were analyzed graphically, using summary data charts and modified Youden plots *(14, 15)*.

2. Materials and Methods

2.1. Laboratories

The operational performance of the ELISAs was monitored in 15 laboratories located in Austria, Belgium, Burkina Faso, Cameroon, Côte d'Ivoire, Ghana, Kenya, Mali, Nigeria, Sudan, Tanzania, Uganda, Zambia, Zanzibar, and Zimbabwe.

2.2. ELISA Reagents and Shipment

Four indirect trypanosomosis antibody (I-TAB) ELISA systems were evaluated. Briefly, they exploited native (AGn) or detergent/heat treated (AGd) antigen preparations: two *T. congolense* (*T.c.*) AG-based indirect ELISAs (I-TAB ELISA (*T.c.*AGn) and I-TAB ELISA (*T.c.*AGd)), as well as two *T. vivax* (*T.v.*) AG-based indirect ELISAs (I-TAB ELISA (*T.v.*AGn) and I-TAB ELISA (*T.v.*AGd)) *(10, 11)*. The antigen-precoated ELISA plates were sealed, packed in plastic bags with silica gel desiccant packets, and stored at 37°C in the original cardboard boxes of the ELISA plate manufacturer until shipment by air freight, without special conditions. The plates were stored at room temperature in counterpart laboratories until used. The frozen biological reagents (control sera and conjugated antibody) were dispatched in vacuum flasks and kept at –20°C until used.

2.3. ELISA Procedure

The ELISAs were performed according to the corresponding standardized FAO/IAEA bench protocols (prototype Version 1.0, November 1998). The assay procedure included the testing of four IQC samples in quadruplicate, referred to as operational performance indicators of the ELISA method: a defined strong antibody positive (C++), a moderate antibody positive (C+), an antibody negative serum sample (C–), and serum diluent buffer as a conjugate control (Cc), as described elsewhere *(12)*.

2.4. Tentative Upper and Lower Control Limits of Raw and Normalized Absorbance

As part of the assay standardization procedure at the FAO/IAEA Agriculture and Biotechnology Laboratory, preliminary IQC upper control limits (UCL) and lower control limits (LCL) were established. Replicates of each IQC (n = 24) were tested in six quadruplicate plates on 15 occasions. For each plate, the optical density (OD) value of each IQC replicate was also expressed as a percentage of the median of four replicates of the C++ OD, according to the FAO/IAEA ELISA data interchange software program (EDI, Version 2.3.1, 1999). For each IQC, the preliminary UCL and LCL of the raw absorbance signal were determined from the overall mean OD value ± 3 standard deviations (SD) of the OD mean values of 90 quadruplicates. Similarly, the tentative UCL–LCL range of the percent positivity (PP) values of each IQC were determined from the overall mean PP value ± 3 SD of PP mean values of 90 quadruplicates.

2.5. ELISA Charting Methods

For the generation of Shewhart-like ELISA control data charts *(13)* and data processing, the spreadsheet software program Microsoft Excel (Microsoft Office 97) was used. The use of ELISA IQC data charting methods at the operator level is shown in **Table 1**. These were then subjected to interlaboratory explorative analysis. The charts examine the agreement of the true operational performance observed under local conditions, with the expected performance determined at the FAO/IAEA Agriculture and Biotechnology Laboratory, to control and monitor the plate-to-plate, day-to-day, and trend performance.

2.6. Detailed and Summary Daily Data Chart

For each laboratory, Shewhart-like control detailed (D) charts and summary daily data (SDD) charts were generated, to plot the daily distribution of the C++ OD values. Similar charts plotted the PP of each IQC from individual plates, expressing the raw OD value as PP relative to the mean of the intermediate OD value (median OD value) of the strong positive control. Shewhart-like control charts plotted the number of plates along the *x*-axis

Table 1
Outline of control data charting of IQC data for monitoring and evaluation of the operational ELISA performance

Explorative data analysis of the operational performance of ELISA using data charting methods

National laboratory generation	[a]Reference laboratory generates
Detailed and summary data charts (Figs. 13.1a, b)	Summary laboratory data chart (Figs. 13.2a, b, 3a, b, 4a, b, 5a, b)
Detailed daily precision charts (Fig. 13.1c)	Summary laboratory precision chart (Figs. 13.2c, 3c, 4c, 5)
Detailed daily proficiency charts (Fig. 13.1d)	Summary laboratory proficiency charts (Figs. 13.2d,3d,4d,5d)

[a]OIE Collaborating Centre for ELISA and Molecular Techniques FAO/IAEA Agriculture and Biotechnology Laboratory, Seibersdorf, Vienna, Austria

against the actual absorbance values or the PP values (*y*-axis), respectively. In addition, the UCL and LCL ranges representing the overall mean OD and PP values ± 3 SD were indicated. The daily IQC results from single plates (mean OD and PP values ± 2 SD) and the overall mean ± 2 SD derived from all plates on one occasion were plotted. Some OD or PP values have been highlighted to illustrate the extremes for the SD.

2.7. Detailed Daily Precision Chart

The intralaboratory analysis of the variation of the IQC replicates within and among plates is referred to as assay repeatability. Detailed daily precision (DDPre) charts plotted the percentage coefficient of variation (CV), which was a measure of relative dispersion of IQC replicates based on the SD. The CV% was calculated by the SD of four PP replicates divided by the corresponding mean for single plates. For this study, the UCL was set as CV = 10%, which was empirically determined and recommended for evaluation of standardized ELISAs *(16)*.

2.8. Detailed Daily Proficiency Chart

The detailed daily proficiency (DDPro) charts plotted the intralaboratory assay proficiency, computing the ratio of antibody binding to antibody non-binding (B/B0) of the median PP of C+/C− from each plate. For calculation, the median of four IQC replicates, rather than the mean, was chosen to approach the true value, rather than the value more biased by dispersion of four replicates. Also, the small difference of antibody activity of C+ compared to C− was considered more suitable to indicate reduced assay proficiency than the higher ratio of C++/C−. The overall mean B/B0 ratio ± 2 SD derived from all plates on one occasion was also plotted. The tentative UCL–LCL range was determined from the overall mean value of C+/C− binding ratios ± 3 SD.

2.9. Interlaboratory Explorative Analysis

For each ELISA system, IQC data were generated under local conditions in laboratories from Africa and Europe. The data were reported to the FAO/IAEA Agriculture and Biotechnology Laboratory, and plotted on summary data and modified Youden plot charts for explorative analysis of the ELISA performance.

2.10. Summary Laboratory Data Charts

The overall mean IQC values of unprocessed (OD) and normalized (PP) absorbance values from each laboratory, representing the true data range, were compared with the tentative UCL–LCL range (overall mean OD and PP values ± 3 SD).

2.11. Modified Youden Plot Analysis

The modified Youden plot analysis identified systematic and random errors among laboratories *(14, 15)*. Briefly, a result obtained by a laboratory on one sample was plotted with respect to the result it obtained on a similar sample. Depending on the relation of the plotted point to the true value, it can be decided whether discrepant results are due to bias, imprecision, or both.

For each laboratory, the overall mean PP values of C+ (*y*-axis) were plotted against those of C– (*x*-axis). A rectangle was formed by the overall laboratory mean PP values ± 1 SD of C+ and C–. Laboratories reporting both IQCs outside the mean ± 1 SD defined quadrant indicated systematic errors (upper right or lower left region). Laboratories revealing random errors for both IQCs were visualized in the upper left or lower right region outside the mean ± 1 SD defined quadrant. Laboratories falling within the vertical or horizontal medium region outside the mean ± 1 SD defined quadrant indicated a random error for one IQC sample.

2.12. Summary Laboratory Precision Chart

For each IQC on single plates and for each individual laboratory, the frequency distribution of the CV values <10% was plotted and compared among laboratories (reproducibility). For each IQC, a box represented the true frequency range based on the overall mean of the frequency ± 1 SD of CV values <10% obtained from all laboratories.

2.13. Summary Laboratory Proficiency Chart

For each laboratory, the overall mean ± 2 SD of binding ratios was plotted to demonstrate the intralaboratory variation of the assay proficiency within the tentative UCL–LCL range (overall mean ± 3 SD). In addition, a range was defined to evaluate the interlaboratory variation of the assay proficiency after computing the overall mean ± 1 SD of pooled B/B0 ratios from single plates of all laboratories.

3. Results

3.1. Determination of Tentative Upper and Lower Control Limits

For each ELISA system, the tentative range of UCL–LCL of IQC absorbance and PP values is demonstrated in **Table 2**. For the I-TAB ELISA (*T.v.*AGn), the preliminary limits of C++ and C+ OD values overlapped, indicating high variation of absorbance for the antibody positive controls, which did not interfere with clear discrimination from C–.

3.2. Explorative Analysis of Intralaboratory ELISA Performance

Shewhart-like data charts for monitoring the ELISA under conditions in Africa are shown in **Fig. 1a–d**. Plots of the IQC data show the dispersion of absorbance values of C++, and PP values of each IQC, respectively, as well as the CV% and B/B0 values. Each plot shown in **Fig. 1a, b** reflects the mean value and its variation in all plates, on various occasions. The bar shows the absolute range of variation of the four replicates to the mean within the measured probability on each plate and on each occasion.

Table 2
Tentative IQC values for LCL and UCL for Cc, C++, C+, C–)

ELISA	Absorbance at 450 nm (average +/– 3SD)			
Controls	Cc	C++	C+	C–
*T.c.*AGn	0.025	1.149	0.413	0.093
LCL–UCL	0.002–0.049	0.887–1.410	0.293–0.534	0.038–0.149
*T.c.*AGd	0.033	1.171	0.507	0.133
LCL–UCL	0.060–0.060	0.818–1.523	0.332–0.681	0.066–0.200
T.v AGn	0.033	1.053	0.538	0.158
LCL–UCL	-0.099–0.165	0.685–1.421	0.292–0.783	0.087–0.228
T.v. AGd	0.032	1.245	0.596	0.161
LCL–UCL	-0.014–0.078	0.852–1.638	0.415–0.778	0.107–0.216
	PP values (average +/– 3SD)			
	Cc	C++	C+	C–
*T.c.*AGn	2.19	99.84	35.9	8.07
LCL–UCL	0.35–4.03	91.16–108.50	30.61–41.19	4.09–12.04
*T.c.*AGd	2.84	100	45.3	11.32
LCL–UCL	0.57–5.10	89.39–110.60	34.6–52.00	7.24–15.39
T.v AGn	3.01	99.86	50.97	15.05
LCL–UCL	-6.86–12.88	90.21–109.50	34.82–67.12	8.46–21.64
T.v. AGd	2.64	99.82	47.88	13.02
LCL–UCL	-1.31–6.58	92.6–107	40.81–54.95	8.00–18.05

For each laboratory, the overall spread of IQC (Cc, C++, C+, C–) data is shown. *n* = number of plates tested. Overall mean and values outside upper and lower control limits set by producer are shown as *bold*

3.3. Explorative Analysis of Interlaboratory ELISA Performance

The data charts reporting the ELISA performance among 15 laboratories are outlined in **Table 1**. The true dispersion of raw and relative absorbance, and B/B0s of IQC data were compared with tentative limits. With respect to the laboratory proficiency testing, the absorbance range expressed as PP values was also explored with reference to the true data range, as computed by the modified Youden plot analysis. The frequency distribution of CV values <10% was analyzed for each IQC, to estimate the expected assay precision under various laboratory conditions.

Explorative data analysis of the operational performance of ELISA using data charting methods	
National laboratory generation	*Reference laboratory generates
Detailed and summary data charts (**Figs 2a and 2b**)	Summary laboratory data chart (**Figs 3a, 3b, 4a, 4b, 5a, 5b, 6a, 6b**)
Detailed daily precision charts (**Fig 2c**)	Summary laboratory precision chart (**Figs 3c, 4c, 5c, 6c**)
Detailed daily proficiency charts (**Fig. 2d**)	Summary laboratory proficiency charts (**Figs 3d, 4d, 5d, 6d**)

Fig. 1. ELISA *T.c.*AGd: (**a**) illustration of daily single and summary plates. (b) illustration of daily single and summary plates. The PP values are plotted on a detailed chart and an SDD chart at a laboratory in Africa (C++, C+, C− and Cc mean PP ± 2 SD). *Lines* represent tentative UCL and LCL (overall mean PP ± 3 SD), as determined at the FAO/IAEA Laboratory. Numbers in *circles* represent examples of alarming PP values. (**c**) illustration of CV% of PP values plotted on DDPre chart at a laboratory in Africa. *Line* represents tentative UCL of CV = 10%. This shows estimates of the relative variation of the plotted means of IQCs from plate to plate. In the example given, the ELISA revealed CV values <10% for C++ and C+, indicating excellent precision. Higher CV% values were generally observed for C− and Cc, as expected, even though CV values <10% were occasionally found. (**d**) C+/C− binding ratios plotted from median PP values of four replicates each, on a daily detailed proficiency chart at a laboratory in Africa. The daily overall mean B/B0 ratio ± 2 SD is also recorded. *Lines* represent tentative UCL and LCL (overall mean ± 3 SD), as determined at the FAO/IAEA Laboratory. The DDPro chart (**Fig.1d**) is an example of the effect of systematic or random errors on the assay performance. The plates tested on day 990118, and two plates tested on day 990125, showed binding ratios below expected limits

3.3.1. I-TAB ELISA (T.c.AGn)

The I-TAB ELISA (*T.c.*AGn) was evaluated in 3 laboratories in Africa and 2 in Europe. The data are shown in **Table 3** and plotted in **Fig. 2a–d**. For each of the four IQCs, expected overall mean absorbance values were observed in two of the 5 laboratories (**Fig. 2a**). Computing the overall mean PP values, 3 of the 5 laboratories demonstrated controlled ELISA performance inside the established tentative limits (**Fig. 2b**). Comparing the assay precision among laboratories (reproducibility), 4 of the 5 laboratories demonstrated similar frequency distribution of CV values <10% of C++ and C+ within the overall mean frequency distribution ± 1 SD: 82.38–101.86 and 61.05–107.46%, respectively (**Fig. 2c**). Assay proficiency with respect to assay accuracy was demonstrated in all the laboratories, as expected (**Fig. 2d**). Among 5 laboratories, 4 laboratories showed similar laboratory proficiency *(7)*.

3.3.2. I-TAB ELISA (T.c.AGd)

The I-TAB ELISA (*T.c.*AGd) was evaluated in 12 laboratories in Africa and 2 laboratories in Europe. The overall mean absorbance and PP values of each IQC at the particular laboratories are shown in **Table 4**. For each of the four IQCs, expected absorbance and PP values were observed in 5 of the 14 laboratories (**Fig. 3a, b**). Similar expected assay precision was found in 12 laboratories, as demonstrated by the frequency distribution of CV values <10% of C++ and C+ within the overall mean frequency distribution ± 1 SD: 73.77–105.60 and 76.87–100.52%, respectively (**Fig. 3c**). The expected assay accuracy was obtained in 12 laboratories (**Fig. 3d**).

Table 3
Operational performance of I-TAB ELISA (*T.c.*AGn)

Laboratory	Absorbance at 450 nm (average +/– 2SD)			
Controls	Cc	C++	C+	C–
Austria (*n* = 80)	0.039	1.266	0.459	0.105
LCL–UCL	0.006–0.072	0.760–1.771	0.218–0.700	0.062–0.148
Belgium (*n* = 6)	**0.090**	**1.301**	**0.471**	**0.127**
LCL–UCL	0.064–0.346	1.031–1.571	0.366–0.577	0.105–0.148
Burkino Fasso (*n* = 20)	**0.061**	**1.422**	**0.515**	**0.133**
LCL–UCL	-0/063–0.555	1.207–1.638	0.307–0.723	-0.038–0.305
Cameroon (*n* = 24)	**0.025**	**1.254**	**0.439**	**0.108**
LCL–UCL	0.010–0.118	0.921–1.587	0.295–0.583	0.008–0.208
Kenya (*n* = 22)	**0.044**	**1.457**	**0.641**	**0.162**
LCL–UCL	0.007–0.244	1.013–1.900	0.344–0.939	0.049–0.274
	PP values (average +/– 2SD)			
Laboratory	**Cc**	**C++**	**C+**	**C–**
Austria (*n* = 80)	**3.09**	**99.53**	**36.09**	**8.38**
LCL–UCL	1.58 4.6	90.05–109	27.14–45.04	5.44–11.32
Belgium (*n* = 6)	**6.89**	**99.00**	**36.12**	**9.69**
LCL–UCL	4.59–9.19	97.56–100.4	33.55–38.7	7.95–11.43
Burkino Fasso (*n* = 20)	**4.18**	**100.00**	**35.99**	**9.20**
LCL–UCL	-3.07–1.42	99.16–100.8	25.08–46.9	-1.59–19.99
Cameroon (*n* = 24)	**1.95**	**99.15**	**34.71**	**8.53**
LCL–UCL	1.10–2.8	89.49–108.8	30.42–39.00	4.35–12.72
Kenya (*n* = 22)	**3.06**	**99.68**	**43.95**	**11.20**
LCL–UCL	1.21–4.91	96.78–102.6	32.55–55.36	5.79–16.61

For each laboratory, the overall spread of IQC (Cc, C++, C+, C–) data is shown. *n* = number of plates tested. Overall mean and values outside upper and lower control limits set by producer are shown as *bold*

3.3.3. I-TAB ELISA (T.v.AGn)

The overall mean absorbance and PP values of IQC data using the I-TAB ELISA (*T.v.*AGn) results from 3 laboratories in Africa and 2 laboratories in Europe are shown in **Table 5**. Out of the 5 laboratories, 2 demonstrated expected absorbance for each of the four IQCs (**Fig. 4a**). The ELISA PP values indicated controlled

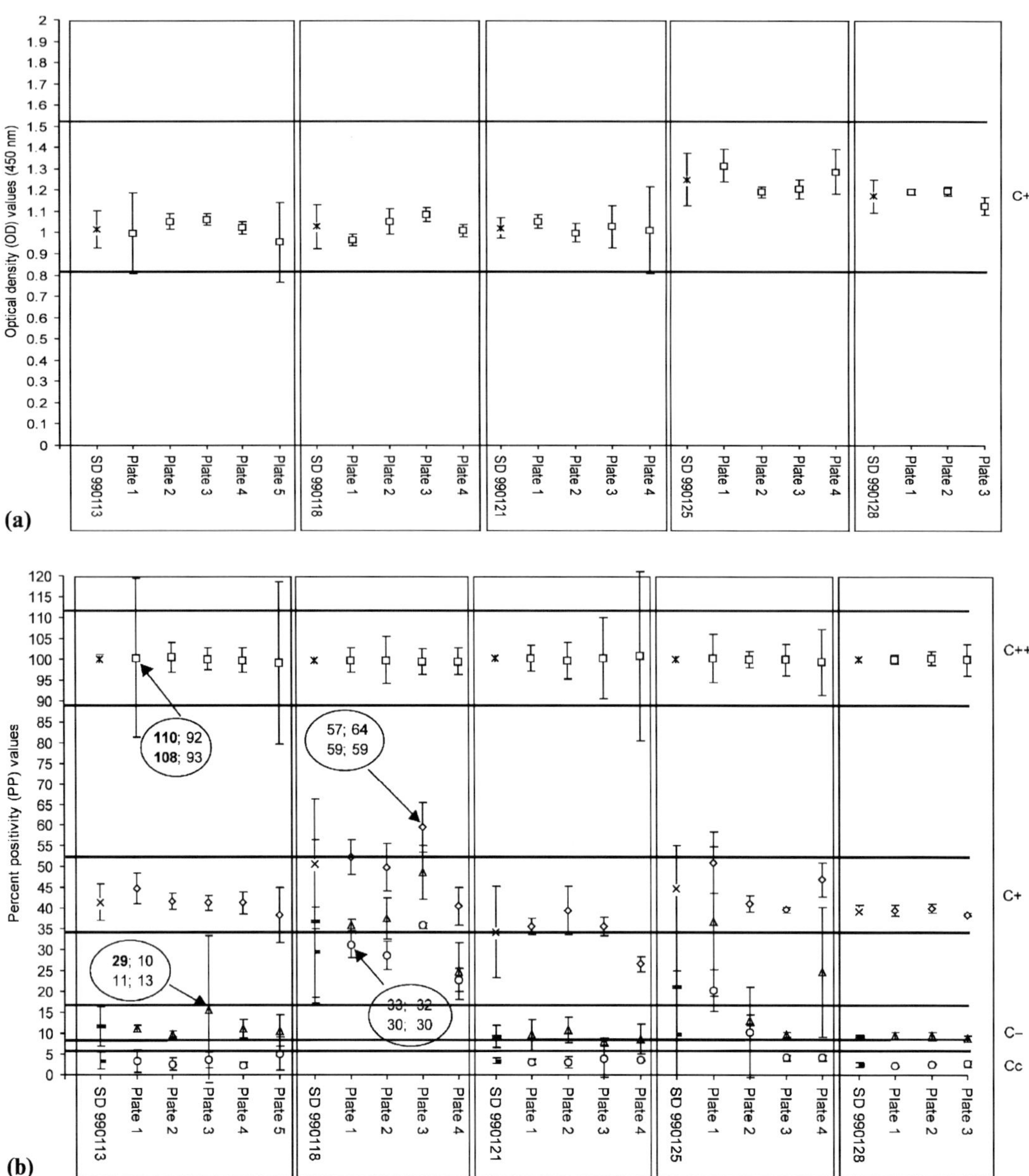

Fig. 2. ELISA *T.c.*AGn: (**a**) summary laboratory data chart plotting IQC values expressed as overall mean OD values. *Boxes* represent tentative range of LCL–UCL (overall mean ± 3 SD). (**b**) summary laboratory data chart plotting IQC values expressed as overall mean PP values. *Boxes* represent tentative UCL–LCL range (overall mean ± 3 SD). (**c**) summary laboratory precision chart illustrating the frequency distribution of CV values <10%. *Broken boxes* represent the true UCL–LCL range (overall mean ± 1 SD) obtained from all laboratories. (**d**) summary laboratory proficiency chart. *Lines* represent tentative UCL–LCL range (overall mean ± 3 SD), as determined at the FAO/IAEA Laboratory. *Broken lines* represent true UCL–LCL range (overall mean ± 1 SD) obtained from all laboratories.

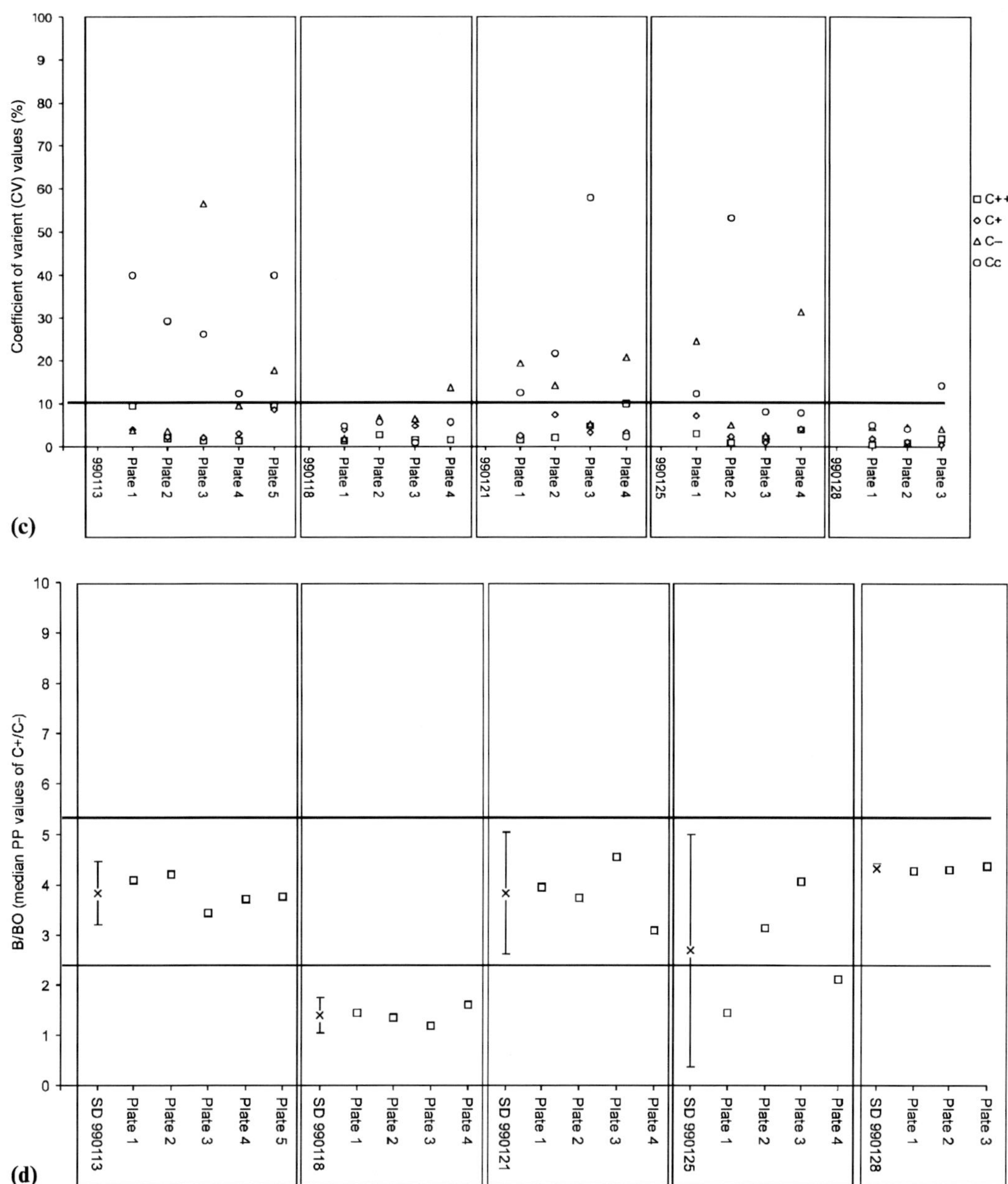

Fig. 2. (continued)

ELISA performance within tentative limits in 4 laboratories (**Fig. 4b**). Expected assay accuracy and assay precision was found in four of the 5 laboratories (**Fig. 4c, d**). These demonstrated a frequency distribution of CV values <10% of C++ and C+ within the overall mean frequency distribution ± 1 SD, namely 74.59–97.81 and 78.55–94.78%, respectively.

3.3.4. I-TAB ELISA (T.v.AGd)

The I-TAB ELISA (*T.v.*AGd) was evaluated in 13 laboratories in Africa and 2 laboratories in Europe. For each the four IQCs,

Table 4
Operational performance of I-TAB ELISA (*T.c.*AGd)

Laboratory	Absorbance at 450 nm (average +/– 2SD)			
	Cc	C++	C+	C–
Austria (n = 80)	0.036	1.237	0.553	0.142
Belgium (n = 6)	**0.70**	1.110	0.475	0.155
B.Fasso (n = 20)	**0.106**	1.097	0.463	0.196
Cameroon (n = 24)	0.037	1.196	0.523	0.128
C. d'Ivoire (n = 12)	0.049	1.256	0.573	**0.206**
Ghana (n = 20)	0.058	**1.649**	**0.853**	**0.291**
Kenya (n = 22)	0.045	1.141	0.502	0.184
Mali (n = 5)	0.020	1.017	**0.742**	**0.045**
Nigeria (n = 16)	0.040	**0.457**	**0.218**	0.077
Tanzania (n = 15)	0.021	1.110	0.473	0.121
Uganda (n = 10)	0.037	1.257	**0.783**	0.193
Zambia (n = 10)	0.047	**1.809**	**0.814**	**0.223**
Zanzibar (n = 20)	0.033	1.499	**0.718**	**0.299**
Zimbabwe (n = 6)	0.052	1.051	0.405	0.130
	PP values (average +/– 2SD)			
	Cc	C++	C+	C–
Austria (n = 80)	3.00	99.73	44.85	11.79
Belgium (n = 6)	**6.37**	100.1	42.83	13.96
B.Fasso (n = 20)	**9.77**	99.92	42.23	13.96
Cameroon (n = 24)	3.17	99.30	43.36	10.78
C. d'Ivoire (n = 12)	4.06	100.18	46.10	**16.61**
Ghana (n = 20)	3.45	99.19	51.42	**17.79**
Kenya (n = 22)	3.87	99.81	46.47	**18.10**
Mali (n = 5)	1.96	100.12	**73.11**	**4.40**
Nigeria (n = 16)	**8.98**	98.97	46.50	**17.18**
Tanzania (n = 15)	1.96	99.94	42.59	10.95
Uganda (n = 10)	2.87	100.64	**60.36**	15.19
Zambia (n = 10)	2.54	100.01	44.51	12.42
Zanzibar (n = 20)	2.22	99.99	47.30	**19.85**
Zimbabwe (n = 6)	4.99	100.13	38.71	12.7

For each laboratory, the overall spread of IQC (Cc, C++, C+, C–) data is shown. n = number of plates tested. Overall mean and values outside upper and lower control limits set by producer are shown as *bold*

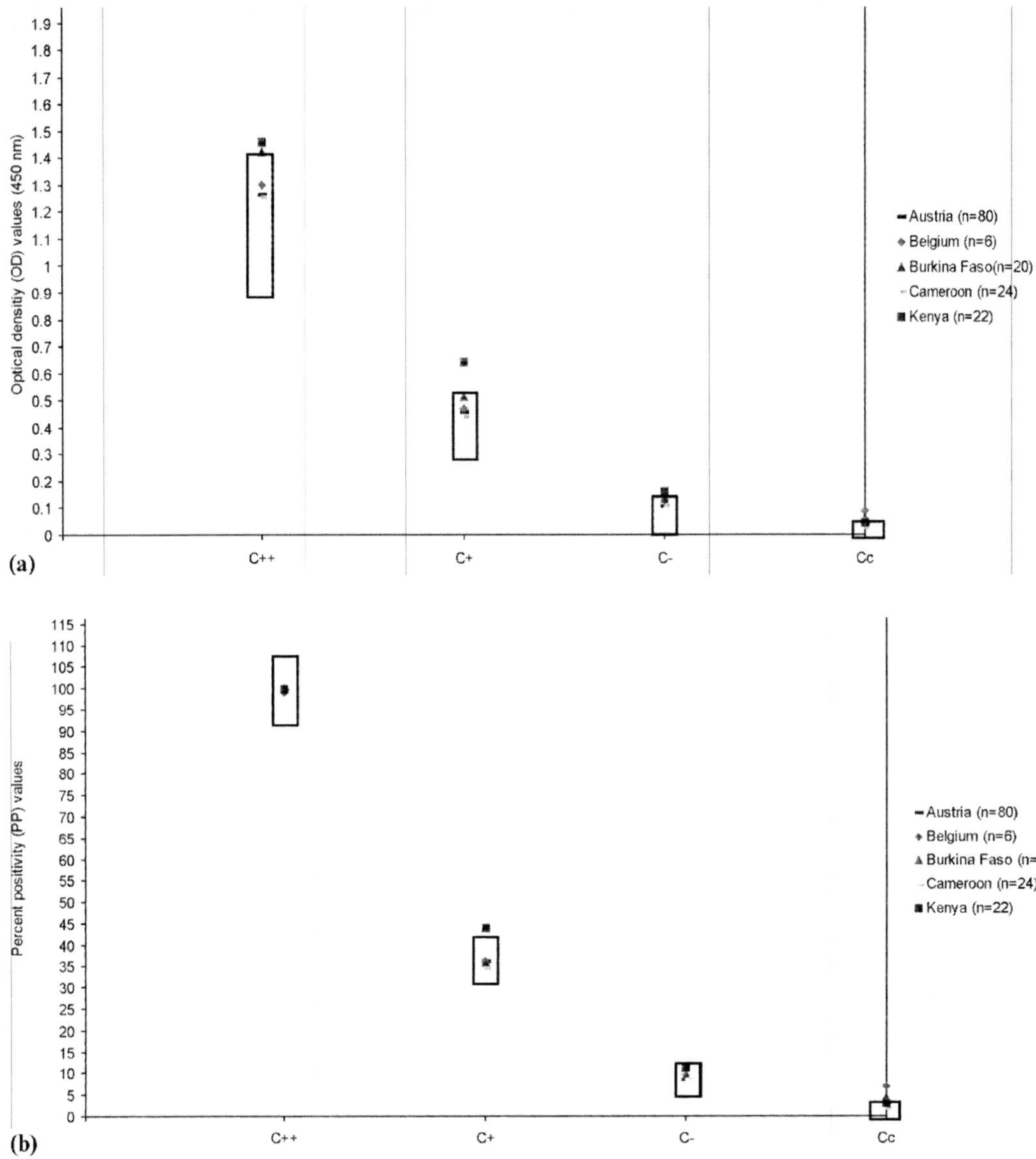

Fig. 3. ELISA *T.c.*AGd: (**a**) summary laboratory data chart plotting IQC values expressed as overall mean OD values. (**b**) summary laboratory data chart plotting IQC values expressed as overall mean PP values. (**c**) summary laboratory precision chart illustrating the frequency distribution of CV values <10%. (**d**) summary laboratory proficiency chart.

expected overall mean absorbance was observed in 8 of the 15 laboratories, and expected PP values were observed in 7 of the 15 laboratories (**Table 6** and **Fig. 5a, b**). Analyzing the inter-laboratory assay precision, 14 and 13 laboratories demonstrated similar frequency distributions of CV values <10% of C++ and C+, respectively, within the overall mean frequency distribution ± 1 C, namely 66.30–106.21 and 56.74–103.96%, respectively

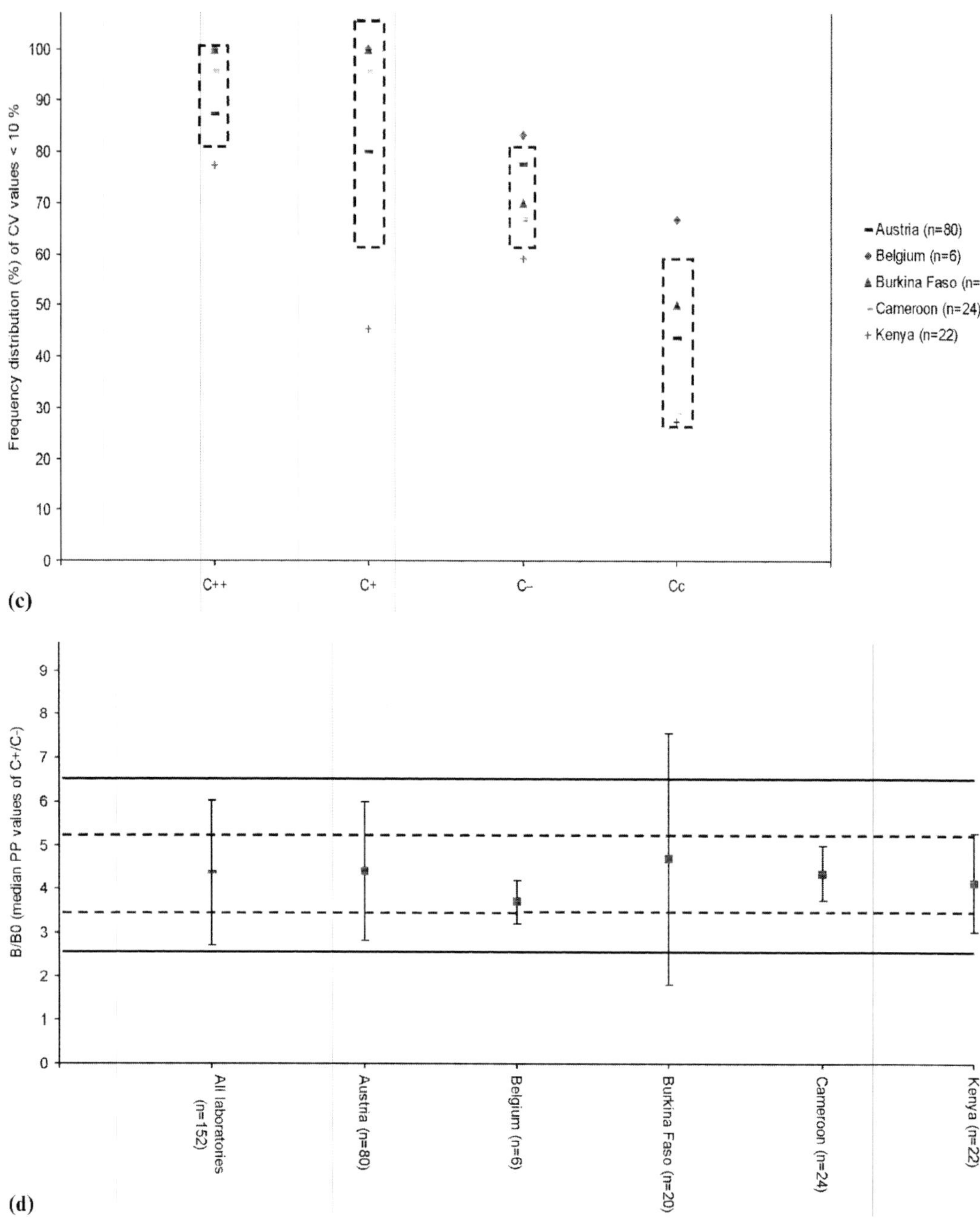

Fig. 3. (continued)

(**Fig. 5c**). Expected assay proficiency was observed in 12 laboratories. Among 15 laboratories, 11 laboratories showed similar laboratory proficiency (**Fig. 5d**).

3.4. Results of Modified Youden Plot Analysis

Using indirect antibody detection ELISAs for trypanosomosis, random and systematic errors in laboratories were identified. For I-TAB ELISA (*T.c.*AGn), I-TAB ELISA (*T.c.*AGd), and I-TAB

Table 5
Operational performance of I-TAB ELISA (*T.v.*AGn)

Laboratory	Absorbance at 450 nm (average +/– 2SD)			
	Cc	C++	C+	C–
Austria (n = 80)	0.59	1.450	0.754	0.207
LCL–UCL	-0.028–0.12	0.857–2.042	0.207–1.300	-0.155–0.569
Belgium (n = 6)	0.089	1.331	0.724	0.245
LCL–UCL	0.065–0.337	0.948–1.014	0.549–0.899	0.193–0.298
B.Fasso (n = 20)	0.028	1.118	0.494	0.151
LCL–UCL	-0.02–0.057	0.602–1.634	0.272–0.717	0.069–0.234
Cameroon (n = 24)	**0.243**	1.280	0.708	0.373
LCL–UCL	-0.178–0.695	0.820–1.741	0.311–1.104	-0.011–0.758
Kenya (n = 22)	0.039	1.101	0.586	0.193
	0.015–0.188	0.859–1.342	0.458–0.714	0.095–0.291
	PP values (average +/– 2SD)			
	Cc	C++	C+	C–
Austria (n = 80)	4.01	99.84	52.06	14.44
LCL–UCL	1.74–6.28	94.52–105.16	31.65–72.47	-3.47–32.64
Belgium (n = 6)	**6.58**	98.40	53.26	18.18
LCL–UCL	5.64–7.51	89.69–107.10	49.09–57.43	15.90–20.46
B.Fasso (n = 20)	**2.47**	99.60	44.45	13.50
LCL–UCL	0.10–2.47	96.42–102.79	34.86–54.03	9.83–17.16
Cameroon (n = 24)	**19.47**	101.59	56.56	**30.09**
LCL–UCL	-3.79–43.28	92.23–109.95	34.22–78.90	5.18–55.01
Kenya (n = 22)	3.5	99.98	53.52	18.01
LCL–UCL	1.19–5.21	98.72	101.24	43.49–63.54

For each laboratory, the overall spread of IQC (Cc, C++, C+, C–) data is shown. n = number of plates tested. Overall mean and values outside upper and lower control limits set by producer are shown as *bold*

ELISA (*T.v.*AGd), data within range overlapped with results from one additional laboratory. The y axes represent values for PP of C+, and the x axes represent values for C– (*see* **Fig. 6a–d**).

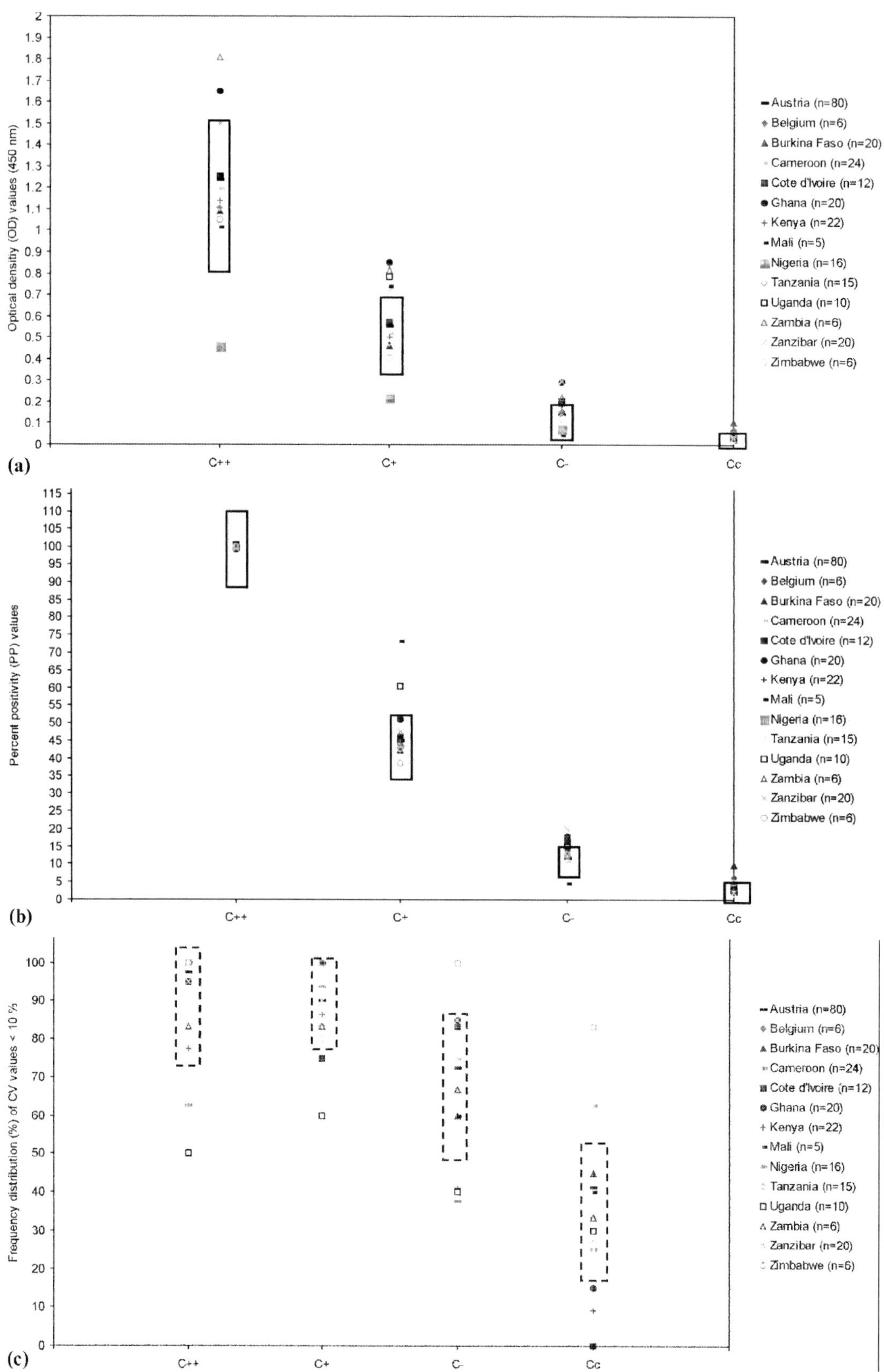

Fig. 4. ELISA *T.c.*AGn: (**a**) summary laboratory data chart plotting IQC values expressed as overall mean OD values. (**b**) summary laboratory data chart plotting IQC values expressed as overall mean PP values. (**c**) summary laboratory precision chart illustrating the frequency distribution of CV values <10%. (**d**) summary laboratory proficiency chart.

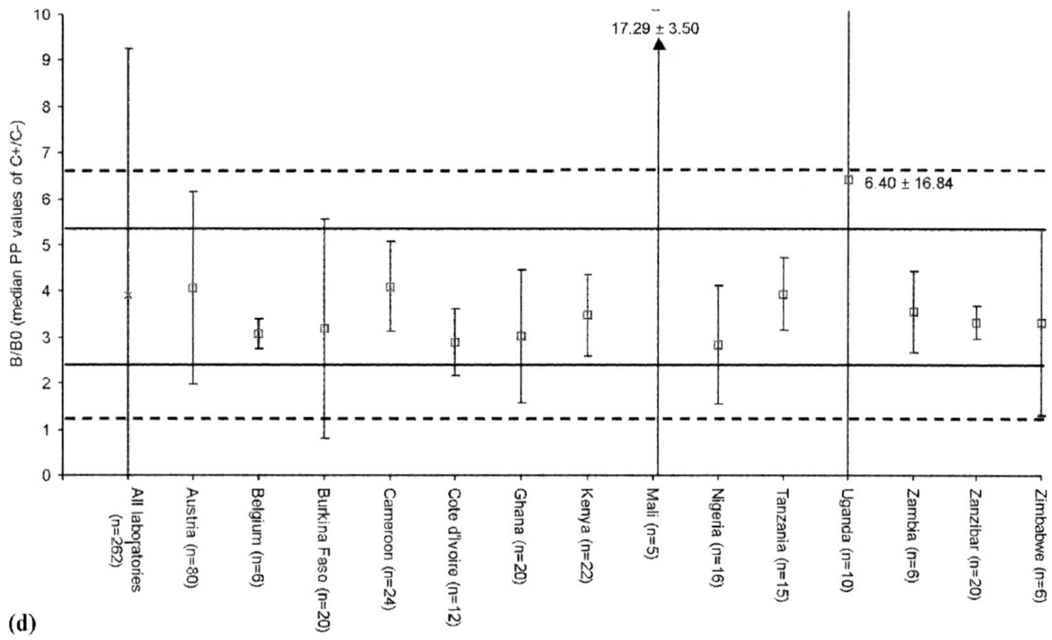

(d)

Fig. 4. (continued)

Table 6
Operational performance of I-TAB ELISA (*T.v.*AGd)

Laboratory	Absorbance at 450 nm (average +/– 2SD)			
	Cc	C++	C+	C–
Austria (n = 80)	0.030	1.401	0.655	0.162
Belgium (n = 6)	**0.085**	1.264	0.562	0.179
B.Fasso (n = 20)	**0.125**	1.199	**0.413**	0.213
Cameroon (n = 24)	0.032	1.044	0.535	0.139
C. d'Ivoire (n = 12)	0.030	1.052	0.513	**0.163**
Ghana (n = 20)	0.052	**0.693**	0.623	**0.229**
Kenya (n = 22)	0.039	1.247	0.609	0.188
Mali (n = 5)	0.051	1.511	**0.509**	**0.209**
Nigeria (n = 16)	0.058	**0.347**	0.184	0.092
Tanzania (n = 15)	0.02	1.119	0.523	0.138
Uganda (n = 10)	0.038	1.228	**0.736**	**0.268**
Zambia (n = 10)	0.028	1.482	0.706	0.199
Zanzibar (n = 20)	0.043	1.285	0.677	**0.234**
Zimbabwe (n = 6)	0.058	0.961	0.609	0.188

(continued)

Table 6 (continued)

Laboratory	Absorbance at 450 nm (average +/– 2SD)			
	PP values (average +/– 2SD)			
	Cc	C++	C+	C–
Austria (n = 80)	2.16	98.99	45.90	11.50
Belgium (n = 6)	**6.68**	98.35	43.60	14.19
B.Fasso (n = 20)	**10.41**	99.77	**34.35**	17.71
Cameroon (n = 24)	3.01	99.65	51.44	13.32
C. d'Ivoire (n = 12)	2.8	99.49	48.75	15.52
Ghana (n = 20)	**8.1**	100.03	**90.11**	**33.17**
Kenya (n = 22)	3.25	100.02	48.81	15.00
Mali (n = 5)	3.41	100.11	**33.69**	13.79
Nigeria (n = 16)	**16.35**	98.97	53.52	**26.18**
Tanzania (n = 15)	1.79	99.74	46.55	12.30
Uganda (n = 10)	3.14	100.62	**58.37**	**20.95**
Zambia (n = 10)	1.86	100.09	47.52	13.45
Zanzibar (n = 20)	3.57	100.28	53.00	**18.66**
Zimbabwe (n = 6)	6.14	99.94	**36.45**	12.05

For each laboratory, the overall spread of IQC (Cc, C++, C+, C–) data is shown. n = number of plates tested. Overall mean and values outside upper and lower control limits set by producer are shown as *bold*

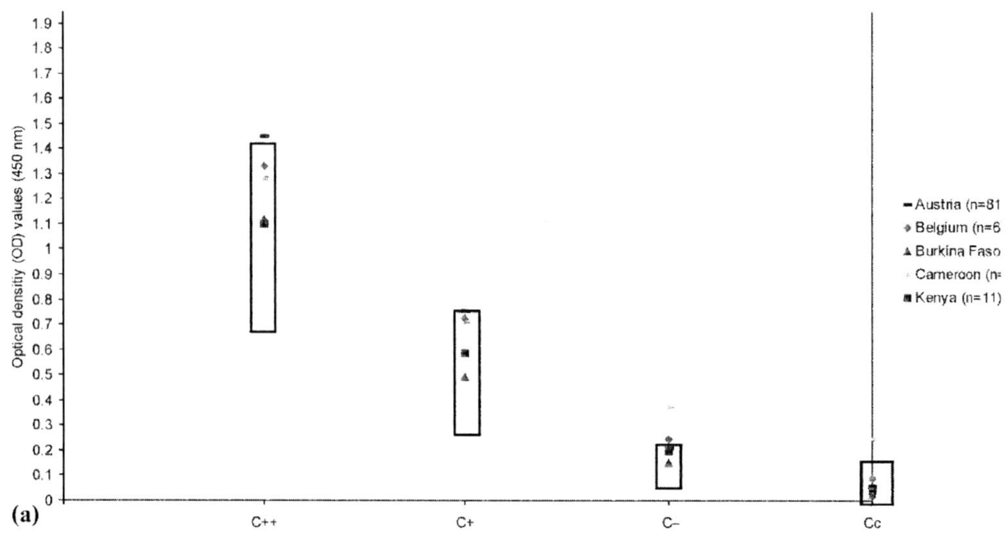

Fig. 5. ELISA *T.c.*AGd: (**a**) summary laboratory data chart plotting IQC values expressed as overall mean OD values. (**b**) summary laboratory data chart plotting IQC values expressed as overall mean PP values. (**c**) summary laboratory precision chart illustrating the frequency distribution of CV values <10%. (**d**) summary laboratory proficiency chart.

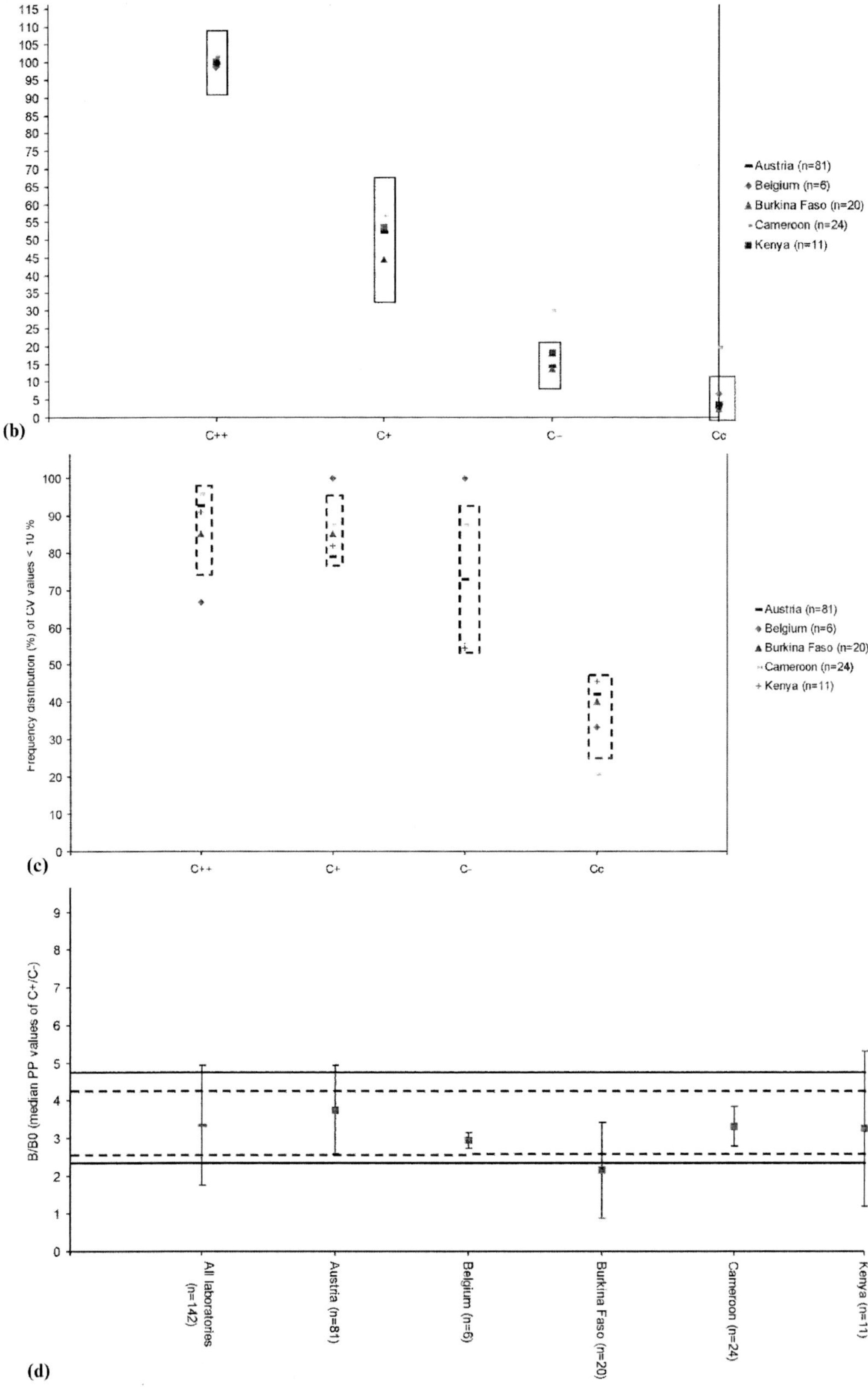

Fig. 5. (continued)

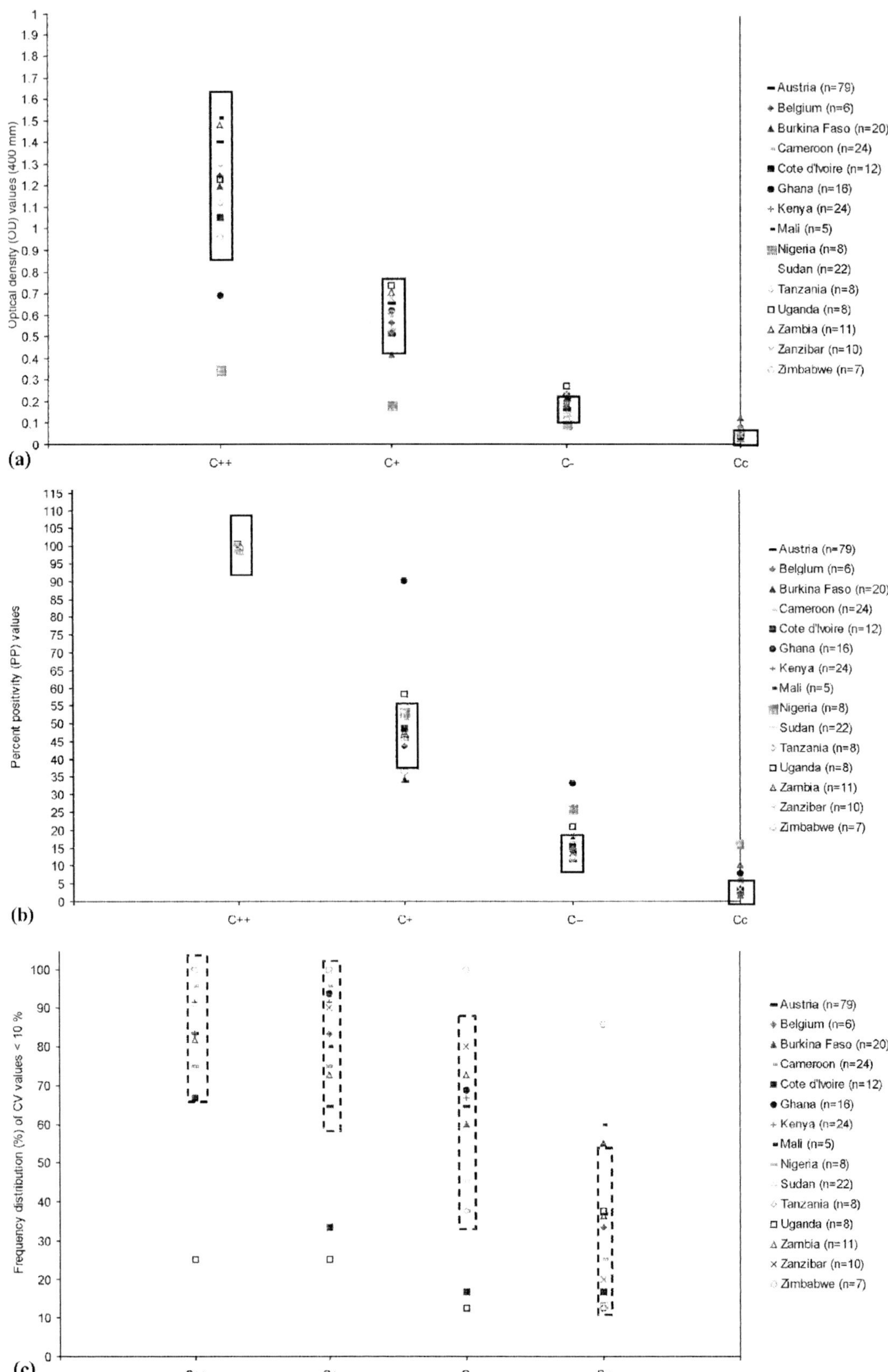

Fig. 6. (**a–d**) Modified Youden plot analyses revealing random and systematic errors in testing.

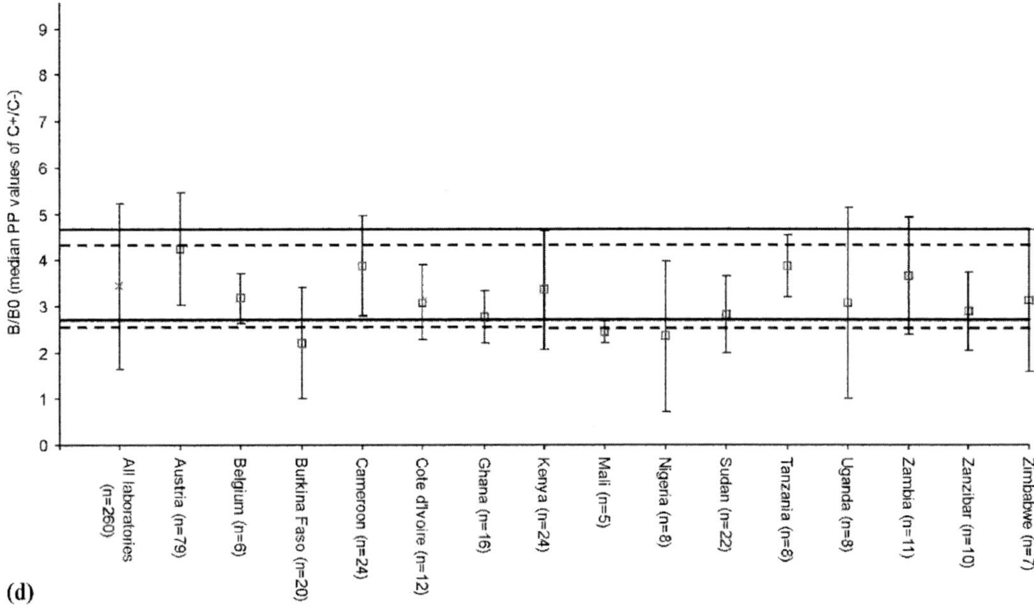

(d)

Fig. 6. (continued)

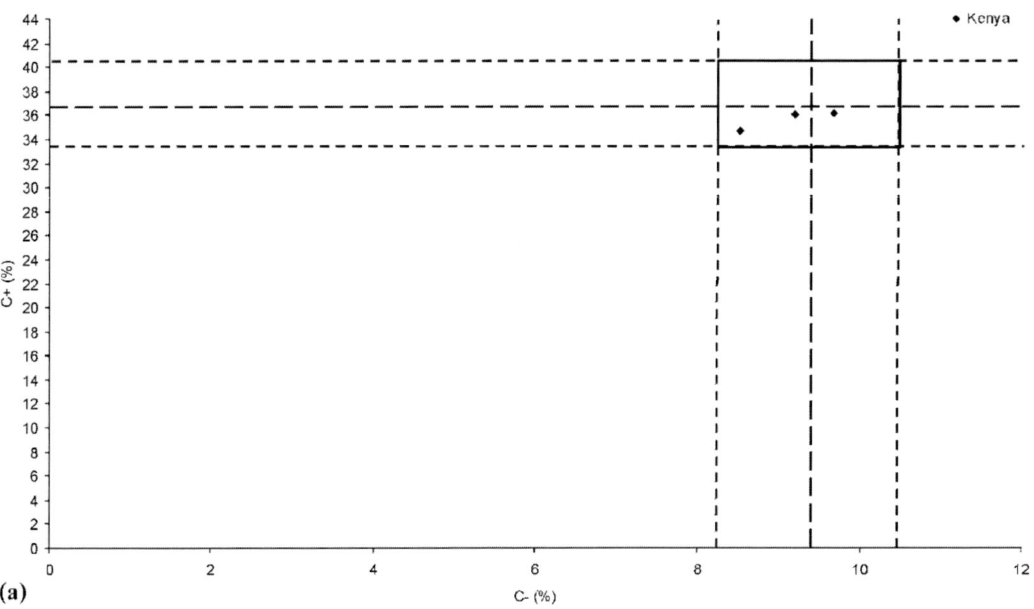

(a)

Fig. 7.

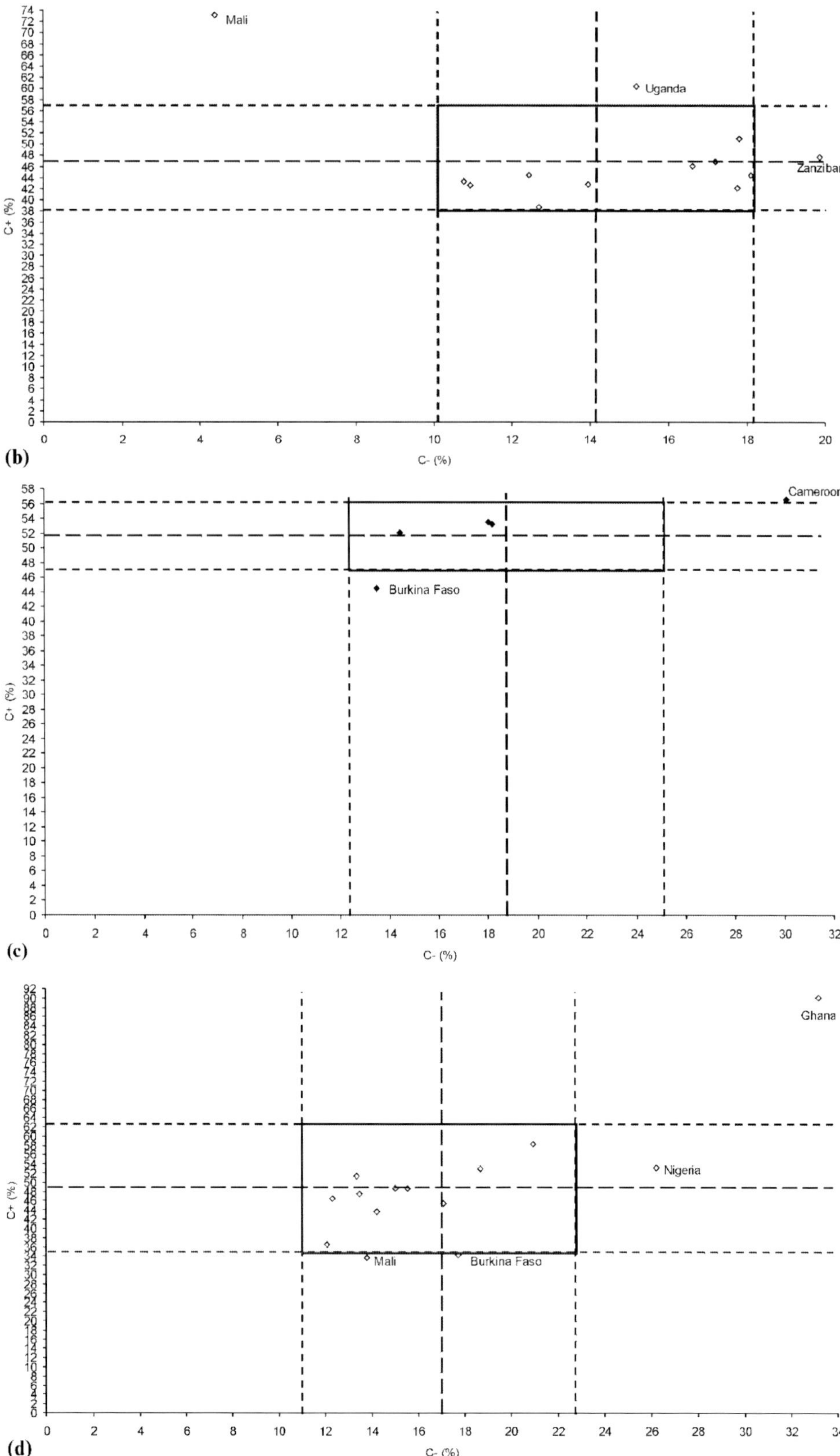

Fig. 7. (continued)

4. Discussion

Charting methods to plot standardized IQC data on Shewhart-like data control charts are useful for monitoring and evaluating the operational performance of ELISA methods. The charting methods: *(1)* kept a constant record of all data; *(2)* monitored the ELISAs from day to day, and week to week; (3) rapidly identified unacceptable results; (4) helped to identify problems with specific reagents; (5) discovered trends in results, e.g., a decrease in performance; (6) noted bias of ELISA performance due to different operators; and (7) fulfilled various criteria for good laboratory practice (GLP).

The detailed plate-to-plate analysis of the replicates of C++, C+, C−, and Cc allowed comparison with the producer-defined data, so that unexpected OD and PP values alerted operators to problems in good time. The discrepancies in the observed and expected absorbance in IQC results could be attributed to errors due to the operator, and to unavoidable random errors inherent in every measurement procedure.

For example, in Ghana, higher than expected IQC absorbance values were obtained. For the C−, the high signal was maintained when analyzing PP values, and it was later reported that the anti-species enzyme-conjugate was used at a dilution of 1/14,000 instead of 1/20,000 *(17)*.

The interpretation of dispersion of OD and PP measurement data with reference to the variability of unavoidable random errors required additional analysis. The frequency distribution of CV values <10% for the C++ and C+ PP values, indicative of the assay precision, were examined, and distribution plots of CV% values of C− and Cc PP values were considered useful for monitoring overall longitudinal changes of performance; however, they were less meaningful for final judgment of the assay precision on single occasions, because their mean values approached zero.

The method of using binding ratios of C+/C− was analyzed, to allow comparison of the analytical sensitivity with respect to the accuracy of assessing that a sample was positive, both within and among tests in laboratories. For both the precision and proficiency assay criteria, it was shown that the assays performed reasonably well within the true range represented by the overall mean value ± 1 SD of all laboratories, irrespective of disparate amounts of dispersion of OD and PP values reported from the laboratories. This suggested that the ELISAs were affected by uncertainties occurring at individual laboratories that were out of the control of the producer of the ELISAs.

It should be noted that IQC performance indicators are different from defined reference control sera originating from local cattle populations. Therefore, IQC results such as reduced binding ratios do not automatically control the assay proficiency with reference to the diagnostic sensitivity and specificity. Here, retesting of test serum samples would be recommended or, even better, the consistent plate-to-plate analysis of locally-defined antibody positive and negative reference sera representing the studied population *(18)*. Moreover, the routine testing of these reference sera locally is strongly recommended, to ensure similar assay proficiency after receipt of new batches of assay reagents.

For interlaboratory analysis of the IQC data, the modified Youden plot analysis proved useful in helping to identify laboratory proficiencies. For example, it was found that the counterparts in Mali were doing the ELISA differently, as compared to other laboratories, and this was suspected because of systematic errors noted for both the C+ and C–. This was later confirmed, as the C++ had been replaced by a locally collected serum sample *(19)*.

In conclusion, a quality control procedure was established for evaluation of the operational performance of indirect trypanosomosis ELISA methods within and among laboratories. From the data, it became evident that the sole use of the IQC absorbance range did not truly reflect the potential operational ELISA performance and should, therefore, not be used as the only decision criterion for plate acceptance or rejection. It is better to examine the distribution of the coefficients of variation, and binding ratios, which can be easily recorded on Shewhart-like data charts at individual laboratories. For interlaboratory evaluation of the ELISA performance and refinement of the producer defined (tentative) UCL and LCL, data should be reported to a reference laboratory. The data charting methods also provided a measure of confidence in the reliable use of trypanosomal antibody detection ELISAs, exploiting antigen-precoated plates, with reference to controlled operational assay performance in diagnostic laboratories in Africa and Europe.

References

1. Luckins, A.G. 1992. Methods for diagnosis of trypanosomiasis in livestock. *World Anim. Rev.* 70/71, pp. 15–20.
2. Luckins, A.G. 1977. Detection of antibodies in trypanosome-infected cattle by means of a microplate enzyme-linked immunosorbent assay. *Trop. Anim. Health Prod.* 9, pp. 53–62.
3. Iagbone, I.F., Staak, C. and Reinhard, R 1989. Fractionation of trypanosome antigens for species-specific sero-diagnosis. *Vet. Parasitol.* 32, pp. 293–299.
4. Greiner, M., Kumar, S. and Kyeswa, C. 1997. Evaluation and comparison of antibody ELISAs for serodiagnosis of bovine trypanosomosis. *Vet. Parasitol.* 73, pp. 197–205.
5. Hopkins, J.S., Chitambo, H., Machila, N., Luckins, A.G., Rae, P.F., van den Bossche, P. and Eisler, M.C. 1998. Adaptation and validation of antibody ELISAs using dried blood spots on filter paper for epidemiological surveys of tsetse-transmitted trypanosomosis in cattle. *Prev. Vet. Med.* 37, pp. 91–99.
6. Nantulya, V.M. and Lindqvist, K.J. 1989. Antigen-detection enzyme immunoassays for the diagnosis of *Trypanosoma vivax*, *T. Congolense* and *T. brucei* infections in cattle. *Trop. Med. Parasitol.* 40, pp. 267–272.
7. OIE, 1997. Manual of Standards for Diagnostic Tests and Vaccines, 3rd Edition. Office International des Epizooties, Paris, pp. 660–664.
8. Rebeski, D.E., Winger, E.M., Lelenta, M., Colling, A., Robinson, M.M., Ndamkou, C., Aigner, H., Dwinger, R.H. and, Crowther, J.R. 1998. Comparison of precoated and freshly coated microtitre plates using denatured antigen for the detection of antibodies against *Trypanosoma congolense* by indirect

enzyme-linked immunosorbent assay. In: Proceedings of the Ninth International Conference of the AITVM, Vol. 1, Harare, Zimbabwe, 14–18 September 14–18, 1998. AITVM (Association of Institutions of Tropical Veterinary Medicine), Harare, Zimbabwe, pp. 376–386.

9. Rebeski, D.E., Winger, E.M., Rogovic, B., Robinson, M.M., Crowther, J.R. and Dwinger, R.H. 1999. Improved methods for the diagnosis of African trypanosomosis. *Mem. Inst. Oswaldo Cruz* 94, pp. 249–253.

10. Rebeski, D.E., Winger, E.M., Okoro, H., Kowalik, S., Bürger, H.J., Walters, D.E., Robinson, M.M., Dwinger, R.H. and Crowther, J.R. 2000. Detection of *Trypanosoma congolense* antibodies with indirect ELISAs using antigen-precoated microtitre plates. *Vet. Parasitol.* 89, pp. 187–198.

11. Rebeski, D.E., Winger, E.M., Robinson, M.M., Gabler, C.M.G., Dwinger, R.H. and Crowther, J.R. 2000. Evaluation of antigen coating procedures of enzyme-linked immunosorbant assay method for detection of trypanosomal antibodies. *Vet. Parasitol.* 90, pp. 1–13.

12. Wright, P.F., Nilsson, E., van Rooij, E.M.A., Lelenta, M. and Jeggo, M.H. 1993. Standardisation and validation of enzyme-linked immunosorbent assay techniques for the detection of antibody in infectious disease diagnosis. *Rev. Sci. Tech. Off. Int. Epiz.* 12, pp. 435–450.

13. Shewhart, W.A. 1931. Economic Control of Quality of Manufactured Product. Van Nostrand, New York (republished by ASQC Quality Press, Milwaukee, WI, 1980).

14. Skendzel, L.P. and Youden, W.J. 1970. Systematic versus random error in laboratory surveys. *Am. J. Clin. Pathol.* 54, pp. 448–450.

15. Youden, W.J., 1960. The sample, the procedure, and the laboratory. *Anal. Chem.* 13, pp. 23–37.

16. Jacobson, R.H. 1998. Validation of serological assays for diagnosis of infectious diseases. *Rev. Sci. Tech. Off. Int. Epiz.* 17, pp. 469–486.

17. Doku, C.K. and, Seidu, I.B.M. 2000. Validation of an improved enzyme-linked immunosorbent assay for the diagnosis of trypanosomal antibodies in Ghanaian cattle. In: R.H. Dwinger (Ed.), Animal Trypanosomosis: Diagnosis and Epidemiology, Results of a FAO/IAEA Co-ordinated Research Programme on the Use of Immunoassay Methods for Improved Diagnosis of Trypanosomosis and Monitoring Tsetse and Tryanosomosis Control Programmes. Backhuys, Leiden, pp. 85–91.

18. Greiner, M., Shivarama Bhat, T., Patzelt, R.J., Kakaire, D., Schares, G., Dietz, E., Böhning, D., Zessin, K.-H. and Mehlitz, D. 1997. Impact of biological factors on the interpretation of bovine trypanosomosis serology. *Prev. Vet. Med.* 30, pp. 61–73.

19. Diall, O., Bocoum, Z. and, Sanogo, Y. 2000. Evaluation of an antibody-detection ELISA using pre-coated plates in the diagnosis of *Trypanosoma congolense* and *T. vivax* infections in cattle in Mali. In: R.H. Dwinger(Ed.), Animal Trypanosomosis: Diagnosis and Epidemiology. , Results of a FAO/IAEA Co-ordinated Research Programme on the Use of Immunoassay Methods for Improved Diagnosis of Trypanosomosis and Monitoring Tsetse and Trypanosomosis Control Programmes. Backhuys, Leiden, pp. 99–104.

Chapter 14

Immunochemical Techniques

The scope of this book does not allow a complete description of the many techniques available for purification and treatment of reagents for facilitating immunoassays in general. There is a large amount of literature covering techniques, and this can be consulted for specific problems. The examination of many of the catalogs produced by commercial companies is useful as they often include good technical sections describing methods using their products. This chapter contains the practical basics of conjugation (a large field in itself), and details other immediately useful techniques that might be first desired in starting an ELISA. The book *Antibodies: A Laboratory Manual (1)* should be regarded as definitive in the laboratory because it is extremely "digestible" and covers a large field of methods, all of which are relevant to ELISA.

1. Labeling Antibodies with Enzymes

Antibodies can be readily labeled by covalent coupling to enzymes *(2–7)*. The ideal product for any coupling reaction should have a 1:1 ratio of antibody to enzyme with no loss of specific activity of either reactant, but this is technically unachievable. However, owing to the amplification of the signal by the enzyme action, even relatively poor conjugates have the required sensitivities. A large number of enzymes have been used to label antibodies. The most commonly used are horseradish peroxidase (HRP), alkaline phosphatase (AP), and β-galactosidase. The ideal enzyme considerations are cost, stability, size, and ease of conjugation. The enzyme should have a high catalytic activity and a range of substrates that yield both soluble and insoluble products (for immunoblotting and immunocytochemical techniques). The purchasing

John R. Crowther, *Methods in Molecular Biology, The ELISA Guidebook, Vol. 516*

DOI: 10.1007/978-1-60327-254-4_14

of enzyme-linked reagents from commercial sources is recommended but for laboratory-produced specific reagents, such as monoclonal antibodies (mAbs) or affinity-purified antibodies, conjugates will need to be prepared in the laboratory.

1.1. Coupling Antibodies to HRP

Two general methods are used for the preparation of antibody peroxidase conjugates: the two-step glutaraldehyde method and the periodate method. Good batches of HRP can be determined by measuring the ratio of the HRP absorbance at 403 and 280 nm (RZ = OD 403 nm/OD 280 nm). This ratio should be at least 3.0. Good reagents designed for coupling are available commercially.

1.1.1. Glutaraldehyde Coupling

In the two-step glutaraldehyde method, glutaraldehyde is first coupled to pure HRP via the relatively few reactive amino groups available on the enzyme. By performing this step in high gluaraldehyde concentrations, very few HRP-HRP conjugates are formed. The HRP-glutaraldehyde mixture is then purified and added to antibody in solution. This method has a low coupling efficiency, so the HRP-antibody conjugates need to be separated from unconjugated material for optimum sensitivity. The HRP must be pure to minimize cross-linking of enzyme molecules to contaminating proteins during the first step of the procedure.

1. Dissolve 10 mg of HRP in 0.2 mL of 1.25% glutaraldehyde (electron microscopic grade) in 100 mM sodium phosphate (pH 6.8). *Caution:* glutaraldehyde is hazardous. Work in a fume hood.
2. After overnight incubation at room temperature, remove excess free glutaraldehyde by gel filtration. To do this, use a gel matrix with an exclusion limit of 20,000–50,000 for globular proteins. Use medium-sized beads (~100 μm in diameter). Prepare a column with 5 mL of bead volume according to the manufacturer's instructions. To make the column easier to load and run, first add 20 μL of glycerol and 20 μL of 1% xylene cylanol. The column should be prerun with a minimum of 10 column vol of 0.15 M NaCl. Allow the column to run until the buffer level drops just below the top of the bed resin. Stop the flow of the column. Carefully load the column with the glutaraldehyde-treated HRP. Release the flow and allow the HRP to run into the column. Just as the level of the HRP solution drops below the top of the column, carefully add 0.15 M NaCl. Run the column with 0.15 M NaCl. Pool the fractions that look brown. These contain the active enzyme.
3. Concentrate the enzyme solution to 10 mg/mL (1 mL final volume) by ultrafiltration or by dialysis against 100 mM sodium carbonate/sodium bicarbonate buffer (pH 9.5) containing 30% sucrose. Change the buffer to 100 mM sodium carbonate–bicarbonate (pH 9.5) either by dialysis or by washing on the ultrafiltration membrane.

4. Add 0.1 mL of antibody (5 mg/mL in 0.15 M NaCl) to the enzyme solution and check that the pH is > 9.0.
5. Incubate at 4°C for 24 h.
6. Add 0.1 mL of 0.2 M ethanolamine (pH 7.0). Incubate at 4°C for 2 h. At this stage there will be present in the solution, the uncoupled HRP, the uncoupled antibody, and the HRP-antibody conjugate. For some assays, no further purification is necessary. In these cases, the uncoupled HRP will not bind to any antigen and will be lost during any washes prior to enzyme detection. Further purification will require separation based on the differences among the three species. The easiest separation will be between the uncoupled HRP and the two antibody-containing fractions. If the antibody binds to protein A, the antibodies can be removed simply, by low pH treatment. Separation between the two antibody fractions can be achieved by gel filtration (a 50-mL S300, or equivalent) or affinity chromatography on a concanavalin A column (eluted with 0.2 M glucose or methylmannoside). Alternatively, the whole separation can be achieved on the basis of size by gel filtration. Column eluates can be assayed by enzyme activity, absorbance at 403 nm, or absorbance at 280 nm.

1.1.2. Periodate Coupling

Periodate treatment of carbohydrates opens the ring structure and allows them to bind to free amino groups. Coupling antibodies and HRP with periodate linkage is an efficient method. This method is based on **ref. 4** and **5**.

1. Resuspend 5 mg of HRP in 1.2 mL of water. Add 0.3 mL of freshly prepared 0.1 M sodium periodate in 10 mM sodium phosphate (pH 7.0).
2. Incubate at room temperature for 20 min.
3. Dialyze the HRP solution against 1 mM sodium acetate (pH 4.0) at 4°C with several changes overnight.
4. Prepare an antibody solution of 10 mg/mL in 20 mM carbonate.
5. Remove the HRP from the dialysis tubing and add to 0.5 mL of the antibody solution.
6. Incubate at room temperature for 2 h.
7. The Schiff's bases that have formed must be reduced by adding 100 μL of sodium borohydride (4 mg/mL in water). Incubate at 4°C for 2 h.

Nakani and Kawaoi (4) Method of Enzyme Activation

1. Dissolve the HRP (HRPO, Sigma Type VI, RZ = 3) in 1.0 mL of freshly prepared
2. 0.3 M sodium bicarbonate, pH 8.1 (should be this pH on making up). Note the milligrams/milliliter on the bottle of HRPO.
3. Add 0.1 mL of a 1% solution (v/v) of fluorodinitrobenzidine in absolute ethanol. Mix for 1 h (leave on bench and gently swirl every 10 min).

4. Add 1.0 mL of 0.08 M sodium periodate ($NaIO_4$) in distilled water. Mix gently for 30 min at room temperature (swirl every 5 min).
5. Add 1.0 mL of 0.16 M ethylene glycol (ethanediol) in distilled water. Mix gently (as in **step 3**) for 1 h.
6. Dialyze against 0.01 M sodium carbonate/bicarbonate buffer, pH 9.5, at 4°C (three changes using 500–1,000 mL each change).

Conjugation

1. Add the IgG (or other protein) dialyzed against 0.01 M carbonate/bicarbonate buffer, pH 9.5) at a ratio of 5 mg of IgG (protein) to 1.33 mg of activated enzyme. (Note: You know the volume of your activated enzyme and know the original milligrams/milliliter, and, therefore you know the effective concentration of the activated enzyme and can add so many milligrams in a certain volume. Mix and stand at room temperature for not less than 3 h (overnight is suitable).
2. Add 1 mg of sodium borohydride ($NaBH_4$)/mg of enzyme used. Make the $NaBH_4$ up fresh to about 200 mg/mL and add a relevant volume containing the correct number of milligrams.
3. Dialyze against phosphate-buffered saline (PBS).
4. You may wish to separate the free enzyme by methods already described, but in most ELISAs this is not necessary.

1.2. Coupling Antibodies to AP

Conjugation of antibodies to AP can be made using a one-step procedure with glutaraldehyde. The conjugates retain good immunological and enzymatic activity but can be large and heterogeneous in nature. The major drawbacks are the high cost of the enzyme and the need to use very concentrated solutions of enzyme and antibody.

1. Mix 10 mg of antibody with 5 mg of AP in a final volume of 1 mL. AP is usually supplied as a suspension in 65% saturated ammonium sulfate, which should be centrifuged at 4,000 × *g* for 30 min (5 min in a microfuge). The antibody solution can then be added to resuspend the enzyme pellet.
2. Dialyze the mixture against four changes of 0.1 M sodium phosphate buffer (pH 6.8) overnight. This is essential to remove free amino groups present in the ammonium sulfate precipitate.
3. Transfer the enzyme-antibody mixture to a container suitable for stirring small volumes. In a fume hood add a small stir bar and place on a magnetic stirrer. Slowly, with gentle stirring add 0.05 mL of a 1% solution of electron microscopy, grade glutaraldehyde. *Caution:* Glutaraldehyde is hazardous.
4. After 5 min, switch off the stirrer and leave for 3 h at room temperature. Add 0.1 mL of 1 M ethanolamine (pH 7.0).

5. After an additional 2 h of incubation at room temperature, dialyze overnight at 4°C against three changes of PBS.
6. Centrifuge at 40,000 × *g* for 20 min.
7. Store the supernatant at 4°C in the presence of 50% glycerol, 1 mM $ZnCl_2$, 1 mM $MgCl_2$, and 0.02% sodium azide.

The procedure may be scaled down to the 1-mg antibody level if the antibody and enzyme concentration is reduced by a factor of 10. Here, the time allowed for coupling should be increased to at least 24 h. The yield of conjugate may be reduced.

1.3. Avidin–Biotin Systems in ELISA

The specific binding between avidin (an egg white protein) and biotin (a water-soluble vitamin) has been exploited in ELISA. Avidin is a tetramer containing four identical subunits, each of which contains a very high-affinity binding site for biotin. The binding is not disturbed by extremes of salt, pH, or chaotropic agents such as guanidine hydrochloride (up to 3 M). The avidin–biotin system is well suited for use as a bridging or sandwich system in association with antigen/antibody reactions. The biotin molecule can be easily coupled to either antigens or antibodies, and avidin can be conjugated to enzymes (and other immunological markers such as fluorochromes, colloidal markers, and ferritin). This section deals briefly with applications of the biotin–avidin system to ELISA. An excellent outline of reagents and biotin/protein-labeling methods (biotinylation) can be found in (**ref.** *8)*. Three basic systems are outlined.

1.3.1. LAB System

An antigen immobilized on a microtiter well is detected by incubation with a primary antibody. After washing, this is detected by incubation with an antispecies antibody that is biotinylated (linked to biotin molecule[s]). Again, after washing, the complex is detected by the addition of avidin that is linked to the enzyme followed by the addition of the relevant substrate.

1.3.2. BRAB System

The BRAB system is essentially the same as the LAB system except that the avidin is not conjugated to an enzyme. Here, the avidin acts as a bridge to connect the biotinylated secondary antibody and biotinylated enzyme. Since the avidin has multiple biotin binding sites, this system allows more biotinylated enzyme to be complexed with a resulting amplification of signal, thus making the system potentially more sensitive than the LAB system.

1.3.3. ABC System

The ABC system is almost identical to the BRAB system except that it requires preincubation of biotinylated enzyme with avidin to form large complexes that are then incubated with the secondary antibody. In this way, there is a large increase in signal owing to the increase in enzyme molecules.

1.4. Methods for Labeling with Biotin

There are many biotinylated commercial reagents designed for use in ELISA. Avrameas and Uriel *(7)* will illustrate the various methods for the introduction of biotin into reagents for use in ELISA using a variety of chemicals. **Table 1** illustrates the versatility of labeling methods for proteins, carbohydrates, and nucleic acids.

2. Preparation of Immunoglobulins

About 10% of serum proteins are immunoglobulins (Igs). After immunization, the specific antibodies produced are about 1–5% of this fraction, so the required Ig (in ELISA) may be from 0.1 to 2.5% of the total protein in a serum. Some assays are favored by the relatively crude fractionation of serum to obtain Igs, e.g., for use in binding to plates in trapping (sandwich assays) to avoid competition for plastic binding sites by other serum proteins. Several methods for separation of Igs are available for use in ELISA. These procedures are suitable for polyclonal antibodies but not necessarily for mAbs. The isolation of total Igs as compared to the purification of specific Igs, is relatively simple.

2.1. Salt Fractionation

Two salts are used for selective Ig precipitation: ammonium sulfate and sodium sulfate. The concentration of ammonium sulfate is expressed as a percentage of saturation whereas the concentration of

Table 1
Biotinylating reagents

Biotinylation reagent	What the reagent is reactive against
NHS-LC-biotin	Primary amines
NHS-biotin	Primary amines
SULFO-NHS-biotin	Primary amines
NHS-LC-biotin	Primary amines
NHS-SS-biotin	Primary amines
Photoactivatable	Nucleic acids
Biotin-HPDP	Thiols
Iodoacetyl-LC-biotin	Thiols
Biotin hydrazide	Carbohydrates
Biotinylaed	Anti-mammalian IgG Protein A

sodium sulfate is expressed as percentage (w/v). The concentration of salt at saturation depends on temperature, particularly for sodium sulfate (five times less at +4°C). The isolation of mammalian IgG and IgA by ammonium sulfate precipitation depends on the volume of the serum being processed. For large volumes, the salt is added directly, whereas for small volumes, the salt is added as a concentrated solution. As already indicated, proteins are precipitated by different amounts of ammonium sulfate. This is a method that can be used to obtain samples of sufficient purity for most ELISAs. The initial volume of serum given here is 10 mL. Adjust the volumes accordingly to suit the starting volume of your serum.

1. To 10 mL of serum add 2.7 g of $(NH_4)_2SO_4$. Add a small quantity in steps. Stir constantly at room temperature.
2. Incubate at room temperature for 1 h while stirring.
3. Centrifuge at ~5,000 × *g* at 4°C for 10–15 min.
4. Discard the supernatant fluid.
5. Dissolve the pellet in 2–3 mL of distilled water.
6. Add 0.5 g of $(NH_4)_2SO_4$, and stir constantly at room temperature.
7. Centrifuge as in **step 3**.
8. Dissolve the pellet in 10 mL of distilled water or PBS.
9. Dialyze against the appropriate buffer for use in ELISA or dialyze against distilled water and then freeze-dry.

2.2. Ion-Exchange Chromatography

After salt fractionation, IgG can be purified further on DEAE-cellulose, DEAE-Sephadex A-50, or DEAE-Sephacel. Such methods are not described in this book, but much literature is available.

2.3. Protein A

Protein A (SpA) is isolated from the cell walls of Cowan 1 or other strains of *Staphylococcus aureus.* It consists of a single polypeptide chain (mol wt of ~42,000). Protein A has a high affinity ($K = 10^8$ L/mol) for the Fc of most mammalian IgGs and can be used for their isolation. A genetically engineered recombinant form of protein A (mol wt 32,000) is marketed, in which most of the nonessential regions have been removed, leaving four IgG binding domains intact.

Although protein A as used in immunoassays has little practical use in detecting sheep, bovine, and goat IgGs, they can be purified when the protein A concentrations are high, as in the commercially available protein A-Sepharose or protein A conjugated to Affi-gels (Bio-Rad) or glass beads. Such reagents are quite useful in rapid separation of most mammalian IgGs. Briefly, 5 mL Protein A columns are equilibrated with PBS. Serum or crude IgG is then added and elution with PBS is maintained.

The IgG attaches to the column (via reaction to the protein A bound to the inert matrix), and the other serum proteins pass through the column. The bound IgG is then eluted by using a 0.9% sodium chloride solution containing 0.6% acetic acid or by adding a solution of sodium thiocyanate (2–5 M). Such methods are particularly useful in the purification of mouse IgGs from mAb ascites preparations.

2.4. Protein G

Protein G is isolated from group G *Streptococcus* sp. The protein is similar to protein A in that it binds to a variety of mammalian Igs through their Fc region, but generally with a higher affinity. Unlike protein A, protein G binds strongly with bovine, ovine, and caprine IgGs.

2.5. Protein A/G

Protein A/G is a genetically engineered protein produced by a gene fusion product from a nonpathogenic *Bacillus* strain. The protein is engineered to have four Fc binding domains of protein A and two of protein G per molecule. The product binds to all classes of mouse IgG, but not with IgA or IgM.

3. Immunosorbents

A breakthrough in the ease of use of immunosorbents was made with the availability of reagents such as *n*-Hydroxysuccinimide-derivatized agarose (Bio-Rad). This gel can be washed three times in cold distilled water and then used to covalently attach any protein, merely by incubation of that protein(s) in a wide variety of buffers (such as 0.1 m sodium carbonate buffer). Blocking of unreacted active sites on the gel is achieved by the addition of ethanolamine or by merely leaving the gel overnight. Such gels are thus quite easy to prepare. Antisera can then be added in neutral buffers, and the addition of some detergents (e.g., 0.5% Tween-80) minimizes nonspecific adsorption of serum proteins. Desorption of bound antibodies can then be achieved by the addition of chaotropic ions (sodium thiocyanate), organic acids with low surface tension or pH extremes. Thus, such affinity techniques can be used to remove unwanted cross-reactions from sera. For example, if a serum has anti-bovine IgG activity, this can be adsorbed out by passing that serum over an affinity column with bound bovine serum or IgG. In this case, the antibodies passing through the column will be free from anti-bovine activity.

Other immunosorbents are available commercially, based on beaded agarose or glass. A wide variety of proteins such as whole serum or IgG can be purchased attached covalently to beads and are extremely convenient (but expensive) for, e.g., the removal of unwanted cross reactive antibodies from small volumes of antisera. The beads are simply added to an antiserum and after a short incubation are separated by centrifugation (in a microfuge at 10,000 × *g* for 10–30 s). The agarose beads thus capture any unwanted antibodies on the solid phase, leaving the antiserum free of that contaminant. This method has the advantage over blocking by addition of high levels of specific protein (against which the unwanted antibodies react) because there is complete separation of immune complexes, which may interfere with ELISAs. Such reagents can be reused by eluting the immunologically bound protein using similar methods (e.g., low pH), followed by extensive washing. The section on immunoaffinity purification in **ref.** *1* should be consulted for extensive practical details of methods.

4. Production of Antisera

The raising of antisera in laboratory animals could fill a manual in itself. The variability in immune response within and between species and the various antigens used means that no brief rules can be given, and reading of the relevant scientific literature is essential. Generally, the administration of a nonreplicating agent requires the addition of an adjuvant, whose effect is to stimulate the immune system so that efficient presentation of the antigen takes place.

4.1. Immunization

The purpose of immunization is to obtain high-titer antisera that bind strongly to antigen (high avidity). The properties of antisera are determined by the genetic composition of the animal injected (particularly the Ir genes). This means that there can be great variation in the quantitative and qualitative aspects of antisera from among species and even among individuals of the same species. This should be borne in mind when considering the use for which the serum is being made. In preparing sera one should (1) always obtain a preimmunization serum, and (2) never automatically pool sera. Point (2) is particularly important if a defined property of an antiserum is required (e.g., in discrimination of antigens).

Up to a certain degree, an increase in the dose (weight) of antigen will increase antibody titer; however, this may also increase cross-reactivity. Adjuvants also increase the immunogenicity of proteins. Haptens should be labeled with carrier proteins to elicit an immune response. The carrier protein should be foreign to the host to be recognized by the T-cells. For most immunogens, the interaction of T- and B-cells is essential for antibody production.

The animal species chosen can be important. The animal species most often used in laboratories are rabbits, goats, guinea pigs, pigs, sheep, and rats. Commercial companies may favor horses and donkeys for large-scale preparations. Many animals contain cross-reactive antibodies in their serum before immunization; this could complicate their use in ELISA, and some simple absorption technique may be required (or may have been performed in commercial preparations) to block such reactions. Another point to remember is that many smaller animals can be immunized as compared to only a few larger animals, owing mainly to cost considerations. Because of the variations in sera from the previously mentioned animals, smaller animals offer advantages in which relatively small volumes of serum are required.

For most immunization regimes, the immunogen (at about 2 mg/mL) is mixed vigorously with an equal volume of Freund's complete or incomplete adjuvant in an isotonic salt solution, to obtain an emulsion that is stable in water. It is essential that the antigen be added in small aliquots in a stepwise fashion to the adjuvant, with vigorous mixing between each addition (e.g., using a vortex mixer). On complete addition of the antigen, the emulsion must be tested for stability. This is easily done by placing a drop of the emulsion on to the surface of some distilled water in a beaker. This should spread out over the surface. However, a second drop added (or sometimes a third) should not spread and remain as a distinct drop, and the edges of the drop should show no signs of dissolution.

4.2. Immunogen Dose

The amount of immunogen needed to induce an immune response depends on the exact nature of the antigen and the host species used. A typical dose/ response is sygmoidal in nature, whereby very large and very small doses of material elicit a weak or no response. Generally, the lowest effective dose of an antigen is preferred when raising antisera for immunoassays since this tends to elicit antibodies of the highest affinity and produce polyclonal sera of high avidity. General values can be given; however, a range of concentrations of antigen is often needed to allow an estimation of its potency. Rabbits and guinea pigs usually require ~100 µg of protein with an adjuvant, whereas doses of between 500 and 1,000 µg are required for larger animals. Generally, subsequent booster doses are lower and given without adjuvant.

4.3. Improving Antigenicity of Antigens

Adjuvants are substances that enhance the immune response. A range of adjuvant methodologies is available, including the following:

1. Water-in-oil emulsions such as Freund's complete adjuvant, Freund's incomplete adjuvant. The complete adjuvant contains heat-killed *Mycobacterium tuberculosis* bacteria whereas the incomplete does not. Both have the basis of an immune modulator, e.g., branched glucose polymers or methylated bovine serum albumin (Pierce's AdjuPrime™)

2. Minerals in which the antigen can be absorbed on aluminum hydroxide, bentonite, or quaternary ammonium salts.
3. Bacterial species such as Bacille Calmette-Guérin, *Bordetella pertussis*, or *Corynebacterium parvum*.
4. Bacterial products such as endotoxins, lipopolysaccharides, and liposomes.
5. Polynucleotides such as poly I-poly C, and poly (A-U).

The adjuvant actions generally stimulate immune responses nonspecifically by increasing antigen presentation and the number of collaborating cells involved. This effectively reduces antigen doses required and enhances immunogenicity of proteins. The adjuvant may alter the spectrum of antibodies produced in terms of both isotypes and specificities. Adjuvants also act to produce depots of antigen that are released slowly, thereby promoting continuous stimulation of the immune system. In addition, adjuvants may protect the immunogen from rapid removal and cleavage from host enzymes (*see* **ref. 9** for review of adjuvants).

In cases in which there is no response in animals after multiple injections, alternative animal species should be tried and the dose of antigen(s) increased. If this does not succeed, then attempts to enhance the antigenicity by direct modification methods can be tried. An excellent practical description of these techniques is found in ref. 7. Common methods include the following:

1. The addition of small modifying groups such as dinitrophenol or arsenate.
2. Denaturation of antigen by heat treatment and/or sodium dodecyl sulfate treatment.
3. Coupling of antigen to small synthetic peptides that are sites for T-cell receptor class II protein binding.
4. Coupling of antigens to large particles such as sheep red blood cells or agarose beads.
5. Purification of antigens with other antibodies and injection of immune complexes.

References

1. Harlow, E. and Lane, D, eds. (1988) *Antibodies. A Laboratory Manual.* Cold Spring Harbor Laboratory Press, Cold Spring Harbor, NY.
2. Avrameas, S. (1972) Enzyme markers: their linkage with proteins and use in immunohistochemistry. *Histochem. J.* **4**, 321–330.
3. Farr, A. G. and Nakane, P. K. (1981) Immunochemistry and enzyme labeled antibodies: a brief review. *J. Immunol. Methods* **47**, 129–144.
4. Nakane, P. K. and Kawaoi, A. (1974) Peroxidase-labelled antibody: a new method of conjugation. *J. Histochem. Cytochem.* **22**, 1084–1091.
5. Tijssen, P. and Kurstak, E. (1984) Highly efficient and simple methods for the preparation of peroxidase and active peroxidase-antibody conjugates for enzyme immunoassays. *Anal. Biochem.* **136**, 451–457.
6. Avrameas, S. and Ternynck, T. (1969) The cross-linking of proteins with glutaraldehyde and its use for the preparation of immunoadsorbents. *Immunochemistry* **6**, 53–66.
7. Avrameas, S. and Uriel, J. (1966) Methode de marquage d'antigen et anticorps avec des

enzymes et son application en immunodiffusion. *Cr. Acad. Sci. D* 262, 2543–2545.

8. Crowther, J. R. (2001) *Immunogens, Ag/Ab Purification, Antibodies, Avidin–Biotin, Protein Modification: PIERCE Immunotechnology Catalog and Handbook, Volume 1*. Pierce and Warriner, UK.
9. Spier, R. andGriffiths, J. B. 1985 *Adjuvants in Animal Cell Biotechnology*, vols. 1 and 2. Academic, New York.

Chapter 15

Test Questions

This chapter consists of a test concerning ELISA and the sciences needed to perform assays. The test can be used to gage knowledge on ELISA. Suggested points are given for the benefit of educators. Of course, the test can be adapted. All the answers can be obtained by reading this book. It may be useful to test oneself before and after referring to the book. Answers follow the test as a guide to marking.

1. Questions

1. What does ELISA stand for?
2. Name two substrates used in ELISA.
3. What is H_2O_2?
4. What is a blocking buffer?
5. Name three enzymes commonly used in ELISA.
6. What is IgG?
7. Complete the following list, filling in gaps in words, according to units in decreasing weight series:

   gram, milligram, ______, nanogram, ______, ______
8. Draw a diagram representing an indirect ELISA.
9. Draw a diagram representing a sandwich ELISA involving the same antibody.
10. Name a use for sulfuric acid in ELISA.
11. Name four immunoglobulin classes.
12. Name the method of titrating two reagents against each other.

John R. Crowther, *Methods in Molecular Biology, The ELISA Guidebook, Vol. 516*

DOI: 10.1007/978-1-60327-254-4_15

13. What does OPD stand for?
14. What does the washing step do in ELISA?
15. How many microliters are in a liter of liquid?
16. What is meant by a competition ELISA?
17. What is the process of internal monitoring of a test called?
18. Name three agents added to solutions to make blocking buffers.
19. What is the most commonly used solid phase in ELISA?
20. Why do you need to tap plates when you add coating reagents?
21. Give three advantages of rotation during the incubation phase of ELISA as compared with stationary conditions.
22. Draw a diagram representing a sandwich ELISA involving an indirect method of detecting the second antibody.
23. Give three reasons why there might be *no* or hardly any color development after the addition of substrate/chromogen in an ELISA.
24. Calculate the following (give the answers in microliters):
    (a) You need a 1/500 dilution of serum in 12 mL of buffer. How much undiluted serum must I add?
    (b) You need a 1/500 dilution of serum in 12 mL. The serum given is already diluted 1/10. How do you do this?
    (c) You need 110 mL of a reagent at 1/20,000. The reagent is already at 1/50. How do you do this?
25. What is an antigen?
26. Give two differences between monoclonal and polyclonal antibodies.
27. Give the substrate and name two chromogens for horseradish peroxidase enzyme.
28. What term describes the region of the antibody molecule that binds to an antigen?
29. What is a conformational epitope?
30. What is meant by the following terms?
    (a) EQA
    (b) SD
    (c) Mean
31. What is meant by the term *stopping*?
32. The plate OD values given below show a checkerboard titration of antigen against a specific conjugate. Antigen is diluted from 1/50 from column 1 to 11 in a twofold dilution range. Conjugate is diluted from row A to G from 1/200 in a twofold range.

	1	2	3	4	5	6	7	8	9	10	11	12
A	2.2	2.3	2.2	2.1	2.0	2.0	1.9	1.6	1.5	1.3	0.8	0.6
B	2.2	2.0	1.9	2.0	1.9	1.8	1.7	1.5	1.3	0.8	0.5	0.3
C	2.1	2.0	1.9	1.9	1.8	1.7	1.6	1.5	1.2	0.7	0.5	0.3
D	1.9	1.9	1.7	1.8	1.5	1.2	1.0	0.7	0.5	0.3	0.2	0.1
E	1.8	1.8	1.7	1.5	1.3	1.1	0.8	0.6	0.5	0.3	0.2	0.1
F	1.3	1.3	1.2	1.2	1.1	0.8	0.6	0.5	0.3	0.2	0.1	0.1
G	0.7	0.7	0.7	0.6	0.6	0.5	0.3	0.2	0.1	0.1	0.1	0.1
H	0.3	0.2	0.1	0.1	0.1	0.1	0.1	0.1	0.1	0.1	0.1	0.1

Answer the following questions based on the data.

(a) Why is color (OD) similar in A1–A5?

(b) Explain possibly why the OD in A12 is high?

(c) Where would you assess the optimal antigen concentration for coating wells expressed as a dilution?

(d) What is the optimal dilution of conjugate? Give an approximate range here.

33. An antiserum is already diluted in blocking buffer to 1/50. You need to make a volume of 90 mL of this antiserum at 1/12,500. Show a calculation to perform this dilution.

34. Explain the following titrations where whole serum is used as a capture antibody compared with the IgG fraction of the serum shown in **Diagram 1**:

35. Define the following terms:
(a) Epitope
(b) Fab fragment
(c) Affinity
(d) Avidity
(e) Monoclonal antibody

36. How could you remove antibodies against bovine serum proteins from an antiserum, in which these are causing problems of cross-reactivity?

37. You require 1 mL of a dilution of reagent at 1/1,000,000. How could you make this using only 3 mL of diluent?

38. What is the main difference between a heterogeneous and homogeneous ELISA?

39. What is an anamnestic response?

40. What does 492 nm refer to?

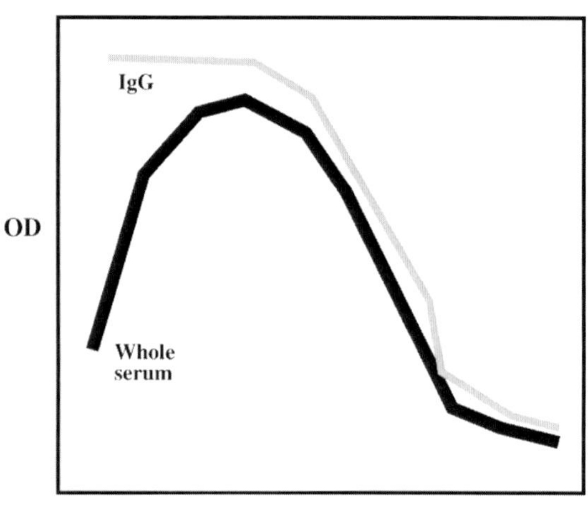

Diagram. 1.

2. Answers

1. Enzyme-linked immunosorbent assay. *(2 points only for completely correct answer)*
2. Hydrogen peroxide or H_2O_2; *p*-nitrophenylphosphate or pnpp; or ortho nitrophenyl β-galactosidase. *(2 points for each correct answer, maximum 4 points)*
3. Hydrogen peroxide. Also allow substrate for horseradish peroxidase conjugates. *(2 points)*
4. Buffered solution to which substances are added to preventing nonspecific adsorption of reagents in ELISA. *(2 points)*
5. Horseradish peroxidase, alkaline phosphatase, β-galactosidase, ABTS, urease. *(2 points for each correct answer, maximum of 6 points)*
6. A class of immunoglobulin from serum, immunoglobulin G. *(2 points)*
7. Gram, milligram, microgram, nanogram, femtogram, attogram. *(2 points for each correct answer)*
8. Must contain a solid phase, attached antigen (coating), antibody-detecting antigen and anti-species conjugate. Allow symbols or drawings such as the following: (**Diagram 2)**

I-Ag + Ab + Anti-Ab + Anti-Abconjugate

(6 points for complete answer)

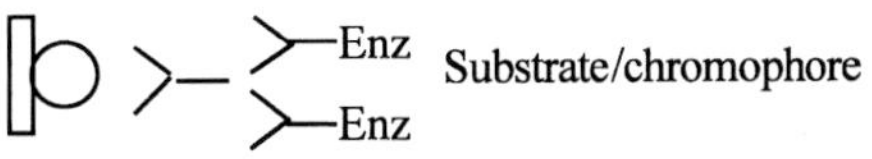

Enz
Enz
Substrate/chromophore

Diagram. 2.

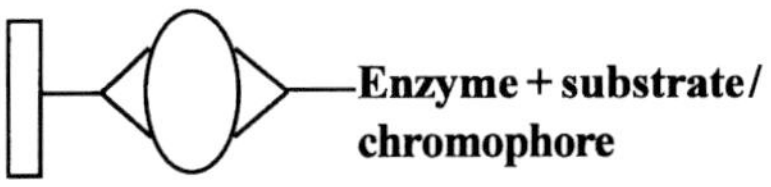

Enzyme + substrate/
chromophore

Diagram.3.

9. Must contain a solid phase, capture antibody, antigen, detecting antibody labeled with conjugate, and chromophore/substrate. Allow symbols or drawings such as the following: (**Diagram. 3**)

   I-Ab + Ag + Ab-enzyme + substrate/chromophore

   (2 points for complete answer)
10. As a stopping reagent – to stop enzymatic reaction. *(2 points)*
11. IgG, IgM, IgA, IgD, or IgE. *(1 point, up to 4 maximum)*
12. Allow chessboard or checkerboard titrations. *(2 points)*
13. *Ortho*-phenylenediamine. *(3 points)*
14. Separates bound and free reagents. *(3 points)*
15. One million (1,000,000). *(3 points)*
16. When a pretitrated system is challenged by the addition of a substance that competes for binding. *(3 points)*
17. Internal quality control or IQC. *(3 points)*
18. Proteins generally, BSA, gelatin, milk powder, detergents, sodium dodecyl sulfate. *(2 points for each correct answer, maximum 6 points)*
19. 96-well microtiter plates. *(2 points, allow 1 point for plastics)*
20. To ensure mixing and adequate entry of reagents. *(2 points)*
21. Ensures mixing; reduces viscosity effects; reduces temperature effects on reaction rates owing only to diffusion mixing; avoids irregular heating effects of stationary conditions owing to insulation by plastic; allows stacking of plates; or reduces time needed for incubation under stationary conditions. *(2 points for each correct answer, maximum of 6 points)*
22. Should contain a solid phase, capture antibody, antigen, detecting antibody and anti-species conjugate with the addition

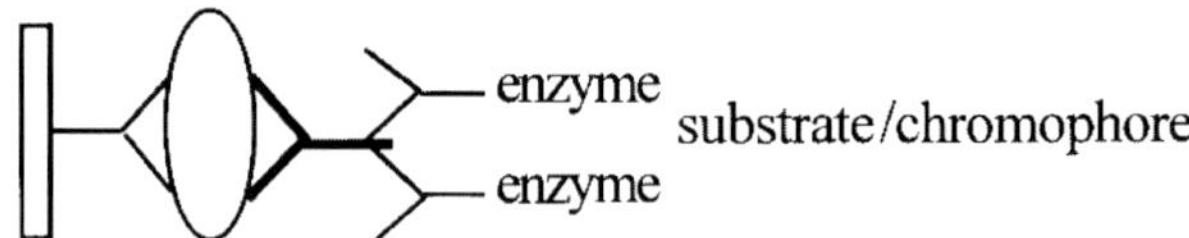

Diagram 4.

of substrate/chromphore. Allow symbols or drawings such as the following: (**Diagram 4**)

I-Ab + Ag + AB + Anti-AB-Enzyme + substrate/chromphore

(6 points)

23. No conjugate added; no substrate added; one other reagent omitted; conjugate activity destroyed; or wrong plates used. *(2 points for each correct answer, maximum of 6 points)*
24. (a) 12 mL = 12,000 μL, 1/500 of 12,000 is 24 μL. The answer is 24 μL. *(2 points)*
    (b) 12 mL = 12,000 μL. If serum was undiluted you would need 12,000/500 = 24 μL, but since it is diluted 1/10, you need ten times more: 10 × 24 μL = 240 μL. The answer is 240 μL. *(3 points)*
    (c) 110 mL = 110,000 μL. If the reagent was not prediluted, you would require 1/20,000 of this: 110,000/20,000 μL = 5.5 μL. Since the reagent is diluted 1/50, you need 50 times more: 50 × 5.5 μL = 275 μL. The answer is 275 μL. *(3 points)*
25. A substance that when injected into an animal elicits antibody production. *(3 points)*
26. mAbs are single affinity reagents; mAbs are homologous population of antibodies; or mAbs react with a single epitope. *(2 points each for reasonable answers, maximum of 4 points)*
27. Hydrogen peroxide is the substrate (allow H_2O_2). Chromogens are HRPO or horseradish peroxidase, ABTS, TMB, AS, or 5-AS. *(2 points for substrate, 2 points each per correct chromogen, maximum of 4 points)*
28. Allow antibody-combining site, paratope, or Fab. *(4 points)*
29. An epitope that relies on a distinct three-dimensional relationship of the same or different proteins to allow interaction with antibodies, or an antigenic site that is denaturable. *(4 points for a reasonable answer)*
30. (a) External quality assurance *(2 points*
    (b) standard deviation *(2 points)*
    (c) average of a set of data. *(2 points)*

31. The process by which enzymatic development of color is stopped before reading data in a spectrophotometer. *(3 points)*

32. (a) The antigen although diluted gives the same color. Thus, there is excess antigen added here as detected with constant 1/200 dilution of conjugate. *(2 points)*

    (b) Here the conjugate is at 1/200 and is sticking nonspecifically where there is no antigen as compared with later dilutions C12, D12, and so on). Thus, three is a high conjugate background. (2 points)

    (c) 1/3,200 to 1/6,400. (2 points)

    (d) 1/200 to 1/400. (2 points)

33. If antiserum was not diluted, I would need 90 mL, i.e., 90,000 μL/12,500 = 7 μL. However, it is already diluted 1/50, and so we need 50 times more: 50 × 7 = 450 μL. Answer is 450 μL. *(5 points)*

34. The whole serum contains other proteins that block the immunoglobulins involved in capture. The IgG is separated from such proteins and can attach to plastic. The whole serum thus has a prozone of poor capture activity. When the serum is diluted, the effect of the other proteins is negated and where high concentrations of IgG are contained, maximal capture can occur. The IgG shows a plateau of activity where IgG is in excess. *(6 points)*

35. (a) Another name for an antigenic site though better defined as an entity through monoclonal antibodies. *(3 points)*

    (b) A fragment of immunoglobulin molecule resulting from digestion. This is the single antibody-combining site of the molecule. *(3 points)*

    (c) Defines force between antibody and antigen. Affinity refers strictly to interaction between one species molecule and single site. *(3 points)*

    (d) Represents sum of all affinities of antibody molecules. *(3 points)*

    (e) A single population of antibody molecules against a single epitope. *(3 points)*

36. Use affinity reagents consisting of bovine serum or bovine IgG attached to the solid phase, columns, use of addition of excess bovine serum. *(4 points)*

37. Dilute 10 μL into 1 mL, mix, take 10 μL of this and add to 1 mL of diluent, and mix. Take 10 μL of this and add to 1 mL of diluent. Each diution step is 10 μL in 1,000 μL = 1/100. Three dilution steps of 1/100 = 1/1,000,000. *(3 points)*

38. Heterologous ELISAs have a washing step to separate bound and free reactants, whereas homogeneous assays do not. *(2 points)*
39. The response to a second injection of an antigen. The primary response involves a delay in antibody production whereas the anamnestic response is immediate, with increasing titer. *(3 points)*
40. This is a wavelength produced by using a filter. It is used to read OPD chromophores with horseradish peroxidase enzyme and hydrogen peroxide substrate. *(3 points)*

INDEX

O

P

Q

R

S

Printed by Books on Demand, Germany